mm Hg

LOGAN'S
MEDICAL AND SCIENTIFIC ABBREVIATIONS

LOGAN'S
MEDICAL AND SCIENTIFIC
ABBREVIATIONS

Carolynn M. Logan
M. Katherine Rice

J. B. LIPPINCOTT COMPANY *Philadelphia*
London *Mexico City* *New York* *St. Louis* *São Paulo* *Sydney*

Acquisitions Editor: Patricia Cleary
Systems Manager/Production: Nora Barry Leary
Manuscript Editor: Tina Rebane
Design Director: Tracy Baldwin
Cover and Interior Design: Anne O'Donnell
Composition: J. B. Lippincott Company
Printer/Binder: R. R. Donnelley and Sons, Inc.

6   5   4   3

Library of Congress Cataloging-in-Publication Data

Logan, Carolynn M.
  Logan's medical and scientific abbreviations.
  Bibliography: p.
  1. Medicine—Abbreviations—Dictionaries. 2. Science
—Abbreviations—Dictionaries. I. Rice, M. Katherine.
II. Title. III. Title: Medical and scientific
abbreviations. [DNLM: 1. Medicine—abbreviations.
2. Science—abbreviations. W 13 L831L]
R123.L8   1987   610'.148   86—14382
ISBN 0-397-54589-4

To L. O. Otterness, M. D.
Carolynn M. Logan

To my parents
with love and thanks
M. Katherine Rice

PREFACE

Over the years, we have become increasingly frustrated by our inability to find a comprehensive reference for the thousands of shortened forms of medical and other scientific terms and expressions. For the venturer outside his or her own specialty, the researcher, or the seeker of historical, arcane terms, this frustration level rises as yet another book of abbreviations must be consulted in the search for that needed, esoteric, pharmaceutical notation; for help in deciphering the handwritten initialization required for a medical biography or other manuscript of historical interest; or to translate the hurried contemporary symbol written by the harried contemporary physician.

All of the ancillary services of medicine at some time require a lucid reference that can be utilized in translating the spoken or written order of the professional medical community. There are also the biology, chemistry, and physics of aerospace medicine, genetics, and industrial and agricultural medicine, to name but a few of over 100 specialties and subspecialties, each of which has its brief forms, both spoken and written, as does any other highly technical field. "Medicine" has drawn from or contributed to nearly every aspect of human health and human endeavor, from agrobiology to zoology. It would be insular, in light of the foregoing, to limit contracted forms merely to the diagnosis and treatment of the individual patient's hospital stay or office visit.

There are those, of course, who insist that they themselves do not use or allow to be used abbreviations in any communications originating from their department. A psychiatrist with whom we spoke was particularly adamant on the subject of abbreviations. We asked, "What about M.D. after your name?" "That's a title", he said. "And you never have used laser, CAT scan, DAP test?" we asked. "Acronyms", he answered. "We follow, scrupulously, the DSM, and *that* is an initialization!"

Acronym, initialization, abbreviation, symbol—all are brief forms for longer terms; and it is these, whatever one wishes to call them, which comprise this book. Used judiciously, they are invaluable; carelessly abused, they waste time and cause misunderstanding. Whatever one's position on brief forms for words and terms, it appears they are here to stay.

Carolynn M. Logan
M. Katherine Rice

ACKNOWLEDGMENTS

Much time and energy have gone into the preparation of this book, and we would like to thank the following people for their efforts in assisting us with its creation:

Mary Pat Milligan, R.R.A, of the University of California, Davis, Medical Center; Michael W. Bennett, Health Sciences Librarian, Kaiser Permanente Medical Center; Cassandra Ancona, C.M.T; Geriann Rueda; Debbie Brown; Tri Thong Dang; and, most particularly, John F. Gummere for his delightful and scholarly contributions to our Latin terminology; and Nora B. Leary, Systems Manager in the Production Services Department of the J. B. Lippincott Company, for painstakingly assisting us with the word-processing/computer formats specifically designed for this project.

We would especially like to thank Patricia L. Cleary, our editor, for her knowledgeable and supportive guidance, humor, and incredible patience.

CONTENTS

INTRODUCTION

This compilation of medical and scientific abbreviations, initializations, acronyms, and symbols has been drawn from over 60 sources: medical dictionaries, "approved" hospital lists, medical journals and texts, submissions from various medical specialties and various other technical listings, and from many hundreds of dictated consultations, history and physical reports, surgeries, and discharge summaries. One obstacle we encountered was the considerable lack of consistency among these sources. As medical specialties multiply and new laboratory, medical, and surgical procedures become established, jargon and unique abbreviations flourish in hospitals, clinics, and medical schools across the country. Often the use of an abbreviation that is permitted in one facility is discouraged or forbidden in another. POMP, CA-BOP, PATCO, AGA, LESA, CABG—the terms increase; they assault us daily.

Our sources were evenly divided on the forms used for metrics: mg., mg, or mgm. for milligram; c.cm., c.c., cc, cu.cm., or cm^3 for cubic centimeter. In a section of abbreviations from the procedures manuals of two university teaching hospitals, consistency was lacking throughout: AU, AS, and AD were approved for (each [or both]) left and right ear; but O.U., O.S., and O.D. (with periods) were required for the same expressions when they concerned the eye; E. R. for emergency room, yet OR for operating room; A.V., AV, A-V, and A/V were the variations for arteriovenous or atrioventricular.

If there is no consistency within a facility's list of "approved" abbreviations and if the "authorities" cannot agree among themselves, one can well understand the consternation such a situation can cause among medical journalists, nurses, medical and legal secretaries, students, attorneys, and hospital medical record and transcription department personnel, as well as among those in state and county agencies who must utilize such medical reports.

It would be futile and wasteful in terms of time and expense for the hospital and clinic to suggest that no abbreviations be allowed, for we are a nation of "short-cutters." While it has been recommended that hospital medical records committees define their own "approved" lists of abbreviations and that hospital personnel utilize and abide by the individual committee's decisions, this seems to have regionalized many terms which otherwise would have been clearly understood and accessible nationwide.

We were interested in the suggestion by some institutions that there be only one definition allowed for each abbreviation. One might applaud this concept within a single department where a single abbreviation may have multiple definitions in areas that could be extremely confusing, for example, AVD standing for aortic valvular disease, arteriovenous difference, and atrioventricular dissociation. However, following this dictum of "one definition per abbreviation" hospitalwide, to which department then shall we "award" the capital letter C? And shall we, thereafter, never abbreviate centigrade, Celsius, coulomb, Culex, the vectorcardiography electrode (between E and A), or any of the other 125 listings from many specialties that also use capital C on a regular basis?

Until such time as there is standardizaton of abbreviations based on that uncommon quality, common sense, and based on a knowledge of the structure and use of these brief forms, the users should have some central source where they may find the terms they see written or hear (spoken or dictated) in order to make sure they have translated them correctly. More importantly, they will be able to **choose**, in many cases, one form from among the many that are currently in use.

Apart from some historically interesting abbreviations that we have included, we have attempted to indicate only those abbreviations that **are** being used and have made but few judgments as to which **should** be acceptable.

No less important is clear and careful pronunciation by the communicator whether orders and instructions are being given directly or over the phone to hospital unit and departmental personnel or through the use of dictating machines for manuscripts and medical reports.

We hope that those of you who have found this book useful might wish to contribute your special and hard-to-find short forms, and their sources, for future editions. A form in the back of this book may be used for that purpose. No matter how numerous or meticulous the proofings, errors do remain undetected. We would welcome such information from you so that we may correct future editions.

USING ABBREVIATIONS

The following suggestions may help to bring consistency to the field of abbreviations and alleviate some of the current confusion when brief forms are written, dictated, or transcribed.

Avoid same-speciality definition for one abbreviation: CC—calcaneocuboid, chondrocalcinosis, coracoclavicular, costochondral, as well as craniocervical. The meaning of the written or dictated abbreviated form must be absolutely clear to the reader/translator.

Capitalization: Periods may be eliminated in most capitalized abbreviations. Although the nonmedical, nontechnical rules dictate that capitalized letters standing for the initial letters of separate words are so indicated by periods between each letter (*i.e.,* U.S.A), excepting acronyms (such as Project HOPE, LASER, and the like), there is nothing to be gained by this practice in a technical field except more awkward and confusing forms to decipher. The purist would be required to write the abbreviation for intravenous pyelogram as IV.P. and that for arteriosclerotic heart disease as AS.H.D.; however, if one has taken the trouble to capitalize such abbreviations (IVP, ASHD), one should be able to identify the phrase without difficulty whether or not it consists of separate words or of combining forms.

A period is not necessary in most cases in which an initial capital indicates an abbreviation (Surg, Ophth). A period should be used, however, in any case where the word might be misconstrued (Anal. Psych, for instance). These abbreviations may be used freely in the intrahospital, intraclinical, or intraoffice setting.

Common laboratory studies: These may be abbreviated; for example, Hct, Hgb (hematocrit and hemoglobin), but H&H (with both numerical values following) for those same tests is confusing to the reader and should be avoided.

Genus and species: The undifferentiated genus, when abbreviated, is usually written lower case with a period (staph., strep.); but when genus **and** species are both indicated, the genus is initially capitalized **and** the species is not abbreviated: *Staph(.) aureus* or *S(.) aureus*.

Greek letters: The typed or written "a" or alpha for α and "B"or beta for the lower-case β are acceptable. In this book, the individual Greek alphabetic symbols are listed under the letter that initiates the anglicized name; that is, γ under "g" as gamma, τ under "t" as tau, and so on (see the list of Greek letters, following the Introduction).

Lower-case abbreviations: Periods between the initials of lower-case abbreviations should be used to prevent them from being misread as an entirely different word or phrase (bid for b.i.d.). It is suggested that standard classical Latin abbreviations, particularly, be so written: long. (longus), lot. (lotio), cap. (capiat). The capitalization of every abbreviation makes copy difficult to read—"MOM PO QS Q4H or PRN"—and tends to give too much importance to standard orders. Metrics, however, appear to be no longer used with periods by about half of the reference books we investigated; that is, cm, kg, and ml.

Narrative reports and material to be published: Reports going to agencies outside the medical field (state and federal agencies, attorneys, private industry) should limit the use of abbreviations. As with articles for publication within the medical field, the abbreviated term or initialization should be written out fully the first time it appears. The abbreviation may then follow (in parentheses) immediately; for example, follicle-stimulating hormone (FSH), mouse unit (MU). Subsequently, the shortened form alone may be used. Of course, the publication's editorial requirements, if different, should be followed.

Orders/instructions: It is helpful to the translator if some type of differentiation is made in the use of a capitalized or lower-case letter when the same initial is used for common but different definitions in the same report. The initial "q" serves for quater (four), quaque (every), and quantum (quantity). Clarity would be served if capital "Q" were used for the "every" term (Qd, Q4h, Qh) and the lower-case "q" were used for the term "four" (q.i.d.). The small "q" (for quantity) is not so easily misread in the lesser-used expressions such as q.s., q.l., or q.p. (sufficient quantity, as much as you like, as much as you please).

Plurals: No plural form need be shown with abbreviations following numbers since the number will indicate whether or not it is more than one; for example, 100 mg, 3 cm. A small "s" immediately following capitalized initializations, no apostrophe (TIAs, EOMs), is acceptable. An apostrophe "s" is necessary following lower-case abbreviations or initializations (w.b.c. 's).

Slang or jargon: If written lower case, these need periods for clarity and to indicate that they are, indeed, abbreviations rather than complete words: subcu., sed. rate, pro. time, verum. (verumontanum). There is a limited but useful place for such terms and they will continue to be used, however much frowned upon.

Symbols: Symbols never take periods, since a symbol is a printed or written sign rather than an abbreviation. An abbreviation is a shortened form of a word or phrase (e.g., ℞, pH). The abbreviations for all elements (K, P, Na, etc.) are considered symbols in chemistry.

When in doubt, write it out: There are over 125 definitions for capital and lower-case A. Unless the meaning of the initial is absolutely clear to the translator, do not use the abbreviation.

Word-processing format: The medical transcriptionist/secretary must accommodate to the word-processing machine and electronic typewriter. In many cases, the valuable and important superscripts and subscripts must be typed on the line (e.g., A2 or A-2 equals P2 or P-2, rather than $A_2 = P_2$) and 10^5 must be typed as "ten to the fifth power". We have made no such accommodation for the hundreds of superscripts and subscripts in the book. Also, certain chemical terms and stereodescriptors use small capital letters, and these may be typed as regular capital letters without confusing the reader.

USING THIS BOOK

Appendices: An alphabetical table of elements; chemotherapy regimens; an overview of tumor, node, metastasis cancer staging; classical Latin abbreviations used in charting and prescription writing; suggested references; and an extensive list of symbols have been included in the appendices for quick reference.

Chemical names: The first entry is the chemical abstract name, alternate, or trivial name, which "matches" the abbreviation. Other names for the same substance appear within the parentheses.

Preference: Listings for both abbreviations and definitions are alphabetical and do not indicate preference. In cases where more than one spelling or word separation was given by two or more reliable sources, each definition is shown.

Titles, degrees, associations: We have, with a few exceptions, excluded titles indicating certification or position, as well as associations, since such a list would have to be selective and might appear to be arbitrary.

GREEK LETTERS

The Greek alphabetic symbols are listed under the letter that initiates the anglicized name; that is, γ under "g" as gamma, τ under "t" as tau, and so on (see below):

Greek Capital	Greek Lower Case	Name	See Under
A	α	alpha	A
B	β	beta	B
X	χ	chi	C and X
Δ	δ	delta	D
E	ϵ	epsilon	E
H	η	eta	E
Γ	γ	gamma	G
I	ι	iota	I
K	κ	kappa	K
Λ	λ	lambda	L
M	μ	mu	M
N	ν	nu	N
O	o	omicron	O
Ω	ω	omega	O
Π	π	pi	P
Φ	ϕ	phi	P
Ψ	ψ	psi	P
P	ρ	rho	R
Σ	σ	sigma	S
T	τ	tau	T
Θ	θ	theta	T
Υ	υ	upsilon	U
Ξ	ξ	xi	X
Z	ζ	zeta	Z

LOGAN'S
MEDICAL AND SCIENTIFIC ABBREVIATIONS

A

abnormal
Absidia (genus)
absolute
absolute temperature
absorbance
Acanthocheilonema (genus)
Acanthopis (genus)
Acarapis (genus)
Acarus (genus)
acceptor
acetate side-chain in pyrrole group (re:
   uroporphyrin)
Acetobacter (genus)
acetone (a ketone body—2-propanone,
   dimethyl ketone, CH_3COCH_3)
acetum (L. vinegar)
acidum (L. acid)
Acinetobacter (genus)
acromion
actin
Actinobacillus (genus)
activity (radiation)
adenine
adenoma
adenosine
adenylic acid
admittance (the reciprocal of
   impedance—re: current and voltage)
adrenaline
adult
Aedes (genus of mosquitoes)
Aerobacter (genus)
(*Aerobacter*) aerogenes
age
akinetic
alanine
albumin
Alcaligenes (genus)
allergist
allergy
alternate
alveolar gas (when written as a
   subscript)
Amblyomma (genus of ticks)
amphetamine
amphophil (affinity for acid or basic
   dyes)
ampicillin
anaphylaxis
Ancylostoma (genus)
androsterone
anesthetic
angle

ångström unit or ångström
annus (L. year)
anode
answer
antagonized
antrectomy
aorta
aqueous
area
area (of heart shadow)
argon
Ascaris (genus)
Aspergillus (genus)
assessment (re: problem-oriented
   medical records)
Asterococcus (genus)
atomic weight
atria
atrium
atrophy
atropine
auricle
auscultation
axilla
axillary
Azotobacter (genus)
electrode placed at left midaxillary line
   (re: vectorcardiography)
haploid set of autosomes
initial negative deflection of retinogram
ocular tension by Goldmann
   applanation tonometer
start of anesthesia
symbol for mass number

A, A.
Actinomyces (genus)
Anopheles (Gr. hurtful—genus of
   mosquitoes)

A, a
acid
acidity, total
action
active
activity
anterior
aqua (L. water)
asymmetric
asymmetry
axial
systemic arterial blood (when written as
   a subscript)

A, a, a.
accommodation (re: Ophth)

1

ampere (SI symbol is A)
anode
anterior
arteria (L. artery)
artery

Å
ångström unit

°A
degree absolute (obsolete, replaced by °K, degrees Kelvin—now Kelvin [K])

Ã
cumulated activity (radiation dose)

A₁
aortic first heart sound

A₂
aortic second heart sound
minor hemoglobin component (2%) in normal human adults

A#1, A#2, etc.
auto number one, auto number two, etc. (re: traffic accident)

AI, AII, AIII
angiotensin (re: polypeptide hormones)

a
acute
ana (Gr. of each)
level of significance (re: statistics)

a.
absorptivity
acceleration
activity (chemical)
anisotrope
anisotropic
ante (L. before)
arterial
arterial blood
arteriole
atto (one quintillion, 10^{-18})
auris (L. ear)
axial
specific absorption coefficient (usually written italic)
symbol for thermodynamic activity

α
alpha (first letter of Greek alphabet)
alpha particle emission (re: radioactive isotopes)
angular acceleration
Bunsen's solubility coefficient
heavy chain of IgA
in organic compounds, refers to the carbon atom which is next to the carbon atom bearing the active group of molecules
in proportion to
Madelung constant (re: ionic crystal calculations; calculating coulomb energy)
optical rotation (re: organic chemistry)
symbol designating first

α-
designates anomer of a carbohydrate
designates one constituent of plasma globulin fraction (e.g., α-fetoprotein)
substituent group of steroid which projects below the plane of the ring

ā
before (L. ante)

a. III
antithrombin (also AT III)

AA
Academic Alertness (test—re: Psychol)
acetic acid
active alcoholic
active-assistive (range of motion excercise—re: PM&R)
acupuncture analgesia
adenylic acid
adjuvant arthritis
adrenocortical autoantibody
aggregated albumin
agranulocytic angina
allergic asthma
alopecia areata
aminoacetone
amino acid(s)
aminoacyl (radical from an amino acid)
amplitude of accommodation (re: Ophth)
amyloid-A protein
anticipatory avoidance
antigen aerosol
aortic amplitude
aortic arch
aplastic anemia
arachidonic acid (5,8,11,14-eicosatetraenoic acid)
arteries
Ascaris antigen
ascending aorta
atlantoaxial
atloaxoid
atomic absorption
Australia antigen (former name for hepatitis B antigen)
auto accident
axonal arborization (re: Neuro)

AA, A.A.
achievement age
Alcoholics Anonymous

AA, A-a
alveolar-arterial (gradient)

A & A
aid and attendance

awake and aware

$\overline{A}\overline{A}$, $\overline{a}\overline{a}$, $(\overline{a}\overline{a})$, $\overset{..}{\overline{a}}\overset{..}{\overline{a}}$, $\overset{..}{a}\overset{..}{a}$, aa.
ana (Gr. of each—indicates same
quantity of two or more ingredients)

aA
azure A

aa.
arteriae (L. arteries)

α-a
alanine

AAA
abdominal aortic aneurysm
abdominal aortic aneurysmectomy
acquired aplastic anemia
acute anxiety attack
amalgam
androgenic anabolic agent
aneurysm of the ascending aorta
anti-actin antibody
aromatic amino acid

aaa.
amalgama (obsolete variant of
amalgam)

AAAD
aromatic amino acid decarboxylase

AAAE
amino acid-activating enzymes

AA-AMP
amino acid adenylate
(adenomonophosphate)

$\alpha_2^A\beta_2^A$
major component of adult hemoglobin

a = A/bc
absorptivity (a = absorbance, b = path
length in cm, c = concentration—re:
light energy absorbed by a solution)

AABS
auto accident, broadside

AAC
antibiotic-associated
(pseudomembranous) colitis
antimicrobial agents and chemotherapy

α_1AC
α_1-antichymotrypsin

AACG
acute angle closure glaucoma (re:
Ophth)

aad, a.a-d, aa-d
adrenalectomized alloxan-diabetic

AAdC
anterior adductor of the coxa

(A-a)D_N
difference in nitrogen tensions between
mixed alveolar air and mixed arterial
blood

A-aDO$_2$, (A-a)D_{O_2}
alveolar-arterial oxygen difference

AADP
amyloid A-degrading protease

AAE
active assistive exercise (re: PM&R)
acute allergic encephalitis

AA ex.
active assisted exercises (re: PM&R)

AAF
acetic-alcohol-formalin (fixing fluid)
2-acetylaminofluorene (a carcinogen)
ascorbic acid factor

AAG
autoantigen

α_1AGp
α_1-acid-glycoprotein, seromucoid
(orosomucoid)

AAH
adrenal androgenic hyperfunction

AAI
acute alveolar injury
Adolescent Alienation Index

AAIN
acute allergic intestinal nephritis

AAK
alloactivated killers

AAL
anterior axillary line

AAM
amino acid mixture

AAME
acetylarginine methyl ester

AAN
α-amino acid nitrogen (alpha-amino
nitrogen)

AAO
amino acid oxidase
awake, alert, and oriented (re:
consciousness)

AAo
ascending aorta (re: pediatric cardiac
catheterization)

$\alpha \mathbf{a}_o$
first Bohr radius of hydrogen

A-aO$_2$
alveolar-arterial oxygen (gradient)

AAOC
antacid of choice

AAP
air at atmospheric pressure

AAPC
antibiotic-associated
  pseudomembranous colitis

A-aP$_{CO2}$, (A-a)P$_{CO2}$
alveolar-arterial carbon dioxide
  difference

AAPF
anti-arteriosclerosis polysaccharide
  factor

AAPMC
antibiotic-associated
  pseudomembranous colitis

AAPS
Arizona Articulation Proficiency Scale
  (re: Psychol)

AAR
antigen-antiglobulin reaction
Australia antigen radioimmunoassay

a.a.r.
against all risks

AARE
auto accident, rear end

AAROM
active assistive range of motion (re:
  PM&R)

AAS
anthrax antiserum
aortic arch syndrome
atomic absorption spectrophotometry

AASH
adrenal androgen stimulating hormone

AASP
acute atrophic spinal paralysis
ascending aorta synchronized pulsation

AAT
Academic Aptitude Test (re: Psychol)
acute abdominal tympany
alanine aminotransferase
alkylating agent therapy
alpha antitrypsin
auditory apperception test

α_1AT
alpha$_1$-antitrypsin

AAU
acute anterior uveitis

AAV
adeno-associated (satellite) virus
adenovirus-associated virus

AAW
anterior aortic wall

AB
abdominal
abnormal
Ace bandage
active bilaterally
Aid to the Blind
air bleed
Alcian blue 8GX (dye)
Alibert-Bazin (syndrome)
antigen binding
apex beat
asbestos body
asthmatic bronchitis

AB, Ab, ab.
antibody(ies)

AB,ab.
axiobuccal (re: Dent)

AB, ab, ab.
abortion

A/B
acid-base (ratio)

A>B
air (conduction) greater than bone
  (conduction—re: Oto)

AB-100
bis(ethyleneimido)phosphorylurethane
  (uredepa— insect sterilant)

A b
anisotropic band

aB
azure B

ab.
about

ABA
abscissic acid
allergic bronchopulmonary aspergillosis
antibacterial activity

A band
anisotropic (in polarized light) band
  (dark-staining zone of striated muscle
  sarcomere; Q bands)

AbAP
antibody against panel

ABB
Albright-Butler-Bloomberg (syndrome)

abbr.
abbreviated
abbreviation

ABC
absolute basophil count
absolute bone conduction
acalculous biliary colic
acid-balance control
aconite, belladonna, chloroform
Adriamycin, BCNU, cyclophosphamide
(re: chemotherapy)
airway, breathing, and circulation (re:
CPR)
alternative birth center
alum, blood, clay
aneurysmal bone cyst
antigen-binding capacity
apnea, bradycardia, cyanosis
aspiration biopsy cytology
Assessment of Basic Competencies (re:
Psychol)
atomic, biological, chemical (re:
warfare)
axiobuccocervical (re: Dent)

A & BC
air and bone conduction

ABCIL
antibody-mediated cell-dependent
immune lympholysis

ABCM
Adriamycin (doxorubicin), bleomycin,
cyclophosphamide, and mitomycin C
(re: chemotherapy)

ABCm
alum, blood, clay method

A.B.C. process
alum, blood, and charcoal (re: water
purification or sewage deodorizer)

ABD
Adriamycin, bleomycin, DTIC
(dacarbazine) (re: chemotherapy)
aged, blind, disabled
average body dose

ABD, Abd, abd.
abdomen
abdominal

ABD, abd.
abduction

abd.
abduct
abductor

ABD HYST, Abd Hyst
abdominal hysterectomy

ABDIC
Adriamycin (doxorubicin), bleomycin,
dacarbazine (DIC), CCNU
(lomustine) (re: chemotherapy)

abdo.
abdomen
abdominal

ABDOM, Abdom, abdom.
abdomen
abdominal

ABD (pad)
abdominal pad

abd. poll.
abductor pollicis

ABDV
Adriamycin, bleomycin, DTIC,
vinblastine (re: chemotherapy)

ABE
acute bacterial endocarditis

abe.
abequose (residue; an unusual sugar—
re: *Salmonella* species)

abend
abnormal end of task (re: computers/
data processing)

aber.
aberrant
aberration

ABG
arterial blood gas
axiobuccogingival (re: Dent)

ABGs
arterial blood gases

α-Bgt
α-bungarotoxin (neuromuscular
investigation tool)

ABI
ankle-brachial index
atherothrombotic brain infarction

ABIC
Adaptive Behavior Inventory for
Children

A bile
bile from common duct

ABK
aphakic bullous keratopathy (re: Ophth)

ABL
acid-base laboratory (studies, tests)
African Burkitt lymphoma
Albright-Butler-Lightwood (syndrome)
α-β-lipoproteinemia (a-beta-
lipoproteinemia)
angioblastic lymphadenopathy

antigen-binding lymphocytes
axiobuccolingual (re: Dent)

ABLB
alternate binaural loudness balance (re:
    Audio)

ABLE
Adult Basic Learning Examination (re:
    Psychol)

ABM
adjusted body mass
alveolar basement membrane
autologous bone marrow

ABMO
antibonding molecular orbital

ABMT
autologous bone marrow
    transplantation

ABN, Abn, abn.
abnormal

AbN
antibody nitrogen

abnor.
abnormal
abnormality

abnorm.
abnormal
abnormality

ABO
abortion
absent bed occupancy
absent bed occupant
antibodies
blood groups (A, AB, B, O)

ABOB
N^1,N^1-anhydrobis(β-hydroxyethyl-
    biguanide (moroxydine—antiviral)

ABO-HD
ABO (blood group) hemolytic disease

Abor, abor.
abortion

ABP
actin-binding protein
Adriamycin, bleomycin, prednisone (re:
    chemotherapy)
androgen-binding protein
antigen-binding protein
arterial blood pressure

ABPA
allergic bronchopulmonary aspergillosis

ABPC
antibody-producing cell

ABPE
acute bovine pulmonary edema
    (emphysema)

ABPS θ
albumin, blood, pus, and sugar negative

ABR
abortus Bang ring (probe, test—for
    brucellosis)
absolute bedrest
auditory brain-stem response

Abr, abr.
abrasions

abras.
abrasions

ABr test
agglutination test for brucellosis

ABS
acute brain syndrome
Adaptive Behavior Scale (re: Psychol)
adult bovine serum
aloin, belladonna, strychnine
anti-B serum
arterial blood sampler
at bedside

Abs
absorption

abs.
absent
absolute
away from

absc.
abscissa (L. torn or wrenched away—
    the x-coordinate value of a point on a
    graph)

abs. config.
absolute configuration

ABSe
ascending bladder septum

abs. feb.
absente febre (L. in the absence of
    fever)

absorp.
absorption

AbSR
abdominal skin reflexes

abst.
abstract

abstr.
abstract

ABT
arteria basilaris thrombus

abt.
about

ABTX
alpha-bungarotoxin (neuromuscular
   investigative tool)

ABU
asymptomatic bacteriuria

ABV
actinomycin D, bleomycin, vincristine
   (re: chemotherapy)
Adriamycin, bleomycin, vinblastine (re:
   chemotherapy)
arthropod-borne virus

ABVD
Adriamycin, bleomycin, vinblastine,
   dacarbazine (re: chemotherapy)

ABW
actual body weight

ABY
acid bismuth yeast (agar)

aby.
antibody

AC
abdominal circumference
abdominal compression
absorption coefficient
absorptive cell
abuse case
acetylcholine
acetylcysteine
acidified complement
Acinetobacter calcoaceticus
aconitine (poisonous alkaloid of
   aconite)
activated charcoal
acute cholecystitis
adenocarcinoma
adenyl cyclase
adherent cell
adrenal cortex
adrenal corticoid
Adriamycin, CCNU (re: chemotherapy)
Adriamycin, cyclophosphamide (re:
   chemotherapy)
air chamber (re: Ophth)
air changes
air conditioning
alcoholic cirrhosis
all culture (broth)
ambulatory controls
anesthesia circuit
angiocellular
anterior column
anterior commissure
anticoagulant
anticomplementary
anti-inflammatory corticoid
   (antiphlogistic corticoid)

antiphlogistic corticoid (anti-
   inflammatory corticoid)
aortocoronary
apophysitis calcanei
arm circumference
Arnold-Chiari (syndrome)
arterial capillary
ascending colon
auriculocarotid

AC, A.C.
air conduction
aortic closure

AC, A.C., A-C, A/C
acromioclavicular

AC, A.C., ac, a/c
alternating current

AC, A.C., ac.
axiocervical

AC, A-C
atriocarotid

AC, A/C, a.c.
anterior chamber (re: Ophth)

AC, ac.
acceleration
acid
acute
anodal closure

AC, a.c., ā.c.
ante cibum (L. before a meal)

A-C
Adriamycin, cyclophosphamide (re:
   chemotherapy)

A/C
albumin-coagulin ratio
anchored catheter

Ac
accelerator (i.e., Ac-globulin)
acetate
acetyl
acryl group
actinium (element)

[228]Ac
mesothorium *II* (actinium isotope)

aC
arabinosylcytosine
azure C (monomethylthionine)

ac.
antecubital

a.c.
ante cibos (L. before meals)

ACA
acute cerebellar ataxia

adenine-cytosine-adenine
adenocarcinoma
ammonia, copper, arsenic
anomalous coronary artery
anterior cerebral artery
anterior communicating aneurysms
anterior communicating artery
anticentromere antibody
anticollagen autoantibody
anticomplement activity
Automatic Clinical Analyzer

AC/A
accommodative convergence-
    accommodation ratio (re: Ophth)

7-ACA
7-aminocephalosporanic acid

ACAC
activated charcoal artificial cell

acac
acetylacetonate

AcAcOH
acetoacetic acid (acetoacetate)

ACAD, acad.
academy

ACAO
acyl coenzyme A oxidase

AC/A ratio
accommodative convergence/
    accommodation ratio (re: Ophth)

ACB
antibody-coated bacteria
arterialized capillary blood

AC/BC
air conduction (time)/bone conduction
    (time)

ACBG
aorta-coronary bypass graft

ACC
acinic cell carcinoma
acute care center
adrenocortical carcinoma
alveolar cell carcinoma
ambulatory care center
anodal closure contraction
antitoxin-containing cell
articular chondrocalcinosis

ACC, Acc
adenoid cystic carcinoma

Acc, acc.
acceleration
accelerator
accident
accommodation

accompany
according

accel.
accelerate(d)
acceleration

AcCh, Ac Ch
acetylcholine

AcChR
acetylcholine receptor

AcCHS
acetylcholinesterase

accid.
accident
accidental

acc. insuff.
accommodative insufficiency (re:
    Ophth)

ACCL, ACCl
anodal closure clonus

AcCoA, Ac Co A
acetylcoenzyme A

accom.
accommodation (re: Ophth)
accompanied
accompany

accum.
accumulated
accumulation
accumulative

accur.
accuratissime (L. most carefully,
    accurately)

ACD
absolute cardiac dullness
absolute claudication distance
actinomycin D
adult celiac disease
allergic contact dermatitis
alpha-chain disease
annihilation coincidence detection
anterior chest diameter
anticoagulant citrate dextrose
area of cardiac dullness

ACD, A.C.D.
acid-citrate-dextrose (solution—citric
    acid, trisodium citrate, dextrose)

AC̄D
alive with disease

AC-DC
bisexual (slang)

AC-DC, ac/dc
alternating current/direct current

ACD sol., ACDsol
acid-citrate-dextrose (solution—citric acid, trisodium citrate, dextrose solution)

Ac, Ds system
Activator-Dissociation system (re: genetics)

ACE
acetonitrile (reaction; Hunt's reaction)
acute coronary event
adrenal cortical extract (adrenocortical extract; corticosteroid; veterinary use for bovine ketosis)
alcohol-chloroform-ether
angiotensin-converting enzyme

ACe
Adriamycin, cyclophosphamide (Cytoxan) (re: chemotherapy)

ace
acentric fragment (re: cytogenetics)

ace.
acetone

ACED
anhydrotic congenital ectodermal dysplasia

ACEH
acid cholesterol ester hydrolase

ACEI
angiotensin-converting enzyme inhibitor

A cells
alpha cells (of pancreas or anterior lobe of hypophysis)

AC Em
actinium emanation (actinon)

Acet, acet.
acetone

acet.
acetum (L. vinegar)

acetab.
acetabulum

AcetylCoA, acetyl-CoA
acetylcoenzyme A

ACF
accessory clinical findings
Acute Care Facility
advanced communications function
area correction factor

ACFn
additional cost of false negatives

ACFp
additional cost of false positives

ACFUCY
actinomycin D, 5-fluorouracil, cyclophosphamide (re: chemotherapy)

ACG
angiocardiography
angle closure
aortocoronary graft
apexcardiogram

AcG, ac-g
accelerator globulin (Factor V)

Ac-globulin
accelerator globulin (Factor V)

ACH
achalasia
active chronic hepatitis
adrenal cortical (adrenocortical) hormone
aftercoming head
arm, chest, height
arm girth, chest depth, hip width (index of nutrition)

ACH, ACh, Ach
acetylcholine

AChE
acetylcholinesterase

ACH index
arm girth, chest depth, hip width index (re: nutrition)

AChR
acetylcholine receptors

AChRAb
acetylcholine receptor antibody

AChRP
acetylcholine receptor protein

AC&HS
ante cibum et hora somni (L. before a meal and at the hour of sleep—at bedtime)

A C hyph.
anterior chamber hyphema

ACI
acoustic comfort index
acute coronary infarction
acute coronary insufficiency
adenylate cyclase inhibitor
adrenal cortical (adrenocortical) insufficiency
anticlonus index
average cost of illness

acid phos.
acid phosphatase

acid PO₄
acid phosphatase

acid p'tase
acid phosphatase

ACIF
anticomplement immunofluorescence

A-c interval
atriocarotid
auriculocarotid

ACIP
acute canine idiopathic polyneuropathy

AC jt.
acromioclavicular joint

ACK
acknowledge (character—re:
    computers/data processing)

ACL
Achievement Check List (re: personality
    test)
Adjective Check List (re: Psychol)
anterior cruciate ligament

ACl
anticlonus (index)

ACLC
Assessment of Children's Language
    Comprehension (re: Psychol)

ACLS
advanced cardiac life support

ACM
acute cerebrospinal meningitis
Adriamycin (doxorubicin),
    cyclophosphamide, and methotrexate
    (re: chemotherapy)
albumin, calcium, magnesium
alveolar capillary membrane
anticardiac myosin
atom connectivity matrix

ACME
Automated Classification of Medical
    Entities

ACMF
arachnoid cyst of the middle fossa

ACMP
alveolar-capillary membrane
    permeability

ACMV
assist-controlled mechanical ventilation

ACN
acute conditioned necrosis

ACO
acute coronary occlusion

alert, cooperative, and oriented (re:
    consciousness)
anodal closing odor

ACO1
aconitase, soluble (aconitate
    hydratase—enzyme)

ACO2
aconitase, mitochondrial (aconitate
    hydratase—enzyme)

ACOP
Adriamycin, cyclophosphamide,
    Oncovin, prednisone (re:
    chemotherapy)

ACOPP, A-COPP
Adriamycin (doxorubicin),
    cyclophosphamide, Oncovin
    (vincristine), procarbazine, and
    prednisone (re: chemotherapy)

ACO-S
aconitase, soluble

acous.
acoustical
acoustics

ACP
acid phosphatase
acyl carrier protein
Animal Care Panel
anodal closing picture
aspirin, caffeine, phenacetin

ACP1
acid phosphatase-1

ACP2
acid phosphatase-2

ACPC
1-aminocyclopentanecarboxylic acid
    (re: amino acid transport studies)

AC-PH
acid phosphatase

ac. phos.
acid phosphatase

ACPP
adrenocorticopolypeptide

ACPS
acrocephalopolysyndactyly

ACR
abnormally contracting regions
absolute catabolic rate
acriflavine
adenomatosis of the colon and rectum
anticonstipating regimen
anticonstipation regimen
axillary count rate

Acr
acrylic

ACS
acrocephalosyndactyly
acute confusional state
anodal closing sound
anticytotoxic serum
antireticular cytotoxic serum
aperture current setting

ACS AO
ascending aorta

ACS grade
American Chemical Society (re:
specifications for chemical purity)

ACSV
aortocoronary saphenous vein

ACSVBG
aortocoronary saphenous vein bypass
graft

ACT
achievement through counseling and
treatment
actinomycin
activated clotting time
activated coagulation time
advanced coronary therapy
advanced coronary treatment
American College Testing (Program)
anterocolic transposition
antichymotrypsin
anticoagulant therapy
anticoagulation therapy
Anxiety Control Training (re: Psychol)
Assessment of Career Development
(re: Psychol)
atropine coma therapy

act.
action
active
activity

=/act, = & act.
equal and active (re: pupils or deep
tendon reflexes)

ACTA Scanner
Automatic Computerized Transverse
Axial Scanner

act-C
actinomycin C

ACTD, act-D
actinomycin D

ACTe
anodal closure tetanus

ACTH
adrenocorticotrop(h)ic hormone

ACTH, big
adrenocorticotrop(h)ic hormone form
produced by certain tumors

ACTH, little
distinguishes conventional
adrenocorticotrop(h)ic hormone when
compared with big
adrenocorticotrop(h)ic hormone

ACTH-RF
adrenocorticotrop(h)ic hormone-
releasing factor

activ.
activity

ACTN
adrenocorticotrop(h)in

ACTP
adrenocorticotrop(h)ic polypeptide

ACTS
acute cervical traumatic sprain
acute cervical traumatic syndrome

ACTS c̄ NRI
acute cervical traumatic syndrome with
nerve root involvement

ACU
acute care unit
agar colony-forming unit
ambulatory care unit
automatic calling unit (re: computers/
data processing)

ACV
acute cardiovascular (disease)
acyclovir
atrial/carotid/ventricular

ACVD
acute cardiovascular disease
atherosclerotic cardiovascular disease

AC/W
acetone/water

ACY1
aminoacylase-1

Acyl-Co A
organic compound—coenzyme A ester

AD
accident dispensary
active disease
acute dermatomyositis
Adair Dighton (syndrome)
addict
adenoid(al) degeneration (virus)
adjuvant disease
admitting diagnosis
adult disease
aerosol deposition
after discharge

alcohol dehydrogenase
Aleutian disease
alveolar duct
Alzheimer's disease
analgesic dose
anodal duration
antigenic determinant
appropriate disability
arthritic dose
atopic dermatitis
atrio dextro (L. in the right atrium)
atrium dextra (L. hall or entrance room + right)
autonomic dysreflexia
autosomal dominant (re: genetics)
average day
average deviation
axis deviation
diphenylchlorarsine (sneezing gas—also Clark I & DA)
drug addict

A/D
analog-to-digital (converter—re: computers)

AD, ad.
axiodistal (re: Dent)

AD, a.d.
auris dextra (L. right ear)

A and D
admission and discharge

A & D
admission and discharge
ascending and descending

Ad
adipocyte
Adrenalin

A d
anisotropic disk

$[\alpha]_D^{25}$
specific optical rotation at 25°C for D (sodium) line (re: organic chemistry)

ad.
adde (L. add)
addetur (L. let there be added)

ADA
adenosine deaminase
anterior descending artery
approved dietary allowance

ADA #
American Diabetes Association diet number

ADA diet
American Diabetes Association diet

ADA-MHA
Alcohol, Drug Abuse, and Mental Health Administration

adB
acceleration decibel

ad baln.
ad balneum (L. to the bath)

ADBC
Adriamycin, DTIC, bleomycin, CCNU (re: chemotherapy)

ADC
Affective Disorders Clinic
Aid to Dependent Children
albumin, dextrose, catalase (medium)
analog-to-digital converter (re: computers)
anodal duration contraction
anterior descending coronary
antral diverticulum of the colon
average daily census
axiodistocervical (re: Dent)

AdC
adrenal cortex

AD capacity
alveolar diffusing capacity

ADCC
antibody-dependent cell-mediated cytotoxicity
antibody-dependent cellular cytotoxicity

ADCON
address constant (re: computers)

ADCP
adenosine deaminase complexing protein

ADD
adenosine deaminase
androstanediene-dione
attention deficit disorder
average daily dose

ADD, add.
adduction

add.
addantur (L. let them be added)
addatur (L. let it be added)
adde (L. add)
addendo (L. by adding)
addendum (L. to be added)
addetur (L. let there be added)
addition
additional
adduct
adductor

add. c. trit.
adde cum tritu (L. add with a rubbing
  [triturition])

ad def. an.
ad defectionem animi (L. to the point of
  fainting)

ad deliq.
ad deliquium (L. to fainting)

addend.
addendum (L. to be added)

ADD-HA
attention deficit disorder with
  hyperactivity

addict.
addiction

addn.
addition

addnl.
additional

add. poll.
adductor pollicis

ad duas vic.
ad duas vices (L. to two doses [for two
  doses])

ADE
acute disseminated encephalitis
antibody-dependent enhancement
apparent digestible energy

Ade
adenine

ad effect.
ad effectum (L. to effect)

ADEM
acute disseminated encephalomyelitis

adenoca.
adenocarcinoma

adeq.
adequate

ad. feb.
adstante febre (L. fever being present)

ADG
atrial diastolic gallop
axiodistogingival (re: Dent)

ad gr. acid.
ad grata aciditatem (L. to an agreeable
  acidity)

ad grat. acid.
ad grata aciditatem (L. to an agreeable
  acidity)

ad grat. gust.
ad gratum gustum (L. to an agreeable
  taste)

ad gr. gust.
ad gratum gustum (L. to an agreeable
  taste)

ADH
alcohol dehydrogenase

ADH, adh
antidiuretic hormone

adh.
adhesions
adhesive

adhes.
adhesions
adhesive

adhib.
adhibendus (L. to be administered)

ADI
acceptable daily intake
allowable daily intake
antral diverticulum of the ileum
autosomal dominant ichthyosis
axiodistoincisal (re: Dent)
axiodistoinclusal (re: Dent)

ad int.
ad interim (L. to meanwhile)

A disk
primary user disk (re: computers/data
  processing)

adj.
adjacent
adjective
adjoining
adjunct
adjust
adjusted
adjutant

ADK
adenosine kinase

ADKC
atopic dermatitis with
  keratoconjunctivitis

ADL
activities of daily living

ADLC
antibody-dependent lymphocyte-
  mediated cytotoxicity (test)

Ad lib., ad lib.
ad libitum (L. freely; at pleasure)

ADM
administrative medicine

Adriamycin (doxorubicin—
    antineoplastic)
apparent distribution mass

ADM, adm.
administrator

AdM
adrenal medulla

Adm
administration

Adm, adm.
admission
admitted

adm.
admit
admove (L. apply; add)

adm. amb.
admitted ambulatory

ad man. med.
ad manus medici (L. [to be delivered]
    into the hands of the [prescribing]
    physician)

Adm Dr
admitting doctor

Admin, admin.
administer
administration

admov.
admove (L. apply; add)
admoveantur (L. let them be added)
admoveatur (L. let there be added; let it
    be applied)

Adm Ph
admitting physician

Adm Phys
admitting physician

ADMR
average daily metabolic rate

adm. w/c
admitted in wheelchair

ADMX
adrenal medullectomy

ADN
aortic depressor nerve

ad naus.
ad nauseam (L. to the extent of
    producing nausea)

ADN-B assay
anti-deoxyribonuclease-B assay (re:
    streptococcus infections)

ad neut.
ad neutralisandum (L. to neutralization)
ad neutrum (L. to neither [neutralize;
    neutralized; neutralization])

ADO
axiodisto-occlusal (re: Dent)

Ado
adenosine (ribofuranosyladenine)

ADOAP
Adriamycin (doxorubicin), Oncovin
    (vincristine), ara-C (cytarabine), and
    prednisone (re: chemotherapy)

Ado-Met
S-adenosylmethionine

ADOP
Adriamycin, Oncovin, prednisone (re:
    chemotherapy)

ADP
acute dermatomyositis and polymyositis
adenopathies
adenosine diphosphate (adenosine 5'-
    diphosphate)
advanced pancreatitis
aminohydroxypropylidene
    diphosphonate
approved drug product
area diastolic pressure
automated data processing
automatic data processing

AdP
adductor pollicis (re: muscles)

ad part. dolent.
ad partes dolentes (L. to the aching
    parts)

ADPase
adenosine diphosphatase (apyrase)

ADPL
average daily patient load

ad pond. om.
ad pondus omnium (L. to the weight of
    the whole)

ADQ
abductor digiti quinti (re: muscles)

adq.
adequate

ADR
Accepted Dental Remedies
adverse drug reaction
adverse drug report
airway dilation reflex

ADR, Adr
Adriamycin (doxorubicin—
    antineoplastic)

Adr, adr.
adrenaline

ad rat.
ad rationem (L. to ratio)

adren.
Adrenalin (adrenaline; epinephrine)

Adria
Adriamycin (antineoplastic)

Adria-L-PAM
Adriamycin, L-phenylalanine mustard
(re: chemotherapy)

ADS
alternate delivery system
anatomical dead space
antibody deficiency syndrome
antidiuretic substance

ad sat.
ad saturandum (L. to saturation)

ad satur.
ad saturandum (L. to saturation)

Adson's M
Adson's maneuver (test)

adst. feb.
adstante febre (L. when fever is
present; while fever is present)

ADT
accepted dental therapeutic(s)
active disk table (re: computers/data
processing)
adenosine triphosphate
A (any), D (what you desire), T (thing)
(re: a placebo)
agar-gel diffusion test
alternate day therapy
alternate day treatment
Auditory Discrimination Test

ADTe
anodal duration tetanus
tetanic contraction

ad tert. vic.
ad tertium vicem (L. to the third time [to
three doses])

ADU
acute duodenal ulcer
automatic dialing unit (re: computers/
data processing)

ad us.
ad usum (L. according to custom)

ad us. ext.
ad usum externum (L. for external use)

ad us. exter.
ad usum externum (L. for external use)

ad us. med.
ad usum medicinalem (L. for medicinal
use)

ad us. propr.
ad usum proprium (L. according to
proper use)

ad us. vet.
ad usum veterinarium (L. for veterinary
use)

ADV
adenovirus
adventitia
Aleutian disease virus

A-DV
arterio-deep venous (difference)

A/DV
arteria/deep venous (difference)
arterio/deep venous (difference)

Adv
advisory

adv.
advanced
adversum (L. against; adverse to;
opposed to)
advice
advise

ad 2 vic.
ad duas vices (L. at two times; for two
doses)

AD virus
adenovirus

ADW
assault with a deadly weapon

A5D5W
alcohol 5%, dextrose 5%, in water

ADX
adrenalectomized

AE
Accurate Empathy (re: Psychol)
acrodermatitis enteropathica
activation energy
adrenal epinephrine
adult erythrocyte
aftereffect
agarose electrophoresis
alcohol embryopathy
alveolar *Echinococcus*
anoxic encephalopathy
anti-epileptic (medication)
apoenzyme
aryepiglottic (re: ENT)
avian (infectious) encephalomyelitis
energy of activation

AE, A.E.
antitoxineinheit (Ger. antitoxic unit)
Antitoxische Einheit (Ger. antitoxic unit)

AE, A-E, A/E
above elbow

A & E
active and equal

A + E
analysis and evaluation

ae.
aetatis (L. of age)

AEA
alcohol, ether, acetone (solution)

AE amp., A/E Amp
above elbow amputation

AEB
acute erythroblastopenia
avian erythroblastosis

A-EB
acquired (non-inherited) epidermolysis
   bullosa acquisita

AEC
at earliest convenience
Atomic Energy Commission

AECD
allergic eczematous contact dermatitis

AED
anti-epileptic drug

AEDP
automated external defibrillator
   pacemaker

AEF
allogenic effect factor
amyloid enhancing factor
aryepiglottic fold (re: ENT)

AEG
air encephalogram

AEG, aeg.
aeger; aegra (L. the sick one [male,
   female])

AEI
arbitrary evolution index
atrial emptying index

AEM
analytical electron microscope
analytical electron microscopy
avian encephalomyelitis

AEN
aseptic epiphyseal necrosis

AEP
acute edematous pancreatitis
artificial endocrine pancreas
auditory evoked potential
average evoked potential

AEq
age equivalent

aeq.
aequales (L. equals)

AER
acoustic evoked response
acute exertional rhabdomyolysis
agranular endoplasmic reticulum
aided equalization response
albumin excretion rate
aldosterone excretion rate
apical ectodermal ridge
auditory evoked response
average electroencephalic response
average evoked response

Aero, aero.
Aerobacter (genus)

AERP
atrial effective refractory period

AES
acetone-extracted serum
anterior esophageal sensor
anti-eosinophil sera
antral ethmoidal sphenoidectomy
aortic ejection sound
Auger's electron spectroscopy

A-esotropia
convergent strabismus (crossed eyes)
   greater in upward than in downward
   gaze

AESP
applied extrasensory perception

AET
absorption-equivalent thickness
β-aminoethylisothiuronium bromide
   hydrobromide (radioprotective agent)
S-(2-aminoethyl)-2-isothiuronium
   bromide hydrobromide
   (radioprotective agent)

aet.
aetas (L. age)
aetatis (L. of age)

aetat.
aetatis (L. of age)

AEV
avian erythroblastosis virus

AF
abnormal frequency
acid-fast (bacilli)

activity front
adult female
afebrile
aflatoxin
albumin-free (tuberculin)
albumose-free (tuberculin)
aldehyde fuchsin
alleged father
amaurosis fugax
amniotic fluid
anchoring fibril
angiogenesis factor
anteflexion
antibody-forming
aortic flow
artificially fed
ascitic fluid
Aspergillus fumigatus
atrial fusion
attenuation factor
auricular fibrillation

AF, Af
atrial flutter

AF, af.
audiofrequency

AF, a.f.
atrial fibrillation

A-F
anterior fontanel
antifibrinogen

AFA
alcohol-formalin-acetic acid

AFB
acid-fast bacillus (bacilli)
aflatoxin B (re: veterinary—a mycotoxin)
aorto-femoral bypass

AFB$_1$
aflatoxin B$_1$ (re: veterinary)

AFC
antibody-forming cell(s)

AFCI
acute focal cerebral ischemia

AFD
accelerated freeze drying

AFDC
Aid to Families with Dependent Children

afeb.
afebrile

aff.
afferent
affinis (L. having an affinity with [but not identical with])

affil.
affiliated

AFG
aflatoxin G (re: veterinary—a mycotoxin)
amniotic fluid glucose
analog function generator (re: computers/data processing)
auditory figure ground

AFH
anterior facial height (re: cephalometrics)

AFI
amaurotic familial idiocy

AFIB, AFib, A fib.
atrial fibrillation

AFIP
Armed Forces Institute of Pathology

AFL
aflatoxicol (re: veterinary)
anti-fatty liver (re: a pancreatic tissue factor)
antifibrinolysin
artificial limb
Aspergillus flavus
atrial flutter

AFLP
acute fatty liver of pregnancy

AFM
aflatoxin M (re: veterinary—a mycotoxin)

AFN
afunctional neutrophil

AFO
ankle-foot orthosis (re: Ortho)

AFP, aFP
alpha$_1$ fetoprotein (alpha-fetoprotein; alphafetoprotein)
anterior faucial pillar (re: ENT)

AfP
affiliate physician

Af Ph
affiliate physician

AFPP
acute fibrinopurulent pneumonia

α-FPT-dec.
flupentixol decanoate

AFQ
aflatoxin Q (re: veterinary)

AFQT
Armed Forces Qualification Test

AFR
antifibrinolysin reaction
ascorbic free radical

AFRD
acute febrile respiratory disease

AFRI
acute febrile respiratory illness

AFS
acquired Fanconi syndrome
adult Fanconi syndrome
antifibroblast serum

AFSP
acute fibrinoserous pneumonia

AFT
active file table (re: computers/data
    processing)
aflatoxin (re: veterinary—a mycotoxin)
agglutination-flocculation test

AFT$_3$
absolute free triiodothyronine

AFT$_4$
absolute free thyroxin(e)

AFTA
autonomous functioning nodule

AFTC
apparent free testosterone
    concentration

AFTN
autonomously functioning thyroid
    nodule

AFTR
atrophy, fasciculation, tremor, rigidity

AFV
amniotic fluid volume

AFX
atypical fibroxanthoma

AG
against gravity
agarose
analytical grade (re: organic chemistry)
antiglobulin
attached gingiva
axiogingival (re: Dent)
azurophilic granule

AG, Ag
antigen

AG, ag
atrial gallop

AG, ag.
antigravity

A-G, A/G
albumin/globulin (ratio)

Ag
argentum (L. silver)

^{105}Ag
radioactive isotope of silver (argentum)

^{110}Ag
radioactive isotope of silver (argentum)

^{111}Ag
radioactive isotope of silver (argentum)

AGA
accelerated growth area
antiglomerular antibody
appropriate for gestational age

Ag-Ab
antigen-antibody (complex)

AGAP
antibody-against panel

AGAS
aerobiospherical genetic adaptational
    system

AGB, a.g.b.
any good brand

AGC
absolute granulocyte count
automatic gain control

AgCl
silver chloride

AGCT
antiglobulin consumption test (Coombs'
    test)
Army General Classification Test

Agcy, agcy.
agency

AGD
agar-gel diffusion
agarose diffusion (method)

AGDD
agar-gel double diffusion

AGE
acrylamide gel
acute gastroenteritis
agarose gel electrophoresis

AGE, ÅGE, A°GE
angle of greatest extension (re: Ortho)

AGED
automated general experimental device

AGF
adrenal growth factor

AGF, ÅGF, A°GF
angle of greatest flexion (re: Ortho)

ag. feb.
aggrediente febre (L. when the fever
increases)

AGG
agammaglobulinemia

AGG, agg.
aggravated

agg.
agglutinate
agglutinated
agglutination
aggregate

aggl.
agglutinate
agglutinated
agglutination

Agglut, agglut.
agglutinate
agglutinated
agglutination

aggrav.
aggravate
aggravation

aggreg.
aggregation

AGGS
anti-gas gangrene serum

AgI
silver iodide

AGIT, agit.
agita (L. shake; stir)

agit.
agitated
agitation

agit. ante sum.
agita ante sumendum (L. shake before
taking)

agit. a. us.
agita ante usum (L. shake before using)

agit. bene
agita bene (L. shake well)

agit. vas.
agitato vase (L. the vial having been
shaken)

AGL
acute granulocytic leukemia
agglutination
aminoglutethimide

AGLMe
N-alpha-acetylglycyl-L-lysine methyl
ester

AGMK
African green monkey kidney

AGMKC
African green monkey kidney cell

AGML
acute gastric mucosal lesion

AGN
acute glomerulonephritis
albumin-globulin (studies)

AGN, agn.
agnosia

AgNO$_3$
silver nitrate

AgNOR
silver-staining nucleolar organizer
region

AGP
acid glycoprotein
agar gel precipitation (test)

AGPI
agar-gel precipitin inhibition

AGPT
agar-gel precipitation test

AGR
anticipatory goal response

A/G ratio
albumin/globulin ratio

AGS
adrenal gland sympathogonioma
adrenogenital syndrome
audiogenic seizure

AGT
abnormal glucose tolerance
activity group therapy (re: Psychol)
acute generalized tuberculosis
antiglobulin test

agt.
agent

AGTH
adrenoglomerulotrop(h)ic hormone

AGTr
adrenoglomerulotrop(h)in

AGTT
abnormal glucose tolerance test

AGV, A.G.V.
aniline gentian violet

19

AH
abdominal hysterectomy
accidental hypothermia
acetohexamide
acid hydrolysis
acute hepatitis
Adie-Holmes (syndrome)
adult home
after-hyperpolarization
alcoholic hepatitis
amenorrhea and hirsutism
aminohippurate
anterior hypothalamus
antihistaminic
antihyaluronidase
arcuate hypothalamus (re: Neuro)
arterial hypertension
artificial heart
ascites hepatoma
autonomic hyperreflexia (re:
  neuromuscular)
axillary hair

AH, Ah, ah
hypermetropic astigmatism (re: Ophth)

Ah
ampere hour

AHA
acetohydroxamic acid (enzyme inhibitor
  [urease])
acquired hemolytic anemia
acute hemolytic anemia
anterior hypothalamic area (re: Neuro)
antiheart antibody
aspartyl-hydroxamic acid
autoimmune hemolytic anemia

AHB
alpha-hydroxybutyric dehydrogenase

α-HBD
α-hydroxybutyrate dehydrogenase

AHC
acute hemorrhagic conjunctivitis
acute hemorrhagic cystitis
antihemophilic Factor C

α-HCH
α-hexachlorocyclohexane

AHCTL
N,-acetylhomocysteinethiolactone (re:
  hepatic disorders)

AHD
acute heart disease
antihyaluronidase
antihypertensive drug
arteriosclerotic heart disease
atherosclerotic heart disease
autoimmune hemolytic disease

AHE
acute hemorrhagic encephalomyelitis

AHEA
Area Health Education Activities

AHEC
Area Health Education Centers

AHES
artificial heart energy system

AHF
acute heart failure
American Hospital Formulary
antihemolytic factor
antihemophilic factor (Factor VIII)
antihemophilic globulin F
Argentinian hemorrhagic fever

AHG
aggregated human globulin
antihemophilic globulin A (Factor VIII)
antihuman globulin

AHGG
aggregated human gamma globulin
antihuman gamma globulin

AHGS
acute herpetic gingival stomatitis

AHH
alpha-hydrazine (analogue of) histidine
arylhydrocarbon hydroxylase (gene
  marker symbol)

αHH
α-hydrazinohistidine

AHI
active hostility index

A & H ins.
accident and health insurance

A-H interval
A-V node impulse conduction measured
  on His bundle electrogram

AHL
apparent half life

AHLE
acute hemorrhagic leukoencephalitis

AHLG
antihuman-lymphocyte globulin

AHLS
antihuman-lymphocyte serum

AHM
ambulatory Holter monitor (re: Cardio)
anterior hyaloid membrane (anterior
  membrana vitrea)

AHMA
antiheart muscle autoantibody

AHMHA
4-amino-3-hydroxy-6-methylheptanoic
acid (statine)

AHO
Albright's hereditary osteodystrophy

AHP
acute hemorrhagic pancreatitis
after hyperpolarization
air at high pressure

AHPO
anterior hypothalamic-preoptic (area)

AHR
antihyaluronidase reaction

AHS
African horse sickness

AHT
antihyaluronidase titer
augmented histamine test
autogenous hamster tumor

AHTG
antihuman thymocytic globulin

AH titer
antihyaluronidase titer

AHTP
antihuman thymocytic plasma

AHTS
antihuman thymus serum

AHU
acute hemolytic uremic (syndrome)
antihyaluronidase
arginine, hypoxanthine, uracil

AHV
avian herpes virus

AI
accidental injury
anaphylatoxin inhibitor
angiogenesis inhibitor
angiotensin I
anxiety index
aortic incompetence
aortic insufficiency
apical impulse
articular index
artificial insemination
artificial intelligence
atherogenic index
atrial insufficiency
autoimmune
axioincisal (re: Dent)

AI, A/I, a.i.
accidentally incurred

A&I
Allergy and Immunology (Service[s])

a.i.
active ingredient

a_i
item discrimination parameter (re:
Psychol; item characteristic curve
[statistics])

AIA
allylisopropylacetamide
amylase inhibitor activity
anti-immunoglobulin antibodies
anti-insulin antibody
aspirin-induced asthma
automated image analysis

AIB
aminoisobutyric (acid)
avian infectious bronchitis

AIBA
aminoisobutyric acid

AIBN
2,2'-azobisisobutyronitrile (industrial
chemical)

AIC
5-aminoimidazole-4-carboxamide

AICA
anterior inferior cerebellar artery
anterior inferior communicating artery

AICAR
5-amino-4-imidazolecarboxamide
ribonucleotide

AICE
angiotensin I converting enzyme

AICF
autoimmune complement fixation

AID
acquired immunodeficiency disease
acute infectious disease
argon ionization detector
artificial insemination—donor
(heterologous)
autoimmune deficiency
autoimmune disease
average interocular difference

AIDS
acquired immune deficiency syndrome

AIE
acute inclusion (body) encephalitis
acute infectious encephalitis

AIEP
amount of insulin extractable (from the)
pancreas

AIF
anemia-inducing factor

anti-inflammatory
anti-invasion factor

AIFD
acute intrapartum fetal distress

AIG
anti-immunoglobulin

A-IGP
activity-interview group psychotherapy

AIH
artificial insemination—husband
  (homologous)

AIHA
autoimmune hemolytic anemia

AIHD
acquired immune hemolytic disease

AIIS
anterior inferior iliac spine

AIL
acute infectious lymphocytosis
angioimmunoblastic lymphadenopathy

AILD
alveolar-interstitial lung disease
angioimmunoblastic lymphadenopathy
  with dysproteinemia

AIM
Artificial Intelligence in Medicine (re:
  computers)
assessment of interactive mode

AIMD
abnormal involuntary movement
  disorder

AIMS
abnormal involuntary movement scale

AIN
acute interstitial nephritides (nephritis)

AINA
automated immunonephelometric
  assay

AINS
anti-inflammatory nonsteroidal

AInsuf, A insuf.
aortic insufficiency

AIO
amyloid of immunoglobulin origin

AIP
acute idiopathic pericarditis
acute infectious polyneuritis
acute intermittent porphyria
aldosterone-induced protein
annual implementation plan
arachidonate-insensitive platelet

automated immunoprecipitation
automated immunoprecipitin (system)
average intravascular pressure

AIR
5-aminoimidazole ribonucleotide
Average Impairment Rating

Air Bronch
air bronchogram

AIRS
Amphetamine Interview Rating Scale

AIS
Abbreviated Injury Scale
androgen insensitivity syndrome
anti-insulin serum

AIT
acute intensive treatment

AITT
arginine insulin tolerance test
augmented insulin tolerance test

AIU
absolute iodine uptake
antigen-inducing unit

AIVR
accelerated idioventricular rhythm

AIVV
anterior internal vertebral vein

AJ, A-J
ankle jerk(s)

AK
acetate kinase
adenylate kinase
artificial kidney

AK, AK, a.k.
above knee

A→K
ankle to knee

AK1
adenylate kinase-1

AK2
adenylate kinase-2

AK3
adenylate kinase-3

AKA
above-knee amputation
alcoholic ketoacidosis
antikeratin antibody

AKA, a.k.a.
also known as

AK amp., A/K Amp, Ak amp.
above-knee amputation

α-KG
alpha-ketoglutarate

AKP
alkaline phosphatase

AKS
auditory and kinesthetic sensation

AL
absolute latency
acinar lumina
acute leukemia
adaptation level
Albright-Lightwood (syndrome)
albumin
annoyance level
antihuman lymphocytic (globulin)
avian leukosis
axial length
axillary loop
axiolingual (re: Dent)

AL, al.
alignment (mark—re: cardiology)

AL, a.l.
auris laeva (L. left ear)

Al
Alfvén number
allergy
aluminum (element)

²⁶Al
radioactive isotope of aluminum

ALA
anterior lip of the acetabulum (re:
Ortho)

ALA, ALa, A La
axiolabial (re: Dent)

ALA, Ala
δ-aminolevulinic acid (δ-
aminolevulinate; aminolevulinic acid)

Ala
alanine (or its mono- or di- radical)

ALAD, ALA-D
abnormal left axis deviation
aminolevulinic acid dehydrase

ALAG, ALaG
axiolabiogingival (re: Dent)

ALAL, ALaL, A La L
axiolabiolingual (re: Dent)

ALAS
aminolevulinic acid synthetase

ALAT
alanine aminotransferase
alanine transaminase

ALB
avian lymphoblastosis

ALB, Alb, alb.
albumin

alb.
albus (L. white)

alb. C
albumin clearance

ALB/GLOB
albumin-globulin ratio

ALC
absolute lymphocyte count
Alternative Lifestyle Checklist
approximate lethal concentration
avian leukosis complex
axiolinguocervical (re: Dent)

Alc, alc.
alcohol

ALCA
anomalous left coronary artery

ALCEQ
Adolescent Life Change Event
Questionnaire

alcoh.
alcohol
alcoholic

AlCr
aluminum crown (re: Dent)

AlcR, Alc R, alcr.
alcohol rub

ALD
adrenoleukodystrophy (Siemerling-
Crentzfeldt disease— re: genetics)
alcoholic liver disease
aldosterone
anterior latissimus dorsi (re: muscles)

ALD, Ald
aldolase

ALDH
aldehyde dehydrogenase

aldo.
aldosterone

ALE
allowable limits of error

ALEP
atypical lymphoepithelioid cell
proliferation

ALF
acute liver failure
anterior long fiber

ALG
Annapolis lymphoblast globulin
antilymphoblastic globulin
antilymphocyte globulin
antilymphocytic globulin
axiolinguogingival (re: Dent)

alg.
algebraic
allergy

ALGOL
algorithmic oriented language (re:
    computers)

algy.
allergy

ALH
anterior lobe hormone
anterior lobe of the hypophysis

align.
alignment

aline.
arterial (line) catheter

aliq.
aliquot (L. some; several)

Alk, alk.
alkaline

Alk phos., alk. phos.
alkaline phosphatase

Alk PO$_4$
alkaline phosphatase

alk. p'tase
alkaline phosphatase

ALL
acute lymphoblastic leukemia
acute lymphocytic leukemia (lymphatic)
Airlifeline

ALL, all.
allergies
allergy

alleg.
alleged
allegedly

allele
allelomorph (re: genetics)

ALLO
atypical Legionella-like organisms

ALM
acral lentiginous melanoma
alveolar lining material

ALME, ALMe
acetyl-L-lysine methyl ester (also acetyl-
    lysine methyl ester)

ALMI
anterior lateral myocardial infarct

ALMV
anterior leaflet of mitral valve

ALN
anterior lymph node

ALO
average lymphocyte output
axiolinguo-occlusal (re: Dent)

A = log$_{10}$(I_0/I)
absorbance (re: ultraviolet and
    spectrophotometry)

ALOMAD
Adriamycin (doxorubicin), Leukeran
    (chlorambucil), Oncovin (vincristine),
    methotrexate, actinomycin D
    (dactinomycin), and dacarbazine (re:
    chemotherapy)

ALOS
average length of stay

ALOX
aluminum oxide

ALP
acute lupus pericarditis
alkaline phosphatase
(pulmonary) alveolar proteinosis
anterior lobe of pituitary
antilymphocyte plasma
argon laser photocoagulation

α-LP
alpha-lipoprotein

A$_1$Lp
α_1-lipoprotein

ALPS
Aphasia Language Performance Scales

ALS
acute lateral sclerosis
Advanced Life Support (System)
afferent loop syndrome (re: Neuro)
amyotrophic lateral sclerosis
amyotrophic lateralizing sclerosis
angiotensin-like substance
anterolateral sclerosis
anticipated life span
antilymphatic serum
antilymphocyte serum
antilymphocytic serum
antiviral lymphocyte serum

ALSD
Alzheimer-like senile dementia

ALT
alanine aminotransferase (also called

GPT, SGPT—[serum] pyruvic
transaminase; alanine transaminase)
alternative
argon laser trabeculoplasty
avian laryngotracheitis

ALT, alt.
altitude

alt.
alternate

ALT:AST
serum alanine aminotransferase to
serum aspartate aminotransferase
(ratio)

ALT/AST ratio
alanine aminotransferase to aspartate
aminotransferase (also called De
Ritis) ratio

ALTB
acute laryngotracheobronchitis

alt. die.
alternis diebus (L. every other day)

alt. dieb.
alternis diebus (L. every other day)

ALTEE
acetyl-L-tyrosine ethyl ester

alt. h.
alternis horis (L. every other hour)

alt. hor.
alternis horis (L. every other hour)

alt. noc.
alterna nocte (L. every other night)

alt. noct.
alterna nocte (L. every other night)

ALTS
acute lumbar traumatic sprain
acute lumbar traumatic syndrome

ALU
arithmetic and logic unit (re: digital
computer)

ALV
Abelson leukemia virus
adeno-like virus
ascending lumbar vein
avian leukemia virus
avian leukosis virus

ALV, alv.
alveolar

ALVAD
abdominal left ventricular assist device

alv. adst.
alvo adstricto (L. when the bowels are
constricted)

Alv-Art, alv-art
alveolar-arterial difference

alv. deject.
alvi dejectiones (L. throwing down of the
bowel— [pertaining to the bowel or
intestine; bowel movement])

ALVF
acute left ventricular failure

Alv PO$_2$, alv. PO$_2$
alveolar oxygen pressure

ALVT
aortic and left ventricular tunnel

alv. vent.
alveolar ventilation

Alvx
alveolectomy

ALW, A.L.W.
arch-loop-whorl (system—re:
fingerprints)

AM
actomyosin
adult monocyte
aerospace medicine
age, mental
alveolar macrophage
alveolar mucosa
amacrine cell
amethopterin
amperemeter
ampicillin
amplitude modulation
anovular menstruation
anterior mitral
antibodies to cardiac myosin
arithmetic mean
arousal mechanism
articular manipulation
aviation medicine
axiomesial

AM, A.M., a.m.
ante meridiem (L. before noon [in the
morning])

AM, A/M
adult male

AM, Am
American

AM, am
ametropia (re: Ophth)
ammeter
amyl

meterangle
myopic astigmatism (re: Ophth)

A-M
Austin Moore (prosthesis—Dr. Austin T. Moore)

A12M1
adenovirus-12 chromosome modification site-1C (re: genetics)

A12M2
adenovirus-12 chromosome modification site-1A (re: genetics)

A12M3
adenovirus-12 chromosome modification site-1B (re: genetics)

A12M4
adenovirus-12 chromosome modification site-17 (re: genetics)

Am
amber suppressor (re: genetics)
americium (element)

^{241}Am
radioactive isotope of americium

a_M
molar absorptivity

$\alpha_2 M$
alpha$_2$-macroglobulin

am.
amplitude

a.m.
ante menstruationem (L. before menstruation)

AMA
actual mechanical advantage
American Medical Association
antimitochondrial antibodies
antimyosin antibody

AMA, a.m.a.
against medical advice

ama, a̤m̤a̤, a̅m̅a̅
as many as
as much as

AMAL
Aero-Medical Acceleration Laboratory

AMAP
as much as possible

AMAT, A-MAT
amorphous material

AMB
amphotericin B
anomalous muscle bundle
avian myeloblastosis

Amb, amb.
ambulance
ambulation
ambulatory

amb.
ambient
ambiguous
ambulate

ambig.
ambiguous

ambul.
ambulate
ambulation
ambulatory

AMC
acetyl methyl carbinol (acetoin—a product of fermentation)
antibody-mediated cytotoxicity
antimalaria campaign
arm muscle circumference
arthrogryposis multiplex congenita
automatic mixture control
axiomesiocervical (re: Dent)

AMCA
4-(aminomethyl)cyclohexane-carboxylic acid (tranexamic acid—hemostatic)

AMCHA
4-(aminomethyl)cyclohexane-carboxylic acid (tranexamic acid—hemostatic)

AMCN
anteromedial caudate nucleus (re: Neuro)

Am & Ct
antibiotic medical and clinical therapy

AMD
acid maltase deficiency
actinomycin D
adrenomyelodystrophy
aeromedical data
Aleutian mink disease
alpha-methyldopa (antihypertensive)
antimorphine dose
axiomesiodistal (re: Dent)

AMDGF
alveolar macrophage-derived growth factor

AME
amphotericin methyl ester

AMegL
acute megakaryoblastic leukemia

Amer
American

AMESLAN
American sign language

AMF
antimuscle factor

AMG
amyloglucosidase (glucoamylase)
antimacrophage globulin
axiomesiogingival (re: Dent)

AMH
anti-müllerian hormone
automated medical history

AMH, AMh, Amh, Am h
mixed astigmatism with myopia
   predominating

AMHT
automated multiphasic health testing

AMHV
age at minimal height velocity

AMHVR
age at minimal height velocity return

AMI
acute myocardial infarction
acute myocardial insufficiency
amitriptyline (hydrochloride)
anterior myocardial infarction
Athletic Motivation Inventory
axiomesio-incisal (re: Dent)

AMIS
aspirin myocardial infarction study

AML
acute monocytic leukemia
acute mucosal lesion
acute myeloblastic leukemia
acute myelocytic leukemia
acute myelogenous leukemia
acute myeloid leukemia
anterior mitral leaflet
Automated Multitest Laboratory

AMLB
alternate monaural loudness balance
   (test)

AMLC
adherent macrophage-like cell
autologous mixed lymphocyte culture

AMLR
autologous mixed lymphocyte reaction
autologous mixed lymphocyte response

AMLS
antimouse-lymphocyte serum

AMLSGA
acute myeloblastic leukemia surface
   glycoprotein antigen

AMM
agnogenic myeloid metaplasia
antibodies to murine cardiac myosin

AMM, amm.
ammonia

AMML
acute monomyelocytic leukemia
acute myelomonocytic leukemia

AMMOL
acute myelomonoblastic leukemia

ammon.
ammonia

αMMT
α-methyl-m-tyrosine (catecholamine
   synthesis inhibitor)

AMN
adrenomyeloneuropathy
anterior median nucleus

AMN, A.M.N.
alloxazine mononucleotide (vitamin B_2
   phosphate [sodium salt]—enzyme
   co-factor vitamin)

AMO
acute mucocutaneous ocular
   (syndrome)
axiomesio-occlusal (re: Dent)

amo.
amorphous

A-mode u.
amplitude modulation unit (re:
   ultrasonography)

AMOL, AMoL
acute monoblastic leukemia
acute monocytic leukemia

AMonoL, A MonoL
acute monocytic leukemia

amor.
amorphous

amorph.
amorphous

AMP
acid mucopolysaccharide
adenosine 5′-monophosphate (adenylic
   acid; adenosine monophosphate—
   nutrient)
2-amino-2-methyl-1-propanol
   (absorbant for acidic gases)
amphetamine
ampicillin
average mean pressure

AMP, amp.
ampule
amputation

A5MP
adenosine 5′-monophosphate

27

3′,5′-AMP
cyclic adenosine monophosphate
(cyclic AMP, cAMP)

amp.
amperage
ampere
amplification
amplitude
ampoule (Brit.)
amputate
amputated

AMPH
amphetamine

amph.
amphoric

amphet.
amphetamine

amp-hr
ampere-hour

ampl.
amplus (L. large)

AMPPE
acute multifocal placoid pigment
epitheliopathy
acute multiple (focal) posterior placoid
epitheliopathy

AMP ~ P ~ P
adenosine triphosphate (ATP)

A-M prosthesis
Austin Moore prosthesis (Dr. Austin T.
Moore)

AMPS
abnormal mucopolysacchariduria
acid mucopolysaccharides

AMP-S
adenylosuccinic acid

α-MPT
α-methyl-*p*-tyrosine (antihypertensive in
pheochromocytoma)

ampt.
amputation
amputee

ampul.
ampulla (L. ampule; ampoule)

AMR
acoustic muscle reflex
activity metabolic rate
alternate motion rate
alternating motion rate
alternating motion reflexes

AMRI
anteromedial rotatory instability (re:
Ortho)

AMRL
Aerospace Medical Research
Laboratories

AMRS
automated medical record system

AMS
abortus, melitensis, suis (re:
veterinary—*Brucella* affecting goats
and swine)
acute mountain sickness
aggravated in military service
ammonium sulfamate (industrial
chemical)
α-amylase (endo-amylase)
amylase
antimacrophage serum
atypical measles syndrome
auditory memory span
automated multiphasic screening
Automicrobic System

ams
amount of a substance

AMSA
acridinylamine methanesulphon-*m*-
anisidide (4′(9-acridinyl-
amino)methane-sulfon-*m*-anisidide;
amsacrine—a neoplastic)

AMT
acute miliary tuberculosis
alpha-methyltyrosine
amethopterin
amitriptyline
amphetamines
Anxiety Management Training (re:
Psychol)

amt, am't
amount

amu
atomic mass unit (occasionally called
dalton)

AmuLV
Abelson murine leukemia virus

AMV
assisted mechanical ventilation
avian myeloblastosis virus

AMVET
American veteran World War II (re: VA
hospitals)

AMVI
acute mesenteric vascular insufficiency

aMVL
anterior mitral valve leaflet

AMX
amoxicillin

AMY, Amy
amylase

AMY1
amylase, salivary

AMY2
amylase, pancreatic

amyl.
amylase

AN
acanthosis nigricans
acoustic neuroma
acoustic noise
administratively necessary
adult normal
ala nasi
amyl nitrate
aneurysm
anomaly
anorexia nervosa
antenatal
anterior
aseptic necrosis
Aspergillus niger
autonomic neuropathy
avascular necrosis

AN, An, A$_n$
normal atmosphere

A/N
as needed

AN1
aniridia, type 1 (re: Ophth)

An
actinon (element)
anatomy (response)
aniridia (re: Ophth)
anisometropia (re: Ophth)
anodal
anode

ANA
acetylneuraminic acid
anesthesia
anesthetic
antinuclear antibody (antibodies)
aspartyl naphthylamide

ANAD
anorexia nervosa and associated
  disorders

Anaes[th]
anaesthesia
anaesthetic

ANAG
acute narrow angle glaucoma

ANAL.
analyst

ANAL., anal.
analysis
analyze

anal.
analgesia
analgesic
analyses

Anal. Psychol
analytical psychology

ANAP
agglutination negative, absorption
  positive

ANAS
anastomosis
auditory nerve-substance activating

Anat, anat.
anatomical
anatomy

anat.
anatomic

anat. align.
anatomical alignment

ANC
absolute neutrophil count
antigen-neutralizing capacity

ANCC, AnCC
anodal closing contraction
anodal closure contraction

AND
administratively necessary days
algoneurodystrophy

AND (&,∧)
a relation whose result is true only if all
  arguments are true; otherwise, the
  result is false (Cf. NAND)

ANDA
abbreviated new drug application

ANDRO
androsterone

AnDTe, An D Te
anodal duration tetanus

Anes, anes.
anesthesia

anes.
anesthesiology
anesthetic

ANESR
apparent norepinephrine secretion rate

anesth.
anesthesia
anesthesiology
anesthetic

AnEx, an. ex., anex.
anodal excitation
anode excitation

ANF
alpha-naphthoflavone
antineuritic factor
antinuclear factor(s)

AN factor
Aspergillus niger factor
(biotin *l*-sulfoxide)

ANG, Ang, ang.
angiogram

ANG I
angiotensin I

ANG II
angiotensin II

Ang, ang.
angle (especially angle of scapula)
angulation

Ang GR
angiotensin generation rate

Angio, angio.
angiography

angio.
angiogram

ang. pect.
angina pectoris

anh.
anhydrous

anhyd.
anhydrous

ANI
acute nerve irritation

ANIA
automated nephelometric
immunoassay

A-N interval
atrial (deflection) and nodal (potential)
(time between the onset of)

aniso.
anisocytosis

Anisometr
anisometropia (re: Ophth)

ANIT
alpha-naphthylisothiocyanate (1-
naphthylisocyanate)

ank.
ankle

ANL
acute nonlymphoblastic leukemia
acute nonlymphocytic leukemia

ANLI
antibody-negative (mice) with latent
infection

ANLL
acute nonlymphoblastic leukemia
acute nonlymphocytic leukemia

Ann, ann.
annals
annual

Annls
annals

annot.
annotation

ANoA
antinucleolar antibodies

ANOC, AnOC, AnOc
anodal opening contraction

ANOV
analysis of variance (re: statistics)

ANOVA
analysis of variance (re: statistics)

ANP
acute necrotizing pancreatitis
A-norprogesterone

ANRI
acute nerve root irritation

ANRL
antihypertensive neutral renomedullary
lipids

ANS
anterior nasal spine
antineutrophilic serum
anti-rat neutrophil serum
arteriolonephrosclerosis
atrial (depolarization) not sensed (re:
Cardio)
autonomic nervous system

ans.
answer

ANSI
American National Standards Institute

ANT
acoustic noise test

2-amino-5-nitrothiazole (Enheptin—re:
   veterinary medicine)

ANT, ant.
anterior

ant.
antenna
antimycin

Ant A
antimycin A

antag.
antagonism
antagonistic

ant. ax.
anterior axillary (line)

ant. ax. line
anterior axillary line

anthro.
anthropologist
anthropology

Anthrop
anthropology

anthropom.
anthropometry

anti-coag
anticoagulant

anti-GBM
antiglomerular basement membrane
   (antibodies)

anti-HAA
antibody hepatitis-associated antigen

anti-HBsAg
antibody to hepatitis B surface antigen

anti-log
antilogarithm

anti-S
anti-sulfanilic acid

ant. jentac.
ante jentaculum (L. before breakfast)

ant. long. ligs.
anterior longitudinal ligaments

Ant pit., ant. pit.
anterior pituitary (anterior lobe of
   pituitary)

ant. prand.
ante prandium (L. before dinner)

ANTR
apparent net transfer rate

ant. sup. sp.
anterior superior spine

Ant sup. spine, ant. sup. spine
anterior superior spine (of ilium)

ant. tib.
anterior tibial

ANTU
alpha-naphthylthiourea (a powerful
   rodenticide)

ANUG
acute necrotizing ulcerative gingivitis

anx.
anxiety
anxious

AO
abdominal aorta
achievement orientation
acid output
acridine orange (test)
ankle orthosis
anodal opening
anterior oblique (muscle)
aortic opening
ascending aorta
atomic orbital (contour)
atrioventricular (valve) opening
auriculoventricular (valve) opening
average optical (density—re:
   absorbance)
avoidance of others (re: Psychol)
axio-occlusal (re: Dent)

AO, Ao
aorta

A-O
acoustic-optic

A/O
alert, oriented

a/o
angle of

AOA
average orifice area

AOAA
aminooxoacetic acid

AOB
accessory olfactory bulb
alcohol on breath

AOC
abridged ocular chart
anodal opening contraction

AOCL, AOCl
anodal opening clonus

AOD
adult-onset diabetes
arterial occlusive disease
arterial oxygen desaturation
arteriosclerotic occlusive disease
auriculo-osteodysplasia

AO diag.
acridine-orange diagnosis

AODM
adult-onset diabetes mellitus

AODT
Animal and Opposite Drawing
    Technique (re: Psychol)

1α-OHCC
1α-hydroxycholecalciferol

17α-OHP
17α-hydroxyprogesterone

AOL
acro-osteolysis

AOM
acute otitis media

AoMP
aortic mean pressure

AOO
anodal opening odor

AOP
anodal opening picture
aortic pressure

A.O.P.
21-acetoxypregnenolone (anti-arthritic)

AoP
left ventricle to aorta pressure gradient

AoPW
aortic posterior wall

AOQL
average outgoing quality limit

AOR
Academic Orientation (scale)
auditory oculogyric reflex

aort. regurg.
aortic regurgitation

aort. sten.
aortic stenosis

AOS
accessory optic tract
anodal opening sound

AOT
anti-ovotransferrin

AOTe
anodal opening tetanus

AO tech.
acridine-orange technique

AOU
apparent oxygen utilization

AoV
aortic valve

AOW
admitted from other ward

AP
acid phosphatase
acinar parenchyma
action potential
active pepsin
acute phase
acute pneumonia
adolescent population
after parturition
alkaline phosphatase
aminopeptidase
angina pectoris
anterior pituitary (gland)
antidromic potential
antiparkinsonism
antipyrine
antral peristalsis
apical pulse
appendectomy
appendix
apurinic acid
area postrema (re: Neuro)
arithmetic progression
arterial pressure
artificial pneumothorax
aspiration pneumonia
association period
atherosclerotic plaque
atrial pacing
atrium pace
axiopulpal (re: Dent)

AP, A-P
abdominal-perineal (resection)
alum precipitated (re: vaccines)
anteroposterior
aortic pulmonary

AP, A/P
ante partum (before the onset of labor—
    re: the mother)
antepartum (re: OB—before parturition
    with reference to the mother)

AP, AP̄
aortic pressure

AP, Ap, ap.
apothecary

A-P
analytic-psychologic
anterior-posterior

A/P
ascites/plasma (ratio)
assessment and plan

A & P
active and present (re: reflexes)
anatomy and physiology
anterior and posterior
assessment and plan
auscultation and palpation

A & P, A + P
auscultation and percussion

↑ AP
anteroposterior (chest) measurement
   increased

↓ AP
anteroposterior (chest) measurement
   decreased

3 AP, 3-AP
3-acetylpyridine (a nicotinic antagonist)

$A_2 > P_2$
aortic second sound is greater than
   pulmonic second sound

$A_2 < P_2$
aortic second sound less than pulmonic
   second sound

$A_2 P_2$
aortic second sound less than pulmonic
   second sound

ap
attachment point (re: genetics)

a p.
a priori (L. first; before)

a.p.
ante prandium (L. before dinner)

a&p
abdominal and perineal

APA
action potential amplitude
aldosterone-producing adenoma
aminopenicillanic acid
antiparietal antibody
antipernicious anemia (factor—vitamin
   B_{12})

6-APA
6-aminopenicillanic acid

APAF
antipernicious anemia factor (vitamin
   B_{12})

APAP
N-acetyl-p-aminophenol (analgesic;
   antipyretic)

A-pattern
eso- or exotropic eye deviation pattern

APB
abductor pollicis brevis (muscle)
atrial premature beat(s)
auricular premature beat(s)

APC
acetylsalicylic acid, phenacetin, and
   caffeine
adenoidal-pharyngeal-conjunctival
   (virus)
all-purpose capsule
alternative patterns of complement
AMSA (amsacrine; 4'-(9-
   acridinylamino)methane-sulfon-m-
   anisidide), prednisone, chlorambucil
   (re: chemotherapy)
antigen-presenting cell
antiphlogistic corticoid
aperture current
apneustic center (re: Neuro)
apparent partition (distribution)
   coefficient (re: chromatography)
aspirin, phenacetin, and caffeine
atrial premature contraction(s)

APCC
activated prothrombin complex
   concentrate

APCC, APC C, APC-C
aspirin, phenacetin, caffeine, with
   codeine

APCD
adult polycystic kidney disease

APCF
acute pharyngoconjunctival fever

APCG
apexcardiogram

APCs
atrial premature contractions

APC tabs
aspirin, phenacetin, and caffeine

APC virus
adenoidal, pharyngeal, conjunctival
   virus

APD
action potential duration
acute polycystic disease
adult polycystic disease
afferent pupillary defect
atrial premature depolarization
autoimmune progesterone dermatitis

A-PD, A-P D
anteroposterior diameter

APDI
adult personal data inventory

APE
acetone powder extract
acute polioencephalitis
airway pressure excursion
aminophylline, phenobarbital, ephedrine
anterior pituitary extract
avian pneumoencephalitis

APELL
Assessment Program of Early Learning
  Levels

APF
acidulated phosphofluoride
anabolism-promoting factor
animal protein factor
antiperinuclear factor

APG
acid-precipitable globulin
animal pituitary gonadotrop(h)in

APGL
alkaline phosphatase (activity of the)
  granular leukocytes

APH
adrenal regeneration hypertension
alcohol-positive history
ante partum hemorrhage (L. before
  onset of labor—re: the mother)
antepartum hemorrhage (L. before
  onset of childbirth— re: the mother)
anterior pituitary hormone

APH, aph.
aphasia

APHP
anti-*Pseudomonas* human plasma

API
alkaline protease inhibitor
atmospheric pressure ionization

α_1PI
human α_1 proteinase inhibitor

APIVR
artificial pacemaker-induced ventricular
  rhythm

APKD
adult-onset polycystic kidney disease
adult polycystic kidney disease

APL
abductor pollicis longus (muscle)
accelerated painless labor
acute promyelocytic leukemia
animal placental lactogen

anterior pituitary-like (hormone—
  chorionic gonado- trop[h]in)
anterior pituitary-like (substance)

AP&Lat
anteroposterior and lateral

A-P & Lat
anterior-posterior and lateral

APLS
Adult Performance Level Survey

APM
acid-precipitable material
alternating pressure mattress
anterior papillary muscle
anteroposterior movement
aspartame

APN
acute pyelonephritis
average peak noise

APNPS
N^4-acetyl-N^1-(p-
  nitrophenyl)sulfanilamide
  (sulfanitran— antibacterial; poultry
  coccidiostat)

APO
adductor pollicis obliquus (muscle)
Adriamycin, prednisone, Oncovin
  (vincristine) (re: chemotherapy)
aphoxide (triethylenephosphoramide—
  antineoplastic)
apomorphine

Apo
apolipoprotein

APORF
acute postoperative renal failure

Apoth, apoth.
apothecary

APP
acute phase protein
Advanced Placement Program (re:
  psychological testing)
alum-precipitated protein
alum-precipitated pyridine
antiplatelet plasma
aqueous procaine penicillin
automated physiologic profile
avian pancreatic polypeptide

APP, app.
appendix

app.
apparatus
apparent
apparently
appears
applied

appointment
appropriate

AP:PA
anteroposterior:posteroanterior (ratio)

appar.
apparatus
apparent

APPG
aqueous procaine penicillin G

appl.
appliance
application
applied

applan.
applanatus (L. flattened; flat)

applic.
application

applicand.
applicandus (L. to be applied)

appoint.
appointment

appos.
apposition

appr.
approximate(ly)

Approx, approx.
approximate(ly)

approx.
approximation

Appt, appt.
appointment

Appx
appendix

APPY, Appy, appy
appendectomy

APR
abdominal-perineal resection
acute phase reactant
amebic prevalence rate
anterior pituitary reaction
anterior primary rami
auropalpebral reflex (re: ENT/Neuro)

apr.
apraxia

aprax.
apraxia

A-P repair
anterior-posterior repair

APRL hand
Army Prosthetics Research Laboratory
(APRL-Sierra hook—re: physiatry)

AProL, A ProL
acute promyelocytic leukemia

A/P & R/P
apical pulse and radial pulse

APRT, A-PRT
adenine phosphoribosyltransferase

APS
acute physiology score
adenosine phosphosulfate

APSGN
acute poststreptococcal
glomerulonephritis

APT
alum-precipitated toxoid

APTA
aneurysm of persistent trigeminal artery

APTT, aPTT
activated partial thromboplastin time

APTX
acute parathyroidectomy

APUD
amine precursor uptake, decarboxylase
amine precursor uptake (and)
decarboxylation (system/cells)

APV
abnormally posterior vector

APW
artificial pond water

AQ
accomplishment quotient
any quantity
aphasia quotient

AQ, A.Q.
achievement quotient

AQ, aq.
aqua (L. water)
aqueous (watery)

aq. astr.
aqua astricta (L. frozen water)

aq. bul.
aqua bulliens (L. boiling water)

aq. bull.
aqua bulliens (L. boiling water)

aq. cal.
aqua calida (L. hot water)

aq. com.
aqua communis (L. common water)

aq. comm.
aqua communis (L. common water)

aq. dest.
aqua destillata (L. distilled water)

aq. ferv.
aqua fervens (L. boiling water)

aq. fluv.
aqua fluvialis (L. flowing water [river water])

aq. font.
aqua fontis (L. spring water [fountain water])

aq. frig.
aqua frigida (L. cold water)

aq. mar.
aqua marina (L. sea water)

aq. menth. pip.
aqua menthae piperitae (L. peppermint water)

aq. niv.
aqua nivalis (L. snow water)

aq. pen.
aqueous penicillin

aq. pluv.
aqua pluvialis (L. rain water)

aq. pur.
aqua pura (L. pure water)

AQS
additional qualifying symptoms

aq. tep.
aqua tepida (L. lukewarm water)

aqu.
aqueous
water solution

AQVN
average quasivalence number (re: statistics)

AR
abnormal record
achievement ratio
actinic reticuloid
active resistance (exercises)
acute rejection
adherence ratio
Admitting Room
airway reactivity
airway resistance
alarm reaction
alcohol related

alkali reserve
allergic rhinitis
amplitude ratio
analytic reaction
androgen receptor
aortic regurgitation
aortic root
apical rate
Argyll Robertson (pupil—Dr. Douglas Moray Cooper Lamb Argyll Robertson—re: Ophth)
arsphenamine
articulare (craniometric point)
artificial respiration
assisted respiration
atrial regurgitation
at risk
atrophic rhinitis (of swine)
attack rate
augmentation reaction
auricular rate
autoradiography
autosomal recessive (re: genetics)

AR, A.R.
analytical reagent (grade—degree of purity of chemicals)

AR, A-R
active resistive (exercise—re: PM&R)

AR, A-R, A/R
apical radial (pulse)

A&R
advised and released

Ar
argon (element)
aryl (an organic radical)

^{37}Ar
radioactive isotope of argon

ar.
aromatic

ARA
acetylene reduction activity
antireticulin antibody
aortic root angiogram

Ara
arabinose (or its mono- or di- radical)

Ara-A, ara-A
adenine arabinoside (vidarabine)

araC, ara-C
arabinosylcytosine (cytosine arabinoside [cytarabine]—antineoplastic; antiviral)

ara-C-HU
cytosine arabinoside and hydroxyurea (re: chemotherapy)

ara-CTP
arabinosylcytosine triphosphate (re:
    chemotherapy)

ara-FC
arabinosyl-5-fluorocytidine (re:
    chemotherapy)

ARAS
ascending reticular activating system
    (re: Neuro)

ara-U
arabinosyluracil (re: chemotherapy)

ARB
adrenergic receptor binder
any reliable brand

ARBOR
arthropod-borne (virus)

ARC
accelerating rate calorimeter
AIDS-related condition
antigen reactive cell
arcuate nucleus (re: Neuro)

ARC, A.R.C.
anomalous retinal correspondence (re:
    Ophth)

ARCA
acquired red cell aplasia

Arch
archives

ARCO
antigen reactive cell opsonization

ArCO—
aromatic acyl radical

ARCOS
Automated Reports and Consolidated
    Orders System

ARD
absolute reaction of degeneration
acute respiratory disease
adult respiratory disease
AIDS-related disease(s)
allergic respiratory disease
all related data
anorectal dressing
arthritis and rheumatic diseases
atopic respiratory disease

ARDS
acute respiratory distress syndrome
adult respiratory distress syndrome
AIDS-related diseases

ARE
active-resistive exercises (re: PM&R)

ARES
antireticulo-endothelial serum

ARF
acute renal failure
acute respiratory failure
acute rheumatic fever
Adjective Rating Form (re: Psychol)

ARFC
active rosette-forming T cell

Arg, arg.
arginine

arg.
argentum (L. silver)

Arg-Rob
Argyll Robertson (Dr. Douglas Moray
    Cooper Lamb Argyll Robertson—re:
    Ophth)

ARI
acute respiratory infection
airway reactivity index
anxiety reaction, intense

ARIA
automated radioimmunoassay

ARIMA
autoregressive integrated moving
    average

ARL
average remaining lifetime

ARM
adrenergic receptor material
aerosol rebreathing method
allergy relief medicine
anorectal manometry
anxiety reaction, mild
arteria radicularis magna
artificial rupture of membranes
atomic resolution microscope

AROA
autosomal recessive ocular albinism
    (re: genetics)

AROM
artificial rupture of membranes

AROM, A(ROM)
active range of motion (re: Ortho)

arom.
aromatic

ARP
absolute refractory period
Advanced Research Projects
Aptitudes Research Project (re:
    Psychol)
assay reference plasma

assimilation regulatory protein
at risk period

ARPES
angular resolved photoelectron
  spectroscopy

ARPPRN
adenine-*D*-ribose-phosphate-
  phosphate-*D*-ribose-nicotinamide
  (nadide—alcohol and narcotic
  antagonist)

A-R pulse
apical-radial pulse

arr.
arrested (re: disease status)

ARS
Academic Readiness Scale (re:
  Psychol)
acquiescent response scale
alizarin red S (re: histology)
antirabies serum

Ars, ars.
arsphenamine

ARSA
arylsulfatase A

ARSB
arylsulfatase B

ARSM
acute respiratory system malfunction

ART
absolute retention time (an automated
  reagin test)
Achilles tendon reflex test
acoustic reflex test
algebraic reconstruction technique (an
  algorithm)
Anturane reinfarction trial
autologous-reactive T cell
automated reagin test

ART, art.
artery

Art, art.
arterial

art.
article
articulation
artificial

arth.
arthritic
arthritis

arthr.
arthrotomy

arthrot.
arthrotomy

ARTI
acute respiratory tract illness

artic.
articular
articulation

artic. manip.
articular manipulation

artif.
artificial

art. insem.
artificial insemination

Art pO$_2$, art. pO$_2$
arterial oxygen pressure

ARU
audio response unit (re: computers)

ARV
anterior right ventricular (wall)

ARVD
arrhythmogenic right ventricular
  dysplasia

AS
acetylstrophanthidin
acidified serum
activated sleep
active sarcoidosis
active sleep
adolescent suicide
aerosol steroid
affective style
alveolar sac
alveolar space
amyloid substance
anal sphincter
androsterone sulfate
ankylosing spondylitis
annulospiral
antiserum to somatostatin
antisocial
antistreptolysin
antral spasm
anxiety state
aortic sounds
aortic stenosis
aqueous solution
aqueous suspension
artificial sweetener
asthma astrocyte
atherosclerosis
atrial sense
atrial septum
atrial stenosis
atropine sulfate
audiogenic seizure

AS, A.S., a.s.
auris sinistra (L. left ear)

AS, A-S
Adams-Stokes (disease or syndrome)
arteriosclerosis

AS, As, as.
astigmatism

A-S
ascendance-submission
ascendancy-submission

As
arsenic (element)

A$_s$
atmosphere, standard

^{72}As
radioactive isotope of arsenic

^{74}As
radioactive isotope of arsenic

^{76}As
radioactive isotope of arsenic

^{77}As
radioactive isotope of arsenic

a.s., a-s
ampere second (ampere-second)

ASA
acetylsalicylic acid (aspirin)
active systemic anaphylaxis
Adams-Stokes attack
American Standards Association
antibody-to-surface antigen
argininosuccinic acid
arylsulfatase-A
aspirin-sensitive asthma

ASA, a͞s͞a͞, asa
as soon as

Asa
β-carboxyaspartic acid

ASAC
acidified serum, acidified complement

ASAP, asap
as soon as possible

ASAS
argininosuccinate synthetase

ASAT
aspartate aminotransferase

A-S attack
Adams-Stokes attack

ASB
Anxiety Scale for the Blind

Aptitude Tests for School Beginners (re:
   Psychol)
asymptomatic bacteriuria

asb
apostilb (re: luminance)

ASC
N-acetylsulfanilyl chloride (re:
   preparation of sulfanilamide and its
   derivatives)
adenosine-coupled spleen cell
altered state of consciousness
antigen-sensitive cell
ascorbic acid
asthma symptom checklist

ASC, asc.
arteriosclerosis

asc.
anterior subcapsular
arteriosclerotic
ascending

ASCAD
arteriosclerotic coronary artery disease

A-scan
ultrasound instrument emitting VHF
   waves

ASC AO, AscAo
ascending aorta

ASCII
American Standard Code for
   Information Interchange
   (re: computers)

Ascit Fl
ascitic fluid

ascr.
ascriptum (L. ascribed to)

ASCT
autologous stem cell transplantation

ASCVD
arteriosclerotic cardiovascular disease
arteriosclerotic coronary artery disease
atherosclerotic cardiovascular disease

AS & CVD
arteriosclerotic and cardiovascular
   disease

ASD
accouchement sans douleur (Fr.
   childbirth without pain)
aldosterone secretion defect
Alzheimer's senile dementia
arthritis syphilitica deformans
atrial septal defect
atrioseptal defect

ASD2
atrial septal defect, secundum type

ASDH
acute subdural hematoma

ASE
axilla, shoulder, elbow (bandage)

ASES
Adult Self-Expression Scale

asex.
asexual

ASF
African swine fever
aniline, sulfur, formaldehyde (re:
   microscopy)

ASG
advanced stage group

ASH
aldosterone-stimulating hormone
ankylosing spinal hyperostosis
antistreptococcal hyaluronidase
asymmetric septal hypertrophy
asymmetrical septal hypertrophy

ASH, AS H, AsH, As.H
hypermetropic astigmatism (re: Ophth)
hyperopic astigmatism (re: Ophth)

A & SH, a & sh
arm and shoulder

ASHCVD
arteriosclerotic hypertensive
   cardiovascular disease

ASHD
arteriosclerotic heart disease
atrial septal heart defect
atrioseptal heart defect

ASHN
acute sclerosing hyaline necrosis

ASI
Addiction Severity Index
anxiety status inventory

ASIS
anterior superior iliac spine
anterosuperior iliac spine
aromatic solvent-induced shift

ASIS→IM
anterior superior iliac spine to internal
   malleolus

ASIS→MM
anterior superior iliac spine to medial
   malleolus

A site
amino acid attachment site (re: protein
   synthesis)

ASK
antistreptokinase

ASL
ankylosing spondylitis, lung
antistreptolysin
argininosuccinate lyase
average speech level

ASLC
acute self-limited colitis

ASLO, ASL-O
antistreptolysin-O

ASLO titer
antistreptolysin-O titer

ASL-titer
antistreptolysin titer

ASM
airway smooth muscle

ASM, AS M, AsM, As.M.
myopic astigmatism

ASMA
antismooth muscle antibody

ASMC
arterial smooth muscle cell

ASMD
atonic sclerotic muscle dystrophy

ASMI
anteroseptal myocardial infarct(-ion)

ASMR
age-standardized mortality ratio

asmt.
assessment

ASN
alkali-soluble nitrogen
arteriosclerotic nephritis

Asn, asn.
asparagine (or its mono- or di- radical)

ASO
antistreptolysin-O
arteriosclerosis obliterans

ASOR
asialo-orosomucoid

ASOT
antistreptococcal antibody titer
antistreptolysin-O titer

ASO titer
antistreptolysin-O titer

ASP
African swine pox
alkali stable pepsin
antisocial personality
aortic systolic pressure
arachidonate-sensitive platelet
area systolic pressure
asymmetric (multi)processing
   (system—re: computers/data
   processing)
attached support processor (re:
   computers)

Asp, asp.
asparaginase
aspartic acid (or its radical forms)

asp.
aspartate
aspect
aspirate(d)
aspiration

ASPAT
antistreptococcal polysaccharide A test

ASPG
antispleen cell globulin

ASPS
alveolar soft part sarcoma

ASPVD
arteriosclerotic peripheral vascular
   disease

ASQ
abbreviated symptom questionnaire
Anxiety Scale Questionnaire
Attitude to School Questionnaire (re:
   Psychol)

ASR
aldosterone secretion rate
aldosterone secretory rate
antistreptolysin reaction
atrial septal resection
automatic send/receive (re: computers/
   data processing)

ASS
argininosuccinate synthetase

ASS, A.S.S.
acute spinal stenosis
anterior superior spine

assby.
assembly

assim.
assimilate(d)

assist.
assistance
assistant

Assn, assn.
association

Assoc, assoc.
associate(d)
association

assocd.
associated (with)

assoc'd
associated

ASSR
adult situation stress reaction

Asst, asst.
assistant

asst.
assist

AST
allergy serum transfer
angiotensin sensitivity test
anterior spinothalamic tract
antistreptolysin test
antistreptolysin titer
aspartate aminotransferase
audiometry sweep test

AST, Ast, ast.
astigmatism

ASTA
anti-alpha-staphylolysin

A sten., Asten
aortic stenosis

Astg
astigmatism

Asth, asth.
asthenopia

asth.
asthenia
asthma

ASTI
antispasticity index

Astigm
astigmatism

ASTO
antistreptolysin-O (titer)

As tol., as tol.
as tolerated

ASTZ
antistreptozyme

ASV
anodic stripping voltametry
antisiphon valve

antisnake venom
avian sarcoma virus

ASV, A-SV, A/SV
arterio-superficial venous (difference)

ASVAB
Armed Services Vocational Aptitude
  Battery

ASVIP
atrial-synchronous ventricular-inhibited
  pacemaker

ASW
artificial seawater

asw, a. sw.
artificially sweetened

Asx
symbol for asparagine (Asn) or aspartic
  acid (Asp)

asx.
asymptomatic

asym.
asymmetrical
asymmetry

asym-
asymmetrical
unsymmetrical

AT
abdominal tympany
Achard-Thiers (syndrome)
achievement test
Achilles tendon
adaptive thermogenesis
adenine and thymine
adjunctive therapy
air temperature
air trapping
alt Tuberculin (Ger. old tuberculin)
aminotransferase
aminotriazole
amitriptyline
anaerobic threshold
anaphylatoxin
anterior tibial (pulse)
antithrombin
antitrypsin
antral transplantation
applanation tension
applanation tonometry
atmosphere
atraumatic
atresia, tricuspid
atrial tachycardia
atropine
attenuated
attenuation
autoimmune thrombocytopenia
axonal terminal (re: Neuro)
tibialis anticus (muscle)

AT, A-T
ataxia telangiectasia (Louis-Bar
  syndrome)

AT, at.
airtight
atom

AT I, AT II
angiotensin I, angiotensin II

AT III, AT-III
antithrombin

AT–7
hexachlorophene

AT 10, AT$_{10}$, A.T. 10
anti-tetany substance 10
  (dihydrotachysterol—calcium
  regulator)

At
acidity, total
astatine (element)

At, a.t.
ampere turn (re: magnetomotive force
  unit)

α-T
alpha-tocopherol

α-T-3
alpha-tocotrienol

at.
atomic

a.t.
additional term

ATA
alimentary toxic aleukia
aminotriazole (herbicide)
antithyroglobulin antibody
anti-*Toxoplasma* antibodies
atmospheres of absolute pressure
aurintricarboxylic acid

ATA, ata
atmosphere absolute (at sea level)

ATB
atrial tachycardia with block
atypical tuberculosis

ATC
activated thymus cells
around the clock
4-thiazolidinecarboxylic acid
  (timonacic—choleretic)

ATCC
American Type Culture Collection

ATCD
antecedents

ATCS
active trabecular calcification surface
anterior tibial compartment syndrome

ATD
Alzheimer-type dementia
anthropomorphic test dummy
antithyroid drugs
asphyxiating thoracic dystrophy

ATDP
Attitudes Toward Disabled Persons (re:
   Psychol)

ATE
acute toxic encephalopathy
adipose tissue extract
autologous tumor extract

ATEM
analytic transmission electron
   microscope

ATEN
atenolol (beta adrenergic blocker)

A tetra P
adenosine tetraphosphate

ATF
ascitic tumor fluid

ATFC
alternative temporal forced choice

At Fib, at. fib.
atrial fibrillation

ATG
adenine, thymine, guanine
antihuman thymocyte globulin
antithymocyte globulin
antithyroglobulin

ATGAM
antithymocyte gamma globulin

**AT/GC ratio, AT:GC (ratio), (A + T)/
(G + C) ratio**
adenine + thymine/guanine + cytosine
   (base ratio)

ATHC
3α-allotetrahydrocortisol (one of the
   allopregnones; Kendall's
   compound C)

ATHSC, Athsc, athsc.
atherosclerosis

ATK
alt Tuberkulin Koch (Ger. Koch's old
   tuberculin)

ATL
Achilles tendon lengthening
adult T-cell leukemia/lymphoma
anterior tricuspid leaflet (re: Cardio)

anti-tension line
atypical lymphocytes

ATLA
adult T-cell leukemia antigen

ATLS
advanced trauma life support

ATLV
adult T-cell leukemia virus

ATM
abnormal tubular myelin
acute transverse myelitis
acute transverse myelopathy

ATM, atm.
atmosphere
atmospheric

atmos.
atmosphere
atmospheric

ATN
acute tubular necrosis

ATNC
atraumatic, normocephalic

at. no.
atomic number

ATNR
asymmetric tonic neck reflex

ATP
adenosine triphosphate (adenosine 5'-
   triphosphate)
ambient temperature and pressure
autoimmune thrombocytopenic purpura

At P
attending physician

AT-PAS
aldehyde-thionine-periodic acid-Schiff
   (method)

ATPase, At P'ase
adenosine triphosphatase

ATPD
ambient temperature and pressure, dry
   (re: gas volume)

ATP (D,S)
ambient temperature and pressure (dry,
   saturated—re: gas volume)

At Phys
attending physician

ATPS
ambient temperature and pressure,
   saturated (re: gas volume)

ATP'tase
adenosine triphosphatase

ATPTX
acute thyroparathyroidectomy

ATR
Achilles tendon reflex
attenuated total reflection

α_1 **Tr**
alpha$_1$-antitrypsin

atr.
atrophy

ATR FIB, atr. fib.
atrial fibrillation

atrop.
atropine

ATS
acid test solution
administrative terminal system
  (re: computers)
anti-rat thymocyte serum
antithymocyte serum
arteriosclerosis
atherosclerosis

ATS, A.T.S.
antitetanic serum
antitetanus serum
anxiety tension state

ATT
arginine tolerance time
aspirin tolerance time

att.
attending

AT type
adenine and thymine type (re:
  pentosenucleic acids)

ATV
Abelson virus transformed (cells)
avian tumor virus

AtV
arteriovenous
assisted ventilation
atrioventricular

at. vol.
atomic volume

at. wt.
atomic weight

ATx
adult thymectomy

atyp.
atypical

ATZ
atypical transformation zone

AU
antitoxin unit (diphtheria)
atomic unit
6-auridine (antineoplastic)

AU, A.U.
ångström unit (10^{-10}m)
arbitrary units

AU, A.U., a.u.
aures unitae (L. both ears together)
aures utrae (L. both ears)
auris utraque (L. each ear)

AU, Au
Australia antigen

Au
aurum (L. gold—element)

^{195}**Au**
radioactive isotope of gold (aurum)

^{198}**Au**
radioactive isotope of gold (aurum)
radiogold colloid

^{199}**Au**
radioactive isotope of gold (aurum)

Au(1)
Australia antigen

a.u.
ad usum (L. according to custom)

Au Ag, AuAg
Australia antigen

Au antigen
Auberger antigen (re: Auberger blood
  group)

Au(1) antigen
hepatitis-associated antigen

AUB
abnormal uterine bleeding

AUC
area under (the plasma concentration
  time) curve

AUC ∞
area under (the plasma concentration
  time) curve

auct.
auctorum (L. of authors)

AUD
arthritis of unknown diagnosis

aud.
auditory

Aud Comp
auditory comprehension

AUFS
absorbance units full scale

AUG
acute ulcerative gingivitis
adenine, uracil, guanine
adenine, uridine, guanosine

aug.
augere (L. to increase)

AUHAA
Australia hepatitis-associated antigen

AUI
Alcohol Use Inventory

AUL
acute undifferentiated leukemia

AUM
asymmetric unit membrane

AUO
amyloid of unknown origin

AuP
Australia antigen protein

aur.
aures (L. ears)
auricle
auricular
auris (L. ear)
aurum (L. gold)

AUR FIB, aur. fib.
auricular fibrillation

auric.
auricle
auricular

aurin.
aurinarium (L. ear cone)

aurist.
auristillae (L. ear drops)

aus.
auscultation

Aus antigen
hepatitis-associated antigen (Australia)

AUSC, ausc.
auscultation

auscul.
auscultation

AuSH, AuSh
Australia serum hepatitis

Au/SH-AG
Australia serum hepatitis antigen

Aus & Perc
auscultation and percussion

aux.
auxiliary

AV
Adriamycin (doxorubicin) and vincristine
    (re: chemotherapy)
alveolar duct
anterior-ventral
(nucleus) anterior, (pars) ventralis (re:
    thalamus)
anteversion
anteverted
antivirin (virus-inhibiting factor produced
    by certain cells [HeLa-S_3, human
    embryo lung, etc.])
aortic valve
arteriolar-venular
assisted ventilation
atrioventricular
audiovisual
augmented vector
auriculoventricular

AV, A-V
arteriovenous
atrioventricular (block, node)

AV, Av
air velocity

AV, Av, av.
average
avoirdupois

A/V
arterial/venous
artery-to-vein ratio

av.
avulsion

AVA
activity vector analysis
antiviral antibody
aortic valve area
aortic valve atresia
arteriovenous anastomosis
auditory vocal automatic (test)

AV-AF, AV/AF
anteverted, anteflexed

AVB
atrioventricular block

AVBR
automated ventricular brain ratio

AVC
aberrant ventricular conduction
allantoin vaginal cream
associative visual cortex
atrioventricular canal
automatic volume control

AVCN
anteroventral division of cochlear
  nucleus

AVCS
atrioventricular conduction system

AVD
aortic valve disease
aortic valvular disease
apparent volume of distribution
arteriovenous difference
atrioventricular dissociation

AV Dis
atrioventricular dissociation

AVDO$_2$
arteriovenous oxygen content difference

AvDP
average diastolic pressure

avdp.
avoirdupois

AVE
all-valence-electron (method)
aortic valve echocardiogram

aver.
average

AVF
antiviral factor
arteriovenous fistula

AVF, aVF
augmented V (unipolar) lead, left leg
  (re: EKG)

av. fx.
avulsion fracture

avg.
average

AVH
acute viral hepatitis

AVHD
acquired valvular heart disease

AVI
air velocity index

A-V interval
time from beginning of atrial systole to
  beginning of ventricular systole (re:
  cardiology)

AVJ
atrioventricular junction

AVJR
atrioventricular junctional rhythm

AVJT
atrioventricular junctional tachycardia

AVK
antivitamin K

AVL
anterior vein of the leg

AVL, aVL
augmented V (unipolar) lead, left arm
  (re: EKG)

AVM
arteriovenous malformation
atrioventricular malformation
avermectins (broad-spectrum
  antiparasitic agents)

AVN
atrioventricular node

AVNFRP
atrioventricular node functional
  refractory period

AVO
atrioventricular opening

avoir.
avoirdupois

AVP
actinomycin D (dactinomycin),
  vincristine, and Platinol (cisplatin) (re:
  chemotherapy)
antiviral protein
arginine vasopressin (8-arginine
  vasopressin)

AVR
accelerated ventricular rhythm
anomalous venous return
aortic valve replacement
arteriovenous ratio

AVR, aVR
augmented V (unipolar) lead, right arm
  (re: EKG)

AVr
antiviral regulator

a/v ratio
ratio of size of arterioles to venules

AVRB
added viscous resistance to breathing

AVRP
atrioventricular refractory period

AVS
aneurysm of (membranous) ventricular
  septum
aortic valve stenosis
arteriovenous shunt
auditory vocal sequencing

AVSD
atrioventricular septal defect

AV shunt, A-V shunt
arteriovenous shunt

AVSV
aortic valve stroke volume

AVT
Allen vision test
area ventralis of Tsai (re: Neuro)
arginine vasotocin (8-arginine-oxytocin)

AVTB
absolute volume of trabecular bone

AV3V
anteroventral third ventricle

AVZ
avascular zone

AW
above waist
alcohol withdrawal
aluminum wafer
alveolar wall
alveolar wash
anterior wall
atomic warfare

A.W.
atomic weight

A & W
active and well
alive and well

A/W
able to work
(in) accordance with

aw, aw.
airways

a.w.a., a̐w̐a̐, a̅w̅a̅
as well as

A wave
atrial depolarization seen as deflection
   in bundle of His electrocardiogram

a wave
jugular venous pulsation
measurement in electroretinogram (part
   of ERG action potential—re: Ophth)

AWBM
alveolar wall basement membrane

AWDW
assault with a deadly weapon

AWF
adrenal weight factor (a corticotrop[h]in
   in ACTH)

AWI
anterior wall infarction

AWL
absent with leave

AWMI
anterior wall myocardial infarction

AWO
airway obstruction

AWOL
absent without leave

AWP
airway pressure

AWRS
anti-whole rabbit serum

AWRU
active wrist rotation unit

AWU, awu
atomic weight unit

AX, Ax, ax.
axis

Ax
axis of cylindrical lens

Ax, ax.
axilla
axillary

ax.
axial
axon

ax. grad.
axial gradient

AXL
axillary lymphoscintigraphy

AXT
alternating exotropia (re: Ophth)

Ax temp.
axillary temperature

AYA
acute yellow atrophy (liver)

AYF
antiyeast factor

AYP
autolyzed yeast protein

AYV
aster yellow virus

A.-Z., Az
Aschheim-Zondek (pregnancy test)

Az
Azotobacter (genus)
azote (Fr. nitrogen)

5-Aza
5-azacytidine (antineoplastic)

5-azaC
5-azacytidine (antineoplastic)

azan stain
Azokarmin B and Anilinblau W
   (Heidenhain's azan stain)

5-AzC
5-azacytosine

5-AzCdR
5-aza-2'-deoxycytidine

5-AzCR
5-azacytidine (antineoplastic)

AZG, azg.
azaguanine (re: leukemia in mice)

AZQ
aziridinylbenzoquinone (antineoplastic)

AZR
alizarin red
Aschheim-Zondek (pregnancy) reaction

AZS
automatic zero set

AZT
Aschheim-Zondek (pregnancy) test

AZ test
Aschheim-Zondek (pregnancy) test

AzU
6-azauracil (antineoplastic)

5-AzU
5-azauracil (antineoplastic)

6-AzU
6-azauracil (antineoplastic)

AZUR, AzUR
6-azauridine (antineoplastic)

5-AzUR
5-azauridine (antineoplastic)

6-AzUR
6-azauridine (antineoplastic)

B

B
Bacillus
bacitracin
bacterium
Bacteroides (genus)
Balantidium (genus)
barometric (secondary symbol)
barometric pressure (when written as a
    subscript)
Bartonella (genus)
base (re: chemical formulae)
base (of prism)
baseline
Basidiobolus (genus)
basophil
bath
behavior
behavioral (contents—re: Psychol;
    Aptitudes Research Project testing
    within structure of intellect model)
bel (acoustic or electric power intensity)
benzoate
Bertiella (genus of tapeworms)
beta (when Greek β not available)
bicuspid
black
Blastomyces (genus)
blood
blue
body (re: Psychol—all the body except
    the nervous system)
bone
bone-marrow derived (lymphocytes)
Bordetella (genus)
boron (element)
Borrelia (genus)
bound
breakfast
Brewster (unit in photo-elastic work)
bronchial
brother
Brugia (genus of filarial worms)
bruit
buccal
Bucky (film in cassette in Potter-Bucky
    diaphragm)
bursa cells (of thymus or lymph nodes)
bypass (or shunt)
gauss (SI symbol—Gs is preferred)
large positive deflection of
    electroretinogram
magnetic induction
tomogram with oscillating Bucky
whole blood

B, B.
bacillus
Baumé scale
Benois scale (obsolete scale—
    measured x-ray penetrability)
Brucella (genus)

B, b.
balneum (L. bath)
base (of any substance)
bis (L. twice, two times)
boils at (when followed by a figure
    designating degrees)
born

B$_1$, B$_2$, B$_3$, etc.
first, second, third, etc., backcross
    generations (re: genetics)

B4
before

β
beta (second letter of the Greek
    alphabet)
symbol denoting second

β+
positron (re: radioactive isotopes)

β−
an anomer of a carbohydrate
beta particle (re: radioactive isotopes)
beta plasma protein fraction constituent
carbon separated from carboxyl by one
    other carbon in aliphatic compounds
substituent of a steroid group that
    projects above the plane of the ring

b
barn (unit of nuclear cross-section; this
    area is now written as 100 fm^2—re:
    nuclear physics)
blood (when written as a subscript)
break (re: cytogenetics)
byte (re: computers)

BA
bacillus abortus (*Brucella abortus*)
background activity
bacterial agglutination
balneum arenae (L. sand bath)
basilar artery
basion (craniometric point)
basket axon (re: Neuro)
best amplitude

betamethasone acetate
bile acid
biliary atresia
biologic activity
Biological Abstracts
blocking antibody
blood agar
blood alcohol
bone age
bongkrekic acid
bovine albumin
brachial arterial (pressure)
brachial artery
branchial artery
breathing apparatus
bronchial asthma
bronchoalveolar
buccoaxial (re: Dent)
buffered acetone

BA, B/A
backache
boric acid

B & A
brisk and active (re: reflexes)

B>A
bone (conduction) greater than air
(conduction—re: Audio)

Ba
barium (element)

^{131}Ba
radioactive isotope of barium

^{133}Ba
radioactive isotope of barium

^{140}Ba
radioactive isotope of barium

β-a
β-alanine (3-aminopropanoic acid)

BAA
branched-chain amino acid

BAB
blood agar base

Bab
Babinski (reflex)

BAC
bacterial adherent colonies
bacterial antigen complex
blood alcohol concentration
blood alcohol content
bronchoalveolar cells
buccoaxiocervical (re: Dent)

Bac, bac.
bacillus

bacitracin
an acronym from Bacillus + Tracy
(named for patient)

BaCl
barium chloride (abbreviation
commonly used for $BaCl_2$)

$BaCl_2$
barium chloride

BACOD
bleomycin, Adriamycin, Cytoxan,
Oncovin, dexamethasone (Decadron)
(re: chemotherapy)

BACON
bleomycin, Adriamycin (doxorubicin),
CCNU (lomustine), Oncovin
(vincristine), and nitrogen mustard
(re: chemotherapy)

BACOP
bleomycin, Adriamycin (doxorubicin),
cyclophosphamide, Oncovin
(vincristine), and prednisone (re:
chemotherapy)

BACT
BCNU, ara-C, cyclophosphamide, 6-
thioguanine (re: chemotherapy)

BACT, Bact
Bacterium (genus no longer used in
bacteriology; all species under this
genus transferred to other genera)

bact.
bacteria
bacterial
bacteriologist
bacteriology
bacterium

bacti.
bacteriology

BAD
biological aerosol detection

BADS
black (locks), (oculocutaneous)
albinism, deafness (of sensorineural
type) syndrome

BAE
bovine aortic endothelium

BaE
barium enema

BaEn
barium enema

Ba enem.
barium enema

BAEP
brain-stem auditory evoked potential

BAER
brain-stem auditory evoked response

BAG
buccoaxiogingival (re: Dent)

BAGG
buffered azide glucose glycerol (broth)

BAI
basilar artery insufficiency

BAIB, B-AIB, β-AIB
beta-aminoisobutyric acid

BAIF
bile acid independent flow
bile acid independent fraction

BAIT
bacterial automated identification
technique

BAL
blood alcohol level
British anti-lewisite (dimercaprol)
bronchoalveolar lavage

BAL, bal.
balance(d)
balneum (L. bath)
balsam

bal. arenae
balneum arenae (L. sand bath)

BALB
binaural alternate loudness balance
(test)

Bal exonuclease
Brevibacterium albidum exonuclease
(re: genetics)

BALL, B-ALL
B-cell acute lymphoblastic leukemia

bal. mar.
balneum maris (L. salt or sea-water
bath)

BALS
bile acid-losing syndrome

bals.
balsamum (L. balsam)

bal. vap.
balneum vaporis (L. steam or vapor
bath)

BAM
basophil-associated mononuclear
bronchoalveolar macrophage

BAm
mean brachial artery (pressure)

BaM
barium meal

BAMON
bleomycin, Adriamycin (doxorubicin),
methotrexate, Oncovin (vincristine),
and nitrogen mustard (re:
chemotherapy)

BAN
British approved name

bands
banded neutrophils

BANS
back, arm, neck, and scalp

BAO
basal acid output
baseline acid output
brachial artery output

BAO-MAO
basal acid output to maximal acid
output (ratio)

BAP
bacterial alkaline phosphatase
basic adaptive process
Behavior Activity Profile (re: Psychol)
blood agar plate
bovine albumin in phosphate (buffer)
brachial artery pressure

BAPI
barley alkaline protease inhibitor

BAPS
bovine albumin phosphate saline

BAPV
bovine alimentary papilloma virus

BAQ
Brain-Age Quotient

BAR
buffer address register (re: computers)

bar.
barometer
barometric

Barb, barb.
barbiturate

BARN
bilateral acute retinal necrosis

BARSA
billing, accounts receivable, sales
analysis (re: computers/data
processing)

BARSIT
Barranquilla Rapid Survey Intelligence
  Test

BART
blood-activated recalcification time

BAS
benzyl analog of serotonin (benanserin
  hydrochloride—serotonin antagonist)
benzyl antiserotonin
boric acid solution

bas.
basilar
basophil(s)

BASH
body acceleration synchronous with
  heart beat

BASIC
beginner's all-purpose symbolic
  instruction code (a programming
  language—re: computers)

baso.
basophil(s)

basos.
basophils

Ba swallow
barium swallow

BAT
Basic Aid Training
benzilic acid 3α-tropanyl ester
best available technology
brown adipose tissue

batt.
battery

BAVIP
bleomycin, Adriamycin (doxorubicin),
  vinblastine, imidazole carboxamide
  (dacarbazine), and prednisone (re:
  chemotherapy)

BAW
bronchoalveolar wash (fluids)
bronchoalveolar washing

BB
bad breath
bed bath
Bellevue bridge (re: scrotal elevation)
Besnier-Boeck (syndrome)
beta blocker
blanket bath
blood bank
blood buffer (base)
blue bloaters (emphysema)
Bogdän-Buday (disease)
breakthrough bleeding
breast biopsy
brush border
buffer base
bundle branch
Busse-Buschke (disease)
isoenzyme of creatine kinase that
  contains two B subunits

BB, bb
bed boards
both bones (re: fractures)

bb.
ball bearing

BBA
born before arrival

BBB
blood buffer base
bundle branch block

BBB, B.B.B.
blood-brain barrier

BBBB
bilateral bundle branch block

BBC, B.B.C.
α-bromobenzyl cyanide (war gas)

BBE
bacteroides bile esculin (agar)

BBF
bronchial blood flow

BBI
Bowman-Birk (soybean) inhibitor

B bile
bile from gallbladder

BBM
brush border membrane

BB to MM
belly button to medial malleolus (exam)

BBMV
brush border membrane vesicle

BBN
broad band noise

BBOT
2,5[bis-2-(5-t-butylbenzoxazolyl)]
  thiophene

BBR
babybird® (baby Bird, Baby Bird)
  respirator
benzbromarone (uricosuric)

B bridge
Bellevue bridge (re: scrotal elevation)

BBRS
Burks' Behavior Rating Scale (for
  Organic Brain Dysfunction)

BBS
bashful bladder syndrome
Besnier-Boeck-Schaumann (syndrome)
bombesin (a neuropeptide)

B/B/S
bilateral breath sounds (equal[ly])

BBT
basal body temperature
Bingham Button Test (re: Psychol)

B.B.U.
(α-bromoisovaleryl)urea (sedative,
　hypnotic)

β-BuTX
β-bungarotoxin (neuromuscular tool)

BB/W
biobreeding/Worcester (rats)

B Bx
breast biopsy

BC
back-cross (backcross—re: genetics)
background counts
bactericidal concentration
basal cell
basket cell (re: Neuro)
battle casualty
bicarbonate
biliary colic
bipolar cell
birth control
blastic crisis
blood cardioplegia
blood center
blood count
blood culture
Blue Cross
bone conduction (hearing test)
Bowman's capsule (re: Uro)
brachiocephalic
bronchial carcinoma
buccal cartilage
buccocervical
Budd-Chiari (syndrome)
buffy coat

BC, b.c.
back care

B/C, b/c
breathed and cried (re: newborn)

B & C
bed and chair (rest)
biopsy and curettage

B & C, b & c
breathed and cried (re: newborn)

b/c
because

BCA
blood color analyzer
breast cancer antigen

BCAA
branched-chain amino acid

BCAT
brachiocephalic arterial trunk

BCAVe, B-CAVe
bleomycin, CCNU (lomustine),
　Adriamycin (doxorubicin), Velban
　(vinblastine) (re: chemotherapy)

BCB
brilliant cresyl blue

BCBR
bilateral carotid body resection

BC/BS
Blue Cross/Blue Shield

BCC
basal cell carcinoma
biliary cholesterol concentration
birth control clinic

β-CCE
ethyl β-carboline-3-carboxylate (re:
　study of benzodiazepine receptors)

BCCI
Barclay Classroom Climate Inventory
　(re: Psychol)

BCCP
biotin carboxyl carrier protein

BCD
binary coded decimal
bleomycin, cyclophosphamide,
　dactinomycin (re: chemotherapy)

BCE
basal cell epithelioma
B cell enriched
before the common era
bubble chamber equipment

B cell
beta cells (of pancreas or anterior lobe
　of hypophysis)
bone marrow-derived lymphocyte
bone marrow or bursa of Fabricius-
　derived cell

B-cells
bursal equivalent (bursa fabricii)
　lymphocytes

BCF
basophil chemotactic factor
bioconcentration factor
breast cyst fluid

BCFP
breast cyst fluid protein

BCG
Bacille bilié de Calmette-Guérin (used
   in preparation of BCG vaccine)
bacille Calmette-Guérin
bacillus Calmette-Guérin
ballistocardiogram
ballistocardiograph
bicolor guaiac (test)
bromcresol green (a pH indicator)

β_{1c} globulin
third component (C3) of complement

BCG test
bicolor guaiac test

BCG vaccine
bacille Calmette-Guérin vaccine

BCH
basal cell hyperplasia
basal cell hypoplasia

BChL
bacteriochlorophyll

B-CHOP
bleomycin, Cytoxan,
   hydroxydaunomycin (Adriamycin),
   Oncovin, prednisone (re:
   chemotherapy)

BCKA
branched-chain keto acids

BCL
basic cycle length

B-CLL
B-cell chronic lymphatic leukemia

BCLS
Basic Cardiac Life Support (System)

BCM
birth control medication
1,6-bis(2-chloroethylamino)-1,6-dideoxy-
   D-mannitol dihydrochloride
   (mannomustine—antineoplastic)
body cell mass

bcm
billion cubic meters

BCME
bis(chloromethyl) ether (sym-
   dichloromethyl ether—a carcinogen)

BCMF
bleomycin, cyclophosphamide,
   methotrexate, and 5-fluorouracil (re:
   chemotherapy)

BCN
bilateral cortical necrosis

BCNS
basal cell nevus syndrome (re: Derma)

BCNU
N,N-bis(2-chloroethyl)-N-nitrosourea
   (carmustine; BiCNU—an
   antineoplastic)

BCO
biliary cholesterol output
binary-coded octal (re: computers)

B comp.
B complex (re: vitamins)

BCOP
BCNU (carmustine),
   cyclophosphamide, Oncovin
   (vincristine), and prednisone (re:
   chemotherapy)

BCP
BCNU (carmustine),
   cyclophosphamide, prednisone (re:
   chemotherapy)
birth control pill
bromcresol purple
5-n-butyl-1-cyclohexyl-2,4,6-
   trioxoperhydropyrimidine (anti-
   inflammatory)

BCP-D
bromcresol purple deoxycholate

BCPS
battery-charging power supply

BCPV
bovine cutaneous papilloma virus

BCR
B-cell reactivity
birth control regimen
bulbocavernosus response (re: Uro)

BCRx, BC℞
birth control medication
birth control treatment

BCS
battered child syndrome
blood cell separator
Budd-Chiari syndrome

BCSI
breast cancer screening indicator

BCT
brachiocephalic trunk

BCT1
branched-chain amino acid
   transferase-1

BCT2
branched-chain amino acid
   transferase-2

BCtg
bovine chymotrypsinogen

BCTR
bovine chymotrypsin

BCU
block control unit (re: computers/data processing)

BCV
basal cell vigilance

BCVP
BCNU (carmustine), cyclophosphamide, vincristine, and prednisone (re: chemotherapy)

BCVPP
BCNU (carmustine), cyclophosphamide, vinblastine, procarbazine, and prednisone (re: chemotherapy)

BCW
biological and chemical warfare
buffer control word (re: computers)

BCYE
buffered charcoal yeast extract

BD
base deficit
base (of prism) down (re: Ophth)
basophilic degeneration
Batten's disease
Baudelocque's diameter (external conjugate—re: OB)
behavioral disorder
Behçet's disease
belladonna
Best delay (re: Audio)
bile duct
binocular deprivation
birth date
Black Death (bubonic plague— pandemic in Europe and Asia after 1353 A.D.)
Blackfan-Diamond (syndrome)
block design (test)
blue diaper (syndrome)
borderline dull (IQ)
bottle drainage
bound
brain damage
brain death
bronchodilator
buccodistal (re: Dent)
bundle

BD, Bd, bd.
board

BD, b.d.
bis die (L. twice a day)

B&D
bondage and discipline

bd.
band

BDAE
Boston Diagnostic Aphasia Examination

BDC
burn dressing change

BDE
bile duct examination
bile duct exploration

BDG
buffered deoxycholate glucose (broth)

BDI
Beck Depression Inventory (re: Psychol)

BDID
bystander dominates initial dominant (re: Psychol)

BDL
below detectable limits
bile duct ligation
bundle

B-DOPA
bleomycin, DTIC, Oncovin, prednisone, Adriamycin (re: chemotherapy)

BDP
bilateral diaphragm paralysis

BDPE, B.D.P.E.
α-bromo-α,β-diphenyl-β(p-ethylphenyl)ethylene (broparoestrol—dermatological estrogen)

BD prism
base-down prism (re: Ophth)

BDR
background diabetic retinopathy

BDS
biological detection system

b.d.s.
bis in die summendus (L. to be taken twice a day)

BDUR
bromodeoxyuridine

BDW
buffered distilled water

BE
bacillary emulsion
bacterial endocarditis
barium enema
Barrett's esophagus

base excess
below elbow
bile esculin
bovine enteritis
brain edema
brain encephalitogen
breast examination
broncho-enterology
broncho-esophagology

BE, B.E.
Bacillen Emulsion (Ger.—re: tuberculin)

BE, Be, Bé
Baumé (specific gravity scale)

B & E
brisk and equal

B ↑ E
both upper extremities

B ↓ E
both lower extremities

Be
beryllium (element)

°Bé
degree Baumé

^{7}Be
radioactive isotope of beryllium

^{10}Be
radioactive isotope of beryllium

BEA
below-elbow amputation

Be^a antigen
Becker antigen

BEAM
brain electrical activity map

BE AMP, B/E Amp, BE amp.
below-elbow amputation

BECF
blood extracellular fluid

BECSAG
Barclay Early Childhood Skill
   Assessment Guide

BEE
basal energy expenditure

bef.
before

beg.
began
begin
beginning

β_{1E} globulin
fourth component (C4) of complement

beh.
behavior
behaviorism

BEI
back-scatter electron imaging
butanol-extractable iodine (obsolete
   procedure— replaced by thyroxin[e]
   assays)

BEIR
biological effects of ionizing radiation
   (re: genetics)

BEL
bell character (re: computers/data
   processing)
bovine embryonic lung

BELIR
beta-endorphin-like immunoreactivity

bellig.
belligerent

ben.
bene (L. well)

BENZ, Benz, benz.
benzidine

benz.
benzoate

Benz test
benzidine test

BEP
- bleomycin, etoposide, Platinol (re:
   chemotherapy)
brain-evoked potential

BEPI
beta-endorphin immunoreactivity

BEPTI, bepti
bionomics, environment, plasmodium,
   treatment, and immunity (re: malaria
   epidemiology)

BER
basic electrical rhythm
blood ethanol response

BERA
brain-stem electric response
   audiometry
brain-stem evoked response
   audiometry

BES
balanced electrolyte solution

BESM
bovine embryo skeletal muscle

BESP
bovine embryonic spleen cell

BET
benign epithelial tumor
Brunauer-Emmet-Teller (method)

bet.
between

BEV
baboon endogenous virus
bleeding esophageal varices

BEV, BeV, Bev, beV, bev
billion electron volts (energy—10^9—
　　used USA—now called giga electron
　　volts, GeV)

bev.
beverage

BEVI
baboon M7 virus replication

BF
bentonite flocculation (test)
bile flow
blastogenic factor
blister fluid
blocking factor
blood flow
body fat
Bolivian (hemorrhagic) fever
breakfast fed
breast feed
buccofacial
buffered
burning feet (syndrome)
butterfat
properdin factor B (a highly basic serum
　　protein)

BF, B/F
black female

BF, bf
bouillon filtrate (Fr. bouillon filtrate
　　tuberculin; Denys' tuberculin)

B/F
bound/free (ratio—re:
　　radioimmunoassay)

BFB
biological feedback

BFC
benign febrile convulsion

BFD
bias flow down

BFDI
bronchodilation following deep
　　inspiration

BFDT
Bekesy Functionality Detection Test (re:
　　Audio)

BFE
blood flow energy

β_{1F} globulin
fifth component (C5) of complement

BFL
bird-fancier's lung

BFO
balanced forearm orthosis
ball-bearing forearm orthosis
blood-forming organ
buccofacial obturator

BFP
biologic false positive
biological false positive
biologically false positivity

BFPO
bis(dimethylamido)phosphoryl fluoride
　　(dimefox— a pesticide)

BFPR
biologic false-positive reactor
biological false-positive reaction

BFR
biologic false-positive reactor
blood flow rate
bone formation rate

BFR sol.
buffered Ringer's solution

BFS
blood-fasting sugar

BFSW
buffered filtered sea water

BFT
bentonite flocculation test
biofeedback training
bladder flap tube

BFU
burst-forming unit

BFU-E, BFU$_e$
burst-forming unit-erythroid

BFU-M/E
burst-forming unit, myeloid/erythroid

BFV
bovine feces virus

BG
Barré-Guillain (syndrome)
basic gastrin
Bender Gestalt (test—re: Neuro/
　　Psychol)
Bertolotti-Garcin (syndrome)
beta-galactosidase
Beurmannn-Gougerot (disease)
bicolor guaiac (test)

blood glucose
bone graft
brilliant green
buccogingival (re: Dent)
Buerger-Grütz (syndrome)

BG, B-G
Bordet-Gengou (bacillus)

b/g
began

BGA
blue-green algae (re: photosynthesis)

BGAg
blood group antigen

BGAV
blue-green algal virus

BGC
blood group class

BGCA
bronchogenic carcinoma

BGD
blood group-degrading (enzymes)

BGG
bovine gamma globulin

BGH
bovine growth hormone

BGLB
brilliant green lactose broth

BGlu
blood glucose

BGP
beta-glycerophosphatase
beta-glycerophosphate

BGS
balance, gait, and station
blood group substance

BGSA
blood granulocyte-specific activity

BGT
basophil granulation test
Bender-Gestalt Test (Visual Motor
  Gestalt Test [VMGT]— re: Psychol/
  Neuro)
bungarotoxin

BGTT
borderline glucose tolerance test

BH
benzalkonium and heparin
Bernard-Horner (syndrome)
bill of health
birth history
Bolton-Hunter (reagent)

borderline hypertensive
both hands
brain hormone
breath holding
bronchial hyperactivity
bronchial hyperreactivity
bundle of His

BHA
benign hilar adenopathy
γ-benzene hexachloride (lindane; HCH;
  γ-BHC—insecticide; scabicide)
bilateral hilar adenopathy
bound hepatitis antibody
butylated hydroxyanisole (food anti-
  oxidant)

BH-AC
N(4)-behenoyl-1-β-D-
  arabinofuranosylcytosine
  (enocitabine—antineoplastic)

BHAT
beta (blocker) heart attack trial

BHb
bovine hemoglobin

BHBA
β-hydroxybutyric acid (β-
  hydroxybutyrate—re: ketone bodies)

BHC
benzene hexachloride (insecticide and
  scabicide)

BHD
BCNU (carmustine), hydroxyurea, and
  dacarbazine (re: chemotherapy)

BHDV, BHD-V
BCNU (carmustine), hydroxyurea,
  dacarbazine, and vincristine (re:
  chemotherapy)

BHF
Bolivian hemorrhagic fever

BHI
biosynthetic human insulin
brain-heart infusion (agar)

BHI-ac
brain-heart infusion (broth with) acetone

BHIB
beef heart infusion broth

BHIBA
brain-heart infusion blood agar

BH interval
bundle of His deflection time (re:
  cardiology)

BHIRS
brain-heart infusion and rabbit serum

BHIS
beef heart infusion supplemented (broth or agar)

BHK
baby hamster kidney
type B Hong Kong (influenza virus)

BHL
bilateral hilar lymphadenopathy
bilateral hilar lymphoma syndrome
biological half-life

BHN
bephenium hydroxynaphthoate (anthelmintic)
Brinell hardness number (re: metal)

BHP
benign hypertrophic prostatitis

BHR
basal heart rate

BHS
beta hemolytic streptococcus
breath-holding spell

BHT
breath hydrogen test
butylated hydroxytoluene (food anti-oxidant)

BHU
basic health unit

BHV
bovine herpes virus

BH/VH
body hematocrit-venous hematocrit (ratio)

BI
background interval
bacterial index
bactericidal index
bacteriological index
base (of prism) in (re: Ophth)
biological indicator
bodily injury
bone injury
bowel impaction
brain injured
burn index

BI, B-I
bi-ischial
body injury

Bi
biceps
biot (unit of current in electromagnetic centimeter- gram-second system, equal to 10 amperes)
bismuth (element)

input blocking factor (re: computers/data processing)

^{206}Bi
radioactive isotope of bismuth

^{207}Bi
radioactive isotope of bismuth

b_i
difficulty parameter (re: Psychol; item character-curve [statistics])

BIA
bacteria inhibition assay (of Guthrie)
bioimmunoassay

Bi antigen
Bile's antigen

BIB
brought in by

bib.
bibe (L. drink)

biblio.
bibliography

BIC
blood isotope clearance

bic.
biceps

bicarb.
bicarbonate

BiCNU
N,N-bis(2-chloroethyl)-N-nitrosourea (carmustine; BCNU— antineoplastic)

BID
brought in dead

b.i.d.
bis in die (L. twice daily; twice a day)

BIDLB
block in the posteroinferior division of the left branch (re: Cardio)

bigem.
bigeminy

BIGGY
bismuth glycine glucose yeast (agar)

BIH
benign intracranial hypertension

bihor.
bihorium (during two hours [perhaps a contraction of Latin bis = twice + horium = hourly])

BII
butanol insoluble iodine

Bi Isch, bi isch
between ischial tuberosities

BIL
basal insulin level
brother-in-law

BIL, Bil, bil.
bilateral

BIL, bil.
bilirubin

BIL/ALB
bilirubin-to-albumin (ratio)

bilat.
bilateral

BILAT SLC, bilat. SLC
bilateral short leg cast

BILAT S&O
bilateral salpingo-oophorectomy

BILAT SXO
bilateral salpingo-oophorectomy

bili.
bilirubin

bili. D/I
bilirubin, direct and indirect

bilirub.
bilirubin

Bili (t/d)
bilirubin (total/direct)

BIM
beginning of information marker (re:
   computers/data processing)

BIMAG
bistable magnetic core (re: computers)

b.i.n.
bis in noctus (L. twice a night)

bind.
binding

Biochem
biochemical
biochemistry

biochem.
biochemist

BIOD
bony intraorbital distance

bioeng.
bioengineering

Biol, biol.
biology

biol.
biological
biologist

Biophys
biophysics

BIP
Background Interference Procedure
bacterial intravenous protein
biparietal diameter (of skull)
brief infertile period

BIP, B.I.P.
bismuth iodoform paraffin (Morison's
   method [obsolete] of treating wounds)

BIPP
bismuth iodoform paraffin paste
   (Morison's method—an obsolete
   method of treating wounds)

BI prism
base-in prism (re: Ophth)

BIQ
hexadecamethylene-1,16-
   bis-(isoquinolinium chloride) (topical
   antifungal)

BIR
basic incidence rate

BIS
Brain Information Service
(sodium) bicarbonate in invert sugar

bis in 7d.
bis in septem diebus (L. twice a week)

BISp, BiSP, Bi sp.
between ischial spines

bisp.
bispinous or interspinous diameter

bisp. diam.
bispinous diameter

BIT
binary digit (re: computers)

BIT, Bi T
bitrochanteric

BITCH
Black Intelligence Test of Cultural
   Homogeneity

bitroch.
bitrochanteric

BIU
barrier isolation unit

biw.
bi-weekly

BJ
Bence Jones (protein—Dr. Harry Bence
   Jones)
biceps jerk
Bielschowsky-Jansky (syndrome)

BJ, B/J
bone and joint

B&J
bone and joint

BJM
bones, joints, muscles

BJP
Bence Jones protein (Dr. Harry Bence
   Jones)

BJ protein
Bence Jones protein (Dr. Harry Bence
   Jones)

BK
Bassen-Kornzweig (syndrome)
below knee
bradykinin
Koch's bacillus (*Mycobacterium
   tuberculosis, Vibrio cholerae*)

Bk
berkelium (element)

bk.
back
black

BKA
below-knee amputation

BK-A
basophil kallikrein of anaphylaxis

BK amp., B/K amp.
below-knee amputation

bkd.
baked

bkf.
breakfast

bkfst.
breakfast

bkft.
breakfast

bkg.
background

BKLY, bkly.
backlying

B-K mole
a type of melanocytic nevi (B-K are
   initials of patients' surnames)

BKS
beekeeper serum

BKTT
below knee to toe

BKWP
below-knee walking plaster (cast)

BL
Barré-Liéou (syndrome)
basal lamina
baseline
Bessey-Lowry (units)
black light
blind loop
blood loss
body lean
bone (marrow derived) lymphocyte
borderline lepromatous
bronchial lavage
buccolingual (re: Dent)
Burkitt's lymphoma

BL, bl.
bleeding
blood

Bl, bl.
black
blue

B-l
bursa (equivalent) lymphocyte

bl.
bland

b.l.
balneum luti (L. mud bath)

BLa
buccolabial

BLAD
borderline left axis deviation (re: Cardio)

BLAT
Blind Learning Aptitude Test

BLB
Bessey-Lowry-Brock method (acid
   phosphatase assay method)
black light blue
black light bulb
Boothby, Lovelace, Bulbulian (mask)

bl. & blue
black and blue

BL = BS
bilateral equal breath sounds

BLB unit
Bessey-Lowry-Brock unit (re:
   measurement of enzyme activity)

BLC
beef liver catalase

BLC, BL C, BIC
blood culture

bl. cult.
blood culture

BLD
basal (cell) liquefactive degeneration
beryllium lung disease

Bld, bld.
blood

Bld Bnk
blood bank

BLE
both lower extremities

bleed.
bleeding

BLEO, Bleo
bleomycin

BLEO-COMF
bleomycin, cyclophosphamide, Oncovin
(vincristine), methotrexate, and 5-
fluorouracil (re: chemotherapy)

bleph.
blepharoplasty

BLESS
bath, laxative, enema, shampoo, and
shower

BLFD
buccolinguofacial dyskinesia

BLG
beta-lactoglobulin

blk.
black

BLL
below lower limit

BLM
basolateral membrane
bilayer lipid membrane
bimolecular liquid membrane
black lipid membrane
bleomycin
buccolinguomasticatory

BL min.
blood loss, minimal

BLN
bronchial lymph nodes

BLNAI
Barclay Learning Needs Assessment
Inventory

BLOBS, bl. obs.
bladder observation

BLP, BLp
β-lipoprotein

BIP
blood pressure

β-LPH
β-lipotropin hormone

BL PR, bl.pr.
blood pressure

BLQ
both lower quadrants

BLRA
beta-lactamase resistant antimicrobial

BLS
basic life support (systems)
blind loop syndrome
blood and lymphatic systems

BIS, BI S
blood sugar

BLSD
bovine lumpy skin disease

BLST
Bankson Language Screening Test

BLT
blood-clot lysis time

BLT, BIT, BI T
blood type

BLT, BI T
blood test

bl. time
bleeding time

BLU
Bessey-Lowry units

BLV
blood volume
bovine leukemia virus

BI vol.
blood volume

bl. x
bleeding time

BM
Bamberger-Marie (syndrome)
basal medium
basal metabolism
basement membrane
basilar membrane
Batten-Mayou (syndrome)
betamethasone
biomedical

Bird Mark (re: Resp)
blind matching (re: Parapsychol)
blood monocyte
body mass
bone marrow
Brailsford-Morquio (syndrome)
breast milk
buccal mass (re: Dent)
buccomesial (re: Dent)

BM, B.M.
bowel movement

BM, B.M., b.m.
balneum maris (L. sea-water bath)

BM, B/M
black male

B2M, β2m
beta-2-microglobulin (beta$_2$
   microglobulin)

BMA
bone marrow arrest

BMAP
bone marrow acid phosphatase

BMC
blood mononuclear cell
bone marrow cell
bone mineral content

BMD
bone marrow depression
bovine mucosal disease

BME
basal medium, Eagle's
biundulant meningoencephalitis
brief maximal effort (re: PM&R)

BMG
benign monoclonal gammopathy

BMI
body mass index

BMK, bmk
birthmark

BML
bone marrow lymphocytosis

BMLM
basement membrane-like material

BMMP
benign mucous membrane pemphigoid

BMN
bone marrow necrosis

BMNR
bone marrow neutrophil reserve

BMO
bonding molecular orbital

BMOC
Brinster's medium for ovum culture

B-mod
behavior modification (re: Psychol)

B-mode
brightness mode (re: echocardiography)
brightness modulation (re:
   echocardiography)

B-mode u.
brightness modulation unit (re:
   echocardiography)

B-MOPP
bleomycin, nitrogen mustard, Oncovin,
   procarbazine, prednisone (re:
   chemotherapy)

BMP
BCNU, methotrexate, procarbazine (re:
   chemotherapy)
bone morphogenic protein

BMPI
bronchial mucous proteinase inhibitor

BMPP
benign mucous membrane pemphigus

BMR
basal metabolic rate

BMS
betamethasone

BMST
Bruce maximal stress test

BMT
basement membrane thickening
basement membrane thickness
benign mesenchymal tumor
bone marrow transplant

BM & T
bilateral myringotomy and tubes

BMU
basic metabolic unit (of bone)
basic multicellular unit

BMZ
basement membrane zone

BN
Babinski-Nageotte (syndrome)
boron nitride
brachial neuritis
bronchial nodes
brown Norway (rat)
bucconasal

B.N.
bladder neck

BNA
Basle Nomina Anatomica

BNB
blood-nerve barrier

BND
barely noticeable difference

BNDD
Bureau of Narcotics and Dangerous
   Drugs

b.n.e.
but not exceeding

BNF
Backus normal form (re: computers)
British National Formulary

BNG
6-bromo-2-naphthyl-beta-galactoside

BNGase
6-bromo-2-naphthyl-beta-galactosidase

BNGF
beta nerve-growth factor

BNO
bladder neck obstruction
bowels not open

BNPA
binasal pharyngeal airway

BNS
benign nephrosclerosis

BNT
brain neurotransmitter

BO
base (of prism) out (re: Ophth)
belladonna/opium
body odor
Bolton (craniometric point)
bowel obstruction
bowels open
bucco-occlusal (re: Dent)

BO, bo.
bowel

B & O
belladonna and opium

BOA
born on arrival
born out of asepsis

BOAP
bleomycin, Oncovin, Adriamycin,
   prednisone (re: chemotherapy)

BOBA
beta-oxybutyric acids

BOC
t-butoxycarbonyl (former abbrev BOC,
   Boc now used—*tert*-
   butoxycarbonyl—re: peptide
   synthesis)

BOD
biological oxygen demand

BOD, B.O.D.
biochemical oxygen demand

Bod U
Bodansky units

BOD Unit
Bodansky unit

BodUnits
Bodansky units

BOEA
ethyl biscoumacetate (anticoagulant)

BOFA
beta-oncofetal antigen
   (carcinoembryonic antigen)

boil.
boiling

bol.
bolus (L. pill)

BOLD
bleomycin, Oncovin (vincristine),
   lomustine, and dacarbazine (re:
   chemotherapy)

BOLT
Basic Occupational Literacy Test

BOM
bilateral otitis media

BOMA
bilateral otitis media, acute

BONP
bleomycin, Oncovin, Natulan
   (procarbazine hydrochloride),
   prednisolone (re: chemotherapy)

BOP
BCNU, Oncovin, prednisone (re:
   chemotherapy)
Buffalo orphan prototype (re: viruses)

BOPAM
bleomycin, Oncovin (vincristine),
   prednisone, Adriamycin (doxorubicin),
   mechlorethamine (nitrogen mustard),
   and methotrexate (re: chemotherapy)

BOPP
BCNU, Oncovin, procarbazine,
   prednisone (re: chemotherapy)

BO prism
base-out prism (re: Ophth)

BOR
basal optic root
bowels open regularly

BORR
blood-oxygen release rate

BOT
beginning of tape (re: computers)

Bot, bot.
botanical
botany

bot.
bottle

BOW
bag of waters (amniotic sac and fluid—
a commonly used vulgarism)

BP
back pressure
Bard-Pic (syndrome)
barometric pressure
basal (state), post (absorptive)
basic protein
bathroom privileges
behavior pattern
benzo[a]pyrene (3,4-benzpyrene;
formerly called 1,2-benzpyrene)
bioequivalence problem
biotic potential
biparietal (diameter of head)
bipolar
birthplace
body plethysmography
bronchopleural
buccopulpal (re: Dent)
building privilege
bullous pemphigoid
bullous pemphigus
bypass

BP, B.P.
blood pressure
British Pharmacopoeia

BP, bp.
bedpan

BP, bp, b.p.
boiling point (boils; boils at; boiling at
[always followed by a figure denoting
temperature])

↑ BP
blood pressure elevated or increasing

↓ BP
blood pressure low or falling

bp, b.p.
base pair (re: nucleic acid molecules)

BPA
blood pressure assembly
bovine plasma albumin
bronchopulmonary aspergillosis
burst-promoting activity (re: EEG)

BPAM
basic partitioned access method (re:
computers/data processing)

BPAS
N-benzoyl-p-aminosalicylic acid
(tuberculostatic antibacterial)

BPB
bromphenol blue

BPC
Behavior Problem Checklist (re:
Psychol)
bile phospholipid concentration
blood pressure cuff
British Pharmaceutical Codex
bronchial provocation challenge

BPD
biparietal diameter
blood pressure decrease(d)
bronchopulmonary dysplasia

BPE
bacterial phosphatidylethanolamine

BPEC
bipolar electrocoagulation

BPF
bradykinin potentiating factor
bronchopleural fistula
burst-promoting factor (re: EEG)

BPG
benzathine penicillin G
blood pressure gauge
bypass graft

BPH
benign prostatic hyperplasia
benign prostatic hypertrophy

BPh
buccopharyngeal

BPh, B Ph
British Pharmacopoeia

BPheo
bacteriopheophytin

BPI
Basic Personality Inventory
beef-pork insulin
Bipolar Psychological Inventory
bits per inch (re: computers)
blood pressure increase(d)

BPL
benign proliferative lesion

benzylpenicilloyl polylysine
bone phosphate of lime
β-propiolactone

BPLA
blood pressure, left arm
β-propiolactone

BP 120/62 lar
blood pressure 120 (systolic), 62
(diastolic), left arm reclining or
recumbent (rar—right arm reclining,
etc.)

BPM
bipiperidyl mustard (obesifying agent in
mice)
births per minute
breaths per minute
brompheniramine maleate
(antihistaminic)

BPM, BpM
beats per minute

BPMS
blood plasma measuring system

BPN
brachial plexus neuropathy

BPO
basal pepsin output
benzylpenicilloyl (re: penicillin allergy
diagnostic aid)
bile phospholipid output

BPO$_2$
benzoyl peroxide ($C_{14}H_{10}O_4$;
($C_6H_5CO)_2O_2$—keratolytic)

BPO-HSA
benzylpenicilloyl human serum albumin

BPP
bovine pancreatic polypeptide
bradykinin-potentiating peptide
breast parenchymal pattern

BP & P
blood pressure and pulse

BPPV
bovine paragenital papilloma virus

BPR
blood per rectum
blood pressure recorder
blood production rate

BPRA
blood pressure, right arm

BPRN
Burn/Plastic (department) resident note

BPRS
brief psychiatric rating scale
brief psychiatric reacting scale

BPS
beats per second
bovine papular stomatitis
brain protein solvent
breaths per second

BPS, bps
bits per second (re: computers/data
processing)

BPTI
basic pancreatic trypsin inhibitor
basic polyvalent trypsin inhibitor

BPV
benign paroxysmal vertigo
benign positional vertigo
bioprosthetic valve
bovine papilloma virus

Bq
becquerel (SI unit of radioactive activity;
approved by CGPM, May 1975)

BQA
Bureau of Quality Assurance

BQC sol.
2,6-dibromoquinone-4-chlorimide
solution (a reagent)

BR
bacteriorhodopsin (biological energy
transduction research tool)
baseline recovery
bathroom
bedrest
bedside rounds
bilirubin
biological response
bowel rest
brachialis
breathing rate
breathing reserve
British Revision (of Basle Nomina
Anatomica—re: anatomical
nomenclature)
bronchus

BR, Br
bronchitis
Brucella (genus)

BR, b.r.
boiling range

Br
breech
bridge (re: Dent)
British
bromine (element)

Br, Br.
brown

Br⁻
bromide

⁷⁷Br
radioactive isotope of bromine

⁸²Br
radioactive isotope of bromine

br.
brachial
branch
breath
breathe
broiled
brother
bruit

BRA
brain
β-resorcylic acid (spot test; reagent for
    iron)

BRAC
basic rest-activity cycle

brach.
brachial

brady.
bradycardia

BRAO
branch retinal artery occlusion

BRAP
burst of rapid atrial pacing

BrAP
brachial artery pressure

BRAT
bananas, rice, apples, toast (diet)
bananas, rice cereal, applesauce, tea
    (diet)

BRAT diet
banana, rice, and tea diet (for diarrhea
    in children)

BRB
bright red blood

BRBA
Brucella (genus)

BRBC
bovine red blood cells

BRBNS
blue rubber-bleb nevus syndrome

BRBPR
bright red blood per rectum

BR c̄ BRP
bedrest with bathroom privileges

br. bx
breast biopsy

BRCM
below right costal margin

BRD
bladder retraining drills

BrdU
5-bromodeoxyuridine

BrdUrd
bromodeoxyuridine

BRH
benign recurrent hematuria

BRI
Bio-Research Index

BRIC
benign recurrent intrahepatic
    cholestasis

Brit
Britain
British

Brkf, brkf.
breakfast

brkt.
breakfast

BRM
biological response modifiers
biuret reactive material (derivative of
    urea)

BRMP
Biological Response Modification
    Program

brn.
brown

BRO
bronchoscopy

bro.
brother

brom.
bromide

Bron
bronchial

Bronch
bronchoscopic
bronchoscopist

Bronch, bronch.
bronchoscope
bronchoscopy

bronch.
bronchitis
bronchogram
bronchus

bronchiect.
bronchiectasis

BRP
bilirubin production

BRP, b.r.p.
bathroom privileges

BRPH, Brph, brph.
bronchophony

BR priv.
bathroom privileges

BRR
baroreceptor reflex response
breathing reserve ratio

Br sounds, br. sounds
breath sounds

BRT
Brook Reaction Test (re: Psychol)

brt.
bright

brth.
breath

BrU
bromouracil

Bruc
Brucella (genus)

BRVO
branch retinal vein occlusion

BS
Bacillus subtilis
Baehr-Schiffrin (disease)
base strap
Batten-Steinert (syndrome)
Behçet's syndrome
bile salt
Binet-Simon (test)
bismuth subsalicylate
blasticidin S (re: agricultural chemical)
Bloch-Sulzberger (syndrome)
Bloom's syndrome (re: genetics)
Blue Shield
borderline schizophrenia
Boyd-Stearns (syndrome)
breaking strength
Brill-Symmers (syndrome)
Brown-Séquard (syndrome)
Brown-Symmers (disease)
British Standard
buffered saline
Bureau of Standards
standard bicarbonate (plasma)

BS, B.S.
blood sugar

BS, B.S., b.s.
breath sounds

BS, B/S
broadside (re: impact of motor vehicle
accident)

BS, bs.
bedside

BS, b.s.
bowel sounds

B-S
Björk-Shiley (mitral valve prosthesis)

B/S
bits per second (re: computers)

B & S, B&S
Bartholin and Skene's (glands—re: OB-
GYN)

@bs.
at bedside

BSA
benzenesulfonic acid
bismuth-sulfite agar
bis-trimethylsilylacetamide (reagent—
re: gas chromatography)
body surface area
bovine serum albumin
bowel sounds active

BSAB
Balthazar Scales of Adaptive Behavior

BSAM
basic sequential access method (re:
computers/data processing)

BSAP
brief short-action potential

BSB
body surface burned

BSBC
buffer-soluble binding component

BS = BL
breath sounds equal bilaterally

BSC
bedside care
bedside commode
Bench scale calorimeter
bile salt concentration

B-scan
ultrasound B-mode (brightness
modulation) scan

BSCP
bovine spinal cord protein

BSD
baby soft diet
bedside drainage
block-surface distance

BSDLB
block in the anterosuperior division of
the left branch (re: Cardio)

BSDT
Bryant-Schwan Design Test (re:
Psychol)

BSE
bacillus species enzyme
bilateral(ly) symmetrical and equal
breast self-examination

BSER
brain-stem electric response
brain-stem evoked response

BSF
back-scatter factor (re: radiation
interference)

B.S.G.
bismuth subgallate (astringent; antacid)

B&S glands
Bartholin and Skene('s) glands (re: OB-
GYN)

BSH
benzenesulfohydrazide (industrial
agent)

BSI
Behavior Status Inventory
bound serum iron
British Standards Institution

BSICF
bile salt independent canalicular
fraction

BSID
Bayley Scales of Infant Development

BSIF
bile salt independent fraction

BSL
benign symmetric lipomatoses
blood sugar level

BS ↓ L base
breath sounds diminished, left base

BSM
bile salt metabolism

BSN
bowel sounds normal

BSNA
bowel sounds normal and active

BSO
bilateral sagittal osteotomy
bilateral salpingo-oophorectomy
bile salt output

BSP
body segment parameter
brom(o)sulfophthalein
(sulfobromophthalein)
Bromsulphalein Sodium™
(sulfobromophthalein sodium)

BSp
bronchospasm

BSPM
body surface potential map

BSQ
Behavior Style Questionnaire

BSR
basal skin resistance
blood sedimentation rate
bowel sounds regular
brain stimulation reinforcement

BSS
Balanced Salt Solution
black silk suture(s)
buffered salt (saline) solution

BSSE
bile salt-stimulated esterase

BSSI
Basic School Skills Inventory

BSSL
bile salt-stimulated lipase

BST
bacteriuria screening test
biceps semitendinosus
blood serologic(al) test
brief stimulus therapy (re: Psychol)

BSTFA
bis-trimethylsilyltrifluoroacetamide
(reagent—re: gas chromatography)

BSU
British Standard Unit

BSV
Batten-Spielmeyer-Vogt (syndrome)
binocular single vision

BSVM
bovine seminal vesical microsomal
(preparation)

BT
Bacillus thuringiensis (microbial
insecticide)
base of tongue
bedtime
bitemporal (diameter of head)

bitrochanteric
bladder tumor
bleeding time
blood transfusion
blood type
blue tetrazolium (stain)
body temperature
borderline tuberculoid
bowel tones
brain tumor
breast tumor

β-T
β-tocopherol

β-T-3
β-tocotrienol

BTA
N-benzoyl-L-tyrosyl-p-aminobenzoic
   acid (BTPABA; bentiromide—a
   diagnostic aid; re: pancreatic
   function)

BTAM
basic telecommunications access
   method (re: computers/ data
   processing)

BTB
breakthrough bleeding
bromothymol blue (also bromthymol—
   an indicator)

BTBL
bromthymol blue lactose

BTC
basal temperature chart

Bt₂cAMP
$N^6,O^{2'}$-dibutyryladenosine 3':5'-cyclic
   phosphate (re: cAMP—a dibutyryl
   derivative of)

BTDS
O-benzoylthiamine disulfide
   (bisbentiamine—vitamin B_1 source)

BTE
benzilic acid 3α-tropanyl ester
bovine thymus extract

BTFS
breast tissue frozen section (re: tumors)
breast tumor frozen section

BTg
bovine trypsinogen

β-TGdR
β-2'-deoxythioguanosine

BTH
butylated hydroxytoluene

BThU, B Th U, B.Th.U
British thermal unit

BTL
bilateral tubal ligation

BTM
benign tertian malaria

BTMD
Batten-Turner muscular dystrophy

BTP
biliary tract pain

BTPABA
N-benzoyl-L-tyrosyl-p-aminobenzoic
   acid (diagnostic aid—re: pancreatic
   function)

BTPD
body temperature and (ambient)
   pressure, dry (re: Resp)

BTPS
body temperature, (ambient) pressure,
   saturated (re: Resp)
body temperature, pressure (prevailing
   atmospheric), and saturation (water
   vapor) (re: Resp)
gas volume (symbol, as if) saturated
   with water vapor at body temperature
   and at the ambient barometric
   pressure (re: lung volume
   measurement)

BTR
Bezold-type reflex
biceps tendon reflex

BT & R
biceps, triceps, and radialis (muscles)

BTr
bovine trypsin

BTS
brady-tachy syndrome (re: Cardio)

BTSH, B-TSH
beef thyroid-stimulating hormone
bovine thyroid-stimulating hormone

BTU, B.T.U., Btu
British thermal unit

BTW
back to work

BTX
benzene, toluene, xylene
brevetoxins (re: neurochemical
   research tools)
bungarotoxin (krait venom used as
   experimental tool— re:
   neuromuscular processes)

BTX-B
brevetoxin-B (re: neurochemical
   research)

BU
base (of prism) up (re: Ophth)
Bodansky units
bromouracil
Burn Unit

Bu
butyl

BUA
blood uric acid

Bucc
buccal

BUDR, BUdR
5-bromo-2'-deoxyuridine (a thymidine analog)

BUE
both upper extremities
built-up edge

BUG
buccal ganglion

BUI
brain uptake index

bul.
bullet

bull.
bulletin
bulliant (L. let them boil)
bulliat (L. let it boil)
bulliens (L. boiling)

BUN
blood urea nitrogen

bun. br. blk.
bundle branch block (re: Cardio)

BUO
bilateral ureteral occlusion
bleeding of undetermined origin
bruising of undetermined origin

buphth.
buphthalmos

BU prism
base-up prism (re: Ophth)

BUQ
both upper quadrants

Bur
buried

bur.
bureau

Burd
Burdick suction

BUS
Bartholin's, urethral, and Skene's (glands—re: OB-GYN)
busulfan (Myleran—re: chemotherapy)

BUT
breakup time

but.
butyrum (L. butter)

BUTE
phenylbutazone (anti-inflammatory)

BuTX, BuTx
bungarotoxin (krait venom used as experimental tool— re: neuromuscular processes)

BV
bacitracin V
basilic vein
billion volts
biologic(al) value
blood vessel
blood volume
bronchovesicular (breath sounds)

b.v.
balneum vaporis (L. vapor bath)

BVAP
BCNU (carmustine), vincristine, Adriamycin (doxorubicin), and prednisone (re: chemotherapy)

BVCPP
BCNU (carmustine), vinblastine, cyclophosphamide, procarbazine, and prednisone (re: chemotherapy)

BVD
bovine viral diarrhea

BVDS
bleomycin, Velban, doxorubicin (Adriamycin), streptozotocin (re: chemotherapy)

BVDT
brief vestibular disorientation test (re: Neuro)

BVE
binocular visual efficiency
blood vessel endothelium
blood volume expander
blood volume expansion

BVH
biventricular hypertrophy

BVI
blood vessel invasion

BVIN
BALB virus induction, N-tropic

B vit. compl.
B vitamin complex

BVIX
BALB virus induction, xenotropic

BVL
bilateral vas ligation

BVM
bronchovesicular markings

BVMGT
Bender Visual-Motor Gestalt Test (re: Neuro/Psychol)

BVO
branch vein occlusion
brominated vegetable oil

BVP
blood vessel prosthesis
blood volume pulse
burst of ventricular pacing

BVPP
BCNU, vincristine, procarbazine, prednisone (re: chemotherapy)

BVR
baboon virus replication

BVRT
Benton Visual Retention Test (re: Psychol)

BVS
blanked ventricular sense

BVU
(α-bromoisovaleryl)urea (bromisovalum—a sedative, hypnotic)

BVV
bovine vaginitis virus

BVX
bacitracin V and X

BW
bacteriological warfare
bed waiting
below waist
biological warfare
biological weapons
birth weight
black and white (re: milk of magnesia and cascara)
bladder washout
blood Wassermann
body water
body weight

BWA
bed waiting admission

BWAS
Barron-Welsh Art Scale (a figure of preference test— re: Psychol)

b-wave
part of ERG (electroretinogram) wave (sharp upward action potential—re: Ophth)

BWD
bacillary white diarrhea (in chicks)

BWG
Bland-White-Garland (syndrome)

BWS
battered woman syndrome

BWST
black widow spider toxin

BWSV
black widow spider venom

BWt
birth weight

BX
bacitracin X

BX, Bx, bx
biopsy

B$_x$
para-aminobenzoic acid

BXO
balanitis xerotica obliterans

By antigen
a low frequency blood group (found only in members of very few families)

BYE
Barile-Yaguchi-Eveland (medium)

BZ
benzodiazepine (tranquilizer)
dl-form of 3-quinuclidinol benzilate ester (re: chemical warfare; hypotensive; cholinergic)

BZ, Bz
benzoyl

BZD
benziodarone (vasodilator)
benzothiazide (diuretic; antihypertensive)

BzH
benzaldehyde (manufacturing chemical; solvent)

BZL
benzol (benzene; medicinal and industrial chemical— re: veterinary— destroys screwworm larvae in wounds)

BzOH
benzoic acid

BZQ
benzquinamide (tranquilizer; anti-emetic)

C

c
calculus
calorie (large)
Calymmatobacterium (genus)
Campylobacter (genus)
Candida (genus)
canine
canine tooth (permanent)
carbohydrate
carbon (element—L. charcoal)
cardiac
carrier
cathodal
cathode
Catholic
Caucasian
Caulobacter (genus)
cellule
Celsius
centigrade
cerebrospinal fluid
certified
cervical (re: vertebral formulae)
cesarean section (caesarean)
chest
chest lead (re: EKGs; C = precordial
    chest lead)
Chilomastix (genus)
Chlamydia (genus)
chloramphenicol
cholesterol
Chromobacterium (genus)
Cimex (genus of bedbugs)
Citrobacter (genus)
Cladosporium (genus)
classes (products—re: Psychol;
    Aptitude Research Project testing
    within structure of intellect model)
clear
clearance (re: renal function tests—
    when followed by a subscript)
clearance rate
clonus
Clostridium (genus)
closure (of an electrical circuit)
clubbing
coarse (re: bacterial colonies)
cocaine
Coccidioides (genus)
coefficient of outflow (re: tonography)
color
colored
color sense
complement

complete
complex
compliance (of lungs—when followed
    by subscripted L)
component
compositus (L. compound)
compound
concentration (when followed by
    subscript)
concentration of gas in blood
conditioned
conditioning
condyle
congius (L. gallon)
constant
consultation
content (of gas in blood phase)
contingency coefficient
contraction
contracture (placed after grade or
    movement in manual muscle
    evaluation—re: physiatry)
control (re: a group in an experiment)
contusus (L. bruised)
convergence
correct
cortex
Corynebacterium (genus)
costa (L. rib)
costal
coulomb (practical and SI unit of
    charge)
Coxiella (genus)
coxsackie (virus)
Cryptococcus (genus)
crystalline enzyme
cubitus
Culex (genus of mosquitoes)
cuspid (permanent)
cuticular
cyanosis
cylinder
cylindrical
cylindric lens
cysteine
cytidine (ribosylcytosine)
cytochrome
cytosine
haploid amount of DNA
heat capacity
millicurie strength of a source (re:
    nuclear medicine)
vectorcardiography electrode (between
    E and A)

C, c
capacitance
central
cubic

C, c, c.
capacity

C, c.
candle
cast
centum (L. one hundred)
cibus (L. meal)
circa (L. about)
contact
cup
curie (the SI symbol Ci is preferred)
cycle(s)

$\overline{C}$, c, c., $\overline{c}$
cum (L. with)

C′
former symbol for complement (re: biochemistry)

C♀
Caucasian female

C♂
Caucasian male

C_1, C_2, C_3, etc.
cytochromes 1, 2, 3
ribs (costa 1, costa 2, etc.)

C-1, C-2, etc., through C-9
nine discrete protein components of complement system

C-1, C-2, etc.
sounds below middle C (re: Audio)

C-1, C-2, C_1, C_2, etc. through C-7, C_7
cervical vertebrae

C#1, C#2, etc.
car number one, car number two, etc. (re: accident)

CI, CII, C-I, C-II, C_I, C_{II}, etc., through C-XII
first cranial nerve, second cranial nerve, etc.

C2
complement component-2 (re: genetics)
C2-deficiency (re: genetics)

C_3 (population)
physically and mentally deficient persons who are products of imperfect development

C′-3
component of complement (C′ is former symbol for complement) in serum

C4
complement component-4 (re: genetics)
C4-deficiency (re: genetics)

C10
decamethonium bromide (skeletal muscle relaxant)

^{11}C
carbon-11 (cyclotron-produced, positron-emitting radioisotope)

^{12}C
carbon-12 (98.89% of natural carbon)

^{13}C
carbon-13 (a natural isotope)

^{14}C
carbon-14 (widely used as metabolic tracer and to date carbonaceous-containing relics)

c
blood capillary (when written as a subscript)
capacity, specific heat
concentration by volume (after optical rotations only— re: organic chemistry)
cuspid (deciduous)
molar concentration

c
speed of light (symbol for constant)

c, c.
capillary
capillary blood
centi- (prefix—100)
centimeter
velocity of light (in a vacuum—re: nuclear medicine)

c.
calorie (small)
canine tooth (deciduous)
cornu (L. horn)
cup
current
cyclic

c′
symbol for coefficient of partage (re: Lab)

c-1, c-2, c-3, etc.
sounds above middle C (re: Audio)

CA
anterior commissure
calcium antagonist
Candida albicans
caproic acid
carbonic anhydrase
cardiac arrest
cardiac arrhythmia

carotid artery
catecholamine
celiac axis
cervicoaxial
cervicoaxillary
Chemical Abstracts (Service)
chemotactic activity
cholic acid
chronological age
citric acid
clotting assay
coagglutination (test—conglutination)
coefficient of absorption
cold agglutination
cold agglutinin
collagenolytic activity
colloid antigen
commissural association (re: Neuro)
common antigen
community acquired
compressed air
conceptual age
conditioned abstinence
conditioned air
coronary artery
corpora allata (re: endocrine function in
    insects)
corpora amylacea
corpus albicans (atretic corpus
    luteum—re: GYN)
corpus alienum (foreign body)
cortisone acetate
Council Accepted (American Medical
    Association)
cricoid arch
cross-sectional area
croup-associated (virus)
cytosine arabinoside
cytotoxic antibody

CA, C/A
Caucasian adult

CA, Ca
cathode

CA, Ca, ca.
cancer
carcinoma

C/A
Clinitest/Acetest

CA^{++}
Factor IV calcium

C&A
Clinitest and Acetest

C of A
coarctation of aorta

Ca
calcium (L. calx; limestone—[element])

carpal (amputation level, upper limb—
    re: Ortho)
cathodal

Ca^{2+}
calcium ion

^{45}Ca, Ca 45
radioactive calcium (calcium-45)

^{47}Ca
radioisotope of calcium

ca.
candle
circa (L. about, approximately)

CAA
carotid audiofrequency analysis
computer-aided assessment
computer-assisted assessment
constitutional aplastic anemia

CAAT
computer-assisted axial tomography

CAB
captive air bubble
cellulose acetate butyrate (re: hard
    contact lenses)
Comprehensive Ability Battery (re:
    Psychol)
coronary artery bypass

CABG
coronary artery bypass graft(ing)

CABGS
coronary artery bypass graft surgery

CABOP, CA-BOP
Cytoxan (cyclophosphamide),
    Adriamycin (doxorubicin), bleomycin,
    Oncovin (vincristine), and prednisone
    (re: chemotherapy)

CABP, CaBP
calcium-binding protein

CABS
CCNU, Adriamycin, bleomycin,
    streptozotocin (re: chemotherapy)
coronary artery bypass surgery

CAC
cardiac accelerator center
cardiac arrest code
carotid artery canal
circulating anticoagulant

CACC, CaCC
cathodal closure contraction

CaCl2
calcium chloride

CaCO₂
content of carbon dioxide in arterial blood

CaCTe
cathodal closure tetanus

CACX, CaCx
cancer of the cervix

CAD
compressed air disease
computer-aided design
computer-aided diagnosis
computer-assisted diagnosis
computerized assisted design
coronary artery disease
cyclophosphamide, Adriamycin, dacarbazine (re: chemotherapy)
cytosine arabinoside (cytarabine) and daunorubicin (re: chemotherapy)

CAD, Cad
cadaver

CADL
Communicative Abilities in Daily Living

CADTe, CaDTe
cathodal duration tetanus

CAE
cellulose acetate electrophoresis
contingent aftereffects
coronary artery embolization

CAE1
cataract, zonular pulverulent
zonular cataract (re: genetics)

CaE
calcium excretion

CaEDTA, CaEdTA
calcium disodium edetate (edathamil calcium disodium; calcium disodium ethylenediaminetetraacetate)

CaEDTE
calcium disodium edetate (edathamil calcium disodium; calcium disodium ethylenediaminetetraacetate)

caerul.
caeruleus (L. sky blue)

CAF
Caucasian adult female
cell adhesion factor
citric acid fermenters
cyclophosphamide (Cytoxan), Adriamycin (doxorubicin), and 5-fluorouracil (5-FU) (re: chemotherapy)

CaF
correction of area factor

caf.
caffeine

CAFP
cyclophosphamide (Cytoxan), Adriamycin (doxorubicin), 5-fluorouracil, and prednisone (re: chemotherapy)

CAFVP
cyclophosphamide (Cytoxan), Adriamycin (doxorubicin), 5-fluorouracil, vincristine (Oncovin), and prednisone (re: chemotherapy)

CAG
cholangiogram
chronic atrophic gastritis
coronary angiogram

Ca gluc.
calcium gluconate

CAH
central alveolar hypoventilation
chronic active hepatitis
chronic aggressive hepatitis
combined atrial hypertrophy
congenital adrenal hyperplasia
congenital adrenogenital hyperplasia
cyanoacetohydrazide (cyanoacetic acid hydrazine; antitubercular—human; anthelmintic [lungworm]— animals)

CAHD
coronary arteriosclerotic heart disease
coronary atherosclerotic heart disease

CAI
computer-aided instruction
computer-assisted instruction
confused artificial insemination
Cultural Attitude Inventories

c-a interval
cardio-arterial interval

CAL
calcium test (re: Dent)
calculated average life
chronic airflow limitation
computer-aided learning
computer-assisted learning

Cal
large (kilogram) calorie (now called kilocalorie—kcal)

cal
calorie (unit of heat in centigram-gram-second system)

cal.
caliber
gram calorie
microcalorie
small calorie

C alb, C_alb, C. alb.
albumin clearance

calc.
calculate
calculated

calCd, calcd.
calculated

calcif.
calcification

Cal Ct, cal. ct.
calorie count

CALD
chronic active liver disease

calef.
calefac (L. make warm)
calefactus (L. warmed)

CALGB
cancer and leukemic group B

cALL
common (null cell) acute lymphoblastic
   leukemia

CALLA
common acute lymphoblastic leukemia
   antigen

CAM
calf aortic microsome
Caucasian adult male
cell-associating molecule
chorioallantoic membrane
   (chorio-allantoic)
computer-aided myelography
computer-assisted myelography
content addressable memory (re:
   computers)
contralateral axillary metastasis
cyclophosphamide (Cytoxan),
   Adriamycin (doxorubicin), and
   methotrexate (re: chemotherapy)

CaM
calmodulin (calcium-dependent
   regulator protein distributed in
   eukaryotic cells)

C_am
amylase clearance

CAMAC
computer automated measurement and
   control

CAMB
Cytoxan (cyclophosphamide),
   Adriamycin (doxorubicin),
   methotrexate, bleomycin (re:
   chemotherapy)

CAMELEON
cytosine arabinoside (cytarabine),
   methotrexate, Leukovorin (citrovorum
   factor), and Oncovin (vincristine) (re:
   chemotherapy)

CAMEO
cyclophosphamide, Adriamycin,
   methotrexate, etoposide, Oncovin (re:
   chemotherapy)

CAMF
cyclophosphamide (Cytoxan),
   Adriamycin (doxorubicin),
   methotrexate, and folinic acid
   (citrovorum factor) (re:
   chemotherapy)

CAmg
cortical amygdaloid nucleus (re: Neuro)

CAMP
Christie, Atkins, Munch-Peterson (test,
   factor)
computer-aided menu planning
computer-assisted menu planning
Cytoxan (cyclophosphamide),
   Adriamycin (doxorubicin),
   methotrexate (MTX), procarbazine
   hydrochloride (Matulane) (re:
   chemotherapy)

CAMP, cAMP, c AMP
cyclic adenosine monophosphate
   (3′:5′-cyclic phosphate; cyclic AMP)

c. amplum
cocleare amplum (L. [spoon shaped like
   a snail's shell] heaping spoonful; also
   spelled cochleare)

CAMS
computer-aided monitoring system
computer-assisted monitoring system

CaMV
cauliflower mosaic virus

CAN
Candida (genus)

CA/N
child abuse and neglect

Can
cancer

can.
cannabis

canc.
cancel(ed)
cancellation

CANP
calcium-activated neutral protease

CANS
central auditory nervous system

CAO
chronic airflow obstruction
chronic airway obstruction
coronary artery occlusion
cyclophosphamide, Adriamycin,
Oncovin (re: chemotherapy)

CaO
calcium oxide (L. calx, quicklime [plus
oxide])

CaO$_2$
arterial oxygen content

CaOC, CáOC
cathodal opening contraction

CaOCl
cathodal opening clonus

CAOD
coronary artery occlusive disease

CAOM
chronic adhesive otitis media

CaOTe
cathodal opening tetanus

ca. ox.
calcium oxalate

CAP
captopril (inhibits angiotensin-
converting enzyme)
catabolite (gene) activator protein (re:
genetics)
cell-attachment protein
cellulose acetate phthalate
central apical portion
chloramphenicol
chloroacetophenone (riot-control agent)
chronic alcoholic pancreatitis
compound action potential
coupled atrial pacing
cyclic AMP-binding protein
cyclophosphamide (Cytoxan),
Adriamycin (doxorubicin), and Platinol
(cisplatin) (re: chemotherapy)
cyclophosphamide (Cytoxan),
Adriamycin (doxorubicin), and
prednisone (re: chemotherapy)
cystine aminopeptidase

CAP, Cap, cap.
capsula (L. a little chest—capsule)

CAP, cap.
capiat (L. let the patient take)

CAP-I
cyclophosphamide (Cytoxan),
Adriamycin (doxorubicin), and Platinol
(cisplatin) (re: chemotherapy)

CAP-II
cyclophosphamide (Cytoxan),
Adriamycin (doxorubicin), and high
dose Platinol (cisplatin) (re:
chemotherapy)

cap.
capacity
caput (L. head)

CAPA
cancer-associated polypeptide antigen
coffee, alcohol, pepper, aspirin

CAP-BOP
cyclophosphamide (Cytoxan),
Adriamycin (doxorubicin),
procarbazine (Matulane), bleomycin,
Oncovin (vincristine), and prednisone
(re: chemotherapy)

CAPD
continuous ambulatory peritoneal
dialysis

capiend.
capiendus (L. to be taken)

cap. moll.
capsula mollis (L. soft capsule)

CAPP
Clinical Appraisal of Psychosocial
Problems

CAPPS
Current and Past Psychopathology
Scales

cap. quant. vult
capiat quantum vult (L. let [the patient]
take as much as he wants)

caps.
. capsula (L. a little box—capsule)
capsule(s)

capsul.
capsula (L. a little box—capsule)

caput. med.
caput medusae (cirsomphalos; also
seen in absolute glaucoma)

CAQ
Change Agent Questionnaire (re:
psychological testing)
Classroom Atmosphere Questionnaire
(re: psychological testing)
Clinical Analysis Questionnaire (re:
psychological testing)

CAR
central apparatus room (re: computers)
channel address register
chronic articular rheumatism
computer-assisted research
conditioned avoidance response

car.
carotid

CARA
chronic aspecific respiratory ailment

CARB, carb.
carbohydrate

carb.
carbonate

carbo.
carbohydrate

carbon tet.
carbon tetrachloride

CARD, card.
Cardiology (Service)
cardiology

card.
cardiac

card. insuff.
cardiac insufficiency

cardio.
cardiology

CARDIOL, Cardiol, cardiol.
Cardiology (Service)
cardiology

cardiol.
cardiologist

cardio-resp
cardiorespiratory

CARE
Computerized Adult and Records
    Evaluation System (re: medical
    records)

CARS
childhood autism rating scale
Children's Affective Rating Scale (re:
    Psychol)

cart.
cartilage

CARTOS
computer-aided reconstruction by
    tracing of serial sections
computer-assisted reconstruction by
    tracing of serial sections

CAS
calcarine sulcus
Cancer Attitude Survey
carbohydrate-active steroid
cardiac adjustment scale
cardiac surgery
carotid artery system
cerebral arteriosclerosis

cold-agglutination syndrome
Concept-Specific Anxiety Scale (re:
    Psychol)
control adjustment strap
coronary artery spasm
Creativity Attitude Survey (re:
    psychological testing)
Cultural Attitude Scales (formerly called
    Tri-Cultural Attitude Scale [without
    Mexican-American scale])

Cas
casualty

CASA
computer-aided self-assessment
computer-assisted self-assessment

CASH
corticoadrenal-stimulating hormone

CASHD
coronary arteriosclerotic heart disease

CASMD
congenital atonic sclerotic muscular
    dystrophy

CAST
Children of Alcoholism Screening Test

C-AST
cytoplasmic aspartate aminotransferase

CAT
California Achievement Test (re:
    psychological testing)
capillary agglutination test
catalase
catecholamines
cellular atypia
Children's Apperception Test
chlormerodrin accumulation test
choline acetyltransferase test
chronic abdominal tympany
classified anaphylatoxin
Cognitive Abilities Test
College Ability Test
computed abdominal tomography
computed axial tomography
computer-aided tomography
computer-assisted axial tomography
computerized axial tomography
Computer of Average Transients
cytosine arabinoside, Adriamycin, 6-
    thioguanine (re: chemotherapy)

cat.
catalyst
cataplasma (L. a poultice)
cataract

CAT-A-KIT
catecholamines radioenzymatic assay
    kit

cat. c̄ II
cataract with intraocular lens

CATH, Cath, cath.
catharticus (L. cathartic)
catheter
catheterize

CAT-H
Children's Apperception Test-Human

Cath
Catholic

cath.
cathartic
catheterization
cathode

cathar.
cathartic

CAT-MET
catecholamine and metabolites

CATSCAN
computerized axial tomography scanner

CAT scan
computerized axial tomography scan

CaTT
calcium tolerance test

Cau
Caucasian

Cauc
Caucasian

Caud
caudal

caut.
cauterization
cauterize
cautiously

CAV
congenital absence of vagina
congenital adrenal virilism
croup-associated virus
cyclophosphamide (Cytoxan),
    Adriamycin (doxorubicin), and
    vincristine (Oncovin) (re:
    chemotherapy)
Cytoxan, Adriamycin, Velban (re:
    chemotherapy)

cav.
cavity

CAVC
complete atrioventricular canal

CAVD
completion, arithmetic (problems),

vocabulary, (following) directions (re:
    psychological testing)

C(a-VDO₂)
arteriovenous oxygen difference

CAVe, CA-Ve
CCNU (lomustine), Adriamycin
    (doxorubicin), and Velban
    (vinblastine) (re: chemotherapy)

CA virus
croup-associated virus

CAW
central airways

CB
carbenicillin
carbobenzoxy chloride
carbonated beverage
catheterized bladder
chronic bronchitis
circumflex branch
color blind
conjugated bilirubin
contrast baths (re: physical therapy)
coracobrachialis
Cruveilhier-Baumgarten (syndrome)

CB, C/B
chest-back (re: EKG lead)

C&B
chair and bed (rest)

CB 11
phenadoxone (narcotic/analgesic)

Cb
columbium (element—now called
    niobium)

C3b
product that results when complement
    C3 breaks down upon storage

cb.
cardboard (or plastic film holder without
    intensifying screens)

CBA
carcinoma-bearing animal
chronic bronchitis with asthma
competitive-binding assay
cost benefit analysis

CBAB
complement-binding antibody

CB agar
chocolate blood agar

C banding
centromeric or constitutive
    heterochromatin banding (re:
    chromosome banding)

CBB
communications in behavioral biology
Coomassie brilliant blue

CBC
Camelot Behavioral Checklist
cerebrobuccal connective
child behavior characteristics

CBC, c.b.c.
complete blood count

CBCN
carbenicillin

CBD
carotid body denervation
closed bladder drainage
common bile duct
community-based distribution

CBDC
chronic bullous disease of childhood

CBDE
common bile duct exploration

CBF
capillary blood flow
cerebral blood flow
ciliary beat frequency
coronary blood flow
cortical blood flow (re: Uro)

CBFP
chronic biological false-positive
(seroreactions for syphilis)

CBG
capillary blood gas
coronary bypass grafting
corticosteroid-binding globulin
(transcortin)
cortisol-binding globulin

CBH
chronic benign hepatitis
cutaneous basophilic hypersensitivity

CBI
close-binding-intimate

C bile
bile from hepatic duct

CBL
circulating blood lymphocyte
cord (umbilical) blood leukocytes

Cbl
cobalamin (vitamin B_{12}—re: all of the
molecules except the cyano group)

CBM
capillary basement membrane

CBMMP
chronic benign mucous membrane
pemphigus

CBMT, CBM(T)
capillary basement membrane
(thickness)

CBMW
capillary basement membrane width

CBN
cannabinol
central benign neoplasm

CBO
carbobenzoxy- (benzyloxycarbonyl-)

CBOC
completion (of) bed occupancy care

CBP
carbohydrate-binding protein
chlorobiphenyls
cobalamin-binding protein

CBPA
competitive protein-binding assay

CBR
carotid bodies resected
chemical, bacteriological, and
radiological (warfare)
chemically bound residue
chronic bedrest
complete bedrest
crude birth rate

C3BR
complement component-3b receptor
(re: genetics)

CBS
chronic brain syndrome
conjugated bile salts

CB3S
coxsackie B3 virus susceptibility (re:
genetics)

CBSP
clearance (of) bromsulfophthalein

CBT
cognitive behavior therapy
computed body tomography
Curschmann-Battern-Steinert
(syndrome)

CBV
capillary blood (flow) velocity
central blood volume
cerebral blood volume
circulating blood volume
corrected blood volume
coxsackie B virus

CBVD
CCNU, bleomycin, vinblastine, dexamethasone (re: chemotherapy)

CBW
chemical and biological warfare
critical band width (of noise)

CBX
computer-based examination

Cbz
carbobenzoxy

Cbz, CB$_z$
carbobenzoxy chloride (carbobenzoxy, benzyloxycarbonyl)

CC
calcaneo-cuboid
calcium cyclamate
cardiac catheterization
cardiac cycle
carotid cavernous (fistula)
case coordinator
Caucasian child
caval catheterization
cell culture
cellular compartment
central compartment
cerebral commissure
cerebral cortex
Céstan-Chenais (syndrome)
chest circumference
cholecalciferol
chondrocalcinosis
choriocarcinoma
ciliated cell
circulation
circulatory collapse
classical conditioning
clean catch (re: urine)
clindamycin
clinical course
closing capacity
coefficient of correlation
colony count (re: urine culture)
color and circulation
colorectal cancer
commission certified (re: stains)
common cold
compound cathartic
computer calculated
congenital cardiopathy
contractile component
contrast cystogram
coracoclavicular
cord compression
coronary collaterals
corpora cardiaca
corpus callosum (re: Neuro)
costochondral
craniocervical
creatinine clearance
critical care

critical condition
crus cerebri
current complaint(s)
cylinder cast

CC, C.C.
chief complaint

CC, Cc
concave

C & C
cold and clammy

cc, c.c.
cubic centimeter

cc, c.c., c̄c
cum correctione (L. with correction—re: Ophth)

CCA
N-(2-carboxyphenyl)-4-chloroanthranilic acid (lobenzarit; antirheumatic)
cephalin cholesterol antigen
chick cell agglutination (unit)
chimpanzee coryza agent (respiratory syncytial virus)
choriocarcinoma
circumflex coronary artery
colitis colon antigen
common carotid artery

C-C-A
cytidyl-cytidyl-adenyl

CCAS
Comprehensive Career Assessment Scale (re: psychological testing)

CCAT
Canadian Cognitive Abilities Test (re: psychological testing)
conglutinating complement absorption test

CCAU
chick cell agglutination unit

CCBV
central circulating blood volume

CCC
calcium cyanamide (carbimide) citrated (citrated calcium carbimide [anti-alcoholic])
cathodal closing contraction
cathodal closure contraction
central counteradaptive changes
chronic calculous cholecystitis
comprehensive care clinic
consecutive case conference
covalently closed circular (re: DNA)
critical care complex

CCCC
centrifugal countercurrent
  chromatography

CCCL, CCCI
cathodal closure clonus

CCCR
closed chest cardiac resuscitation

CCCS
condom catheter collecting system

CCCU
comprehensive cardiovascular care unit

CCD
calibration curve date
charge coupled device
childhood celiac disease
computer-controlled display
contracurrent distribution
cortical collecting duct
countercurrent distribution
cumulative cardiotoxic dose

CCD #1
chronic cystic disease, grade 1

CCE
carboline-carboxylic (acid) ester
chamois contagious ecthyma
clear-cell carcinoma (re: endothelium)
clubbing, cyanosis, or edema
countercurrent electrophoresis
cyanosis, clubbing, and edema

C cells
a cell of pancreatic islets of guinea pig
  (re: thyroid)
gamma cells of pancreas
parafollicular cell (re: thyroid)

CCF
cancer coagulative factor
cardiolipin complement fixation
carotid cavernous fistula
cephalin-cholesterol flocculation
compound comminuted fracture
congestive cardiac failure
crystal-induced chemotactic factor

CCFA
cefoxitin-cycloserine-fructose agar
  (medium)

CCG
cholecystogram

CCGC
capillary column gas chromatography

CCGG
cytosine-cytosine-guanine-guanine

CCH
C-cell hyperplasia
chronic cholestatic hepatitis

CCHD
cyanotic congenital heart disease

CCHS
congenital central hypoventilation
  syndrome

CCI
chronic coronary insufficiency
College Characteristics Index
  (institutional profile perceived by its
  students)
corrected count increment

CCIM
coronary care, intensive, medical

CCK
cholecystokinin

CCK-GB
cholecystokinin cholecystography—
  gallbladder

CCKLI
cholecystokinin-like immunoreactivity

CCK-PZ
cholecystokinin-pancreozymin

CCL
carcinoma cell line
critical carbohydrate level
critical condition list

C & Cl, c. & cl.
coitus and climax

CCLI
composite clinical and laboratory index

CCM
congestive cardiomyopathy
contralateral competing message
critical care medicine
cyclophosphamide (Cytoxan), CCNU
  (lomustine), and methotrexate (re:
  chemotherapy)

c.cm.
cubic centimeter

CCMS
clean catch midstream

CCMSU
clean catch midstream urine

CCMT
catechol methyltransferase

CCMU
critical care medicine unit

CCN
caudal central nucleus
coronary care nursing
critical care nursing

CCNS
cell cycle nonspecific (antitumor agent)

CCNU
N-(2-chloroethyl)-N'-cyclohexyl-N-nitrosourea (chloroethyl cyclohexylnitrosourea [lomustine—not a combination]—antineoplastic)

CCOF
chromosomally competent ovarian failure

CCOT
cervical compression overloading test

CCP
chronic calcifying pancreatitis
ciliocytophthoria (re: Resp)

CCPD
continuous cyclic peritoneal dialysis

CCPDS
centralized cancer patient data system

CCPR
crypt cell production rate

C_{CR}, CCr, C Cr, C.Cr., C cr, C_{cr}
creatinine clearance

CCRS
carotid chemoreceptor stimulation

CCS
casualty clearing station
cell cycle specific (antitumor agent)
cholecystosonography
cloudy cornea syndrome
concentration camp syndrome
costoclavicular syndrome

CC&S
corneae, conjunctivae, and sclerae

CCSA
central chemosensitive area

C_{CSF}
cerebrospinal fluid (drug) concentration

CCT
carotid compression tomography
central conduction time
chocolate coated tablet
coated compressed tablet
combined cortical thickness
composite cyclic therapy
controlled cord traction
cranial computed tomography
crude coal tar
cyclocarbothiamine (oral thiamine therapy)

C ct.
colony count

cct.
circuit

CCTe
cathodal closure tetanus

CCTM
color, circulation, temperature, and movement

CCTP
Coronary Care Training Program

CC-TV
closed-circuit television

CCU
Cardiac Care Unit
cardiovascular care unit
Cherry-Crandall units
color-changing units
community care unit
Coronary Care Unit
Critical Care Unit

CCUP
colpocystourethropexy

CCV
channel catfish virus
conductivity cell volume

CCV-AV
CCNU (lomustine), cyclophosphamide (Cytoxan), vincristine (Oncovin) alternating with Adriamycin (doxorubicin) and vincristine (re: chemotherapy)

CCVD
chronic cerebrovascular disease

CC-Virus
common cold virus

CCVPP
CCNU, cyclophosphamide. Velban, procarbazine, prednisone (re: chemotherapy)

CCW
Central Colony (in) Wisconsin (institution for mentally retarded where major genetic study was made)

CCW, ccw
counterclockwise

Ccw
chest wall compliance

CD
cadaver donor
canine distemper
canine dose
carbon dioxide (CO_2)
carbonate dehydratase

cardiac disease
cardiac dullness
cardiac dysrhythmia
cardiovascular disease
Carrel-Dakin (fluid)
cat dander (test)
celiac disease
cell dissociation
central deposition
cesarean delivered
character disorder
chemotactic difference
childhood disease
chronotropic dose
circular dichroism (re: wavelength of
   light)
civil defense
Clostridium difficile
colloid droplet
combination drug
common duct
communication deviance
complete diagnosis
completely denatured
conduct disorder
conjugate diameter
consanguineous donor
constant drainage
contact dermatitis
contagious disease
control diet
conventional dialysis
convulsive disorder
convulsive dose
corneal dystrophy
covert dyskinesia
Crohn's disease
curative dose
cutdown
cystic duct

CD, C.D.
communicable disease

CD, C-D
cervicodorsal

CD, Cd, cd
caudal
drug coefficient

CD, cd
candela (L. candle—SI base unit of
   luminous intensity)

CD, c.d.
conjugata diagonalis (L. diagonal
   conjugate—diameter of pelvic inlet)

C/D, C/d
cigarettes per day

C/D, C:D
cup-to-disc ratio (re: Ophth)

C&D
curettage and dessication
cystoscopy and dilatation
cystoscopy and dilation

CD$_{50}$
median curative dose

Cd
cadmium (element)
color denial
cord

^{109}Cd
radioactive isotope of cadmium

^{115}Cd
radioactive isotope of cadmium

Cδ
constant region for immunoglobulin

CDA
cetyldimethylethylammonium bromide
   (topical antiseptic)
chenodeoxycholic acid (re: dissolving
   gallstones)
ciliary dyskinesia activity
complement-dependent antibody
completely denatured alcohol
congenital dyserythropoietic anemia

CDAA
α-chloro-*N,N*-diallylacetamide
   (herbicide)

CDAI
Crohn's disease activity index

CDAO
caudal portion of the dorsal accessory
   olive (re: Neuro)

C & DB
cough and deep breathe
cough and deep breathing

CDC
calculated date of confinement
call direction code (re: computers)
cancer detection center
capillary diffusion capacity
cardiac diagnostic center
cell division cycle
Centers for Disease Control
chenodeoxycholate (acid)
chenodeoxycholic (acid—re: dissolution
   of cholesterol gallstones)
child development clinic
Communicable Disease Center
complement-dependent cytotoxicity
Crohn's disease of the colon

CD-C
controlled drinker-control

CDCA
chenodeoxycholic acid

CDCF
Clostridium difficile culture filtrate

CDD
certificate of disability for discharge
chronic degenerative disease
chronic disabling dermatosis
critical degree of deformation

C-DDP
cis-diamminedichloroplatin (*cis*-
platinum, cisplatin, or Platinol; also
platinum diamminodichloride)

CDE
canine distemper encephalitis
chlordiazepoxide (tranquilizer)
common duct exploration

CDE antigen
Rh blood group (Fisher-Race
nomenclature)

CDEC
2-chloroallyl diethyldithiocarbamate
(herbicide)
Comprehensive Developmental
Evaluation Chart

CDF
chondrodystrophia fetalis
ciliary dyskinesia factor

CDFR
cumulative duration of the first
remission

CDH
ceramide dihexoside (a glycolipid)
chronic disease hospital
congenital diaphragmatic hernia
congenital dislocation of the hip
congenital dysplasia (of the) hip
congenitally dislocated hip
congenitally dysplastic hip

CDI
cell-directed inhibitor
Children's Diagnostic Inventory
chronic diabetes insipidus

CDILD
chronic diffuse interstitial lung disease

CDL
chlorodeoxylincomycin (7(S)-chloro-7-
deoxylincomycin; clindamycin—
antibacterial)
Copying Drawings with Landmarks

CDLE
chronic discoid lupus erythematosus

CDM
Career Decision-Making (re:
psychological testing)
chemically defined medium
N′-(4-chloro-2-methylphenyl)-*N*,*N*-
dimethylmethanimidamide
(chlordimeform—acari-, insecticide)

cDNA
complementary DNA

CDP
chronic destructive periodontitis
collagenase-digestible protein
constant distending pressure
continuous distending pressure
coronary drug project
cytosine diphosphate (cytidine 5′-
diphosphate—a nucleoside
diphoshate)

CDPC
cytidine diphosphate choline

Cd-probe
cadmium probe

CDPS
common duct pigment stones

CDR
calcium-dependent regulator protein
(calmodulin)
Chronological Drinking Record
complementary determining region (re:
protein)
computerized digital radiography
correct delayed reaction

C3DR
complement component-3d receptor
(re: genetics)

CDRS-R
Children's Depression Rating Scale-
Revised (re: Psychol)

CDS
cervicodorsal syndrome
cul-de-sac (Fr. bottom of a sack—a
blind pouch)
cumulative duration of survival

CdS
cadmium sulfide (re: dermatology)

CDSS
clinical decision support system

CDT
carbon dioxide therapy
Clostridium difficile toxin
combined diphtheria tetanus

CDTe
cathode duration tetanus

CdTe
cadmium telluride

CDV
canine distemper virus

Cdyn, C dyn.
dynamic compliance (re: Resp)

CDZ
chlordiazepoxide (sedative; minor tranquilizer)

CE
California encephalitis
Camurati-Engelmann (syndrome)
capital epiphysis
cardiac enlargement
cardioesophageal
cell extract
Charcot-Erb (syndrome)
chemical energy
chick embryo
cholesterol esters
chorioepithelioma
chromatoelectrophoresis
ciliated epithelium
clinical emphysema
columnar epithelium
conjugated estrogens
constant error
continuing education
contractile element (of skeletal muscle)
converting enzyme
crude extract
cytopathic effect
cytopathogenic effect

CE, C-E
Carpentier-Edwards (valve)
chloroform-ether (mixture)

C & E
consultation and examination
cough and exercise

Ce
celeriter (L. quickly)
cerium (element)

^{139}Ce
radioactive isotope of cerium

^{141}Ce
radioactive isotope of cerium

^{143}Ce
radioactive isotope of cerium

^{144}Ce
radioactive isotope of cerium

C_ϵ
constant region for immunoglobulin

CEA
carcinoembryonic antigen

cholesterol esterifying activity
cost effectiveness analysis
crystalline egg albumen (L. egg white; the pure protein is spelled albumin, and commercial egg white—albumen)

CE angle
capital epiphysis angle (re: Ortho)

CEBD
controlled extrahepatic biliary drainage

CEC
cefaclor
ciliated epithelial cells
contractile electrical complex

CECT
contrast-enhanced computed tomography

CEE
central European encephalitis
chick embryo extract

CEEB
College Entrance Examination Board (test)

CEEC
calf esophagus epithelial cell

CEENU, CeeNU
chloroethyl cyclohexyl nitrosourea (lomustine—an antineoplastic)

CEEV
central European encephalitis virus

CEF
centrifugation extractable fluid
chick embryo fibroblast

CEFT
Children's Embedded Figures Test (re: Psychol)

CEG
chronic erosive gastritis

CEH
cholesterol ester hydrolase

CEHC
calf embryonic heart cell

CEI
Character Education Inquiry (situational test—re: Psychol)
converting enzyme inhibitor
corneal epithelial involvement

CEID
crossed electroimmunodiffusion

CEJ, cej, c.e.j.
cement-enamel junction (re: Dent)

CEL, Cel
Celsius (temperature scale; originally
zero represented melting point of ice
and boiling point of water was 100°.
Christen inverted the scale in 1743,
but it is still called Celsius. Also called
centigrade)

CELI
Carrow Elicited Language Inventory (re:
psychological testing)

cell.
celluloid (re: Dent)

CELO
chicken embryo lethal orphan (virus)

CELOV
chicken embryo lethal orphan virus

Cels
Celsius (temperature scale—Although
Christen inverted scale in 1743, it is
still called Celsius; also centigrade)

CEM
conventional transmission electron
microscope

cemf
counterelectromotive force

C.E. mixture, C-E mixture
chloroform and ether mixture
(anesthetic—rarely used)

cen
centromere (re: cytogenetics)

cen.
center
central

CENT, Cent, cent.
centigrade

cent.
centimeter
central

centi.
centigrade

centihg
centimeters of mercury (sometimes
used—re: pressure; pronounced with
silent "h")

CEO, c.e.o.
chick embryo origin

CEOT
calcifying epithelial odontogenic tumor

CEP
CCNU, etoposide (VP-16-213),
prednimustine (re: chemotherapy)

congenital erythropoietic porphyria
cortical evoked potential (re: Neuro)
countercurrent electrophoresis
counterelectrophoresis

CEPA
2-chloroethanephosphonic acid
(ethephon; CEPHA—plant growth
regulator)

CEPB
Carpentier-Edwards porcine
bioprosthesis (re: Cardio)

ceph.
cephalic

CEPHA
2-chloroethanephosphonic acid
(ethephon; CEPA—plant growth
regulator)

ceph-chol. floc.
cephalin cholesterol flocculation

**CEPH FLOC, Ceph Floc, Ceph floc.,
ceph. floc., ceph-floc**
cephalin flocculation

CER
conditioned emotional response
conditioned escape response
control electrical rhythm
cortical evoked response

CER, Cer
ceramide (a sphingolipid class)

cer.
cervical

CERA
continuous electrical response activity

cerat.
ceratum (L. wax ointment)

CERD
chronic end-stage renal disease

cereb.
cerebral

CERT, Cert, cert.
certificate
certified

cerv.
cervical
cervix

cerv. ser.
cervical series (re: Radio)

CES
chronic electrophysiological study
Classroom Environment Scale (re:
psychological testing)

CES, c.e.s.
central excitatory state (re: Neuro)

CESD
cholesterol ester storage disease

C1 esterase inhibitor
an inhibitor of the complement system
that blocks C1s (a subunit of the first
protein to act in the complement
system)

CET
controlled environment treatment

CETE
central European tick-borne
encephalitis

CEU
continuing education unit

CEV
California encephalitis virus

CEZ
cefazolin (antibacterial)

CF
calf (blood) flow
calibration factor
cancer free
carbolfuchsin (carbol-fuschin; Ziehl's
stain)
carbon filtered
cardiac failure
carotid foramen
carrier free
Carworth Farms (mice—Webster strain)
case file
cephalothin (broad-spectrum antibiotic)
characteristic frequency
chemotactic factor
chest and left leg (re: EKG leads)
Chiari-Frommel syndrome
chick fibroblast
choroid fissure
Christmas factor (blood coagulation
Factor IX)
citrovorum (folinic acid) factor
climbing fiber
clotting factor
colicin factor
collected fluid
colonization factor
colony forming
color and form
column of fornix
complement fixation
completely follicular
constant frequency
contractile force
coronary flow
cough frequency
count(s) fingers
coupling factors

court files
crystal field
cycling fibroblast

CF, C.F.
cystic fibrosis

CF, C/F
Caucasian female
counting fingers

CF, C'F
complement fixing

CF, cf, cf.
confer (L. compare, confer, bring
together, compare with, or refer to)

Cf
californium (element)
iron (ferrum) carrier

252Cf
californium-252 (neutron radiation
source— antineoplastic)

cf
centrifugal force

CFA
colonization factor antigen
colony-forming assay
complement-fixing antibody
complete Freund's adjuvant
cryptogenic fibrosing alveolitis

CFA/I
colonization factor antigen I

C factor, C-factor
cleverness factor (re: Psychol)

CFB
central fibrous body

CFC
capillary filtration coefficient
capillary-forming capacity (cell)
chlorofluorocarbon
colony-forming cell
continuous flow centrifugation

CFCL
continuous flow centrifugation
leukapheresis

CFC-S
colony-forming cells—spleen

CFD
cephalofacial deformity
craniofacial dysostosis

CFF
critical flicker frequency
critical flicker fusion (test)
cystic fibrosis factor

CFF, c.f.f.
critical fusion (flicker) frequency

CFFA
cystic fibrosis factor activity

Cf-Fe
carrier-bound iron (ferrum)

CFI
cardiac function index
chemotactic-factor inactivator
complement fixation inhibition (test)

CFIT
Culture Fair Intelligence Test (Cattell)
Culture Free Intelligence Test (former
   name for Culture Fair Intelligence
   Test [Cattell])

C'Fix
complement fixation test (C' is former
   symbol for complement)

CFM
chlorofluoromethane (fluorocarbon)
Corometrics Fetal Monitor

cfm, cf/m
cubic feet per minute

CFNS
chills, fever, night sweats

CFP
chronic false positive
cyclophosphamide (Cytoxan), 5-
   fluorouracil, and prednisone (re:
   chemotherapy)
cystic fibrosis of the pancreas
cystic fibrosis patients
cystic fibrosis protein

CFPD
critical frequency of photic driving (re:
   EEG)

CFPS
continuous flow plasmapheresis system

CFR
case-fatality ratio
citrovorum-factor rescue
complement fixation reaction
correct fast reaction

CFS
call for service
cancer family syndrome
craniofacial stenosis

cfs
cubic feet per second

CFSE
crystal field stabilization energy

CFT
cardiolipin flocculation test
clinical full time
complement fixation test
complement-fixing titer
Complex Figure Test (re: Psychol)
continuous flow tub

CF TEST, C-F test
complement fixation test

CFU
colony-forming unit(s)

CFU-C
colony-forming unit—culture

CFU-E
colony-forming unit—erythroid
   (precursors of erythrocytes)

CFU$_{EOS}$
colony-forming unit—eosinophil
   (precursors of eosinophils)

CFU-F
colony-forming unit—fibroblast

CFU-GM
colony-forming unit—granulocyte
   macrophage

CFU-L
colony-forming unit—lymphoid

CFU-M
colony-forming unit—megakaryocyte

CFU$_{MEG}$
colony-forming unit—megakaryocyte
   (precursors of megakaryocytes)

CFU/mL
colony-forming units per milliliter

CFU$_{NM}$
colony-forming unit—neutrophil-
   monocyte (precursors of neutrophils)

CFU-S
colony-forming unit—spleen (myeloid
   stem cell)
colony-forming unit—stem (cell)

CFW
Carworth Farm Webster (strain of mice)

CFWM
cancer-free white mouse

CFX
circumflex (coronary artery)

CFZ
capillary-free zone

CFZC
continuous-flow zonal centrifugation

CG
Cardio-Green™ (indocyanine green)
Ceelen-Gellerstedt (syndrome)
central gray (matter of brain)
(chrome violet) CG (aurin tricarboxylic
   acid)
choking gas (phosgene)
choriogenic gynecomastia
chorionic gonadotrop(h)in
chronic glomerulonephritis
cingulate gyrus (re: Neuro)
colloidal gold
control group
cryoglobulin
cryoglobulinemia
cystine guanine

CG, c.g.
center of gravity

Cg, cg, cg.
centigram

Cγ
constant region for immunoglobulin

cg.
chemoglobulin

CGA
catabolite gene activator (re: genetics)

CGD
chromosomal gonadal dysgenesis
chronic granulomatous disease

CGDE
contact glow discharge electrolysis

CGFH
congenital fibrous histiocytoma

CGH
chorionic gonadotrop(h)ic hormone

CGI
carbimazole
chronic granulomatous inflammation
clinical global impression
clinical global inventory

CGL
chronic granulocytic leukemia

c gl, c. gl.
correction with glasses

CGM
central gray matter (of spinal cord)

cgm, cgm.
centigram

CGMMV
cucumber green mottle mosaic virus

cGMP
cyclic guanosine 3,5′-monophosphate

CGN
chronic glomerulonephritis

CGNB
composite ganglioneuroblastoma

CG/OQ
cerebral glucose oxygen quotient

CGP
choline glycerophosphatide
chorionic growth (hormone)-prolactin
circulating granulocyte pool
Comparative Guidance and Placement
   Program (re: psychological testing)

CGPM
Conférence Générale des Poids et
   Mesures

CGRS
Clinician's Global Rating Scale

CGS
cardiogenic shock
catgut suture

CGS, cgs, c.g.s.
centimeter gram second (metric
   system)

CGT
chorionic gonadotrop(h)in

CGTT
cortisol glucose tolerance test

CGTT, C-GTT
cortisone glucose tolerance test

CH
case history
chain
(wheel)chair
Chédiak-Higashi (syndrome)
chiasma
Chinese hamster
chirugia (L. surgery)
chloral hydrate
cholesterol
Christchurch chromosome
chronic hepatitis
chronic hypertension
Clarke-Hadfield (syndrome)
common hepatic (duct)
communicating hydrocele
Community Health
complete healing
congenital hyp othyroidism
Conradi-Hünermann (syndrome)
continuous heparinization

CH, C-H
crown-heel (length of fetus)

CH, Ch, ch.
chapter

chest
chief

C&H
cocaine and heroin

C$_H$1, C$_H$2, C$_H$3
constant regions (of IgA or IgG)

CH$_{50}$
(total serum) hemolytic complement

Ch
chordae (tendineae—re: Cardio)

Ch, ch.
child

Ch.
check
Chido (antibodies)
choline

Ch^1
Christchurch chromosome

cH$^+$
hydrogen ion concentration

ch.
chopped
chronic

CHA
chronic hemolytic anemia
common hepatic artery
congenital hypoplastic anemia
continuous heated aerosols
cyclohexyladenosine
cyclohexylamine

ChA
choline acetylase

CHAC, ChAc
choline acetyltransferase

CHAD
cyclophosphamide (Cytoxan),
hexamethylmelamine, Adriamycin
(doxorubicin), and *cis*-
diamminedichloroplatinum (cisplatin)
(re: chemotherapy)

CHAID
chi-squared automatic interaction
detection (re: statistics)

CHAI-virus
cytopathic human auto-interfering virus

CHAL
chronic haloperidol

CHAMP
Childrens' Hospitals' Automated
Medical Program (re: medical
records)

CHAMPUS
Civilian Health and Medical Programs
for Uniformed Services

chap.
chapter

CHAR
character (re: computers/data
processing)

char.
character
characteristic
characterized

CHART, Chart, chart.
charta (L. paper [a powder in paper])

chart.
chartula (L. a small [medicated] paper)

chart. bib.
charta bibula (L. blotting paper)

chart. cerat.
charta cerata (L. waxed paper;
parchment paper)

CHAT
choline acetyltransferase

CHB
complete heart block

CHBA
congenital Heinz body (hemolytic)
anemia

C & H breathing
coarse and harsh breathing

CHD
Chédiak-Higashi disease
childhood disease
chronic hemodialysis
compensated heart disease
congenital heart defects
congenital heart disease
congenital hip disease
congenital hip dislocation
congestive heart disease
constitutional hepatic dysfunction
cyanotic heart disease

CHE, ChE
cholinesterase

CHE2
cholinesterase (serum)-2

CHEF
Chinese hamster embryo fibroblasts

CHEM, Chem, chem.
chemotherapy

chem.
chemical
chemist
chemistry

chemo.
chemotherapy

chems
chemistries

CHESS
Cornell High Energy Synchrotron
   Source

CHEST
Chick Embryotoxicity Screening Test

CHEX-UP, ChexUP, Chex-Up
cyclophosphamide,
   hexamethylmelamine, 5-fluorouracil,
   Platinol (re: chemotherapy)

CHF
chick heart fibroblast
congenital hepatic fibrosis
congestive heart failure
cyclophosphamide,
   hexamethylmelamine, 5-fluorouracil,
   (re: chemotherapy)

CHFD
controlled high flux dialysis

chg.
change

chg'd
changed

chg's
changes

CHH
cartilage-hair hypoplasia (autosomal
   recessive disease)

X, χ
chi (the 22nd letter of the Greek
   alphabet)

CHI
closed head injury
creatinine-height index

chi
chimera (re: cytogenetics)

CHINA
chronic infectious neuropathic agent
chronic infectious neurotropic agent

CHIP
cis-dichlorotrans-hydrox-*bis*-iso-
   propylamine platinum IV

chirurg.
chirurgicalis (L. surgical)

CHL
Chinese hamster lung
chlorambucil
chloramphenicol

Chl, chl.
chloroform

chl.
chloride

CHLA
cyclohexyl linoleic acid

Chl-A
chimpanzee leukocyte antigen

Chlb
chlorobutanol (industrial chemical;
   pharmaceutical aid; dental analgesic)

CHLD
chronic hypoxic lung disease

chlor.
chloroform

CHMD
clinical hyaline membrane disease

CHN
carbon, hydrogen, nitrogen
central hemorrhagic necrosis
Child Neurology

Chng
change

CHO
carbohydrate
Chinese hamster ovary
chorea
cyclophosphamide (Cytoxan),
   hydroxydaunomycin (doxorubicin),
   and Oncovin (vincristine) (re:
   chemotherapy)

CH$_2$O
formaldehyde gas

Cho
choline

CHOB
cyclophosphamide, Adriamycin,
   Oncovin, bleomycin (re:
   chemotherapy)

CHOI
(considered) characteristic (of)
   osteogenesis imperfecta

CHOL, Chol, chol.
cholesterol

c̄hold
withhold

CHOL E
cholesterol esters

chole.
cholecystectomy

cholecyst.
cholecystectomy

cholelith.
cholelithiasis

choles.
cholesterol

CHOL EST, Chol est., chol. est.
cholesterol esters

cholest.
cholesterol

CHOP
cyclophosphamide,
    hydroxydaunomycin/doxorubicin
    (Adriamycin), Oncovin, prednisone
    (re: chemotherapy)

CHOP-BLEO
cyclophosphamide,
    hydroxydaunomycin/doxorubicin
    (Adriamycin), Oncovin, prednisone,
    bleomycin (re: chemotherapy)

CHO, P, F
carbohydrates, proteins, and fats

CHOR
cyclophosphamide, hydroxydaunomycin
    (doxorubicin), Oncovin (vincristine),
    and radiation therapy (re:
    chemotherapy)

chord. chirurg.
chorda chirurgicalis (L. surgical cord—
    re: suture)

CHP
capillary hydrostatic pressure
charcoal hemoperfusion
child psychiatry
comprehensive health planning
coordinating hospital physician
cutaneous hepatic porphyria

chpx., ch. px.
chickenpox

CHQ
chlorquinol (topical anti-infective)

CHR
Cercarien-Hüllen-Reaktion (test for
    Schistosoma mansoni)

CHR, Chr.
Chromobacterium (genus)

CHR, chr.
chronic

c hr
candle hour
curie hour

Chr^a antigen
low frequency blood group antigen

Chrbac
Chromobacterium (genus)

ChrBrSyn, Chr Br Syn
chronic brain syndrome

Chr B Synd
chronic brain syndrome

CHRIS
Cancer Hazards Ranking and
    Information System

Chron, chron.
chronological

chron.
chronic
chronology

CHRS
cerebrohepatorenal syndrome

CHS
Chédiak-Higashi syndrome
cholinesterase
chondroitin sulfate
contact hypersensitivity

CHT
contralateral head turning

cht.
chartula (L. a small [medicated] paper)

ChTg
chymotrypsinogen

ChTK
chicken thymidine kinase

CHTZ
chlorothiazide

Chu
centigrade heat unit

CHV
canine herpes virus

CHVP
cyclophosphamide, hydroxydaunomycin
    (doxorubicin), VM-26 (teniposide),
    and prednisone (re: chemotherapy)

CH1VPP, Ch1VPP
chlorambucil, vinblastine, procarbazine,
    prednisone (re: chemotherapy)

CI
cardiac index
cardiac insufficiency
cell inhibition
cellular immunity
cephalic index
cerebral infarction
chemical ionization
chemotactic index
chemotherapeutic index
chromatid interchange
chronically infected
clinical impression
clinical investigator
clonus index
closure index
coefficient of intelligence
colloidal iron
colony inhibition
color index
complete iridectomy
confidence interval
contamination index
continuous infusion
coronary insufficiency
corrected (count) increment
crystalline insulin
cytotoxic index

Ci
curie (radioactivity unit)

c_i
chance-response parameter ("guessing parameter"—re: psychological testing; item characteristic curve theory [statistics])

CIA
canine inherited ataxia
CCNU (lomustine), isophosphamide, and Adriamycin (doxorubicin) (re: chemotherapy)
chymotrypsin inhibitor activity
colony-inhibiting activity
congenital intestinal aganglionosis

cib.
cibus (L. food; meal)

CIBD
chronic inflammatory bowel disease

CIBHA, CIB HA
congenital inclusion body hemolytic anemia

CIC
cardiac inhibitor center
cardiac inhibitory center
cardio-inhibitor center
circulating immune complexes
constant initial concentration
Crisis Intervention Clinic

CICA
cervical internal carotid artery
collagen-induced coagulant activity

CICU
cardiac intensive care unit
Cardiology Intensive Care Unit
Cardiovascular Inpatient Care Unit
Coronary Intensive Care Unit

CID
central integrative deficit
chick infective dose
combined immunodeficiency disease
cytomegalic inclusion disease

CIDEP
chemically induced dynamic electron polarization

CIDNP
chemically induced dynamic nuclear polarization

CIDS
cellular immunodeficiency syndrome

CIE
cellulose ion exchanger
Commission International de l'Eclairage (re: standardized measurement of colors)
countercurrent immunoelectrophoresis
counterimmunoelectrophoresis

CIE-C
counterimmunoelectrophoresis— colorimetric

CIE-D
counterimmunoelectrophoresis— densitometric

CIE observer
hypothetical observer having color vision sensitivity (recommended in 1931 by Commission Internationale de l'Eclairage [C.I.E.])

CIEP
counterimmunoelectrophoresis

CIES
Correctional Institutions Environment Scales (re: psychological testing)

CIF
clone-inhibiting factor
cloning inhibiting factor
cloning inhibitory factor

CIG
cigarette use
cold-insoluble globulin (a fibronectin)

CIg
cytoplasmic immunoglobulin

cIgM
cytoplasmic immunoglobulin M

CIH
carbohydrate-induced
  hyperglyceridemia

Ci-hr
curie-hour

CII
Carnegie Interest Inventory (re:
  Psychol)

CIIA
common internal iliac artery

CIIP
chronic idiopathic intestinal pseudo-
  obstruction

CIM
cimetidine
cortically induced movement

CIMS
chemical ionization mass spectrometry
clinical information scale
Conflict in Marriage Scale (re: Psychol)

CIN
central inhibitory (state)
cerebriform intradermal nevus
cervical intra-epithelial neoplasia
chronic interstitial nephritis

C_{IN}, C_{in}, c.in.
inulin clearance (re: Uro)

$\bar{c}$ in
within

CINE
chemotherapy-induced nausea and
  emesis

C1 INH
C1 (esterase) inhibitor

$\bar{c}$ in NL
within normal limits

C.I. number
Colour (color) Index number

CIOF
chromosomally incompetent ovarian
  failure

CIP
chronic inflammatory polyneuropathy
Comprehensive Identification Process
  (re: psychological testing)

CIPD
chronic inflammatory

polyradiculoneuropathy,
  demyelinating
chronic intermittent peritoneal dialysis

CIPF
clinical illness promotion factor

CIPM
Conférence International des Poids et
  Mesures

CIR, cir.
circuit
circular
circulation
circulatory
circumcised
circumcision

cir.
circumference
circumferential

CIRC, Circ, circ.
circumcision

Circ
circuit
circulating
circumcised

Circ, circ.
circular
circulation
circulatory

circ.
circumference
circumferential

circ. & sen.
circulation and sensation

circ. & sens.
circulation and sensation

circum.
circumflex

cir. meas.
circumferential measurements

CIRP
Cooperative Institutional Research
  Program (re: psychological testing)

CIS
carcinoma in situ
catheter-induced spasm
Chemical Information System

CIS, c.i.s.
central inhibitory state

CiS
cingulate sulcus

cis-
stereochemical opposite of *trans-*

CISCA, CisCA
cisplatin, Cytoxan, Adriamycin (re: chemotherapy)

***cis*-DDP**
cis-diamminedichloroplatinum (cisplatin; *cis*-platinum II—antineoplastic)

***Cis*-platinum**
cis-diamminedichloroplatinum (Platinol; cisplatin)

CIT
combined intermittent therapy

cit.
citrate

cito disp.
cito dispensetur (L. let it be dispensed quickly)

CIV
common iliac vein

CIXU
constant infusion excretory urogram

CJD
Creutzfeldt-Jakob disease

CK
calf kidney
chicken kidney
cholecystokinin
choline kinase
contralateral knee
creatine kinase
cytokinin (re: botany)

CK, ck.
check(ed)

CK_1, CK_2, CK_3
isoenzymes of creatine kinase

ck.
cook

CKBB
creatine kinase, BB isozyme

CKC
cold knife conization

ckd.
checked
cooked

CKG
cardiokymograph(y)

CKMB, CK-MB
MB isoenzyme of creatine kinase

ckw.
clockwise

CL
capacity of lung
capillary lumen
cardinal ligament
cardiolipin
center line
(nucleus) centralis lateralis (thalami)
chemiluminescence
chest and left arm lead (re: EKG)
cholelithiasis
cholesterol-lecithin (test)
chronic leukemia
clamp lamp
clear liquid
cleft lip
complex loading
composite lymphoma
confidence level
contact lens
continence line
cricoid lamina
criterion level
critical list
cutis laxa (re: Derma)
cycle length
cytotoxic lymphocyte

CL, C_L
compliance, lung

CL, Cl
Clostridium (genus)
colistin

CL, Cl, cl.
clinic

Cl, cl.
clavicle
clinical
clonus
closure

CL, cl., c.l.
corpus luteum

C_L
constant (light chain)

C/L
clear liquid (diet)

Cl
chloride (Cl^-)
chlorine (element—Gr. chloros, green)

^{36}Cl
radioactive isotope of chlorine

^{38}Cl
radioactive isotope of chlorine

cl
centiliter

cl.
clean
clear
cleared
close(d)
cloudy

CLA
cervicolinguoaxial
communications line adapter (re:
   computers)
cyclic lysine anhydride

CLAH
congenital lipoid adrenal hyperplasia

C lam.
cervical laminectomy

CLAS
congenital localized absence of skin

class.
classification

CLASSI
Cornell Learning and Study Skills
   Inventory (re: Psychol)

classif.
classification
classified

clav.
clavicle

CLB
chlorambucil
curvilinear body

CLBBB
complete left bundle branch block

ClB technique
crossover suppressor (an inversion), a
   lethal (mutation), and the dominant
   marker **B**ar eye (re: sex-linked and
   viable mutations in *Drosophila
   melanogaster*)

CLC
Charcot-Leyden crystal
colchicine

CL/CP
cleft lip and cleft palate

CLD
chronic liver disease
chronic lung disease
congenital limb deficiency

cld.
cleared
closed
colored

CLDM
clindamycin

cldy.
cloudy

CLE
centrilobular emphysema

CLED
cystine-lactose electrolyte deficient

CLF
cardiolipin fluorescence (antibody)
crystal ligand field

CLH
chronic lobular hepatitis
corpus luteum hormone

CLI
corpus luteum insufficiency

CLIF
cloning inhibitory factor

CLIN, Clin, clin.
clinic
clinical

Clini
Clinitest

Clin Path, Clin path.
clinical pathologist
clinical pathology

Clin proc.
clinical procedures

CLIP
cerebral lipidosis (without visceral
   involvement/with onset of disease
   past infancy)
corticotrop(h)in-like intermediate lobe
   peptide

c/liq.
clear liquids(s)

CLK
clock (re: computers/data processing)

CLL
cholesterol-lowering level
cholesterol-lowering lipid
chronic lymphatic leukemia
chronic lymphocytic leukemia

Cl Lab
Clinical Laboratory

CLLE
columnar-lined lower esophagus

Cl liq.
clear liquid(s)

CLML
Current List of Medical Literature

CLMW
cauliflower mosaic virus

CLO
cod liver oil

CLOF
clofibrate

Clon
Clonorchis (genus—liver fluke)

Clostr
Clostridium (genus)

CLP
chymotrypsin-like protein
Clinical Pathology

CL ± P
cleft lip ± palate

Cl Pal, Cl pal., cl. pal.
cleft palate

clr.
clear

cl. rd.
closed reduction (re: Ortho)

CLS
confused language syndrome
Consultation-Liaison Service (re:
    psychiatry)

CLSH
corpus luteum-stimulating hormone

CLSL
chronic lymphosarcoma (cell) leukemia
chronic lymphosarcomatous leukemia

CLT
chronic lymphocytic thyroiditis
clot-lysis time
communication line terminal (re:
    computers)
computer language translator (re:
    computers)

CLT, Cl T
clotting time

CL$_{TB}$
total body (drug) clearance

cl. time
clotting time

C & L trx
cervical and lumbar traction

cl. vd.
clean voided (specimen—re: urine)

CL VOID, Cl void
clean voided (specimen—re: urine)

CIVPP
chlorambucil, vinblastine, procarbazine,
    prednisone (re: chemotherapy)

CLX
cloxacillin

CM
California mastitis (test)
capreomycin
carboxymethylcellulose
cardiac muscle
cardiomyopathy
carpometacarpal
causa mortis (L. cause of death)
cell membrane
(nucleus) centrum medianum
    (centromedianus—re: thalamus)
cerebral mantle
cervical mucus (re: GYN)
chemotactic migration
Chick-Martin (coefficient)
chloroquine-mepacrine
chondromalacia
chopped meat (medium)
circular measure
circular muscle
circumferential measurement
clindamycin
clinical medicine
coccidioidal meningitis
cochlear microphony (microphonia—re:
    Oto)
complete medium (re: microbiology)
computer module (re: computers)
conditioned medium
congenital malformation
congestive myocardiopathy
continuous murmur
contrast media
contrast medium
control mark (re: computers)
cow's milk
cytoplasmic membrane

CM, C/M
Caucasian male

CM, Cm, cm.
complications

CM, cm
centimeter

CM, c.m.
costal margin

C/M
counts per minute

CM—
carboxymethyl radical

C&M
cocaine and morphine (mixed)

Cm
communality (re: California
  Psychological Inventory test)
curium (element)

Cm, C$_m$
maximal clearance (re: urea clearance
  test)
maximum clearance (re: urea clearance
  test)

Cμ
constant region for immunoglobulin

^{242}Cm
radioactive isotope of curium

^{244}Cm
radioactive isotope of curium

cM
centimorgan

c.m.
cras mane (L. tomorrow morning)

cm^2
square centimeter

cm^3
cubic centimeter

CMA
Candida metabolic antigen
chronic metabolic acidosis
cultured macrophages

c. magnum
cocleare magnum (L. [spoon shaped
  like a snail's shell] large spoonful—
  also spelled cochleare)

CMAmg
corticomedial amygdaloid (nucleus—re:
  Neuro)

CMAP
compound muscle action potential

CMB
carbolic methylene blue
p-chloromercuribenzoate (PCMB,
  *p*CMB)

CMC
carboxymethylcellulose (sodium—
  pharmaceutic aid)
carpometacarpal
cell-mediated cytolysis
cell-mediated cytotoxicity
chronic mucocutaneous candidiasis
critical micellar concentration
critical micelle concentration
cyclophosphamide, methotrexate,
  CCNU (re: chemotherapy)

CMCC
chronic mucocutaneous candidiasis

CM-cellulose
carboxymethylcellulose (sodium)

CMC-VAP
cyclophosphamide (Cytoxan),
  methotrexate, CCNU (lomustine),
  vincristine (Oncovin), Adriamycin
  (doxorubicin), and procarbazine (re:
  chemotherapy)

CMD
childhood muscular dystrophy
count median diameter (of particles)

CME
cervical mediastinal exploration
cervical mucous extract (re: GYN)
continuing medical education
crude marijuana extract
cystoid macular edema

c. medium
cocleare medium (L. a half spoonful)

CMF
calcium and magnesium free
catabolite modular factor
chondromyxoid fibroma
cold mitten friction (re: physical therapy)
cortical magnification factor
craniomandibulofacial
Cytoxan (cyclophosphamide),
  methotrexate, 5-fluorouracil (5-FU)
  (re: chemotherapy)

CMF/AV
cyclophosphamide (Cytoxan),
  methotrexate, 5-fluorouracil,
  Adriamycin (doxorubicin), and
  Oncovin (vincristine) (re:
  chemotherapy)

CMFAVP
cyclophosphamide, methotrexate, 5-
  fluorouracil, Adriamycin, vincristine,
  prednisone (re: chemotherapy)

CMFE
calcium and magnesium free plus EDTA

CMFP, CMF-P
cyclophosphamide (Cytoxan),
  methotrexate, 5-fluorouracil, and
  prednisone (re: chemotherapy)

CMFT
cardiolipin microflocculation test (VDRL
  test)
cyclophosphamide, methotrexate, 5-
  fluorouracil, tamoxifen (re:
  chemotherapy)

CMFVAT
cyclophosphamide, methotrexate,

5-fluorouracil, vincristine, Adriamycin, testosterone (re: chemotherapy)

CMFVP
Cytoxan, methotrexate, 5-fluorouracil, vincristine (Oncovin), prednisone (re: chemotherapy)

CMG
canine myasthenia gravis
chopped meat glucose (agar)
congenital myasthenia gravis
cooked meat glucose
cyanmethemoglobin
cystometrogram
cystometrography

CMGN
chronic membranous glomerulonephritis

CMGT
chromosome-mediated gene transfer

CMH
congenital malformation of heart

CMHC
community mental health center

cm H₂O
centimeters of water pressure

CMI
carbohydrate metabolism index
Career Maturity Inventory (re: Psychol)
cell-mediated immunity
cell multiplication inhibitory (activity)
cellular-mediated immune (response)
chronic mesenteric ischemia
circulating microemboli index
computer-managed instruction
Cornell Medical Index—Health Questionnaire

CMID
cytomegalic inclusion disease

c.min., c/min, c/min.
cycles per minute

CMIR
cell-mediated immune response

CMJ
carpometacarpal joint

CML
cell-mediated lymphocytotoxicity
cell-mediated lympholysis
cell-mediated lymphotoxicity
chronic myelocytic leukemia
chronic myelogenous leukemia
chronic myeloid leukemia
count median length
cross midline

CML-BC
blastic crisis of chronic myelogenous leukemia

CMM
cell-mediated mutagenesis
cutaneous malignant melanoma

cmm, c mm
cubic millimeter

CMME
chloromethyl methyl ether (carcinogen at technical grade)

CMMS
Columbia Mental Maturity Scale

CMN
caudal mediastinal node
cystic medial necrosis (of aorta)

CMNAA, CMN-AA
cystic medial necrosis of the ascending aorta

CMND
command (re: computers/data processing)

CMNO
cardiomyopathy, nonobstructive

CMO
calculated mean organism
canonical molecular orbital (method)
cardiac minute output
card made out
comfort measures only

cMo
centimorgan (unit of measure of crossover frequency— re: genetics)

CMoL
chronic monocytic (monoblastic) leukemia

CMOMC
cell meeting our morphologic criteria

CMOP
cyclophosphamide, Oncovin, procarbazine, prednisone (re: chemotherapy)

C-MOPP
cyclophosphamide (Cytoxan), mechlorethamine (Mustargen), Oncovin (vincristine), procarbazine, and prednisone (a modification of standard MOPP chemotherapy regimen in which Cytoxan is substituted for the M [Mustargen]— also called COPP)

101

CMOS
complementary metal oxide
  semiconductor (logic)

CMP
cardiomyopathy
chondromalacia patellae
cytidine monophosphate (cytidine-5'-
  phosphate; cytidylic acid; cytidylate)

2'-CMP
cytidine-2'-monophosphate (2'-cytidylic
  acid)

3'-CMP
cytidine-3'-monophosphate (3'-cytidylic
  acid)

cmpd.
compound

CMPGN
chronic membranoproliferative
  glomerulonephritis

cmps
centimeters per second

CMR
cerebral metabolic rate
common mode rejection
crude mortality ratio

CMRG
cerebral metabolic rate of glucose

CMRL
cerebral metabolic rate of lactate

CMRO
cerebral metabolic rate of oxygen

CMRO$_2$
cerebral metabolic rate of oxygen

CMRR
common mode rejection ratio (re:
  amplifiers)

CMS
cervical mucous solution (re: GYN)
chromosome modification site
circulation, motion, and sensation
circulation, muscle sensation (re:
  PM&R)
click murmur syndrome (re: Cardio)
Clyde Mood Scale
Conflict Management Survey (re:
  psychological testing)
conversational monitor system (re:
  computers/data processing)

c.m.s.
cras mane sumendus (L. to be taken
  tomorrow morning)

cm/s
centimeters per second

cm/sec
centimeters per second

cm/sec^2
centimeters per second per second
  (squared)

CMSS
circulation, motor ability, sensation, and
  swelling

CMT
California mastitis test (re: veterinary
  medicine)
cancer multistep therapy
catechol-O-methyltransferase
cervical motion tenderness
Charcot-Marie-Tooth (disease; atrophy)
chronic motor tic
Concept Mastery Test (re: Psychol)
Current Medical Terminology

CMTD
Charcot-Marie-Tooth disease

CMU
N'-(4-chlorophenyl)-N,N-dimethylurea
  (chlorophenyldimethylurea;
  monuron—an herbicide)
cognition of semantic units (re:
  psychological testing)
complex motor unit
maximal concentration of urea
  (clearance test)

CMV
controlled mechanical ventilation
cucumber mosaic virus
cytomegalovirus

CN
caudate nucleus (re: Neuro)
cellulose nitrate
Charge Nurse
child nutrition
chloroacetophenone (a tear gas; war
  gas)
clinical nursing
cochlear nucleus (re: Neuro)
congenital nephrosis
congenital nystagmus (re: Ophth)
cranial nerve
Crigler-Najjar (disease)
cyanide radical (CN$^-$ or —CN)
cyanogen (a compound of two cyano
  radicals)
cyanosis neonatorum

C/N
carbon to nitrogen (ratio)

CN II, CN III, etc.
cranial nerves

Cn
color naming

C_n
n-fold proper rotation axis (re: symmetry operation)

cn.
canned (re: diet)

c.n.
cras nocte (L. tomorrow night)

CNA
calcium nutrient agar

CNAG
chronic narrow angle glaucoma (re: Ophth)

CNAP
cochlear nucleus action potential

CNB
cutting needle biopsy

CNCBL
cyanocobalamin (vitamin B_{12})

CND
cannot determine

CNDC
chronic nonspecific diarrhea of childhood

CNE
chronic nervous exhaustion
concentric needle electrode
could not establish

CNEMG
concentric needle electromyography

CNES
chronic nervous exhaustion state

CNF
chronic nodular fibrositis
congenital nephrotic (syndrome), Finnish

CNH
central neurogenic hyperpnea
community nursing home

CNHD
congenital nonspherocytic hemolytic disease

CNI
chronic nerve irritation

CNL
cardiolipin natural lecithin

CNM
computerized nuclear morphometry

CNO
congenital nephrotic (syndrome), other (types)

CNOH
cyanic acid (C≡NOH; CHNO)

CNP
continuous negative pressure
cranial nerve palsy

CNPsy
consultation, neuropsychiatric

CNPV
continuous negative pressure ventilation

CNRS
citrated normal rabbit serum

CNRU
clinical nutrition research unit

CNS
central nervous system
computerized notation system
cyanide sulfonate (sulfocyanate—the thiocyanate radical, CNS^- or —CNS)

c.n.s.
cras nocte sumendus (L. to be taken tomorrow night)

CNSHA
congenital nonspherocytic hemolytic anemia

CN sign
cranial nerve sign (re: poliomyelitis)

CNS-L
central nervous system leukemia

CNSLD
chronic nonspecific lung disease

CNT
could not test
current night terrors

CNTE
calf thymus nuclear extract

CNV
colistimethate, nystatin, vancomycin
conative negative variation (re: Psychol)
contingent negative variation

CO
candidal onychomycosis
carbon monoxide
cardiac output
castor oil
central office
centric occlusion
cervical orthosis
choline oxidase
coccygeal
Colton (blood group)
compound

CO, Co
coenzyme

CO, C/O
check out

C/O, C/o, c/o
(under the) care of

C/O, c/o
complains of

CO I, CoI
coenzyme I (diphosphopyridine
nucleotide—DPN; nicotinamide
adenine dinucleotide)

CO II, CoII
coenzyme II (triphosphopyridine
nucleotide—TPN; nicotinamide
adenine dinucleotide phosphate)

CO_2
carbon dioxide

Co
cobalt (element)
compliance
condensation (number)
Cowling number (re:
magnetohydrodynamics)

Co.
county

C_o
initial concentration of DNA (re: de- and
renaturing)

^{56}Co
cobalt-56

^{57}Co
cobalt-57

^{58}Co
cobalt-58

^{60}Co
cobalt-60

co.
compositus (L. a compound,
compounded)
cutoff

c/o
complaining of

COA
calculated opening area
condition on admission

COA, CoA, Co A
coenzyme A

CoA5Ac
5-acetyl-coenzyme A

COAB
Computer Operator Aptitude Battery
(re: psychological testing)

COAD
chronic obstructive airway disease

COAG
chronic open angle glaucoma

COAG, coag.
coagulation

coag.
coagulase
coagulate

coag. time
coagulation time

COAP
cyclophosphamide (Cytoxan), Oncovin
(vincristine), ara-C (cytarabine), and
prednisone (re: chemotherapy)

COAP-BLEO
cyclophosphamide (Cytoxan), Oncovin
(vincristine), ara-C (cytarabine),
prednisone, and bleomycin (re:
chemotherapy)

CoAS-
coenzyme A radical or reduced
coenzyme A

CoASH
coenzyme (its acyl group linked to —SH
group)

CoA-SPC
coenzyme A-synthetizing protein
complex

COB
cranky old bastard (re: chart note)

COBOL
common business oriented language
(re: computers)

COBS
cesarean-obtained barrier-sustained
(animals)
chronic organic brain syndrome

COBT
chronic obstruction of biliary tract

COC
cathodal opening clonus
cathodal opening contraction
combination-type oral contraceptive

COC, Coc, coc.
coccygeal

coch.
cochleare (L. [spoon shaped like a snail's shell] by the spoonful)

coch. amp.
cochleare amplum (L. [spoon shaped like a snail's shell] a heaping spoonful)

cochl.
cochleare (L. [spoon shaped like a snail's shell] by the spoonful)

cochl. amp.
cochleare amplum (L. [spoon shaped like a snail's shell] a heaping spoonful)

cochleat.
cochleatum (L. [spoon shaped like a snail's shell] spoonful)

cochl. mag.
cochleare magnum (L. [spoon shaped like a snail's shell] a large spoonful)

cochl. med.
cochleare medium (L. [spoon shaped like a snail's shell] a half spoonful)

cochl. parv.
cochleare parvum (L. [spoon shaped like a snail's shell] a teaspoonful)

coch. mag.
cochleare magnum (L. [spoon shaped like a snail's shell] a large spoonful)

coch. med.
cochleare medium (L. [spoon shaped like a snail's shell] half spoonful)

coch. mod.
cochleare modicum (L. [spoon shaped like a snail's shell] a medium-size spoonful [dessert spoonful])

coch. parv.
cochleare parvum (L. [spoon shaped like a snail's shell] a teaspoonful)

COCL, COCl
cathodal opening clonus

COCM
congestive cardiomyopathy

CO₂ comb.
carbon dioxide combining (power)

Coct, coct.
coctio (L. boiling)

COD
cause of death
chemical oxygen demand
condition on discharge

COD, cod.
codeine

coef.
coefficient

coeff.
coefficient

COEPS
cortically originating extrapyramidal system (re: Neuro)

COF
cut-off frequency

CoF
cobra factor

COFAL test
complement fixation avian leukosis test

COFS
cerebro-oculo-facial-skeletal (syndrome)

COG
clinical obstetrics and gynecology
cognitive (function tests)

cog.
cognate

Cog Disorg
cognitive disorganization

COGTT
cortisone (primed) oral glucose tolerance test

COH
carbohydrate (CH_2O—as a general formula)

COHB, COHb
carboxyhemoglobin

Coher
coherent

COHgB
carboxyhemoglobin

COIB
Crowley Occupational Interests Blank (re: psychological testing)

COL
CircOlectric (bed)

COL, col.
cola (L. filter, strain [imperative])
colony

Col
collagen
cortisol

col.
colatus (L. strained, filtered)
collateral
color
colored
column

colat.
colatus (L. strained, filtered)

COLD
chronic obstructive lung disease

colen.
colentur (L. let them be strained, filtered)

colet.
coletur (L. let it be strained, filtered)

COLI
collagen I (α1 and α2 chains)

coll.
collect
collection
collective
college
colloidal
collyrium (L. eyewash—a soothing eye water; originally any eye preparation—poultice, salve)

collat.
collateral

collat. circ.
collateral circulation

Colles' fx.
Colles' fracture

collun.
collunarium (L. a nose wash)

collut.
collutorium (modified L. col- + past participle of luo-, to wash [lutus]; washed thoroughly [mouthwash])

coll. vol.
collective volume

collyr.
collyrium (L. an eyewash—a soothing eye water; originally any eye preparation—poultice, salve)

color.
coloretur (L. let it be colored)
colorimetry (including spectrophotometry and photometry)

colost.
colostomy

colp.
colporrhaphy

col/temp
color, temperature

COM
chronic otitis media (re: Oto)
computer output microfilm (system—re: medical records)
computer output microfilmer (re: computers/data processing)
cyclophosphamide, Oncovin (vincristine), and MeCCNU (semustine) (re: chemotherapy)
cyclophosphamide, Oncovin, methotrexate (re: chemotherapy)

com.
comminuted
common
communicable

COMA-A
cyclophosphamide (Cytoxan), Oncovin (vincristine), methotrexate/citrovorum factor, Adriamycin (doxorubicin), and ara-C (cytarabine) (re: chemotherapy)

COMB
cyclophosphamide (Cytoxan), Oncovin (vincristine), MeCCNU (semustine), and bleomycin (re: chemotherapy)
Cytoxan, Oncovin, methotrexate, bleomycin (re: chemotherapy)

comb.
combative
combination
combine(d)
combining

COMC
carboxymethylcellulose

COMe
Cytoxan, Oncovin, methotrexate (re: chemotherapy)

COMF
cyclophosphamide (Cytoxan), Oncovin (vincristine), methotrexate, and 5-fluorouracil (re: chemotherapy)

comf.
comfortable

COMLA
cyclophosphamide (Cytoxan), Oncovin (vincristine), methotrexate, leucovorin, ara-C (cytarabine) (re: chemotherapy)

comm.
comminuted
commission
committee
communicable
communication

comm. cer.
commotio cerebri (L. violent movement
of cerebrum— [cerebral concussion])

commin.
comminuted

commn.
commission
commissioner

commun.
communicable (disease)

commun. dis.
communicable disease

COMP
CCNU, Oncovin, methotrexate,
procarbazine (re: chemotherapy)
cyclophosphamide (Cytoxan), Oncovin
(vincristine), methotrexate, and
prednisone (re: chemotherapy)

COMP, comp.
complaint
complication
composition
compound

comp.
comparable
comparative
compare
compensated (heart disease)
compensation (case)
complete
completed
composed (of)
compositus (L. compound,
compounded, compounded [of])
compress
compressible

Comp case
compensation (workers') case

compd.
compound
compressed

compet.
competition

compl.
complains
complaint
complementary
complete
completed
complicated
complications

Complic, complic.
complications

complic.
complicating

compn.
composition

compr.
compressed
compression

comprn.
compression

compt.
competent

COMS
chronic organic mental syndrome

COMT, Comt
catechol-O-methyltransferase

COMTRAC
computer(-based case) tracing

COMUL test
complement fixation murine leukosis
test

CON
certificate of need

con.
contra (L. against)

ConA, Con A
concanavalin A (reagent)

CONC, conc.
concentrated
concentration

conc.
concentrate
concisus (L. cut, brief)
conclusion

concd.
concentrated

concentr.
concentrate
concentrated
concentration

CONCIS, concis.
concisus (L. cut; brief)

concn.
concentrate
concentration

cond.
condensed
condition(s)
conduction
conductivity
conductor

cond. milk
condensed milk

condn.
condition

cond. ref.
conditioned reflex

cond. resp.
conditioned response

conduct.
conductivity
conductor

CONELRAD
control of electromagnetic radiation

conf.
confectio (L. a confection)
conference
confined
confused

confus.
confused

CONG, cong.
congenital

cong.
congested
congius (L. gallon)
congress

congen.
congenital

congr.
congruent

coniz.
conization

conj.
conjunctiva

conjug.
conjugated
conjugation

CONPADRI
cyclophosphamide, Oncovin
   (vincristine), L-phenylalanine
   mustard, and Adriamycin
   (doxorubicin) (re: chemotherapy)

Cons, cons.
consult
consultant
consulting

cons.
conserva (L. keep, save)
consonans (L. sounding with [tinkling])
consonation
consultation

conserv.
conservative (re: treatment)

consol.
consolidation

consperg.
consperge (L. dust, sprinkle
   [imperative])
conspergere (L. to dust or sprinkle)
conspergitur (L. it is being sprinkled)

const.
constant

constit.
constituency
constituent
constitution
constitutional

consult.
consultant
consultation

CONT, cont.
continue

cont.
contain(ed)
containing
contents
continued
continuous
continuously
contra (L. against)
contusus (L. bruised)

contag.
contagion
contagious

cont'd
continued

conter.
contere (L. rub together)

contg.
containing

contin.
continue(d)
continuetur (L. let it be continued)
continuing

contr.
contract
contracted
contraction
contracture

contra.
contraction
contraindicated
contraindication

contralat.
contralateral

cont. rem.
continuentur remedia (L. let the
medicines be continued)

contrit.
contritus (L. broken; ground)

cont. Rx
continue medication

contus.
contusus (L. bruised)

CONV
conventional (rat)

conv.
convalescence
convalescent
conventional
convergence
convulsion

converg.
convergence

conv. strab.
convergent strabismus (re: Ophth)

COOD
chronic obstructive outflow disease

COOH
carboxyl group (characteristic of organic
acids)

coop.
cooperate
cooperation
cooperative

coor.
coordination

coor. AMR
coordination and alternate motion rate

CoOrd, coord.
coordination

COP
capillary osmotic pressure
change of plaster
circumoval precipitin
colloid(al) osmotic pressure
Cytoxan (cyclophosphamide), Oncovin
(vincristine sulfate), prednisone (re:
chemotherapy)

COPA
Cytoxan (cyclophosphamide), Oncovin
(vincristine sulfate), prednisone,
Adriamycin (doxorubicin) (re:
chemotherapy)

COPA-BLEO
cyclophosphamide (Cytoxan), Oncovin
(vincristine), prednisone, Adriamycin
(doxorubicin), and bleomycin (re:
chemotherapy)

COPAC
CCNU (lomustine), Oncovin
(vincristine), prednisone, Adriamycin
(doxorubicin), and cyclophosphamide
(Cytoxan) (re: chemotherapy)

COPB
cyclophosphamide, Oncovin,
prednisone, bleomycin (re:
chemotherapy)

COP-BLAM
cyclophosphamide, Oncovin,
prednisone, bleomycin, Adriamycin,
Matulane (procarbazine) (re:
chemotherapy)

COP-BLEO
cyclophosphamide (or chlorambucil),
Oncovin (vincristine), prednisone,
and bleomycin (re: chemotherapy)

COPD
chronic obstructive pulmonary disease

COPE
chronic obstructive pulmonary
emphysema
Coping Operations Preference Enquiry
(re: psychological testing)

COPP
CCNU, Oncovin, procarbazine,
prednisone (re: chemotherapy)
cyclophosphamide (Cytoxan), Oncovin
(vincristine), procarbazine,
prednisone (re: chemotherapy)

COPRO
coproporphyria
coproporphyrin

COPS
California Occupational Preference
System (also called COPSystem and
COPSystem Inventory—re:
psychological testing)

COQ, CoQ
coenzyme Q (ubiquinone)

coq.
coquatur (L. let it be boiled)
coque (L. boil)

coq. in s.a.
coque in sufficiente aqua (L. boil in
sufficient water)

coq. s.a.
coque secundum artem (L. boil
    properly)

coq. simul
coque simul (L. boil at the same time)

COR
cardiac output recorder
conditioned orientation reflex
corpus (L. body)
corrosive
cortisone
custodian of records

COR, Cor
coronary

CoR, Co R
Congo red

cor.
correct
corrected
correction
corrective

CORA
conditioned orientation reflex
    audiometry

corr.
corrected
correspond
correspondence
corresponding

corresp.
correspond
correspondence
corresponding

cort.
cortex (L. bark, rind)
cortical
cortisone

COS
clinically observed seizure

cos
cosine

cosec
cosecant

Cosm
clearance, osmolarity

cos sites
cohesive end sites (re: genetics)

COSTAR
Computer Stored Ambulatory Record
    (re: medical records)

COT
content of thought

continuous oxygen therapy
contralateral optic tectum
critical off-time

CO$_2$T
carbon dioxide therapy

cot
$C_ot_{1/2}$ (C_o = initial concentration , $t_{1/2}$ =
    re-annealing time [half-reaction time]
    in reassociation kinetics—re:
    molecular genetics)

cot.
cotangent (ctn)

cotan.
cotangent (ctn)

COTD
cardiac output by thermodilution

COTE, COTe
cathodal opening tetanus

c̄ out
without

COV
cross-over value (re: genetics)

CoVF
cobra venom factor

COWS
cold to the opposite, warm to the same
    (Hallpike caloric stimulation
    response—re: audiometry)

COWS of WASP
Commission on World Standards of the
    World Association of Societies of
    Pathology (re: lab values)

CP
capillary pressure
cardiac performance
cardiac pool
cardiopulmonary
cardiopulmonary performance
caudatus putamen (re: Neuro)
cell passage
cerebellopontine
cerebral palsy
ceruloplasmin
cervical probe
chest pain
child psychiatrist
Child Psychiatry
Child Psychology
chloropurine
chloroquine and primaquine
    (chloroquine-primaquine)
chronic pancreatitis
chronic pyelonephritis
cicatricial pemphigoid
circular polarization

cleft palate
Clinical Pathology
clonogenic proliferating (cells)
closing pressure
clottable protein
cochlear potential
code of practice
cold pressor
color perception
combination product
combining power
compensated base
compound
compressed (tablet)
congenital phosphoria
coproporphyria
coproporphyrin
coracoid process
cor pulmonale
cortical plate
Corynebacterium parvum
costal plaque
C peptide
creatine phosphate
cross-linked protein
crude protein
current practice
cyclophosphamide and prednisone (re: chemotherapy)
cystoscopy and pyelogram

CP, cp, cp.
compare

CP, cp.
candle power
chemically pure

C/P
cholesterol-phospholipid ratio

C&P
compensation and pension
complete and pain free (re: range of motion)
cystoscopy and panendoscopy
cystoscopy and pyelogram
cystoscopy and pyelography

Cp
chickenpox
peak concentration
phosphate clearance

C$_p$
constant pressure (re: molar heat capacity)

cP
chronic polyarthritis

cP, cp.
centipoise (1/100th of a poise—measure of dynamic viscosity)

c$_p$
constant pressure (re: specific heat capacity)
plasma drug concentration

CPA
cardiopulmonary arrest
carotid phonoangiography
cerebellopontine angle
chlorophenylalanine
chronic pyrophosphate arthropathy
circulating platelet aggregate
costophrenic angle
cyclophosphamide
cyproterone acetate

C3PA
complement 3 proactivator (convertase)

CPAB
Computer Programmer Aptitude Battery (re: psychological testing)

CPAF
chlorpropamide-alcohol flushing
chlorpropamide-primed alcohol (induced) flushing

CPAH, C$_{PAH}$, Cpah, C$_{pah}$
p-aminohippuric acid clearance

CPAI
central principal axis of inertia

CPAP
constant positive airway pressure
continuous positive airway pressure
continuous pulmonary artery pressure

c. parvum
cochleare parvum (L. [spoon shaped like a snail's shell] a teaspoonful)

CPB
cardiopulmonary bypass
competitive protein-binding

CPBA
competitive protein-binding analysis
competitive protein-binding assay

CPBV
cardiopulmonary blood volume

CPC
capillary packed column
central posterior curve (re: corneal optics)
cerebellar Purkinje cell
Cerebral Palsy Clinic
cetylpyridinium chloride
chronic passive congestion
circumferential pneumatic compression
clinicopathologic conference
committed progenitor cell

CPCL
congenital pulmonary cystic lymphangiectasis

CPCN
capitated primary care network

CPCP
chronic progressive coccidioidal pneumonitis

CPCR
cardiopulmonary cerebral resuscitation

CPCS
clinical pharmacokinetics consulting service

CPD
calcium pyrophosphate deposition
cephalopelvic disproportion
childhood polycystic disease
chorioretinopathy and pituitary dysfunction (syndrome)
chronic peritoneal dialysis
citrate-phosphate-dextrose
congenital polycystic disease
contact potential difference
contagious pustular dermatitis
critical point drying
cyclopentadiene (manufacturing chemical)

CPD, cpd.
compound

CPDA
citrate-phosphate-dextrose-adenine (anticoagulant preservative)

CPDA-1
citrate-phosphate-dextrose-adenine (anticoagulant preservative)

CPD-adenine
citrate-phosphate-dextrose-adenine (anticoagulant preservative)

CPDD
cis-platinum diamminedichloride (*cis*-platinum; Platinol; *cis*-diamminedichloroplatinum —re: chemotherapy)

Cpd E
compound E (cortisone)

Cpd F
compound F (hydrocortisone)

CPDL
cumulative population-doubling level

cpds
compounds

CPE
cardiogenic pulmonary edema

chronic pulmonary emphysema
compensation, pension, and education
complete physical examination
complex partial epilepsy
cytopathic effect (re: distinct virus replication in cell culture)
cytopathogenic effect(s)
cytopathological effect(s)

CPEO
chronic progressive external ophthalmoplegia

CPF
clot-promoting factor

CPFA
contact product-forming activity

CPFV
cucumber pale fruit viroid

CPG
capillary blood gases
complex pregnanediol

CPGN
chronic proliferative glomerulonephritis

CPH
chronic persistent hepatitis

CPH 5
Cutter protein hydrolysate, 5% (in water)

CPHA
Commission on Professional Hospital Activities

CPI
California Psychological Inventory
Cancer Potential Index (re: environmental monitoring)
characters per inch (re: computers/data processing)
congenital palatopharyngeal incompetence
constitutional psychopathia inferior
constitutional psychopathic inferiority
coronary prognostic index

CPIB
ethyl *p*-chlorophenoxyisobutyrate (clofibrate—antihyper-lipoproteinemic)

CPIP
chronic pulmonary insufficiency of prematurity

CPK
creatine phosphokinase

CPK-MB
MB isoenzyme of creatine phosphokinase (CK-MB)

CPL
caprine placental lactogen
conditioned pitch level (re: Audio)
congenital pulmonary lymphangiectasis

C/PL
cholesterol to phospholipid (ratio)

cpl.
complete

CPLM
cysteine-peptone-liver (infusion) media

CPM
cards per minute (re: data processing)
CCNU, procarbazine, methotrexate (re:
    chemotherapy)
central pontine myelinolysis (re: Neuro)
chlorpheniramine maleate
    (antihistaminic)
cognitive-perceptual-motor (re: Neuro)
Colored Progressive Matrices
continuous passive motion
critical path method (re: management
    scheduling method; PERT; network
    analysis)

CPM, cpm, c.p.m.
counts per minute

cpm
cycles per minute

CPMI
central principal moments of inertia

CPMP
computer-patient management
    problems

CPMS
chronic progressive multiple sclerosis

CPMV
cowpea mosaic virus

CPN
chronic polyneuropathy
chronic pyelonephritis

CPNM
corrected perinatal mortality (re:
    statistics)

CPOB
cyclophosphamide, prednisone,
    Oncovin, bleomycin (re:
    chemotherapy)

C₃ pop.
population of imperfectly developed
    persons (physically or mentally)

CPP
canine pancreatic polypeptide
Career Planning Program (re:
    psychological testing)

cerebral perfusion pressure
Conditioned Place Preference (re:
    Psychol)
1,2-cyclopentenophenanthrene

CPPB
constant positive-pressure breathing
continuous positive-pressure breathing

CPPD
calcium pyrophosphate dihydrate

CPPV
continuous positive-pressure ventilation

CPQ
Children's Personality Questionnaire

CPR
cardiac pulmonary reserve
cardiopulmonary reserve
cardiopulmonary resuscitation
centripetal rub
cerebral cortex perfusion rate
chlorophenyl red
cortisol production rate
cumulative patency rate
customary, prevailing, and reasonable

CPRAM
controlled partial rebreathing
    anesthesia method

C/P ratio
cholesterol-phospholipid ratio

CPRS
Children's Psychiatric Rating Scale
Comprehensive Psychiatric Rating
    Scale

CPS
carbamyl phosphate synthetase
cardioplegic perfusion solution
characters per second (re: computers/
    data processing)
Child Personality Scale
Children's Protective Service
chloroquine, pyrimethamine,
    sulfisoxazole (re: malaria)
clinical performance score
clinical pharmacokinetic service
coagulase-positive staphylococci
columns per second (re: computers)
Comrey Personality Scales
constitutional psychopathic state
contagious pustular stomatitis
C-polysaccharide
cumulative probability of success (re:
    statistics)

CPS, cps, c.p.s.
cycles per second

cps
counts per second

CPSCS
California Preschool Social
   Competency Scale (re: psychological
   testing)

CPS-I
carbamyl phosphate synthetase

CPSI
Children's Perception of Support
   Inventory (re: Psychol)

CPT
carotid pulse tracing
chest physiotherapy
ciliary particle transport activity
clinical pharmacokinetics team
cold pressor test
cold pressure test
combining power test
concentration performance test
continuous performance task
continuous performance test
Cooperative Primary Tests (re:
   psychological testing)
Current Procedural Terminology

C & P trx.
cervical and pelvic traction

CPTX
chronic parathyroidectomy

CPU
caudate putamen (re: Neuro)
central processing unit (re: electronic
   data processing)

CPUE
chest pain of unknown etiology

CPV
canine parovirus (re: veterinary
   medicine)
cytoplasmic polyhidrosis virus

CPX, C Px
complete physical examination

CPZ
chlorpromazine

CQ
chloroquine (antimalarial; anti-emetic;
   lupus erythematosus suppressant)
chloroquinine-quinine (antimalarial)
circadian quotient
conceptual quotient

CQE
Comprehensive Qualifying Examination

C1q (radioassay)
a subunit of the complement (protein
   C1) system

CR
Cacchi-Ricci (syndrome)

calculation rate
calculus removed
calorie restricted
cardiac rehabilitation
cardiac resuscitation
cathode ray
centric relation
cephalothin
chest and right arm (re: EKG leads)
chest roentgenogram
chick rectum
chief resident
child resistant
choice reaction
chronic rejection
clinical record(s)
clinical research
closed reduction
clot retraction
coefficient (of fat) retention
colonization resistance
colon resection
colorectal
complement receptor
complete remission
complete responders
complete response
conditioned reflex
conditioned response
Congo red
continuous reinforcement
controlled respiration (re: anesthesia)
conversion rate
cooling rate
corona radiata (re: Neuro)
correct response
corticoid resistant
cortisone resistant
cremaster reflex
cresyl red (an indicator)
critical ratio
cytidine

CR, C-R
cardiorespiratory

CR, C-R, Cr
crown-rump (measurement of embryo
   or fetus)

CR, Cr, cr.
creatinine

Cr
chromium (element)
crown

Cr, cr.
cranial

Cr$_I$, Cr$_{II}$, etc.
first cranial nerve, second cranial nerve,
   etc.

51Cr
radioactive isotope of chromium

cr.
cras (L. tomorrow)
creatine

CRA
central retinal artery
Chinese restaurant asthma
chronic rheumatoid arthritis

CRABP
cellular retinoic acid-binding protein

CRAM
card random-access memory (re:
    computers)

CRAN
chief resident's admitting note

cran.
cranial

crani.
craniotomy

CRAO
central retinal artery occlusion

crast.
crastinus (L. for tomorrow)

CRB
chemical, radiological, and biological
    (warfare)

CRBBB
complete right bundle branch block

CRBC
chicken red blood cell

CRBP
cellular retinol-binding protein

Cr&Br
crown and bridge (re: Dent)

CRC
calomel, rhubarb, colocynth (cathartic)
cardiovascular reflex conditioning
clinical research center
concentrated red (blood) cell
cross-reacting cannabinoids

CR & C
closed reduction and cast

CrCl, Cr$_{cl}$
creatinine clearance

CRCS
cardiovascular reflex conditioning
    system

CRD
childhood rheumatic disease
child restraint device
chorioretinal degeneration
chronic renal disease

chronic respiratory disease
complete reaction of degeneration

CRE
cumulative radiation effect

creat.
creatine
creatinine

C region
carboxyl-terminal region of an Ig chain

crem.
cremasteric

cremas.
cremasteric

crep.
crepitant
crepitation
crepitus

CREST
calcinosis, Raynaud's (phenomenon),
    esophageal (dysfunction),
    sclerodactyly, telangiectasia

CRF
case report form
chronic renal failure
chronic respiratory failure
coagulase-reacting factor
continuous reinforcement
corticotrop(h)in-regulating factor
corticotrop(h)in-release factor
corticotrop(h)in-releasing factor

CRH
corticotrop(h)in (ACTH)-releasing
    hormone

CRHV
cottontail rabbit herpes virus

CRI
Cardiac Risk Index
Caring Relationship Inventory (re:
    psychological testing)
chemical rust-inhibiting (germicide)
chronic renal insufficiency
chronic respiratory insufficiency
cold running intelligibility (re: Audio)
Composite Risk Index
concentrated rust inhibitor
cross-reactive idiotype (re: genetics)

Crit, crit.
hematocrit

crit.
critical

crit. press.
critical pressure

crit. temp.
critical temperature

CRL
complement receptor location
complement receptor lymphocyte
crown-rump length (re: neonate)

CR lead
chest lead, right arm (electrode)

CRM
Certified Reference Materials (re:
    material issued by organizations such
    as National Bureau of Standards)
contralateral remote masking
counting rate meter (re: radiation
    detection)
cross-reacting material
crown-rump measurement (re: neonate)

CRM+
cross-reacting material positive (re:
    blood clotting)

CRM−
cross-reacting material negative (re:
    blood clotting)

Crm
cream

CRN
complement-requiring neutralizing
    (antibody)

cRNA
chromosomal RNA

CRNF
chronic rheumatoid nodular fibrositis

Cr nn
cranial nerves

cr. ns
cranial nerves

CRO
cathode ray oscillograph
cathode ray oscilloscope
centric relation occlusion

CROM
cervical range of motion

CROP
cyclophosphamide, Rubidazone,
    Oncovin (vincristine), and prednisone
    (re: chemotherapy)

CROS
contralateral routing of signal(s)

CRP
chronic relapsing pancreatitis
confluent, reticulate papillomatosis
corneoretinal potential
coronary rehabilitation program
C-reactive protein
cross-reacting protein (re: genetics)

CrP, Cr P
creatine phosphate (phosphocreatine)

CRPA
C-reactive protein antiserum

CRPF
contralateral renal plasma flow

CRS
Chinese restaurant syndrome
    (monosodium glutamate sensitivity)
colon and rectal surgery
colorectal surgery
compliance of the respiratory system
congenital rubella syndrome

CRSM
cherry red spot myoclonus (syndrome)

CRSP
comprehensive renal scintillation
    procedure

Cr Sp
craniospinal

CRST
calcinosis cutis, Raynaud's
    (phenomenon), scleroderma,
    telangiectasis (syndrome)

CRT
cardiac resuscitation team
cathode ray tube
chromium release test
complex reaction time
corrected retention time (re: column
    chromatography)
cortisone-resistant thymocyte

crt.
hematocrit

CRU
cardiac rehabilitation unit
Clinical Research Unit

CRV
central retinal vein

cr. vesp.
cras vespere (L. tomorrow evening)

CRVF
congestive right ventricular failure

CRVO
central retinal vein occlusion

CRVS
California Relative Value Studies

cryo.
cryoprecipitate
cryotherapy

crys.
crystal
crystalline

cryst.
crystal
crystalline
crystallization
crystallized

crystn.
crystallization

CS
calf serum
carcinoid syndrome
cardiogenic shock
carotid sheath
carotid sinus
cat scratch
celiac sprue
Central Service
Central Supply
cerebrospinal
cerebrospinal (fluid)
cervical spine
chemical sympathectomy
chest strap
chief of staff
chondroitin sulfate
chorionic somatomammotropin
Christian Scientist
chronic schizophrenia
cigarette smoker
cigarette smoke (solution)
citrate synthase, (mitochondrial—re:
    cytogenetics)
clinical stage
clinical state
Cockayne's syndrome
Collet-Sicard (syndrome)
completed stroke
completed suicide
concentration strength (solution)
conditioned stimulus
congenital syphilis
conjunctival secretions
contact sensitivity
continue same
continuing smoker
continuous stripping
control serum
convalescent status
coronary sclerosis
coronary sinus
corpus striatum (L. the striate body—re:
    Neuro)
cortical spoking (a type of cataract
    formation)
corticoid sensitive
corticosteroids

cover screen
current smoker
current strength
Curschmann-Steinert (syndrome)
Cushing's syndrome
cycloserine
β,β-dicyano-o-chlorostyrene (riot
    control agent)

CS, C.S., C/S, c/s
cesarean section

CS, Cs
standard of clearance (re: urea
    clearance test)

CS, Cs, cs.
conscious
consciousness

C/S, c/s
culture and sensitivity
cycles per second

C&S
calvarium and scalp
conjunctiva(e) and sclera(e)
cough and sneeze

C&S, C + S
culture and sensitivity

Cs
cell surface (antigen)
cesium (element)

Cs, cs.
case(s)

^{131}Cs
radioactive isotope of cesium

^{132}Cs
radioactive isotope of cesium

^{134}Cs
radioactive isotope of cesium

^{137}Cs
radioactive isotope of cesium

C1s
a subunit of first protein to react in
    complement system

cS
centistoke (measurement of kinematic
    viscosity)

cs
chromosome (re: cytogenetics)

CSA
canavaninosuccinic acid
carbonylsalicylamide (carsalam—
    analgesic)
cell surface antigen
chondroitin sulfate-A

Cognitive Skills Assessment (Battery—
re: psychological testing)
colony-stimulating activity
compressed spectral array
cross-sectional area

CSA, CsA
cyclosporin A

CSAVP
cerebral subarachnoid venous pressure

CSB
chemistry screening battery
Cheyne-Stokes breathing
contaminated small bowel

CSB I & II
Chemistry Screening Batteries I and II

csb
chromosome break (re: cytogenetics)

CSBF
coronary sinus blood flow

CSC
cigarette smoke condensate
collagen sponge contraceptive
corneae, sclerae, and conjunctivae
corticostriatocerebellar
cryogenic storage container

CSC, c.s.c
coup sur coup (Fr. blow upon blow—in
small doses at short intervals)

csc
cosecant

CSCS
Children's Self-Concept Scale

CSD
carotid sinus denervation
cat-scratch disease
combined system disease
conditionally streptomycin dependent
cortically spreading depression
craniospinal defect
critical stimulus duration

CSE
cross-sectional echocardiography

C/sec.
cesarean section
cycles per second

CSECT
control section (re: computers)

C sect.
cesarean section

C. section, C-section
cesarean section

C/S effect
cough/sneeze effect

CSER
cortical somatosensory evoked
response

CSF
cerebrospinal fluid (liquor
cerebrospinalis)
circumferential shortening fraction
colony-stimulating factor
coronary sinus flow

CSFP
cerebrospinal fluid pressure

CSF-WR
cerebrospinal fluid Wassermann
reaction

csg
chromosome gap (re: cytogenetics)

CSGBM
collagenase solubilized glomerular
basement membrane

CSH
chronic subdural hematoma
cortical stromal hyperplasia

CSHEP
constriction, sclerosis, hemorrhage,
exudate, papilledema (re: Ophth)

CSI
calculus surface index
cancer serum index
cavernous sinus infiltration
cholesterol saturation index

CSICU
Cardiac Surgical Intensive Care Unit

CSII
continuous subcutaneous insulin
infusion

CSIIP
continuous subcutaneous insulin
infusion pump

CSIS
clinical supplies and inventory system

CSL
cardiolipin synthetic lecithin
corn-steep liquor

CSLU
chronic stasis leg ulcer

CSM
carotid sinus massage (re: Cardio)
cerebrospinal meningitis
circulation, sensation, motion

color, sensation, motion
corn-soy milk

CSMG
cystosphincterometrogram

CSMP
chloramphenicol-sensitive microsomal
    protein
continuous systems modeling program
    (re: computers)

CSMT
chorionic somatomammotropin

CSM test
convexity-symmetry, maximum test

CSN
cardiac sympathetic nerve
carotid sinus nerve

CSNB
congenital stationary night blindness

CSNRT
corrected sinus node recovery time

CSNS
carotid sinus nerve stimulation
carotid sinus nerve stimulator

CSO
common source outbreak

CSOM
chronic serous otitis media
chronic suppurative otitis media

CSP
carotid sinus pressure
cell surface protein
cerebrospinal pressure
chemistry screening panel
Cooperative Statistical Program
    (re: IUD data)
criminal sexual psychopath

CS-P
chondroitin sulfate-protein

C sp.
cervical spine

C-spine
cervical spine

CSQ
College Student Questionnaires (re:
    psychological testing)

CSR
Central Supply Room
Cheyne-Stokes respirations
continued stay review
corrected sedimentation rate
corrected survival rate (re: statistics)

cortical secretion rate (re: adrenal
    glands)
cortisol secretion rate
cumulative survival rate (re: statistics)

c-src
cellular gene (present in various
    vertebrates) which hydridizes with the
    oncogene of the Rous sarcoma virus

CSRT
corrected sinus node recovery time (re:
    Cardio)

CSS
Cancer Surveillance System (re:
    medical records)
carotid sinus stimulation
Central Sterile Supply
chewing, sucking, swallowing
chronic subclinical scurvy
cranial sector scan

CSSD
Central Sterile Supply Department

CSSQ
College Student Satisfaction
    Questionnaire (re: psychological
    testing)

CST
cavernous sinus thrombosis
central sharp transients (re: Cardio)
Christ-Siemens-Touraine (syndrome)
compliance, static
computer scatter tomography
Conceptual Systems Test
contraction stress test (re: GYN)
convulsive shock therapy

cSt
centistoke (SI centimeter-gram-second
    measurement— Sir George Stokes)

Cstat
static lung compliance

CSU
casualty staging unit
catheter specimen of urine
Central Statistical Unit (re: VDRL, etc.)

CSV
chick syncytial virus
chrysanthemum stunt viroid

CSW
current sleepwalker

CT
calcitonin
calf testis
cardiothoracic (ratio)
carotid tracing
carpal tunnel
catastrophe theory

cellular therapy
center thickness
cerebral thrombosis
cerebral tumor
cervical traction
chemotaxis
chemotherapy
chest tube
chlorothiazide
cholera toxin
cholesterol total
chordae tendineae (re: Cardio)
chronic thyroiditis
chymotrypsin
circulating time
circulation time
classic technique
clear tones
closed thoracotomy
clotting time
coagulation time
coated tablet
cobra toxin
cognitive therapy
coil test
collecting tubule
colon, transverse
combined tumor
compressed tablet
computed tomography
computer (-assisted) tomography
computerized tomography
computer tomography
connective tissue
continue(d) treatment
continuous-flow tub (re: physiotherapy)
contraceptive techniques
contraction time
controlled temperature
Coombs' test
corneal transplant
coronary thrombosis
corrected transposition
corrective therapy
cortical thickness
cough threshold
Courvoisier-Terrier (syndrome)
cover test (re: Ophth)
crest time
crutch training
cystine-tellurite (medium)
cytolytic thymus (derived lymphocyte)
cytotoxic therapy
total content (carbon dioxide)

CT, C-T
cervicothoracic area
cervicothoracic syndrome

C/T
compression-to-traction (ratio)
crossmatch-to-transfusion (ratio)

C & T
color and temperature

C$_{T-1824}$
clearance of Evans blue or T-1824

Ct.
Ctenocephalides (a genus of fleas)

ct
chromatid (re: cytogenetics)

ct.
count

CTA
chemotactic activity
chromotropic acid (a reagent)
cyproterone acetate (anti-androgen)
cystine trypticase agar
cytoplasmic tubular aggregates
cytotoxic assay
(lympho)cytotoxic assay

CTa, Cta, cta.
catamenia (L. according to the month—
    [menstruation])

CTAB, C.T.A.B.
cetyltrimethylammonium bromide
    (cetrimonium bromide— topical
    antiseptic)

CTAL
cortical thick ascending limb

c. tant.
cum tanto (L. with the same amount
    [of])

CTAP
connective tissue-activating peptides

CTAT
computerized transaxial tomography
    (former term for CT—computed
    tomography)

CTB
ceased to breathe

ctb
chromatid break (re: cytogenetics)

CTBS
Canadian Tests of Basic Skills (re:
    psychological testing)

CTC
chlortetracycline (chlorotetracycline—
    re: antibacterial; antiprotozoal)
clinical trial certificate
concentration to control
Creativity Tests for Children (re:
    psychological testing)
cultured T cell

CTCL
cutaneous T-cell lymphoma

ctCO₂
concentration of total carbon dioxide

CTD
carpal tunnel decompression
circulation time, descending
congenital thymic dysplasia
connective tissue disease

CT & DB
cough, turn, and deep breathe

CTE
calf thymus extract
cultured thymic epithelium

CTEM
conventional transmission electron
 microscope

C-terminal
carboxyl terminal

CTF
certificate
Colorado tick fever
cytotoxic factor

CTG
cardiotocogram (re: the record of
 monitored fetal heartbeat during
 labor)
cardiotocography (re: the monitoring of
 the fetal heartbeat during labor)

CT/G
cholesterol/triglyceride ratio

ctg
chromatid gap (re: cytogenetics)

CTGA
complete transposition of the great
 arteries

CTH
ceramide trihexoside (re: glycolipid
 lipidosis)

CTL
cytotoxic thymus (-dependent)
 lymphocyte

C-T-L
cervical, thoracic, lumbar

CTLL
cytotoxic T (thymus-dependent)
 lymphocyte line

CTLSO
cervicothoracolumbosacral orthosis

CTM
cardiotachometer
connective tissue massage (re:
 physiatry)

continuous tone masking
cricothyroid muscle

CTMM
computed tomographic metrizamide
 myelography

CTMM-SF
California Short-Form Test of Mental
 Maturity

CTN
computed tomography number
continuous noise (condition)

ctn
cotangent

C & T N, BLE
color and temperature normal, both
 lower extremities

CTP
California Test of Personality
cytidine triphosphate (cytidine 5'-
 triphosphate)

CTP-³H
cytidine triphosphate, tritium-labeled

C-TPN
cyclic total parenteral nutrition

CTPP
cerebral tissue perfusion pressure

CTPV
coal tar pitch volatiles

CTPVO
chronic thrombotic pulmonary vascular
 obstruction

CTR
cardiothoracic ratio
carpal tunnel release
central tumor registry
computerized tumor registry

ctr.
center

CT ratio
cardiothoracic ratio

C trx.
cervical traction

CTS
carpal tunnel syndrome
Clinical Teaching Support
composite treatment score
computerized topographic scanner
contralateral threshold shift
corticosteroid

CT scan
computerized axial tomography scan

121

CTT
central tegmental tract
compressed tablet triturate
computed transaxial tomography (now
    called computed tomography)
computerized transaxial tomogram
critical tracking task

CTTT
carotid-thyroid transit time

CTU
Cardiac/Thoracic Unit
centigrade thermal unit
constitutive transcription unit

CTV
cervical and thoracic vertebrae

CTW
central terminal of Wilson
combined testicular weight

CTX
cefotaxime (antibacterial)
cerebrotendinous xanthomatosis
chemotaxis
chemotoxins

CTX, Ctx
cyclophosphamide (Cytoxan)

CTx
cardiac transplantation

Ctx-Plat
cyclophosphamide, Platinol (re:
    chemotherapy)

CTZ
ceftezole (antibacterial)
chemoreceptor trigger zone (vomiting
    area in medulla)
chlorothiazide

CT zone
chemoreceptor trigger zone (vomiting
    area in medulla)

CU
cardiac unit
casein unit
cause unknown
chymotrypsin unit
clinical unit
color unit
contact urticaria
Convalescent Unit

Cu
cuprum (L. copper—[an element])

C_u
urea clearance

^{61}**Cu**
radioactive copper

^{64}**Cu**
radioactive copper

^{67}**Cu**
radioactive copper

cu, cu.
cubic

cUA $^-$
concentration of undetermined ions

CuB
copper band (re: Dent)

CUC
chronic ulcerative colitis

cu cm
cubic centimeter

CUD
cause undetermined
congenital urinary tract deformities

CUE
cumulative urinary excretion

CUES
College and University Environment
    Scales (re: psychological testing)

cu ft
cubic foot

CUG
cystidine-uridine-guanidine
cystourethrogram

CuHVL
copper half-value layer

cu in
cubic inch

cuj.
cujus (L. of which, of any)

cuj. lib.
cujus libet (L. of any you please; of
    whatever you please)

cult.
culture (re: bacteriology)

cum.
cumulative (report)

cu m
cubic meter

cu mm
cubic millimeter

cu μ**m**
cubic micrometer

CuO
cupric oxide

CUPS
carcinoma of unknown primary site

CUR
cystourethrorectocele

cur.
curative
current

curat.
curatio (L. a taking care of [a dressing])

CUS
catheterized urine specimen

CuSCN
cuprous thiocyanate

CU spec.
catheterized urine specimen

cu yd
cubic yard

CV
cardiac volume
cardiovascular
cell volume
central venous
cerebrovascular
cervical vertebrae
closing volume
coefficient of variation
color vision
concentrated volume (solution)
conducting veins
conduction velocity
conjugata vera (L. true conjugate
    [diameter of pelvic inlet])
consonant vowel
contrast ventriculography
conventional ventilation
conversational voice
corpuscular volume
costovertebral
coxsackievirus
cresyl violet
crystal violet
cutaneous vasculitis

CV, c.v.
cras vespere (L. tomorrow evening)

C/V
coulomb per volt

Cv
specific heat at constant volume

C$_v$
constant volume (re: molar heat
    capacity)

c$_v$
constant volume (re: specific heat
    capacity)

CVA
cerebrovascular accident (nonspecific
    term for thrombosis, hemorrhage, or
    embolism of cerebral blood supply)
cervicovaginal antibody
chronic villous arthritis
cyclophosphamide, vincristine,
    Adriamycin (re: chemotherapy)

CVA, cva
costovertebral angle

CVA-BMP, CVA + BMP
cyclophosphamide (Cytoxan),
    vincristine, Adriamycin (doxorubicin),
    BCNU (carmustine), methotrexate,
    and procarbazine (re: chemotherapy)

CVAH
congenital virilizing adrenal hyperplasia

CVAT, CVA T
costovertebral angle tenderness

CVA tend.
costovertebral angle tenderness

CVB
CCNU, vinblastine, bleomycin (re:
    chemotherapy)

CVC
central venous catheter
crying vital capacity

CV cath.
central venous catheter

CVCT
cardiovascular computed tomography

CVD
cardiovascular disease
cerebrovascular disease
collagen vascular disease
color vision deviant

CVD, cvd.
curved

CVF
cardiovascular failure
central visual field (re: Ophth)
cervicovaginal fluid
cobra venom factor

CVG
contrast ventriculography
coronary vein graft

CVH
cervicovaginal hood
combined ventricular hypertrophy
common variable
    hypogammaglobulinemia

CVHD
chronic valvular heart disease

CVI
cardiovascular incident
cerebrovascular insufficiency
chronic venous insufficiency
common variable immunodeficiency

CVID
common variable immunodeficiency

C virus(es), C-virus(es)
coxsackievirus(es)

CVL
clinical vascular laboratory

CVM
cardiovascular monitor
cyclophosphamide, vincristine,
    methotrexate (re: chemotherapy)

CVO
central vein occlusion
central venous oxygen
circumventricular organs
conjugata vera obstetrica (L. true
    obstetric conjugate [diameter of
    pelvic inlet])

CVO$_2$
mixed venous oxygen content

CVOD
cerebrovascular obstructive disease

CVP
cardioventricular pacing
cell volume profile
central venous pressure
chlorfenvinphos (insecticide; acaricide)
citrus vitamin P (vitamin P complex, a
    bioflavonoid)
Cytoxan (cyclophosphamide),
    vincristine, prednisone (re:
    chemotherapy)

CVP lab.
cardiovascular-pulmonary laboratory

CVPP
CCNU (lomustine), vinblastine,
    prednisone, and procarbazine (re:
    chemotherapy)
cyclophosphamide, Velban,
    procarbazine, prednisone (re:
    chemotherapy)

CVPP-CCNU
cyclophosphamide, vinblastine,
    procarbazine, prednisone, CCNU (re:
    chemotherapy)

CVR
cardiovascular-renal
cardiovascular resistance
cardiovascular-respiratory (system)
cardiovascular review

cephalic vasomotor response
cerebrovascular resistance

CVRD
cardiovascular renal disease

CVRR
cardiovascular recovery room

CVS
cardiovascular surgery
cardiovascular system
challenge virus strain
chorionic villi sampling
clean-voided specimen
current vital signs

CVSF
conduction velocity of slower fibers

CV status
cardiovascular status

CVS virus
challenge virus standard

CVTR
charcoal vital transport medium

CW
cardiac work
casework
Cavaré-Westphal (syndrome)
cell wall
chemical warfare
chemical weapon
chest wall
children's ward
Christian-Weber (syndrome)
cotton wool
crutch-walking

CW, cw
continuous wave

CW, cw.
clockwise

C/W
compare with
consistent with

c wave
a component in electroretinogram (re:
    Ophth)
a jugular venous pulse wave

CWB
Charcot-Weiss-Baker (syndrome)

CWBTS
capillary whole blood true sugar

CWD
cell wall defective
cell wall deficient

CWDF
cell wall-deficient (bacterial) forms

CWF
Cornell Word Form (re: Psychol)

CWHB
citrated whole human blood

CWI
cardiac work index

CWL
cutaneous water loss

CWOP
childbirth without pain

CWP
childbirth without pain
coal worker's pneumonoconiosis
(anthracosis)

CWS
cell wall skeleton
cold-water soluble
comfortable walking speed

CWT
cold water treatment

cwt
cent (L. centum [+ weight—
hundredweight])

CX
cerebral cortex
chest x-ray
cloxacillin
critical experiment

CX, Cx, cx.
cervix
convex

Cx
cervical
circumflex (coronary artery)
clearance
complex

cx
cylinder axis

CXR
chest x-ray film

CY
calendar year

CY, Cy, cy.
cyanogen

CY, cy.
copy

Cy
cyst
cytarabine

cy.
cyanosis
cyanotic

CYA, CyA
cyclosporin A (cyclosporine,
ciclosporin—re: immunosuppressive)

CyADIC
cyclophosphamide, Adriamycin
(doxorubicin), and DIC (dacarbazine)
(re: chemotherapy)

cyan.
cyanosis
cyanotic

cyath.
cyathus (L. ladle for removing wine from
the bowl [wineglass])

cyath. vin.
cyathus vinarius (L. a wineglass)

cyath. vinos.
cyathus vinosus (L. wineglass)

CYC
cyclophosphamide (Cytoxan)

CYC, cyc.
cyclotron

cyc.
cyclazocine (an analgesic)
cycle

CYCLO, Cyclo
cyclophosphamide

CYCLO, Cyclo, cyclo.
cyclopropane

CYD
cytidine (re: ribonucleosides)

CYE
charcoal yeast extract

CYL
casein yeast lactate (medium)

cyl.
cylinder (cast—re: Ortho)
cylindrical lens

CYN
cyanide
cynarin(e) (choleretic)

CYNAP
cytotoxicity negative, absorption
positive
cytotoxic-negative absorption-positive
(reaction)

CYP
cyanofenphos (insecticide)

CYS
cystoscopy

CYS, Cys
cysteine

Cys
|
Cys, Cys-Cys, Cys-cys
cystine

Cyst-Cys, Cyst-cys
cysteine

|
Cys
half-cystine (or its mono- or di-radical)

Cysto, cysto.
cystoscopic (examination)
cystoscopy

cysto.
cystogram
cystoscope

CYT
cytochrome

Cyt
cytoplasm
cytosine

cytohet
cytoplasmically heterozygous (re: genetics)

cytol.
cytological
cytology

cyt. sys.
cytochrome system

CY-VA-DACT
cyclophosphamide, vincristine, Adriamycin (doxorubicin), and dactinomycin (re: chemotherapy)

CYVADIC, CY-VA-DIC, CyVADIC
Cytoxan (cyclophosphamide), vincristine, Adriamycin, and dimethyl imidazole carboxamide (DTIC = dimethyl triazene imidazole carboxamide; DIC) (re: chemotherapy)

CYVMAD
cyclophosphamide, vincristine, methotrexate, Adriamycin, DTIC (dimethyl triazene imidazole carboxamide; DIC) (re: chemotherapy)

CZ
carzinophilin (antineoplastic)
cefazolin

CZI
crystalline zinc insulin

D

D
absorbed dose
aspartic acid (D form)
dead air space
dead space (when written as a subscript)
dead space gas (secondary symbol)
death
debye (unit of electric dipole moment)
decimal reduction time (re: heat sterilization)
demal (1 gram equivalent of solute per cubic decimeter)
dermatologist
dermatology
Dermatophagoides (genus)
detail response
developed
deviation
Devonian (geologic time division—Paleozoic era)
dextrose
diagnosis
diastole
diathermy
didymium (element—now called praseodymium)
Dientamoeba (genus)
difference
diffuse
diffusing capacity (in general—primary symbol)
diffusion coefficient
diffusion constant
dihydrouridine (re: nucleic acids)
dinner
dioptry
Diphyllobothrium (genus)
Diplococcus (genus)
diplomate
disease
dispense
displacement, electric
divergent production (operation—re: Psychol; Aptitudes Research Project testing within structure of intellect model)
diverticulum
dog (re: veterinary medicine)
dominant
donor
down
Dracunculus (genus—nematode parasite)

drive
drive state
Drosophila (genus—fruit fly)
drug
dual
ductus
duodenum
duration (re: electrodiagnosis)
dwarf
mean dose
vitamin D potency of cod liver oil
vitamin D unit

D, d
date
daughter
day
deceased
degree
dentur (L. let [such] be given)
dextro-
dextrorotatory
divorced
doubtful

D, d, *d*
deuteron (nucleus of deuterium [^{2}H]; heavy hydrogen)

D, d.
da (L. give)
dead
deciduous
density
detur (L. let it be given)
dexter (L. right)
diameter
died
diopter
distal
dorsal (re: vertebral formulae)
dosis (L. dose)
duration

D –
designates configuration of a stereoisomer by comparing its structure with the standard, D-glyceraldehyde

$\overline{\text{D}}$
mean dose

D$_1$
inulin dialysance

D₁, D₂
dorsal nerves 1, 2
dorsal vertebrae 1, 2

D/3
distal third

1-D, 2-D, 3-D
one-dimensional, two-dimensional,
    three-dimensional

2D
second-degree (erythemal) dose

2,4-D
(2,4-dichlorophenoxy)acetic acid (an
    herbicide)

3D
third-degree (erythemal) dose

d
atomic orbital with angular momentum
    quantum number 2 (re: physics/
    chemistry)
the dalton unit (occasionally used for
    atomic mass unit)
days (diurnal)
deci- (prefix)
diarrhea
dies (L. day)
distance, cm^2 (re: nuclear medicine)
diurnal
doctor
ductus
dyne
focal-film distance (re: Radio)
rare-detail response
specific gravity (d_4^{19} specific gravity at
    19° referred to water at 4°)

δ
delta (fourth letter of Greek alphabet)
double bond

d-
dextro (chemical abbreviation for right
    or clockwise— i.e., dextrorotatory)

-d
deutrium-containing compound

/d
daily
per day

1/d
once a day

2/d
twice a day

DA
dark adaptation (re: Ophth)
daunomycin and ara-C (cytarabine) (re:
    chemotherapy)
degenerative arthritis

delayed action (re: drugs)
deoxyadenosine
differential analyzer
differentiation antigen
diphenylchlorarsine (a war gas)
direct agglutination
disability assistance
disaggregated
dopaminergic
drug addict
ductus arteriosus

DA, D.A.
developmental age

DA, Da
dopamine (decarboxylated dopa)

D-A
donor-acceptor

D/A
date of accident
date of admission
digital-to-analog (ratio)
discharge and advise

Da, da.
daughter

(dA)₃₀₀₀
homopolymer chain containing 3000
    deoxyriboadenylate residues (re:
    genetics)

da.
day
deca- (prefix designating 10)

DAA
data access arrangement (re:
    computers/data processing)
dihydroxyaluminum aminoacetate
    (antacid)

2,4-DAA
2,4-diaminoanisole (also called 4-
    methoxy-*m*-phenylenediamine or 4
    MMPD—re: hair dyes)

DAAO
D-amino acid oxidase

DAB
days after birth
p-dimethylaminoazobenzene (test—C.I.
    Solvent Yellow 2)
dysrhythmic aggressive behavior

DAC
digital-to-analog converter (re:
    computers)

DACA
dissecting aneurysm of the coronary
    artery

DACL
Depression Adjective Check List

D/A converter
digital-to-analog converter

DACPM
di-(4-amino-3-chlorophenyl)methane
(also called MOCA— curing agent)

DACS
data acquisition and control system (re:
computers)

DACT
dactinomycin (actinomycin D)

DAD
diffuse alveolar damage
dispense as directed

DADA
dichloroacetic acid
diisopropylammonium salt (vasodilator; hypotensive)

DADDS
N,N'-diacetyl-4,4'-diaminodiphenyl
sulfone (acedapsone—antimalarial;
leprostatic)

DADPS
4,4'-diaminodiphenyl sulfone
(dapsone—antibacterial)

DAE
diving air embolism

DAF
delayed auditory feedback

dag
decagram

DAGT
direct antiglobulin test

DAH, D.A.H.
disordered action of the heart

dal
decaliter

DALA, D-ALA
delta aminolevulinic acid

DALUS-MUS-PG
domestic animal luteolytic-uterine
smooth muscle prostaglandin

DAM
data association message (re:
computers)
degraded amyloid
descriptor attribute matrix (re:
computers)
diacetylmonoxime

diacetylmorphine
discriminant analytic model

dam
decameter

DAMA
discharged against medical advice

DAMP
2-(4,4'-diacetoxydiphenylmethyl)
piridine (cathartic)

dAMP
deoxyadenosine monophosphate
(deoxyadenosine-5'-phosphate;
deoxyadenylic acid—hydrolysis
product of DNA)

dand.
dandus (L. to be given)

DANS
1-dimethylaminonaphthalene-5-sulfonic
acid
1-dimethylaminonaphthalene-5-sulfonyl
chloride

DANT
diallynortoxiferine (dichloride form as
skeletal muscle relaxant)

DAO
diamine oxidase (histaminase)

DAo
descending aorta

DAP
data acquisition processor
delayed after polarization
depolarizing afterpotential
diastolic aortic pressure
1,4-dihydrazinophthalazine
(dihydralazine—anti-hypertensive)
dihydroxyacetone phosphate
direct agglutination pregnancy (test)
(direct latex agglutination pregnancy
test)
dynamic aortic patch

DAP, D-A-P
Draw-a-Person (test—re: Psychol)

DAP-II
dianhydrogalactitol, Adriamycin
(doxorubicin), and Platinol (cisplatin)
(re: chemotherapy)

DAPI
4'6-diamidino-2-phenylindole·2HCl (a
stain)

DAPT, Dapt
2,4-diamino-5-phenylthiazole
(amiphenazole; Daptazole— narcotic
antagonist)
direct agglutination pregnancy test

DAR
death after resuscitation
decision-aiding ranges
dual asthmatic reaction

DARF
direct antiglobulin rosette-forming

DAR factor
differential absorption ratio

DARP
drug abuse rehabilitation program

DAS
dead air space
Death Anxiety Scale (re: Psychol)
dextroamphetamine sulfate (CNS
    stimulant)
digital-analog simulator (re: computers)

DASD
direct access storage device (re:
    computers)

DASE, D.A.S.E.
Denver Articulation Screening
    Examination (re: psychological
    testing)

DASI
Developmental Activities Screening
    Inventory

DASP
double antibody solid phase

DAT
daunomycin, ara-C, 6-thioguanine (re:
    chemotherapy)
delayed action tablet
dementia of the Alzheimer type
desktop analysis tool
O,S-diacetylthiamine (acetiamine,
    vitamin B_1)
diet as tolerated
differential agglutination(s) test
differential agglutination titer
Differential Aptitude Test (re: Psychol)
diphtheria antitoxin
direct agglutination test
direct antiglobulin test

DATC
4,4′-di(isoamyloxy)thiocarbanilide
    (tiocarlide— antibacterial)

DATP
deoxyadenosine triphosphate

DATTA
Diagnostic and Therapeutic Technology
    Assessment

dau.
daughter

DAUNO
daunorubicin (daunomycin;
    rubidomycin; leukaemomycin C;
    antineoplastic)

DAVH
dibromodulcitol, Adriamycin
    (doxorubicin), vincristine, and
    Halotestin (fluoxymesterone) (re:
    chemotherapy)

DAW
dispense as written

DB
Baudelocque's diameter (external
    conjugate diameter of pelvis)
deep breath
dense body
dextran blue
diabetic
diagonal band
Diamond-Blackfan (syndrome)
diet beverage
direct bilirubin
disability
distobuccal (re: Dent)
Dollinger-Bielschowsky (syndrome)
double blind
dry bulb (temperature)
duodenal bulb
Dutch belted (rabbits)

DB, D/B
date of birth

Db
diabetes

D_β
total beta dose

dB, db
decibel

DBA
1,2:5,6-dibenzanthracene (EPA listing
    as carcinogen)

dBa
adjusted decibels (re: computers/data
    processing)

DBC
dibencozide (cobamamide—vitamin B_{12}
    coenzyme)
dye-binding capacity

DBCL
dilute blood clot lysis (method)

DBCP
1,2-dibromo-3-chloropropane (soil
    fumigant)

DBD
definite brain damage

dibromodulcitol (dibromodulcit; mitolactol—antineoplastic)

DBE
dibromoethane (ethylene dibromide, EDB—fumigant)

DBED
N,N'-dibenzylethylenediamine (re: manufacture of penicillin)

DBED penicillin
dibenzylethylenediamine dipenicillin (penicillin G benzanthine—antibacterial)

DBG
dextrose, barbital, gelatin

DBH
dopamine-beta-hydroxylase

DBI
Development at Birth Index
l-phenethylbiguanide (phenformin HCl—oral hypoglycemic; withdrawn from market in 1978)

dBk
decibels above 1 kilowatt

dbl.
double

DBM
diabetic management
dibromomannitol (mitobronitol—antineoplastic)

dBm
decibels above 1 milliwatt

DBMC
4,6-di-*tert*-butyl-*m*-cresol (industrial chemical)
dystrophica bullosa Mendes da Costa

DBMS
data base management system

DBO
distobucco-occlusal (re: Dent)

DBP
demineralized bone powder
diastolic blood pressure
dibutyl phthalate (insect repellent for clothing)
distobuccopulpal (re: Dent)
Döhle body panmyelopathy

DBR
disordered breathing rate

dBrn
decibels above reference noise (re: computers/data processing)

DBS
deep brain stimulation
Denis Browne splint (re: orthopaedics)
despeciated bovine serum
dibromsalicil (antiseptic)
direct bonding system
Division of Biological Standards

DBT
disordered breathing time
dry bulb temperature

DBW
desirable body weight

DC
daily census
data conversion (re: computers)
decimal classification (re: computers)
deep compartment
degenerating cell
deoxycholate
descending colon
design change (re: computers)
detail condition (re: computers)
dextran charcoal
diagnostic center
diagnostic code
differentiated cell
diffuse cortical
digital computer
digit copying
dilatation and curettage
dilation catheter
direct Coombs' (test)
direct coupled (re: computers)
direct cycle (re: computers)
direction cycle (re: computers)
discharged
display console (re: computers)
distal colon
distocervical (re: Dent)
donor's cells (corpuscles)
dressing change
duodenal cap
dyskeratosis congenita

DC, D.C., dc, d.c.
direct current

DC, D/C
damp, cold (re: weather)

DC, D/C, D/c, dc, d/c
discontinue

DC, D/C, dc
discharge

DC, D/C, d/c
decrease

D & C, D&C
dilatation and curettage
dilation and curettage
drug and cosmetic (dyes)

DCA
deoxycholate-citrate agar
deoxycholic acid
deoxycorticosterone acetate
desoxycholate citrate agar
desoxycorticosterone acetate
dichloroacetate
dichloroacetic acid (escharotic)

DCABG
double coronary artery bypass graft

DCAG
double coronary artery graft

DCB
3,3′-dichlorobenzidine (industrial
　　chemical)
dilutional cardiopulmonary bypass

DCBE
double contrast barium enema

DCBF
dynamic cardiac blood flow

DCC
dicyclohexylcarbodiimide (re: peptide
　　synthesis)
dorsal cell column

DCC, DCc, D.Cc.
double concave

DCCI
dicyclohexylcarbodiimide (re: peptide
　　synthesis)

DCCMP
daunorubicin, cyclocytidine, 6-
　　mercaptopurine, and prednisone (re:
　　chemotherapy)

DCD
Dennis Test of Child Development

Dc'd, dc'd
discontinued

dCDP
deoxycytidine diphosphate

DCE
demosterol-to-cholesterol enzyme

DCEE
sym-dichloroethyl ether (soil fumigant)

DCET
O,S-dicarbethoxythiamine (vitamin B_1
　　source)

DCF
2′deoxycoformycin
dopachrome conversion factor

DCF, D.C.F.
direct centrifugal flotation

2′-DCF
2′-deoxycoformycin

d.c.f.
detur cum formula (L. let it be given with
　　set form—"prescribed rule")

DCG
deoxycorticosterone glucoside
desoxycorticosterone glucoside
disodium cromoglycate
dynamic electrocardiography

DCH
delayed cutaneous hypersensitivity

DCI
dichloroisoproterenol (adrenergic agent)

DCL
dicloxacillin
diffuse cutaneous leishmaniasis

DCLS
deoxycholate citrate lactose saccharose
　　(agar)

DCM
dichloromethotrexate (re:
　　chemotherapy)
dyssynergia cerebellaris myoclonia

DCML
dorsal column medial lemniscus

DCMO
2,3-dihydro-5-carboxanilido-6-methyl-
　　1,4-oxathiin (carboxin—systemic plant
　　fungicide)

DCMP
daunorubicin, cytarabine, 6-
　　mercaptopurine, and prednisone (re:
　　chemotherapy)

dCMP
deoxycytidine monophosphate
　　(deoxycytidine-5′-phosphate;
　　deoxycytidylic acid)

DCMX
2,4-dichloro-*m*,5-xylenol
　　(dichloroxylenol— preservative; mold
　　inhibitor)

DCN
Data Collection Network (re: medical
　　records)
delayed conditioned necrosis
dorsal column nucleus
dorsal cutaneous nerve

DCNU
1-(2-chloroethyl)-1-nitroso-3-(D-glucos-
　　2-yl)urea (chlorozotocin—
　　antineoplastic)

D_{CO}
diffusing capacity for carbon monoxide
(re: Resp)

D. colony
dwarf colony

DCP
dicalcium phosphate
dynamic compression plate

DCPC
p,p'-dichlorodiphenylmethyl carbinol
(chlorfenethol— acaricide)

DCPM
di-(*p*-chlorophenoxy)methane (miticide)

DCPU
dorsal caudate putamen

DCR
dacryocystorhinostomy
data conversion receiver (re:
computers)
design change recommendation (re:
computers)
detail condition register (re: computers)
digital conversion receiver (re:
computers)
direct cortical response

DCS
decompression sickness
dense canalicular system
diffuse cerebral sclerosis
disease control serum
dorsal column stimulator

DCT
diastolic control team
direct Coombs' test
distal convoluted tubule (kidney)
diurnal cortisol test
dynamic computed tomography

dct.
decoctum (L. boiled [down to
concentrate or extract an active
principle by boiling thoroughly])

DCTL
direct-coupled transistor logic (re:
computers)

DCTP, dCTP
deoxycytidine triphosphate

DCV
DTIC, CCNU, vincristine (re:
chemotherapy)

DCX
double charge exchange

DCx, D.Cx.
double convex

DD
dangerous drug
data definition (re: computers)
data demand (re: computers)
day of delivery
day dressing
decimal display (re: computers)
degenerative disease
delay driver (re: computers)
delusional disorder
dependent drainage
detrusor dyssynergia
developmental disability
developmentally disabled
died of the disease
differential diagnosis
digestive disease
digital data (re: computers)
digital display (re: computers)
Di Guglielmo's disease
discharge by death
discharge diagnosis
discharged dead
Distortion of Dots
dog dander (test)
double diffusion (test)
dry dressing
Duchenne's dystrophy
Dupuytren's disease
dying declaration

DD, dd
disk diameter(s) (1.5 mm—re: Ophth)

DD I, DD II
detrusor dyssynergia, types I and II

D→D
discharge to duty

Dd
unusual detail response

dD
confabulated detail response (re:
Psychol)

d.d.
de die (L. daily)
detur ad (L. let it be given to)

DDA
digital differential analyzer
digital display alarm
metabolite of DDT excreted in urine

DDAS
digital data acquisition system (re:
computers)

DDAVP
1-desamino-8-D-arginine vasopressin
(desmopressin—antidiuretic)

DDC
diethyldithiocarbamic acid

(diethyldithiocarbamate,
diethyldithiocarbimine—an herbicide)
direct digital control
direct display console

DDD
defined daily dose
degenerative disc disease
dense deposit disease
Denver dialysis disease
dichlorodiphenyldichloroethane (*p,p'*-
DDD—insecticide)
2,4'-dichlorodiphenyldichloroethane
(*o,p'*-DDD; Lysodren; mitotane—re:
chemotherapy)
2,2'-dihydroxy-6,6'-dinaphthyl disulfide
(re: protein-bound sulfhydryl groups;
analytical—not to be confused with
the insecticide)
dihydroxydinaphthyl disulfide (Barrnett-
Seligman histological procedure)
direct distance dialing (re: computers/
data processing)

DDG
deoxy-D-glucose
digital display generator (re: computers)

DDH
dissociated double hypertropia

d. d. in d.
de die in diem (L. from day to day)

DDMP
diamino-
dichlorophenylmethylpyrimidine

DDMS
degenerative dense microsphere

dDNA
denatured DNA

DDP
density-dependent phosphoprotein
diamminedichloroplatinum (cisplatin—
antineoplastic)
digital data processor (re: computers/
data processing)

DDQ
2,3-dichloro-5,6-dicyanobenzoquinone
(oxidizing agent)

DDR
diastolic descent rate (re: Cardio)

DDS
dialysis disequilibrium syndrome
4,4'-diaminodiphenyl sulfone
(dapsone—antibacterial)
digital display scope (re: computers)
disability determination service
disease disability scale
dystrophy-dystocia syndrome

Dds
detail response to small white space

DDSO
4,4'-diaminodiphenyl sulfoxide
(experimental leprotic)

DDST
Denver Developmental Screening Test

DDT
Degos-Delort-Tricot (syndrome)
dichlorodiphenyltrichloroethane
(insecticide; pediculicide)
digital data transmitter (re: computers)
ductus deferens tumor

DDVP
O,O-dimethyl *O*-(2,2-dichlorovinyl)
phosphate (dichlorvos—insecticide)

DDW
double distilled water

D/DW
dextrose in distilled water

D 5 DW, D 5%Dw
dextrose, 5%, in distilled water

DdW
detail response elaborating the whole

DDx.
differential diagnosis

DE
decision element (re: computers)
dendritic expansion (re: Neuro)
deprived eye (re: Ophth)
diagnostic error
digestive energy
digital element (re: computers)
display element (re: computers)
display equipment (re: computers)
division entry (re: computers)
dose equivalent
dream element(s)
drug evaluation
Duchenne-Erb (syndrome)
duodenal exclusion
duration of ejection

D&E
diet and elimination
dilatation and evacuation
dilation and evacuation

2-DE
two-dimensional echocardiography

d.e.
dosis effectiva (L. effective dose)
edge detail

DEA
dehydroepiandrosterone (an androgen)

diethanolamine (alkaline phosphatase
   assay buffer)
Drug Enforcement Adminstration

DEA#
Drug Enforcement Administration
   number (physician's narcotic number)

DEAE
2-diethylaminoethanol
2-diethylaminoethyl (anticholinergic)

DEAE-cellulose
diethylaminoethyl cellulose (*O*-
   (diethylaminoethyl) cellulose—re:
   chromatography and as ion-
   exchange material)

DEAE-D
diethylaminoethyl dextran

dearg. pil.
deargentur pilulae (L. let the pills be
   silvered)

deaur. pil.
deaurentur pilulae (L. let the pills be
   gilded)

3-deazaU
3-deazauridine

DEB
diepoxybutane (prevents microbial
   spoilage)
dystrophic epidermolysis bullosa

deb.
debridement

DEBA
diethylbarbituric acid (sedative;
   hypnotic)

D-EB-B
dominant epidermolysis bullosa Bart
   (re: genetics)

D-EBD-CT
dominant epidermolysis bullosa
   dystrophica Cockayne- Touraine (re:
   genetics)

D-EBD-P
dominant epidermolysis bullosa
   dystrophica albopapuloidea Pasini
   (re: genetics)

D-EBH-DM
dominant epidermolysis bullosa
   herpetiformis Dowling- Meara (re:
   genetics)

debil.
debilitation
debility

DEBS
dominant epidermolysis bullosa simplex
   (re: genetics)

D-EBS-K
dominant epidermolysis bullosa
   simplex, Köbner (re: genetics)

D-EBS-M
dominant epidermolysis bullosa simplex
   with mottled pigmentation (re:
   genetics)

D-EBS-O
dominant epidermolysis bullosa simplex
   Ogna (re: genetics)

deb. spis.
debita spissitudine (L. of the proper
   consistency)

deb. spiss.
debita spissitudo (L. proper
   consistency)

D-EBS-WC
dominant epidermolysis bullosa
   simplex, Weber-Cockayne (re:
   genetics)

DEC
Developmental Evaluation Center
diethylcarbamazine (antifilarial)
dynamic environmental condition
   (cycle)

dec.
decanta (L. pour off)
deceased
deciduous
decimal
decimeter
decoctum (L. boiled [down to extract an
   active principle or to concentrate by
   boiling thoroughly])
decompose(d)
decrease(ed)

DecAo
descending aorta

decd., dec'd
deceased

dec'd
decomposed

decel.
deceleration

decim.
decimeter

DECO
decreasing consumption of oxygen

decoct.
decoctum (L. boiled down [to extract an

135

active principle or to concentrate by boiling thoroughly])

decomp.
decompensated (heart disease)
decompose(d)
decomposition

decompn.
decompensation
decomposition

dec (R)
decrease, relative

decr.
decrease
decreased (diminished)

decub.
decubitus (L. lying down)

DED
date of expected delivery
defined exposure dose
delayed erythema dose

de d. in d.
de die in diem (L. from day to day)

DEEG
depth electroencephalogram
depth electroencephalography
depth electrography

DEF
decayed, extracted, or filled (dental formula—re: permanent teeth)
duck embryo fibroblast

DEF, def.
defecation

Def, def.
deficiency

def.
defecate
deferred
deficient
deficit
define
definite
definition

def, d.e.f.
decayed, extracted, or filled (dental formula— deciduous teeth)

D eff.
dosis efficax (L. efficacious dose)

defib.
defibrillate

defic.
deficiency

deficient
deficit

deform.
deformity

DEG
diethylene glycol (manufacturing chemical)

Deg, deg.
degeneration
degree

degen.
degeneration
degenerative

deglut.
deglutia (L. swallow [imperative])
deglutiatur (L. let it be swallowed)

DEH
dysplasia epiphysealis hemimelica

DEHFT
developmental hand-function test

dehyd.
dehydrated
dehydration

dej.
dento-enamel junction (re: Dent)

DEL
the delete character (re: computers/data processing)

Del, del.
delivery

del
deletion (re: cytogenetics)

del.
deliver
delusion

deliq.
deliquescent

deliquesc.
deliquescent

Delt
deltoid

Δ-G
Gibbs free-energy change (thermodynamic static G)

δ-T
δ-tocopherol

DEM
demodulator (re: computers)
diethylmaleate

DEM, Dem
Demerol (meperidine hydrochloride)

dem.
demonstrate(d)

Demen Prae
dementia praecox

demin.
demineralization

DEMOD
demodulator (re: computers)

DEN
diethylnitrosamine (*N*-nitrosodiethylamine—antioxidant; stabilizer—listed as a carcinogen)

DENA
diethylnitrosamine (*N*-nitrosodiethylamine—antioxidant; stabilizer—listed as a carcinogen)

denat.
denatured

denom.
denominator

Dent, dent.
dental
dentist
dentistry
dentition

dent.
dentate
dentur (L. give; let them be given)

dent. tal. dos.
dentur tales doses (L. let such doses be given)

DEP
diethylpropanediol (2,2-diethyl-1,3-propanediol—a skeletal muscle relaxant)

Dep, dep.
dependents

dep.
deposit
depuratus (L. purified)

DEPA
N-(3-oxapentamethylene)-*N'*,*N"*-diethylenephosphoramide (ODEPA)

DEPC
diethyl pyrocarbonate (esterifying agent)

depr.
depressed
depression

depress.
depressed
depression

DEPS
distal effective potassium secretion

Dept, dept.
department

DEQ
Depressive Experiences Questionnaire (re: Psychol)

DER, DeR, De R
reaction of degeneration

der
derivative chromosome (re: cytogenetics)

deriv.
derivative
derive
derived (of, from)

Derm
dermatitis

Derm, derm.
dermatologist
dermatology

derm.
dermatological
dermatome

DES
dermal-epidermal separation
diethylstilbestrol
diffuse esophageal spasm
disequilibrium syndrome

desat.
desaturated
desaturation

desc.
descendent
descending
descent

Desc AO
descending aorta

descr.
describe

DESI
drug efficacy study implementation

2,4-DES-Na
sodium 2,4-dichlorophenoxyethyl sulfate (disul-sodium— herbicide)

DESP
decaspiride (fenspiride—bronchodilator; antiadrenergic)

desq.
desquamation

DEST
Denver Eye Screening Test
dichotic environmental sounds test

dest.
destilla (L. distil)
destillatus (L. distilled)

destil.
destilla (L. distil)

DET
diethyltryptamine (hallucinogenic)

det.
detur (L. let it be given)
detur (L. give)

determin.
determination

det. in dup.
detur in duplo (L. let twice as much be
given)

det. in 2 plo.
detur in duplo (L. let twice as much be
given)

DET-MS
dihydroergotamine mesylate
(vasoconstrictor)

detn.
detention
determination

detox.
detoxification

d. et s.
detur et signetur (L. let it be given and
labeled)

det. time
detention time

D Ety
disease etiology

DEUC
direct electronic urethrocystometry

DEV
duck egg (embryo) vaccine
duck egg (embryo) virus

dev.
develop(ed)
development
deviate
deviated
deviation

devd.
developed

devel.
developed
development

DEX
dexamethasone

dex.
dexterity
dextrorotatory
Dextrostix

dext.
dexter (L. right)
dexterity
dextra (L. right)
dextro (L. right)

DF
Daae-Finsen (disease)
Debré-Fibiger (syndrome)
decapacitation factor (re: sperm)
decayed and filled (re: permanent teeth)
decontamination factor
deferoxamine (desferrioxamine
    mesylate—chelating agent for iron)
deficiency factor
diabetic father
diaphragmatic function
dietary fiber
digital fluoroscopy
discriminant function
disseminated foci
distribution factor
dome fragment
dorsiflexion
dry (gas) fractional (concentration)

DF, D/F, df, d.f.
degree(s) of freedom (of movement)

DF, df
degree of freedom (re: statistics)

df
decayed and filled (re: deciduous teeth)

DFA
direct fluorescence antibody (test)
dorsiflexion assist

DFB
dinitrofluorobenzene (reagent; hapten)
dysfunctional (uterine) bleeding

DFC
deletion of final consonants
dry-filled capsules

DF caries
decayed or filled (re: index of
    permanent teeth)

df caries
decayed or filled (re: index of deciduous
    teeth)

DFD
defined formula diets

DFDD
difluorodiphenyldichloroethane (contact insecticide)

DFDT
difluorodiphenyltrichloroethane (contact insecticide)

DFE
diffuse fasciitis with eosinophilia

DFECT, D-FECT
dense fibroelastic connective tissue

DFG
direct forward gaze

DFI
disease-free intervals

DFM
decreased fetal movement

DFMC
daily fetal movement count

DFMR
daily fetal movement record

DFO
deferoxamine (desferrioxamine mesylate—iron chelating agent)

DFOM
deferoxamine (desferrioxamine mesylate—iron chelating agent)

D forms
diphtheroid forms
dwarf forms

DFP
diastolic filling period (re: Cardio)
diisopropyl fluorophosphonate (isoflurophate; cholinergic—re: Ophth)

DF^{32}P
diisopropylphosphofluoridate (radiolabeled—re: red cell survival test)

DFS
disease-free survival

DFSP
dermatofibrosarcoma protuberans

DFT
defibrillation threshold
diagnostic function test (re: computers/ data processing)
discrete Fourier transforms

DFT 4, DFT$_4$
dialyzable free thyroxin(e)

DFU
dead fetus in uterus
dideoxyfluorouridine

DG
darkground
dentate gyrus (re: Neuro)
deoxyglucose (deoxy-D-glucose)
   deoxyguanosine (2'-deoxyribosylguanine—re: DNA)
diastolic gallop
diglyceride
distogingival (re: Dent)
Duchenne-Griesinger (disease)

DG, dg
diagnose
diagnosis
diagnostic

2DG, 2-DG
2-deoxy-D-glucose (antiviral agent)

D$_g$
prefix specifying configuration of certain stereoisomers (re: carbon atoms)

D$_\gamma$
total gamma dose

dG
deoxyguanylate

dg
decigram

DGCI
delayed gamma camera image

dge.
drainage

DGF
duct growth factor

DGI
disseminated gonococcal infection

dgm
decigram

dGMP
deoxyguanosine-5'-phosphate (deoxyguanosine monophosphate; deoxyguanosine phosphate; deoxyguanylic acid)

DGN
diffuse glomerulonephritis

DGS
diabetic glomerulosclerosis

DGTP, dGTP
2-deoxyguanosine-5'-triphosphate

dgtr.
daughter

DGV
dextrose, gelatin, veronal (solution)

DGVB
dextrose, gelatin, veronal buffer

DH
daily habits
dehydrocholic acid (a cholerectic)
dehydrogenase
delayed hypersensitivity
dental habits
dermatitis herpetiformis
developmental history
diffuse histiocytic
disseminated histoplasmosis
dominant hand
dorsal horn
ductal hyperplasia

D/H
deutrium to hydrogen (ratio)

DHA
dehydroacetic acid
dehydroascorbic acid
dehydroepiandrosterone
dihydroxyacetone (artificial tanning
   agent)

DHAD
1,4-dihydroxy-5,8-bis[[2-[(2-
   hydroxyethyl)amino]ethyl] amino]-
   9,10-anthraquinone dihydrochloride
   (mitoxantrone hydrochloride—
   antineoplastic)

DHAQ
1,4-dihydroxy-5,8-bis[[2-[(2-
   hydroxyethyl)amino]ethyl] amino]-
   9,10-anthraquinone (mitoxantrone—
   antineoplastic)

DHAS, DHA-S
dehydroepiandrosterone (sodium)
   sulfate (sodium
   dehydroepiandrosterone sulfate—an
   androgen)

DHA-S
dehydroacetic acid sodium salt hydrate
   (fungicide; bacteriocide)

DHB
duck hepatitis B virus

DHBE
3,3'-dihydroxydibutyl ether (choleretic)

DHCA
deep hypothermia and circulatory arrest

1,25-DHCC
1α,25-dihydroxycholecalciferol
   (calcitriol—calcium regulator)

DHE
dihematoporphyrin ether
dihydroergotamine

DHE 45, D.H.E. 45
dihydroergotamine mesylate (re:
   migraine)

DHEA
dehydroepiandrosterone

DHEAS
dehydroepiandrosterone (sodium)
   sulfate (an androgen)

DHEA-SO$_4$
dehydroepiandrosterone (sodium)
   sulfate (an androgen)

DHEW
Department of Health, Education and
   Welfare

DHF
dengue hemorrhagic fever
dorsihyperflexion

DHFR
dihydrofolate reductase

DHFS
dengue hemorrhagic fever shock
   (syndrome)

DHGG
deaggregated human gamma globulin

DHI
dihydroxyindol

DHIA
dehydroisoandrosterol
dehydroisoandrosterone
   (dehydroepiandrosterone; pras-
   terone—re: androgen)

DHIC
dihydroisocodeine

DHL
diffuse histiocytic lymphoma
diffuse histocytic lymphoma

DHM
dihydromorphine (analgesic)

DHMA
3,4-dihydroxymandelic acid

DHO
dihydroergocornine (sympatholytic,
   adrenolytic)

DHP
dehydrogenated polymers
dihydropteridine reductase (variant form
   of phenylalanine)

DHPc
dorsal hippocampus (re: Neuro)

dhPRL
decidual human prolactin

DHR
delayed hypersensitivity reaction(s)

DHS
delayed hypersensitivity
duration of hospital stay

D-5-HS, D/5 HS
dextrose (5%) in Hartmann's solution
    (lactated Ringer's)

DHSM
dihydrostreptomycin (antibiotic)

DHT
dihydrotachysterol (AT-10)
4-dihydrotestosterone (stanolone)
(1,2-dihydroxy-3-propyl)theophylline
    (diphylline; diprophylline; and
    others—smooth muscle relaxant)

DHZ
dihydralazine (an antihypertensive)

DI
defective-interfering
degradation index
desorption ionization
deterioration index
detrusor instability (re: Uro)
diabetes insipidus
diagnostic imaging
diaphragmatic
diphtheria
disability insurance
dispensing information
distal intestine
distoincisal (re: Dent)
dorsal interosseous
dorso-iliacus
drop in
drug information
drug interactions
dyskaryosis index

DI, D/I
date of injury

Di
didymium (now praseodymium, Pr)
Diego blood group

d.i.
inside detail

d$_i$
differences (re: statistics)

DIA
death in action
depolarization-induced automaticity

Di A
Diego antigen

Dia
diabetes

Dia, dia.
diameter
diathermy

DIA-1
NADH-diaphorase

DIA-4
diaphorase-4

diab.
diabetes
diabetic

Diag, diag.
diagnosis

diag.
diagnose
diagnostic
diagonal
diagram

DIAGNO
(differential) diagnosis

DIAL
Developmental Indicators for the
    Assessment of Learning

DIA LW, dia. l.w.
long wave diathermy

diam.
diameter

Di antigen
Diego blood group

diaph.
diaphragm
diaphyseal
diaphysis

DIAR
dextran-induced anaphylactoid reaction

dias.
diastolic

DIA SW, dia. s.w.
short wave diathermy

diath.
diathermy

DIAZ
diazepam

DIB
Diagnostic Interview for Borderlines
disability insurance benefits

DIC
differential interference contrast (re: microscope)
diffuse intravascular clotting
diffuse intravascular coagulation
5(or 4)-(dimethyltriazeno)imidazole-4(or 5)-carboxamide (dacarbazine; DIC; DTIC—antineoplastic)
disseminated intravascular coagulation
disseminated intravascular coagulopathy
drug information center

dic
dicentric chromosome (re: cytogenetics)

DICD
dispersion-induced circular dichroism

dict.
dictate
dictated
dictionary

DID
dead of intercurrent disease
direct inward dialing (re: computers/data processing)
double immunodiffusion (technique)
dystonia-improvement-dystonia

DIDMOAD
diabetes insipidus, diabetes mellitus, optic atrophy, and (nerve) deafness

DIE
died in Emergency Room
direct injection enthalpimetry

dieb. alt.
diebus alternis (L. on alternate days)

dieb. secund.
diebus secundis (L. every second day)

dieb. tert.
diebus tertiis (L. every third day)

DIF
diffuse interstitial fibrosis
direct immunofluorescence
dose increase factor

DIFF, Diff, diff.
differential (blood count)

Diff
differential (leukocyte count)

diff.
difference
different
differential
difficult

diff. diag.
differential diagnosis

DIFP
diffuse interstitial fibrosing pneumonitis
diisopropyl fluorophosphonate (cholinergic, toxic—re: Ophth)

DIG, dig.
digitalis

Dig
digoxin

dig.
digeratur (L. let it be digested)
digest
digestion

DIHE
drug-induced hepatic encephalopathy

DIL
daughter-in-law
drug information log

Dil
Dilantin
dilation

dil.
dilatation
dilate
dilated
dilue (L. dilute or dissolve)
diluted
dilution
dilutus (L. dilute, diluted)

dilat.
dilatation
dilate
dilated
dilation

DILD
diffuse infiltrative lung disease
diffuse interstitial lung disease

dild.
diluted

DILE
drug-induced lupus erythematosus

diln.
dilution

diluc.
diluculo (L. at daybreak)

dilut.
dilute
diluted
dilution
dilutus (L. diluted, dilute)

DIM
divalent ion metabolism
dosis infectiosis media (L. medium infectious dose)

DIM, dim.
dimidius (L. halved)

dim.
dimension
diminished
diminutus (L. diminished)

dimin.
diminished
diminution

DIMS
disorder of initiating and maintaining
   sleep

DIMSA
disseminated intravascular multiple
   systems activation

dim. T
diminished time
diminished tone

DIN
Deutsche Industrie Norm (photographic
   emulsion speed indicator system)

d. in dup.
detur in duplo (L. let twice as much be
   given)

d. in p. aeq.
divide in partes aequales (L. divide into
   equal parts)

diop.
diopter

DIP
desquamative interstitial pneumonia
desquamative interstitial pneumonitis
diisopropylamine (re: organic synthesis)
distal interphalangeal (joint)
drip-infusion pyelogram
dual-in-line package (re: integrated
   circuits)

Dip
diphtheria

DIPA-DCA
diisopropylamine dichloroacetate
   (vasodilator; hypotensive)

DIPC
diffuse interstitial pulmonary
   calcification

DIPF
diisopropyl phosphofluoridate

diph.
diphtheria

diph-tet, diph/tet
diphtheria-tetanus (toxoid)

diph-tox
diphtheria toxoid (plain)

diph. tox. AP
diphtheria toxoid—alum precipitated

DIPJ
distal interphalangeal joint

dipt.
diopter

DIR
disturbed interpersonal relationships
double isomorphous replacement

Dir
director

dir
direct (re: cytogenetics)

dir.
direct
directione (L. by direction)
directions
directory

DIRD
drug-induced renal disease

direct. prop.
directione propria (L. with proper
   direction; with the proper directions)

dir. prop.
directione propria (L. with proper
   direction; with the proper directions)

DIS
Diagnostic Information System

Dis
discharge

dis.
disability
disabled
discomfort
disease
dislocation
distance
distribution

disab.
disability
disabled

disart.
disarticulation

disartic.
disarticulation

DISC, disc.
discontinue(d)

disc.
discharge(d)
discomfort

disch.
discharge(d)

disch. AMA
discharged against medical advice

dischg.
discharge(d)

Disch PHC
discharged to post-hospital care

DISH
diffuse idiopathic skeletal hyperostosis

DISI
dorsal intercalary segment instability

DISL, Disl
dislocate
dislocated
dislocation

disloc.
dislocate
dislocated
dislocation

dism.
dismiss
dismissed

DIS/min
disintegrations per minute

disod.
disodium

disord.
disorder

disp.
dispensa (L. dispense)
dispensary
dispensatory
dispense
dispensetur (L. let it be dispensed)
disposition

displ.
displace
displacement

dissd.
dissolved

dissem.
disseminate
disseminated
dissemination

dissoc.
dissociate
dissociation

dist.
distal
distance
distended
distillation
distilled
distinguish(ed)
distribute(d)
district
disturbance

dist. f.
distinguished from

dist. H$_2$O
distilled water

distill.
distillation

distn.
distillation

distr.
distressed
distribute(d)
distribution

distrib.
distribute(d)
distribution

DIT
diet-induced thermogenesis
drug-induced thrombocytopenia

DIT, DiT
diiodotyrosine (thyroid inhibitor)

div.
divergence
division
divorced

divid.
dividatur (L. divide)

div. in p. aeq.
dividatur in partes aequales (L. let it be
divided into equal parts)

div. in par. aeq.
dividatur in partes aequales (L. let it be
divided into equal parts)

DIVP
dilute intravenous Pitocin

DJ
Dubin-Johnson (syndrome)

DJD
degenerative joint disease

DJOA
dominant juvenile optic atrophy

DJS
Dubin-Johnson syndrome

DK
decay
degeneration of keratinocytes
Déjérine-Klumpke (syndrome)
diabetic ketoacidosis
diet kitchen
diseased kidney
dog kidney

dk.
dark

DKA
diabetic ketoacidosis
didn't keep appointment

DKB
deep knee bends
3',4'-dideoxykanamycin B (dibecacin—
    antibacterial)

dkg
decagram (dag)

dkl
decaliter (dal)

dkm
decameter (dam)

DKP
dikalium phosphate (cathartic)

DKTC
dog kidney tissue culture

DKV
deer kidney virus

DL
danger list
deep lobe
difference limen (threshold)
diffusion lung capacity
direct laryngoscopy (re: ENT)
directed listening
disabled list
distolingual (re: Dent)
dosis letalis (L. lethal dose)

DL, D$_L$
diffusing capacity of the lung

DL, D-L
Donath-Landsteiner (test)

D/L
date of liability
date of loss

DL-, dl-
optically inactive by external
    compensation as contrasted with
    meso- (racemic)

dl
deciliter

DLA, DLa
distolabial (re: Dent)

D-L Ab
Donath-Landsteiner antibody

DLAI, DLaI
distal labioincisal (re: Dent)

DL antibody
Donath-Landsteiner antibody
    (hemolysin)

DLap
distolabiopulpal (re: Dent)

DL & B
direct laryngoscopy and bronchoscopy

DLC
differential leukocyte count
dual lumen catheter

DLCO
diffusing capacity of the lung for carbon
    monoxide

DLCO$_2$
diffusing capacity of the lung for carbon
    dioxide

DLCO-SB, D$_{LCO}$SB
single breath diffusing capacity of the
    lung

D$_{LCO}$SS
steady state diffusing capacity of the
    lung

D$_{LCO}$SS$_1$
measured arterial pCO$_2$

D$_{LCO}$SS$_2$
end-tidal gas

D$_{LCO}$SS$_3$
physiologic dead space

D$_{LCO}$SS$_4$
mixed venous CO$_2$

DLE
delayed light emission
dialyzable leukocyte extract
discoid lupus erythematosus
disseminated lupus erythematosus

DLF
dorsolateral funiculus (re: Neuro)

D-L hemolysin
Donath-Landsteiner hemolysin
    (antibody)

DLI
distolinguoincisal (re: Dent)
double label index

D line
measurement of refraction index or
optical rotation (a bright yellow
doublet in emission spectrum of
sodium)

DLL
dihomo-gammalinoleic acid (precursor,
prostaglandin biosynthesis)

DLLI
dulcitol lysine lactose iron (agar)

DLO
distolinguo-occlusal (re: Dent)

D_{LO_2}
diffusing capacity of the lung for oxygen

DLP
delipidized serum protein
developmental learning problems
direct linear plotting
dislocation of the patella
distolinguopulpal (re: Dent)

DLT
dihydroepiandrosterone loading test

DLV
defective leukemia virus

DLVO
Derjaguin-Landau-Verwey-Overbeek
(theory—re: microbiology)

DLWD
diffuse lymphocytic, well-differentiated

DM
dermatologist
dermatology
dermatomyositis
Descemet's membrane
dextromethorphan
diabetic mother
diastolic murmur
diffuse mixed
distant metastases
dopamine
dorsomedial
dose modification
double membrane
dry matter
duodenal mucosa

DM, D_M
membrane component of diffusion
membrane diffusing capacity

DM, d.m.
diabetes mellitus

dM
decimorgan

dm
decimeter

DMA
dimethyladenosine
dimethylamine (reagent to magnesium)
dimethylarginine
direct memory access (re: computers)
direct memory address (re: computers)

DMAB
p-dimethylaminobenzaldehyde (Erlich's
reagent)

DMABA
p-dimethylaminobenzaldehyde (Erlich's
reagent)

DMAC
N,N-dimethylacetamide (solvent)

DMAE
dimethylaminoethanol (deanol—
antidepressant)

DMARD
disease-modifying antirheumatic drug

DMC
demeclocycline (antibacterial)
p,p'-dichlorodiphenylmethyl carbinol
(dimite—an acaricide)
β,β-dimethylcysteine (penicillamine—
chelating agent)
direct microscopic count

DMCC
direct microscopic clump count

DMCT
demethylchlortetracycline (obsolete
term for demeclocycline—
antibacterial)

DMD
disease-modifying drug
Duchenne's muscular dystrophy

DMDZ
desmethyldiazepam (nordazepam—
tranquilizer)

DME
dimethyl ether (of D-tubocurarine
iodide)
diphasic meningoencephalitis
dropping mercury electrode
drug-metabolizing enzyme
Dulbecco's modified Eagle's (medium)

DMEM
Dulbecco's minimum essential medium
Dulbecco's modified Eagle's medium

DMF
D = number of carious (decayed) teeth;
  M = number of missing teeth;
  F = number of filled teeth
N,N-dimethylformamide (solvent)
diphasic milk fever

DMFA
N,N-dimethylformamide (solvent)

DMF caries
decayed, missing, and filled (re: index of
  permanent teeth)

dmf caries
decayed, missing, and filled (re: index of
  deciduous teeth)

DMFS caries
decayed, missing and filled surfaces
  (re: index of permanent teeth)

dmfs caries
decayed, missing, and filled surfaces
  (re: index of deciduous teeth)

DMFT
decayed, missing, and filled
  (permanent) teeth

DMG
N,N-dimethylglycine

DMGG
N′-dimethylguanylguanidine
  (metformin—cholinergic)

DMI
Defense Mechanism Inventory
Diagnostic Mathematics Inventory (re:
  psychological testing)
diaphragmatic myocardial infarct
direct migration inhibition

DMKA
diabetes mellitus ketoacidosis

DML
distal motor latency

DMM
disproportionate micromelia

DMN
dimethylnitrosamine (anti-oxidant)
dorsal motor nucleus (of vagus nerve)
dorsomedial nucleus

DMNA
dimethylnitrosamine (anti-oxidant)

DMO
5,5-dimethyl-2,4-oxazolidinedione
  (demethadione;
  dimethyloxazolidinedione—
  anticonvulsant)

DMOOC
diabetes mellitus out of control

DMP
diffuse mesangial proliferation
dimercaprol (chelating agent)
dimethylphosphate (of 3-hydroxy-*N*-
  methyl-*cis*-crotonamide;
  monocrotophos—insecticide)
dimethylphthalate (insect repellant;
  solvent)

DMPA
O-(2,4-dichlorophenyl) *O*-methyl
  isopropylphosphoramidothioate
  (herbicide; not to be confused with
  DMPA® dimethylolpropionic acid)
dimethylolpropionic acid (re: water
  soluble alkyl resins; do not confuse
  with herbicide, DMPA)

DMPE
3,4-dimethoxyphenylethylamine (re:
  schizophrenia)

DMPEA
3,4-dimethoxyphenylethylamine (re:
  schizophrenia)

DMPP
dimethylphenylpiperazinium (autonomic
  ganglionic cell stimulant—highly
  selective)

DMPS
2,3-dimercapto-1-propanesulfonic acid
  (antidote to heavy metal poisoning)

DMRF
dorsal medullary reticular formation

DMS
dense microsphere
dermatomyositis
diffuse mesangial sclerosis
dimethyl sulfate (methylating agent—re:
  organic chemicals)
dimethyl sulfoxide (industrial chemical;
  topical anti- inflammatory; proposed
  penetrant to enhance absorption)

dms
double minute sphere

DMSA
disodium monomethanearsonate
  (herbicide)

DMSO
dimethyl sulfoxide (industrial chemical;
  topical anti- inflammatory; proposed
  penetrant to enhance absorption)

DMSO$_2$
dimethyl sulfone (solvent)

DMT
dermatophytosis
dimethyl terephthalate (re: analytical
   chemistry)
N,N-dimethyltryptamine (hallucinogen)

DMTT
3,5-dimethyl-2-thionotetrahydro-1,3,5-
   thiadiazine (dazomet—soil fungicide,
   nematocide)

DMTU
dimethylthiourea

D Mx
maximal dose

DN
Deiters' nucleus
diabetic neuropathy
dibucaine number
dicrotic notch
dinitrocresol (selective herbicide;
   insecticide)

DN, D/N
dextrose-nitrogen (ratio)

D & N, D + N
distance and near (vision)

Dn, dn.
decinem (obsolete term, 1/10 nem—re:
   Peds)
dekanem (obsolete term, 10 nems—re:
   Peds)

DNA
deoxyribonucleic acid
did not answer
did not attend
does not apply

DNA-P
deoxyribonucleic acid phosphorus

DNAse, DNase
deoxyribonuclease
   (desoxyribonuclease)

DNB
dorsal noradrenergic bundle

DNB, D.N.B.
dinitrobenzene (highly toxic industrial
   chemical)

DNBP
dinitrobutylphenol (dinoseb—miti-,
   acara-, fungicide)

DNC
did not come
4,4′-dinitrocarbanilide
dinitrocresol (selective herbicide;
   insecticide)

DNCB
dinitrochlorobenzene (1-chloro-2,4-
   dinitrobenzene; 2,4-dinitro-1-
   chlorobenzene—a reagent to test
   pyridine compounds)
2,6-dinitro-1-chlorobenzene

DND
died a natural death

DNE
group D non-enterococcal
   (streptococci)

DNF
Durand-Nicolas-Favre (disease)

DNFB
2,4-dinitro-1-fluorobenzene (Sanger's
   reagent)

DNIC
diffuse noxious inhibitory control

DNK
did not keep (appointment)

DNKA
did not keep appointment

DNL
lysosomal DNA-ase (re: genetics)

DNLL
dorsal nucleus of lateral lemniscus

DNOC
3,5-dinitro-*o*-cresol (dinitrocresol—
   selective herbicide)

DNOCHP
dinitro-*o*-cyclohexylphenol (insecticide)

DNOCP
dinocap (acaricide; fungicide)

DNP
diisophenol (veterinary; anthelmintic)
do not publish

DNP, Dnp
deoxyribonucleoprotein
2,4-dinitrophenol (a toxic dye)

DNPA
do not publish, adopted

DNPH
2,4-dinitrophenylhydrazine (used to
   determine aldehydes and ketones)

DNPK
do not publish, keeping

DNPT
diethyl-nitrophenyl thiophosphate
   (diethyl-*p*-nitrophenyl
   monothiophosphate; parathion—a
   highly toxic insecticide; acaricide)

DNR
daunorubicin (daunomycin;
    rubidomycin—re: chemotherapy)
did not respond
do not resuscitate
dorsal nerve root

DN/R
dextrose-to-nitrogen ratio

D/N r
(urinary) dextrose-to-nitrogen ratio

D-N ratio, D:N ratio
dextrose-to-nitrogen ratio (in urine)

DNS
deviated nasal septum
diaphragm nerve stimulation
did not show

DNS, Dns
dansyl (a fluorescent reagent)

D5NS, D5/NS, D5 n/s
dextrose 5% in normal saline

D5%/NS
5% dextrose in normal saline

D5¼NS, D5 ¼ NS
dextrose 5% with ¼ normal saline

D5 ½ n/s
5% dextrose in ½ normal saline

D5NSS, D/5NSS, D₅NSS
dextrose 5% in normal saline solution

DNT
did not test

DNTP
diethyl-p-nitrophenyl
    monothiophosphate (parathion—
    insecticide; acaricide)

DNUA
distillable nonurea adductable

DNV
dorsal nucleus of the vagus (re: Neuro)

DO
diamine oxidase (histaminase)
dissolved oxygen
disto-occlusal (re: Dent)
doctor's orders
drugs only

D₀
diffusing capacity of oxygen

D-O
directive-organic

do.
dicto (L. the same, as before, repeat)
ditto

DOA
date of admission
date of admittance
date of arrival
dead on arrival
differential optical absorption
dominant optic atrophy

DOAC
Dubois oleic albumin complex (re:
    bacteriology)

DOAP
daunorubicin, Oncovin (vincristine), ara-
    C (cytarabine), and prednisone (re:
    chemotherapy)

DOB
dangle out of bed
date of birth
doctor's order book

DOC
date of conception
dead of other causes
deoxycholate
deoxycholic (acid)
deoxycorticosterone (11-
    desoxycorticosterone)
died of other causes

doc.
doctor
document
documentation

DOCA
deoxycorticosterone acetate (11-
    deoxycorticosterone acetate;
    desoxycorticosterone acetate)

DOCG
deoxycorticosterone glucoside

DOCS
deoxycorticoids

DOC-SR
desoxycorticosterone secretion rate

DOD
date of death
date of departure
date of dictation
dead of disease
died of disease
direct outward dialing (re: computers/
    data processing)

DOE
date of examination
desoxyephedrine (deoxyephedrine—
    acari-, insecticide)
direct observation evaluation
dyspnea on exercise
dyspnea on exertion

D-O-E
d-deoxyephedrine
   (methamphetamine—central
   stimulant)

DOES
disorders of excessive sleepiness
disorders of excessive somnolence

DOI
date of injury
died of injuries

dol
dolorimetric unit (re: pain intensity)

dol.
dolor (L. pain)

DOM
deaminated-O-methyl metabolite
2,5-dimethoxy-4-methylamphetamine
   (hallucinogen STP)
dissolved organic matter

dom.
domestic

D.O.M.F
dibromohydroxymercurifluorescein
   disodium salt (mercurochrome;
   merbromin—antibacterial;
   veterinary— antiseptic)

DON
6-diazo-5-oxo-L-norleucine (diazo-
   oxonorleucine—antineoplastic)

don.
donec (L. until)

donec alv. sol. ft.
donec alvus soluta fuerit (L. until the
   bowels are open)

donec alv. sol. fuerit
donec alvus soluta fuerit (L. until the
   bowels are open)

DOPA, Dopa
3,4-dihydroxyphenylalanine (levodopa)

DOPAC
dihydroxyphenylacetic acid
   (homogentisic acid)

dopase
dopa oxidase

DOPC
determined osteogenic precursor cell

DOPE
disease-oriented physician education

DOPS
diffuse obstructive pulmonary syndrome

dor.
dorsal

dorm.
dormant

dorna
desoxyribose nucleic acid

dorsi.
dorsiflexion

dorsifl.
dorsiflexion

DORV
double outlet right ventricle

DOS
day of surgery
deoxystreptamine (component of
   certain antibiotics)
disk operation system (re: computers/
   data processing)

dos.
dosage
dosis (L. dose)

DOSC
Dubois oleic serum complex (re: Bact)

DOSS
dioctyl sodium sulfosuccinate (docusate
   sodium—re: industrial chemical; stool
   softener; surfactant)
distal over-shoulder strap

DOT
date of transcription
date of transfer

DOTES
Dosage Record and Treatment
   Emergent Symptom (Scale)

DOX
doxorubicin (re: chemotherapy)

doz.
dozen

DP
data processing
deep pulse
definitive procedure
degradation products
dementia precox (praecox)
dense plate
dental prosthetics
developed pressure
diaphragmatic plaque
diastolic pressure
diffuse precipitation
diffusion pressure
digestible protein
diphosgene (a war gas)
diphosphate

dipropionate
directional preponderance
disability pension
discriminating power
disopyramide phosphate
displaced person
distal pancreatectomy
distal phalanx
distopulpal (re: Dent)
donor's plasma
dorsalis pedis (pulse)
driving pressure
dynamic programming

DP, D.P.
dry pint

DP, dp
degree of polymerization (number of
monometric units in the polymer)

D-P
Depo-Provera (medroxyprogesterone
acetate)

2,4-DP
dichlorprop (herbicide)

Dp
dyspnea

dP
pressure difference

dp.
deltopectoral

d.p.
directione propria (L. with proper
direction)

DPA
Designed Plan Agencies (re: medical
records)
3',4'-dichloropropionanilide (herbicide)
diphenolic acid (industrial chemical)
diphenylamine (re: chemistry analysis
tests)
dipropylacetate (di-n-proplacetic acid;
valproic acid—re: anticonvulsant;
antiepileptic)
dynamic physical activity

DPA reaction
diphenylamine reaction (symptoms
similar to analine but less toxic)

DPB
days postburn

DPC
delayed primary closure
desaturated phosphatidylcholine
diethyl pyrocarbonate (DEPC—re:
esterifying agent; preservative for
wines, soft drinks)

direct patient care
distal palmar crease

DPD
desoxypyridoxine hydrochloride (inhibits
vitamin B_6)
diffuse pulmonary disease
diphenamid (diphenyl-
dimethlyacetamide—herbicide)

DPDL
diffuse poorly differentiated lymphoma

DPDT, dpdt
double-pole double-throw (switch)

dp/dt
ratio of change of ventricular pressure
to change in time (D = change)

DPE
Death Personification Exercise (re:
Psychol)
dipivalyl epinephrine (dipivefrin—
adrenergic; re: Ophth)

DPF
days postfarrowing (re: veterinary
medicine—swine)
diisopropyl fluorophosphate (DFP;
isoflurophate—re: ophthalmic
cholinergic)

DPFR
diastolic pressure-flow relationship

DPG
2,3-diphosphoglycerate (2,3-
bisphosphoglycerate—an
intermediate in glycolysis)
displacement placentogram

1,3-DPG
1,3-diphosphoglycerate

2,3-DPG
2,3-diphosphoglycerate (2,3-
bisphosphoglycerate)

DPGM
diphosphoglycerate mutase
(diphosphoglyceromutase)

DPGN
diffuse proliferative glomerulonephritis

DPGP
diphosphoglycerate phosphatase

DPH
Department of Public Health
diaphragm
diphenylhydantoin (Dilantin; phenytoin)

DPI
daily permissible intake
days post inoculation
dietary protein intake

diphtheria and pertussis immunization
drug prescribing index
Dynamic Personality Inventory

DPIP
2,6-dichlorophenol-indophenol sodium
(Tillman's reagent)

DPJ
dementia paralytica juvenilis

DPL
distopulpolingual (re: Dent)

DPLa
distopulpolabial (re: Dent)

DPM
discontinue previous medication

dpm, d.p.m.
disintegrations per minute

DPN
dermatosis papulosa nigra
diphosphopyridine nucleotide (nadide;
nicotinamide adenine dinucleotide—
alcohol and narcotic antagonist)

DPN+
diphosphopyridine nucleotide, oxidized

DPNase
diphosphopyridine nucleotide
hydrolyzing enzyme

DPNH
diphosphopyridine nucleotide (reduced
form—now called nicotinamide
adenine dinucleotide, reduced)

DPP
differential pulse polarography
2,6-dimethoxyphenylpenicillin sodium
salt (methicillin sodium—
antibacterial; veterinary—
antimicrobial)

DPPD
N,N'-diphenyl-*p*-phenylene-diamine
(anti-oxidant, industrial, agricultural)

DPPH
1,1-diphenyl-2-picrylhydrazyl (free
radical—re: analytic reagent for
reducing substances)

DPR
2,3-diaminopropionic acid (re: the salts
as growth inhibitors for
microorganisms)
doctor population ratio

DPS
dimethyl polysiloxane (simethicone—
antiflatulant)

dps
disintegrations per second

DPST, dpst
double-pole single-throw (switch)

DPT
department
dichotic pitch (discrimination) test
diphtheria, pertussis, tetanus (vaccine)
diphtheric pseudotabes
dipropyltryptamine (hallucinogen)

DPTA
diethylenetriamine penta-acetic acid
(iron-chelating agent)

DPTI
diastolic pressure time index

DPTP
diphtheria, pertussis, tetanus,
poliomyelitis

DPTPM
diphtheria, pertussis, tetanus,
poliomyelitis, measles

dptr.
diopter

DPV
different pulse voltametry

DPW
distal phalangeal width

DQ
deterioration quotient
developmental quotient (re: Ped)

DQ, D.Q.
dry quart

DR
Déjérine-Roussy (syndrome)
deoxyribose
diabetic retinopathy
diagnostic radiology
dining room
distribution ratio
dorsal raphe
dose ratio
drug receptor

DR, D.R.
delivery room
reaction of degeneration (re: muscle
fibers)

DR, dr.
dorsal root (of spinal nerves)

Dr
rare detail response (re: Psychol)

Dr.
doctor

dr
unusual rare detail response (re: Psychol)

dr.
drain
dram (drachm)
dressing

DRA
dextran-reactive antibody
disease-resistant antigen

dr. ap.
drachm (dram) apothecaries' (weight)

DRAT
differential rheumatoid agglutination test

DRB
daunorubicin (re: chemotherapy)

DRBC
dog red blood cell

DRC
damage risk criteria
dendritic reticulum cell
dog red (blood) cell

DRC$_1$, DRC$_2$, etc.
dorsal root, cervical

DRD
dorsal root dilator

DREF
dose reduction effectiveness factor

D reg.
diseased region

DRF
daily replacement factor (of lymphocytes)
dose reduction factor

DRG
diagnostic related group
disease-related group
dorsal respiratory group (re: neurons)
dorsal root ganglion (re: Neuro)

drg.
drainage
draining

DRI
direct rooming-in
Discharge Readiness Inventory

DRID
double radioisotope derivative

dRib
deoxyribose

DRL
differential reinforcement of low (response rates)

DRL #1, DRL #2, DRL$_1$, DRL$_2$, etc.
dorsal root, lumbar

D5RL
dextrose 5% with Ringer's lactate

DRLST
Del Rio Language Screening Test (re: Psychol)

DRMS
drug reaction monitoring system

DRN
dorsal raphe nucleus

drng.
drainage
draining

DRnt
diagnostic roentgenology

DRO
destructive read-out (re: computers)

DRP
digoxin reduction product
dorsal root potential

DRQ
discomfort relief quotient

DRR
dorsal root reflex

DRS
descending rectal septum
Diabetic Retinopathy Study
drowsiness
Dyskinesia Rating Scale

DRS$_1$, DRS$_2$, etc.
dorsal root, sacral

DRSG, drsg.
dressing

DRT$_1$ DRT$_2$, etc.
dorsal root, thoracic

DRTS
Dose Record and Treatment (Emergent) Symptom (scale)

DS
data set (re: computers)
dead (air) space (re: Resp)
Debré-Semelaigne (syndrome)
deep sedative
deep sleep
defined substrate
dehydroepiandrosterone sulfate
Déjérine-Sottas (syndrome)

delayed sensitivity
dendritic spine
density (optical) standard
deprivation syndrome
desynchronized sleep
diaphragm stimulation
difference spectroscopy
differential stimulus
diffuse scleroderma
digit span
digit symbol (test)
dilute strength (of solution)
dioptric strength
discrimination score
discriminative stimulus
disseminated sclerosis
dissolved solids
donor's serum
Doppler's sonography
double strength
double subordinance
Down's syndrome
driving signal
drug store
dry swallow (medication order)
duration of systole

DS, D/S, D/s
dextrose and (in) saline
dextrose and saline

DS, ds
double-stranded (DNA)

D/S
Doerfler-Stewart (test)
dominance and submission

D & S
dermatology and syphilology

D5S, D5/S, D-5-S
dextrose (5%) in saline

Ds
associative detail response to white
    space

D$_s$
symbol (re: carbonyl group)

DSA
digital subtraction angiography
disease-susceptible antigen

DSAP
disseminated superficial actinic
    porokeratosis

DSAS
discrete subaortic stenosis

Dsb
single-breath diffusing (capacity)

DSBL
disabled

DSBT
donor specific blood transfusion

DSC
decussation (of the) superior cerebellar
    (peduncles—re: Neuro)
differential scanning calorimeter
disodium cromoglycate (cromolyn—
    prophylactic antiasthmatic)

DSCB
data set control block

DSCF
Doppler-shifted constant frequency

DSCG
disodium cromoglycate (cromolyn—
    prophylactic antiasthmatic)

DSCT
dorsal spinocerebellar tract

DSD
depressed spectrum disease
depression sine depression
discharge summary dictated
dry sterile dressing

DSDB
direct self-destruction behavior

DSDDT
double sampling dye dilution technique

dsDNA
double-stranded DNA

DSDS
daughter sites of dimer strands

DSF
dry sterile fluff

DSG
dry sterile gauze

Dsg, dsg.
dressing

DSHR
delayed skin hypersensitivity reaction

DSI
Depression Status Inventory

DSIP
delta sleep-inducing peptide (rabbit)

DSL
data-set label (re: computers)

dslv.
dissolved

DSM
dextrose solution mixture
Diagnostic and Statistical Manual of
    Mental Disorders

dihydrostreptomycin (DHSM; DST—
  antibiotic)
dried skim milk
drink skim milk

d.s.n.
detur suo nomine (L. let it be given in
  his/her name)

DSO
distal subungual onychomycosis

DSP
decreased sensory perception
dibasic sodium phosphate (cathartic)

DSp
digit span

D-spine
dorsal spine

DSR
distal splenorenal
double simultaneous recording
dynamic spatial reconstructor

dsRNA
double-stranded ribonucleic acid

DSRS
distal splenorenal shunt

DSS
dengue shock syndrome
dioctyl sodium sulfosuccinate (stool
  softener; sodium salt as surfactant)
disability status scale
docusate sodium (stool softener)

DST
daylight saving time
desensitization test
desensitization time
dexamethasone suppression test
dihydrostreptomycin (DHSM; DSM—
  antibiotic)
disproportionate septal thickening
donor-specific transfusion

D-S test
Doerfler-Stewart test (re: Oto)

DSU
double setup

DSUH
direct suggestion under hypnosis

DSVP
downstream venous pressure

DSW
device status word (re: computers)

DSWI
deep surgical wound infection

DSy
digit symbol

DT
Déjérine-Thomas (syndrome)
delirium tremens
depression of transmission
differently tested
diphtheria-tetanus
diphtheria toxoid
discharge tomorrow
dispensing tablet
distance test (hearing)
dorsalis tibialis
double tachycardia
doubling time (of tumor size)
dye test

DT, D.T.
duration tetany

DT, dT
1-(2-deoxyribosyl)thymine (thymidine;
  thymine deoxyribuonucleoside)

D/T
date of treatment
deaths: total (ratio)

D/T, d.t.
due to

DTA
differential thermoanalysis

D tal. dos.
dentur tales doses (L. let such doses be
  given)

DTBC
D-tubocurarine (muscle relaxant)

DTBP
di-*tert*-butyl peroxide (polymerization
  catalyst)

DTC
day treatment center
differentiated thyroid carcinoma
D-tubocurarine (muscle relaxant)

d.t.d.
dentur tales doses (L. let such doses be
  given)
detur talis dosis (L. give such a dose)
dosis therapeutica die (L. daily
  therapeutic dose)

d.t.d. No. iv
dentur tales doses No. iv (L. let four
  such doses be given)

dTDP
thymidine diphosphate (thymidine 5'-
  diphosphate)

DTE
desiccated thyroid extract

DTF
Debré-de Toni-Fanconi (syndrome)
detector transfer function
9-dicyanomethylene-2,4,7-
    trinitrofluorene (re: aromatic
    hydrocarbons and amines)

DTH
delayed-type hypersensitivity (reaction)

dThd
1-(2-deoxyribosyl)thymine (thymidine;
    thymine deoxyribonucleoside)

DTIC
5(or 4)-(dimethyltriazeno)imidazole-4(or
    5)- carboxamide (dacarbazine; DIC—
    antineoplastic)

DTIC-ACT-D
DTIC (dacarbazine), actinomycin D
    (dactinomycin— re: chemotherapy)

DTICH
delayed traumatic intracerebral
    hemorrhage

D time
dream time

DTL
diode-transistor-logic (re: computers)

DTLA
Detroit Tests of Learning Aptitude

DTM
dermatophyte test medium

DTMC
di(p-chlorophenyl)
    trichloromethylcarbinol (dicofol—
    acaricide)

DTMP, dTMP
deoxythymidine monophosphate
    (thymidine-5′- phosphate; thymidine
    monophosphate; thymidylic acid)
thymidylate (salt or ester of thymidylic
    acid)

DTN
diphtheria toxin, normal

DTO
deodorized tincture of opium

Dtox
dosis toxica (L. toxic dose)

DTP
diethylenetriamine pentaacetic acid
    (pentetic acid; DTPA—iron chelating
    agent)
diphtheria, tetanus, pertussis

DTP, D.T.P.
distal tingling on percussion (Tinel's
    sign)

DTPA
diethylenetriamine pentaacetic acid
    (pentetic acid— chelating agent)

DTPT
dithiopropylthiamine (TPD; vitamin B_1
    propyl disulfide; prosultiamine—
    enzyme co-factor)

DTR
deep tendon reflex(es)
distribution tape reel (re: computers)

dtr.
daughter

DTR = & act.
deep tendon reflexes equal and active

DTR/NL
deep tendon reflexes within normal
    limits

DTRTT
digital temperature recovery time test

DTS
dense tubular system (re: skeletal and
    cardiac sarcolemma)
diphtheria toxin sensitivity

DTs, Dt's, dt's
delirium tremens

DTT
device for transverse traction
diagnostic and therapeutic team
diphtheria-tetanus toxoid
1,4-dithiothreitol (Cleland's reagent)

dTTP
desoxythymidine triphosphate
    (thymidine triphosphate; thymidine
    5′-triphosphate)

DTUS
diathermy, traction, and ultrasound

DTV
due to void

DT-VAC
diphtheria-tetanus vaccine

DTVMI
Developmental Test of Visual Motor
    Integration (re: Neuro)

DTVP
Developmental Test of Visual
    Perception (re: Psychol)

DTX
detoxification

d. tx. US
diathermy, traction, and ultrasound

DTZ
diatrizoate

DU
density (optical) unknown
deoxyuridine
dermal ulcer
diagnosis undetermined
5-diazouracil (re: cancer research)
dog unit (re: adrenal cortical hormones)
dose unit
duodenal ulcer

D$_U$
urea dialysance

du
dial unit

DUA
dorsal uterine artery

DUB
dysfunctional uterine bleeding

dUDP
deoxyuridine diphosphate

DUF
Doppler ultrasonic flowmeter

DUL
diffuse undifferentiated lymphoma

dulc.
dulcis (L. sweet)

DUM
dorsal unpaired median (axon; neuron)

DUMETi
dorsal unpaired median extensor tibia

DUMP, dUMP
deoxyuridine-5′-phosphate
(deoxyuridine monophosphate;
deoxyuridine phosphate)

D unit
unit of x-ray intensity equal to 102
roentgen (obsolete term)

duod.
duodenal
duodenum

dup
duplication (re: cytogenetics)

dup.
duplicate
duplication

DUR
drug use review

dur.
durante (L. duration; during)
durus (L. hard)

dur. dol.
durante dolore (L. while the pain lasts)

dur. dolor.
durante dolore (L. while the pain lasts)

DUSN
diffuse unilateral subacute neuroretinitis
("wipe-out" syndrome)

DUV
damaging ultraviolet

DV
dependent variable
difference in volume
difference of volume
dilute volume (of solution)
distemper virus
divorced
dorsoventral
dorsoventralis
double vision

DV, dv, d.v.
double vibrations

D&V
diarrhea and vomiting
disks and vessels (re: Ophth)
ductions and versions (re: Ophth)

DVA
distance visual acuity
duration of voluntary apnea (test)

D value
decimal reduction time

DVB
cis-diamminedichloroplatinum,
vindesine, bleomycin (re:
chemotherapy)

DVC
divanillalcyclohexanone (cyclovalone—
choleretic; cholagogue)

DVD
dissociated vertical deviation
(alternating sursumduction—re:
Ophth)
double vessel disease

DVDALV
double-vessel disease with abnormal
left ventricle

DVE
duck virus enteritis

DVI
digital vascular imaging
Doppler (systolic) velocity index

DVIS
digital vascular imaging system

dvlp.
develop
development

DVM
digital voltmeter (re: computers)

DVN
dorsal vagal nucleus

DVR
digital vascular reactivity
double valve replacement

DVT
deep vein thrombosis
deep venous thrombosis

DW
daily weight
doing well
dry weight
whole response to detail

DW, D/W
distilled water

D/W
dextrose in water
dry to wet

D5W, D5/W, D₅W, D-5-W, D-5/W
dextrose (5%) in water

D5%/W
5% dextrose in water

D5 & W
dextrose (5%) and water

D10W
10% dextrose in water

D wave
symbol re: electroretinogram

DWD
died with disease

DWDL
diffuse, well-differentiated lymphocytic
(lymphoma)

DWI
driving while intoxicated

DW, impro.
doing well, improving

DWT
deadweight ton
dichotic word test

dwt
denarius weight (L. denarius—a Roman
coin which was also used as a
measure of weight [pennyweight])

DX
dextran
dicloxacillin

DX, Dx, dx.
diagnosis

dx.
difficulties

↑ dx, ↗ dx
increased difficulties

DX.C.
detoxin complex (re: agricultural
chemical)

DXD, dxd.
discontinued

DXM
dexamethasone

DXR
deep x ray
doxorubicin (re: chemotherapy)

DXRT
deep x-ray therapy

DXT
deep x-ray therapy
dextrose

DY
Dyke-Young (syndrome)

Dy
dysprosium (element)

¹⁶⁵Dy
radioactive isotope of dysprosium

dyn
dyne (a centimeter-gram-second unit of
force)

dyn.
dynamics
dynamometer

dysp.
dyspnea
dyspneic

DZ
diazepam
dizygotic (re: cytogenetics)
dizygous (re: cytogenetics)

dizziness
Durand-Zunin (syndrome)

Dz
disease

dz.
dozen

DZAPO
daunorubicin, azacytidine, ara-C
(cytarabine), prednisone, and
Oncovin (vincristine) (re:
chemotherapy)

DZP
diazepam

E

E
air dose
cortisone (compound E)
each
east
Echinococcus (genus)
Echinostoma (genus)
edema
Eikenella (genus)
Eimeria (widespread genus—re: wildlife vertebrates, fowl, domesticated animals)
Einheit (Ger. unit)
einsteinium (element; obsolete abbreviation—Es now used)
elastance
electric(al) affinity
electric field vector
electrode potential
electromotive force
embryon (Gr. embryo)
emmetropia (re: Ophth)
endogenous
Endolimax (genus—nonpathogenic intestinal amoebic parasite)
Endomyces (genus—yeastlike fungus)
endoplasm
enema
energy
Entamoeba (genus)
Enterobacter (genus)
Enterobius (genus)
enterococcus
Enteromonas (genus)
enzyme
eosinophil(e)
epicondyle
Epidermophyton (genus)
epinephrine
error
Erwinia (genus—plant pathogen)
Erysipelothrix (genus)
erythrocyte
erythromycin
Escherichia (genus)
esophagus
esophoria (re: Ophth)
esophoria for distance (re: Ophth)
ester
estradiol
ethanol
ethyl
Eubacterium (genus)
exa- (prefix—attached to SI units)

examiner
exercise
experiment
experimental
experimenter
expiration
expired
expired gas (when written as a subscript [secondary symbol]—re: Resp)
extension
extinction (coefficient)
extraction fraction
extraction ratio
extralymphatic
eye
glutamic acid
glutamine
internal energy
kinetic energy of a particle
mathematical expectation
redox potential (oxidation-reduction potential)
vectorcardiography electrode (midsternal)
vitamin E

E, e
early
electric charge
electron

$\bar{E}$
average beta energy

E′
esophoria for near (re: Ophth)

E−, (*E*)−
entgegen (Ger. opposite— stereodescriptor; equivalent to *trans* in simple cases)

E°
symbol for standard potential

E^1
esophoria, near viewing (re: Ophth)

E$_1$, E$_2$, E$_3$, etc.
those generations following some experimental manipulation (re: genetics)

E$_1$
estrone

E_2
estradiol

E3
lachesine chloride (a muscarine
    agonist—re: Neuro)

E_3
estriol

E_4
estetrol (estrogen produced in fetus)

4E
four plus edema

E_{10}
tocoquinone-10

e
base of Naperian (natural) logarithms
    $(= 2.71828)$
electron charge
elementary charge
symbol for base of natural logarithms

e, e.
ex (L. from, out of)

e^+
symbol for positron

$e-$
internal conversion electron (re:
    radioactive isotopes)

e^-
symbol for a negative electron

ϵ
dielectric constant
epsilon (fifth letter of Greek alphabet—
    lower case)
heavy chain of IgE
molar absorptivity
molar extinction coefficient
    (concentrated in gram moles per liter)
permittivity (dielectric constant)

η
eta (seventh letter of Greek alphabet,
    lower case)
viscosity

EA
early antigen
educational age
egg albumin
elbow aspiration
electric affinity
electroacupuncture
electroanesthesia
electrophysiological abnormality
embryonic antigen
endocardiographic amplifier
enteral alimentation
enteroanastomosis

enzymatic active
erythrocyte antibody
erythrocyte antisera
esterase activity
estivoautumnal (malaria)
ethacrynic acid

E&A
evaluate and advise

E→A
"E to A" (egophony—re: pulmonary
    consolidation— all vowels including
    "e" heard as "ah" through
    stethoscope; Shibley's sign)

E_α
kinetic energy of an alpha particle

ea.
each

EAA
electroacupuncture analgesia
essential amino acid(s)
extrinsic allergic alveolitis

Ea antigens
encoded allogenes (by certain mouse
    genes—re: genetics)

EAB
elective abortion

EABV
effective arterial blood volume

EAC
Ehrlich ascites carcinoma
electroacupuncture
erythema action (spectrum)
erythema annulare centrifugum
erythrocyte antibody complement
erythrocyte coated by antibody and
    complement
eudismic affinity correlation
external auditory canal

EACA
ϵ-aminocaproic acid (hemostatic)

EACD
eczematous allergic contact dermatitis

EAD
extracranial arterial disease

ead.
eadem (L. the same)

EAE
experimental allergic encephalitis
experimental allergic encephalomyelitis
experimental autoimmune encephalitis
experimental autoimmune
    encephalomyelitis

EAG
electroantennogram
electroatriogram

EAHF
eczema, asthma, hay fever (complex)

EAHLG
equine antihuman-lymphoblast globulin

EAHLS
equine antihuman-lymphoblast serum

EAI
erythrocyte antibody inhibition

EAK
ethyl amyl ketone (solvent)

EAM
external acoustic meatus
external auditory meatus

EAMG
experimental autoimmune myasthenia
   gravis

EAN
experimental allergic neuritis

EAO
experimental allergic orchitis

EAP
electroacupuncture
epiallopregnanolone (androgen in
   pregnancy urine)
erythrocyte acid phosphatase
evoked action potential

EAPFS
electron appearance potential fine
   structure

EAQ
eudismic affinity quotient

e-aq
aqueous electron

EAR
electroencephalographic audiometry
expired air resuscitation

EaR, Ea R, Ea. R.
Entartungsreaktion (Ger. reaction of
   degeneration)

EAT
Edinburgh Articulation Test (re: Psychol)
Education Apperception Test
Ehrlich ascites tumor
electroaerosol therapy
epidermolysis acuta toxica
experimental autoimmune thymitis
experimental autoimmune thyroiditis

EATC
Ehrlich ascites tumor cell

EAV
equine abortion virus
extra-alveolar vessel

EAVM
extramedullary arteriovenous
   malformation

EB
east bound (re: motor vehicle accident)
elbow bearing
epidermolysis bullosa
Epstein-Barr (virus)
esophageal body
estradiol benzoate
Evans blue (dye)

EB, E.B.
elementary body (bodies [old term for
   virions, especially largest virus
   particles])

EBA
epidermolysis bullosa atrophicans

EBC
esophageal balloon catheter

EBCDIC
extended binary coded decimal
   interchange code (re: computers)

EBD
epidermolysis bullosa dystrophica

EBDD
epidermolysis bullosa dystrophica
   dominant

EBDGP
epidermolysis bullosa dystrophica
   generalisata Pasini

EBDR
epidermolysis bullosa dystrophica
   recessive

EBF
erythroblastosis fetalis

EBG
electroblepharogram

EBI
emetine and bismuth iodide
   (antiamoebic)
erythroblastic islands
estradiol-binding index

EBK
embryonic bovine kidney

EBL
erythroblastic leukemia
estimated blood loss

EBL/S
estimated blood loss/surgery

EBM
expressed breast milk

EBNA
Epstein-Barr nuclear antigen

E/BOD
electrolytic biological oxygen demand

EBP
epidural blood patch
estradiol-binding protein

EBR
electron beam recording (re:
    computers/data processing)

EBS
elastic back strap
electric brain stimulator
epidermolysis bullosa simplex

EBSS
Earle's balanced salt solution

EBT
p-ethylsulfonylbenzaldehyde
    thiosemicarbazone (subathizone—re:
    antitubercular)
external beam (photon) therapy

EBV
effective blood volume
Epstein-Barr virus

EBVDNA
Epstein-Barr virus-determinated nuclear
    antigen

EBZ
epidermal basement zone

EC
effect of closing (of eyes—re: EEGs)
effective concentration
ejection click
electrochemical
electron capture
Ellis-van Creveld (syndrome)
embryonal carcinoma
emetic center
endothelial cell
enteric-coated (tablets)
entering complaint
enterochromaffin cells
entorhinal cortex
entrance complaint
environmental complexity
Enzyme Commission (of the
    International Union of Biochemistry)
enzyme-treated cell
epidermal cell
epithelial cell
equalization-cancellation

Erb-Charcot (syndrome)
error correcting (re: computers)
Escherichia coli
esophageal carcinoma
ether and chloroform
excitation-contraction
experimental control
expiratory center
external carotid
external conjugate
extracellular
extracellular concentration
extracranial
extruded cell
eye care
eyes closed

E-C
ether-choloroform (mixture)

E/C
endo/cystoscopy
estriol/creatinine
estrogen to creatinine (ratio)

EC #(___)
Empirin with codeine gr.___

EC$_{50}$
median effective concentration

ECA
electrical control activity
electrocardioanalyzer
enterobacterial common antigen
ethacrynic acid (diuretic)
ethylcarboxylate adenosine
external carotid artery

ECAO virus
enteric cytopathogenic avian orphan
    virus

ECB
electric cabinet bath

ECBO
enteric cytopathogenic bovine orphan
    (virus)

ECBO virus
enteric cytopathogenic bovine orphan
    virus

ECBV
effective circulating blood volume

ECC
electrocorticogram
embryonal cell carcinoma
emergency cardiac care
endocervical cone
endocervical curettage
estimated creatinine clearance
external cardiac compression
extracorporeal circulation
extrusion of cell cytoplasm

ECCE
extracapsular cataract extraction (re: Ophth)

E-C coupling
excitation-contraction coupling (re: muscles)

ECCO virus
enteric cytopathogenic cat orphan virus

ECD
electrochemical detection
electrochemical detector
electron capture detector
endocardial cushion defect
enzymatic cell dispersion

ECDB
encourage to cough and deep breathe

EC detector
electron capture detector

ECDEU
early clinical drug evaluation unit

ECDO
enteric cytopathic dog orphan (virus)
enteric cytopathogenic dog orphan (virus)

ECE
equine conjugated estrogen

ECEO virus
enteric cytopathogenic equine orphan virus

ECES
Education and Career Exploration System (re: psychological testing)

ECF
East Coast fever
effective capillary flow
eosinophilic chemotactic factors
erythroid colony formation
Escherichia coli filtrate
extended care facility
extracellular fluid

ECFA, ECF-A
eosinophil chemotactic factor of anaphylaxis

ECF-C
eosinophil chemotactic factor-complement

ECFV
extracellular fluid volume

ECG
electrocardiogram
electrocardiograph

ECGF
endothelial cell growth factor

ECGS
endothelial cell growth supplement

ECHO
echocardiography
enteric cytopathogenic human orphan (virus)
enterocytopathogenic human orphan (virus)
etoposide, cyclophosphamide, hydroxydaunomycin (doxorubicin), and Oncovin (vincristine) (re: chemotherapy)

ECHO, echo
echocardiogram
echoencephalogram (sonoencephalogram)

Echo EG
echoencephalogram

ECHO virus
enterocytopathogenic human orphan virus

ECI
electrocerebral inactivity
extracorporeal irradiation (of blood)

ECIB
extracorporeal irradiation of blood

ECIL
extracorporeal irradiation of lymph

ECK
extracellular kalium (potassium)

ECL
electrogenerated chemiluminescence
emitter-coupled logic
enterochromaffin-like
euglobulin clot lysis

eclamp.
eclampsia

Eclec, eclec.
eclectic

ECLT
euglobulin clot lysis time

ECM
embryo chicken muscle
erythema chronicum migrans (re: Lyme disease)
external cardiac massage
external chemical messenger
extracellular material
extracellular matrix

E-C mixture
ether-chloroform mixture

ECMO
enteric cytopathic monkey orphan
  (virus)
enteric cytopathogenic monkey orphan
  (virus)
extracorporeal membrane oxygenation
extracorporeal membrane oxygenator

ECMP
entero-coated microspheres of
  pancrelipase

E.C. No.
Enzyme Commission Number

ECochG
electrocochleography

ECoG
electrocorticogram
electrocorticography

E coli, E. coli
Escherichia coli

econ.
economic
economics

Eco RI
restriction endonuclease from *E. coli*
  (re: molecular genetics)

Eco RII
restriction endonuclease from *E. coli*
  (re: molecular genetics)

ECP
effector cell precursor
endocardial potential
eosinophil cationic protein
erythrocyte coproporphyrin
erythroid committed precursor
Escherichia coli polypeptides
estradiol 17-cyclopentanepropionate
  (estradiol 17β- cypionate)
estradiol 17β-cyclopentanepropionate
external cardiac pressure
external counterpulsation
free cytoporphyrin in erythrocytes

ECPO
enteric cytopathogenic porcine orphan
  (virus)

ECPOG
electrochemical potential gradient

ECPR
external cardiopulmonary resuscitation

ECR
electrocardiographic response
error cause removal

ECRB
extensor carpi radialis brevis

ECRL
extensor carpi radialis longus

ECRO virus
enteric cytopathogenic rodent orphan
  virus

ECS
elective cosmetic surgery
electrocerebral silence
electroconvulsive shock
extracellular space

ECSO virus
enteric cytopathic swine orphan virus
enteric cytopathogenic swine orphan
  virus

ECSP
epidermal cell surface protein

ECT
electroconvulsive (electroshock)
  therapy
emission computerized tomographic
  (scanner)
enteric-coated tablet
euglobin clot test
euglobulin clot test
extracellular tissue

ect.
ectopic

ECTEOLA-celluose
epichlorhydrine and triethanolamine
  (treated) cellulose (re: anion
  exchange)

ECU
Environmental Control Unit
extended care unit
extensor carpi ulnaris

ECV
extracellular volume
extracorporeal volume

ECVD
extracellular volume of distribution

ECVE
extracellular volume expansion

ECW
extracellular water

ED
early differentiation
ectodermal dysplasia
ectopic depolarization
effective dose
Ehlers-Danlos syndrome
elbow disarticulation
electrodiagnosis
electrodialysis
electron diffraction

elemental diet
embryonic death
Emergency Department
emotional disturbance
entering diagnosis
Entner-Doudoroff (metabolic pathway—
   re: bacterial metabolism)
enzymatic deficiencies
epidural
epileptiform discharge
equilibrium dialysis
erythema dose
ethynodiol (oral contraceptive in
   combination with estrogen; diacetate
   form as a progestin)
evidence of disease
exertional dyspnea
extensor digitorum
external diameter
external dyspnea
extra-low dispersion

ED₅₀
median effective dose

Ed, ed.
editor

E_d
depth dose

ed.
edema
edition

EDA
electrodermal audiometry
electrolyte-deficient agar
electron-donor-acceptor (interaction)

EDAX
energy dispersive x-ray analysis

EDB
early dry breakfast
ethylene dibromide (fumigant)
extensor digitorum brevis

EDBP
erect diastolic blood pressure

EDC
end-diastolic count
estimated date of conception
estimated date of confinement
ethylene dichloride (industrial solvent;
   fumigant)
expected date of confinement
expected delivery, cesarean
extensor digitorum communis

ED&C
electrodesiccation and curettage

EDCI
energetic dynamic cardiac insufficiency

EDCS
end-diastolic chamber stiffness
end-diastolic circumferential stress

EDCT
early distal proximal tubule

EDD
effective drug duration
end-diastolic dimension
enzyme-digested delta (endotoxin)
estimated due date
expected date of delivery

edem. turb.
edematous turbinates

EDEN
Evaluation Disposition (Toward the)
   Environment (re: psychological
   testing)

edent.
edentulous

EDF
extradural fluid

EDG
electrodermography

EDH
extradural hematoma

EDICP
electron-dense iron-containing particle

EDIM
epidemic disease of infant mice
epizootic diarrhea of infant mice

E-diol
estradiol

edit.
editorial

EDL
end-diastolic (segment) length
end-diastolic load
extensor digitorum longus

ED/LD
emotionally disturbed/learning disabled

EDM
early diastolic murmur
extramucosal duodenal myotomy

EDMA
ethylene glycol dimethacrylate
   (hydroxyethyl methacrylate—re:
   optics)

EDN
electrodesiccation

EDOC
estimated date of confinement

EDP
electron dense particles
electronic data processing
end-diastolic pressure

EDPA
2-ethyl-3,3-diphenyl-2-propenylamine
(central stimulant; antihypotensive)

EDQ
extensor digiti quinti

EDR
early diastolic relaxation
effective direct radiation
electrodermal response
electrodialysis (with) reversed (polarity)

EDS
edema disease of swine
Ego Development Scale
Ehlers-Danlos syndrome
energy-dispersive spectrometer
excessive daytime sleepiness
extradimensional shift

EDT
end-diastolic (cardiac wall) thickness

EDTA
ethylenediaminetetraacetic acid
(edathamil; edetic acid— re:
chelating agent)

educ.
education
educational

EDV
end-diastolic volume

EDVI
end-diastolic volume index

EDWGT
emergency drinking water germicidal
tablet

EDWTH
end-diastolic wall thickness

EDX, EDx, E Dx
electrodiagnosis

EDXA
energy-dispersive x-ray analysis

EE
embryo extract
end to end (anastomosis)
end expiration
energy expenditure
Enterobacteriaceae enrichment (broth)
equine encephalitis
expressed emotion
external ear
eye and ear

E-E
erythematous-edematous (reaction)

E & E
eyes and ears

EEA
electroencephalic audiometry
elemental enteral alimentation
end-to-end anastomotic (device)

EEC
ectrodactyly-ectodermal dysplasia-
clefting (ectrodactyly, ectodermal
dysplasia, clefting [syndrome])
enteropathogenic *Escherichia coli*

EECD
endothelial-epithelial corneal dystrophy

EECG
electroencephalogram
electroencephalography

EEDQ
N-ethoxycarbonyl-2-ethoxy-1,2-
dihydroquinoline (re: synthesis of
peptides)

EEE
eastern equine encephalomyelitis
experimental enterococcal endocarditis
external eye exam

EEEP
end-expiratory esophageal pressure

EEE virus
eastern equine encephalomyelitis virus

EEG
electroencephalogram
electroencephalograph

EEGA
electroencephalographic audiometry

EELS
electron energy loss spectroscopy

EEM
erythema exudativum multiforme

EEME
17α-ethynylestradiol 3-methyl ether
(mestranol— oral contraceptive)

EE3ME
17α-ethynylestradiol 3-methyl ether
(mestranol— oral contraceptive)

EEMG
evoked electromyogram

EENT, E.E.N.T.
eye(s), ear(s), nose, throat

EEP
end-expiratory pressure
equivalent effective photon

EEPI
extraretinal eye position information

EER
electroencephalic response
electroencephalographic response

EES, E.E.S.
erythromycin ethylsuccinate

EESG
evoked electrospinogram

EF
ectopic focus
edema factor
ejection factor
ejection fraction
elastic fibril
electric field
elongation factor
embedded figures
embryo-fetal
emotional factor
encephalitogenic factor
endothoracic fascia
endurance factor
eosinophilic factor
epithelial focus
equivalent focus
erythroblastosis fetalis
erythrocyte fragmentation
essential findings
exposure factor
extended field (re: radiotherapy)
extra fine
extra food
extrinsic factor

EF-2
an elongation factor (re: protein
   synthesis)

EFA
essential fatty acids
extrafamily adoptees

EFAD
essential fatty acid deficient

EFC
elastin fragment concentration
endogenous fecal calcium
ephemeral fever of cattle

EFE
endocardial fibroelastosis

EFF
efficiency

eff.
effect

effective
effects
efferent
efficient
effusion

effect.
effective

effer.
efferent

EFFU
epithelial focus-forming unit

EF-G
an elongation factor (re: protein
   synthesis)

EFL
effective focal length
external fluid loss

E. floccosum
Epidermophyton (genus; *floccosum* is
   the only species— re: tinea pedis)

EFM
electronic fetal monitor(ing)
external fetal monitor

EFP
effective filtration pressure
endoneural fluid pressure

EFPS
epicardial fat pad sign

EFR
effective filtration rate

EFS
electric field stimulation
electric foot shock

EFT
Embedded Figures Test (re: Psychol)

EF-T
an elongation factor (re: protein
   synthesis)

EF-Tu
an elongation factor (re: protein
   synthesis)

EFV
extracellular fluid volume

EFVC
expiratory flow-volume curve (re: Resp)

EFW
estimated fetal weight

EG
enteroglucagon
Erb-Goldflam (syndrome)

esophagogastrectomy
external genitalia

EG-1
eukaryote amino acid binder (re: protein
  synthesis)

e.g.
exempli gratia (L. for example)

EGA
estimated gestational age

E-Game
"E" card is used to test visual acuity of
  children or non-English-speaking
  clients

EGAT
Educational Goal Attainment Tests (re:
  Psychol)

EGC
early gastric cancer
epithelioid A globoid cells

EGD
esophagogastroduodenoscopy

EGDF
embryonic growth and development
  factor

EGF
epidermal growth factor

EGFR
epidermal growth factor, receptor (re:
  genetics)

EGF-URO
epidermal growth factor-urogastrone

EGG
electrogastrogram
electrogastrography

EGH
equine growth hormone

EGL
eosinophilic granuloma of the lung

EGLT
euglobulin lysis time

EGM
electrogram
extracellular granular material

EGN
experimental glomerulonephritis

EGOT
erythrocyte glutamic oxaloacetic
  transaminase

EGR
erythrocyte glutathione reductase

EGT
ethanol gelation test

EGTA
esophageal gastric tube airway

EH
early healed
enteral hyperalimentation
environment and heredity
epidermolytic hyperkeratosis
essential hypertension

EH, e.h.
enlarged heart

E&H
environment and heredity (re:
  psychology/psychiatry)

E_h, eH
oxidation-reduction potential (redox
  potential—more commonly used now
  are E_O+ and E^O)

EHAA
epidemic hepatitis-associated antigen

EHB
elevate head of bed

EHBA
extrahepatic biliary atresia

EHBD
extrahepatic bile duct

EHBF
estimated hepatic blood flow
exercise hyperemia blood flow
extrahepatic blood flow
extrahepatic blood flow (clearance)

EHC
enterohepatic circulation
enterohepatic clearance
essential hypercholesterolemia
extended health care
extrahepatic cholestasis

EHD
electrohemodynamics
epizootic hemorrhage disease (re:
  poultry)

EHDP
ethane-1-hydroxy-1,1-diphosphonic acid
  (both free acid and disodium salt;
  etidronic acid; ethane
  hydroxydiphosphate—chelating
  agent; bone cancer regulator)

EHF
epidemic hemorrhagic fever (Far
  Eastern, Korean, Manchurian
  hemorrhagic fever; Korin fever;
  Songo fever)
exophthalmos-hyperthyroid factor

extremely high factor
extremely high frequency

EHL
effective half-life (of radioactive
    substances)
endogenous hyperlipidemia
essential hyperlipidemia
extensor hallucis longus

EHMS
electrohydrodynamic ionization mass
    spectrometry

EHNA
erythro-9-(2-hydroxy-3-nanyl)adenine

EHO
extrahepatic obstruction

EHP
effective horsepower
excessive heat production
extra high potency

EHPH
extrahepatic portal hypertension

EHPT
Eddy hot plate test

EHSDS
Experimental Health Services Delivery
    Systems (re: medical records)

EHT
essential hypertension

EHV
electric heat vector
equine herpes virus

EI
electrolyte imbalance
electron impact
electron ionization
emotionally impaired (re: Psychol)
enzyme inhibitor
eosinophilic index
excretory index
external intervention

E/I
expiration-inspiration (ratio)

EIA
electroimmunoassay
enzyme immunoassay(s)
equine infectious anemia
exercise-induced asthma

EIAB
extracranial-intracranial arterial bypass

EIB
exercise-induced bronchoconstriction
exercise-induced bronchospasm

EIC
elastase inhibitory capacity
enzyme inhibitor complex

EICDT
Ego-Ideal and Conscience
    Development Test

EID
egg-infective dose
electroimmunodiffusion
electronic induction desorption

EIEC
enteroinvasive *Escherichia coli*

EIF
eukaryotic initiation factor (re: protein
    synthesis)

eIF-1, eIF-2, etc.
eukaryotic initiation factors (re: protein
    synthesis)

EIM
excitability-inducing material

EIMS
electron ionization mass spectrometry

EIP
end-inspiratory pause
extensor indicis proprius

EIPS
endogenous inhibitor of prostaglandin
    synthase

EIRnv
extra-incidence rate in nonvaccinated
    (groups)

EIRv
extra-incidence rate in vaccinated
    (groups)

EIS
endoscopic injection sclerosis

EISA
electroencephalogram interval
    spectrum analysis

EIT
erythroid iron turnover

EIV
external iliac vein

EJ, Ej
elbow jerk

EJB
ectopic junctional beat

EJP
excitatory junction potential

ejusd.
ejusdem (L. of the same)

EK
electrokardiogram (electrocardiogram)
enterokinase
erythrokinase

EKC
epidemic keratoconjunctivitis

EKG
electrokardiogram (electrocardiogram)
electrokardiograph (electrocardiograph)

EKV
erythrokeratoderma variabilis

EKY
electrokymogram
electrokymograph

EL
early latent
Eaton-Lambert (syndrome)
egg lecithin
electroluminescence
elopement (status—re: Psychol)
erythroleukemia
exercise limit
external lamina

EL, El, el.
elixir (Arabic via late Latin—elixir)

EL1
elliptocytosis-1 (re: genetics)

El
elastase

el.
elbow

ELA
elastomer lubricating agent
endotoxin-like activity

ELB
early light breakfast
elbow lock billet (re: Ortho)

elb.
elbow

ELBW
extremely low birth weight

ELD
egg lethal dose

El Dx
electrodiagnosis (re: physiatry)

elec.
electric
electrical
electricity

elect.
elective
electric
electuarium (L. electuary—a medium
   which melts in the mouth; a
   confection)

elect. surg.
elective surgery

elem.
elementary

elev.
elevate
elevation
elevator

ELF
elective low forceps

ELH
egg-laying hormone

ELI
exercise lability index (re: asthma)

ELIA
enzyme-labeled immunoassay

ELIEDA
enzyme-linked immuno-electrodiffusion
   assay

ELISA
enzyme-linked immunoadsorbent assay
enzyme-linked immunosorbent assay
enzyme-linked immunospecific assay

elix.
elixir (Arabic via Late Latin—elixir)

ELM
external limiting membrane

ELN
electronic noise

ELP
early labeled peak
elastase-like protein
endogenous limbic potential
Estimated Learning Potential (re:
   Psychol)

ELR
equal listener response (scale—re:
   acoustics)

ELS
Eaton-Lambert syndrome
electron loss spectroscopy
extralobar sequestration

ELT
euglobulin lysis test
euglobulin lysis time

ELU
extended length of utterance

ELV
erythroid leukemia-inducing virus

Elx
elixir (Arabic via late Latin—elixir)

EM
early memory
ejection murmur
electron micrograph
electron microscope
electron microscopy
electrophoretic mobility
emotionally (disturbed)
emphysema
end of medium character (re:
    computers/data processing)
erythema multiforme
erythrocyte mass
erythromycin
esophageal manometry
esophageal motility
excreted mass

EM, Em, em.
emmetropia (normal vision)

EM, em.
electromagnetic

E-M
Embden-Meyerhof ([glycolytic]
    pathway—re: glucose metabolism)

E&M
endocrine and metabolic
endocrine and metabolism

E of M
error of measurement

e/m
ratio of charge (of an electron) to mass

EMA
electronic microanalyzer
epithelial membrane antigen

EMAD
equivalent mean age at death (re:
    statistics)

eman
eman(anation)—equivalent to 10^{-10}
    curie per liter

E^{max}
maximum energy of a beta spectrum

EMB
engineering in medicine and biology
eosin-methylene blue (agar)
ethambutol (antibacterial;
    tuberculostatic)
ethambutol-Myambutol

explosive mental behavior
explosive motor behavior (re: Neuro)

EMB, Emb, emb.
embryology

emb.
embolus
embryo

EMBASE
Excerpta Medica database

embry.
embryology

embryol.
embryology

EMC
electron microscopy
encephalomyocarditis
essential mixed cryoglobulinemia

EMCRO
Experimental Medical Care Review
    Organization

EMC virus
encephalomyocarditis virus

EMD
esophageal mobility disorder

EMEM
Eagle's minimal essential medium

emend.
emendatis (L. emended)

EMER
electromagnetic molecular electronic
    resonance

emer.
emergency

emerg.
emergency

EMF
electromagnetic flowmeter
endomyocardial fibrosis
erythrocyte maturation factor
evaporated milk formula

EMF, E.M.F.
erythrocyte maturation force

EMF, emf
electromotive force

EMG
electromyelography
electromyogram
electromyograph
electromyography
exomphalos, macroglossia, and

giantism (Beckwith- Wiedemann syndrome)
eye movement gauge

EMGN
extramembranous glomerulonephritis

EMI
Electric and Musical Industries (manufacturer of first scanner for CAT)
electromagnetic interference

EMIC
emergency maternity and infant care

EMIT
enzyme-multiplied immunoassay technique
enzyme-multiplied immunoassay test

EMJH
Ellinghausen, McCullough, Johnson, Harris (medium)

EML
effective mandibular length

EMLD
external muscle layer damage(d)

EMM
erythema multiforme major

EMMA
eye-movement measuring apparatus

emot.
emotion
emotional

EMP
electromagnetic pulse
Embden-Meyerhof-Parnas (pathway— Embden-Meyerhof)
Embden-Meyerhof pathway (re: glucose metabolism)
epimacular proliferation
external membrane protein
extramedullary plasmacytoma

Emp
Empirin

emp.
emplastrum (L. a plaster)
employee
employer
employment

e.m.p.
ex modo praescripto (L. in [or] after the manner prescribed; as directed)

Emp comp.
Empirin compound (discontinued from market)

EMPEP
erythrocyte membrane protein electrophoretic pattern

emph.
emphysema

emphys.
emphysema

empl.
employee
employer
employment

EMPP
4'-ethyl-2-methyl-3-piperidino-propiophenone (muscle relaxant)

emp. vesic.
emplastrum vesicatorium (L. a blistering plaster)

EMQ
6-ethoxy-1,2-dihydro-2,2,4-trimethylquinoline (ethoxyquin—anti-oxidant)

EMR
educable mentally retarded
electromagnetic radiation
ethanol metabolic rate
eye movement recording

EMS
early morning specimen
early morning stiffness
electrical muscle stimulation
Emergency Medical Service
emergency medical system
ethyl methanesulfonate (ethyl methanesulfonic acid; ethyl mesylate—re: experimental mutagen)
extramedullary site

EMT
emergency medical team

EMTP
N-ethyl-α-methyl-m-(trifluoromethyl)phenethylamine (fenfluramine—an anorectic)

EMU
early morning urine

EMU, emu
electromagnetic unit

emul.
emulsion

emuls.
emulsio (L. an emulsion)

EMV
eyes, motor, voice (Glascow Coma Scale—1 through 6—re: Neuro)

E$_2$, M$_3$, V$_2$, etc.
eyes, motor, voice (Glasgow Coma
    Scale—1 through 6—re: Neuro)

EMVC
early mitral valve closure

EN
electronarcosis (re: psychiatry)
endocardial
enteral nutrition
erythema nodosum

EN, en.
enema

E 50% N
extension 50% of normal

en.
ethylenediamine (industrial chemical;
    pharmaceutical aid)

ENA
extractable nuclear antigens

END
elective node dissection
enhancement Newcastle disease

end
endoreduplication (re: cytogenetics)

Endo
endocardium
endodontics

endo.
endocardial
endocrine
endocrinology
endotracheal

endocr.
endocrine
endocrinology

Endocrin, endocrin.
endocrinology

ENDOR
electron nuclear double resonance

endos.
endosteal

endost.
endosteal

endo-trach
endotracheal

ENE, E.N.E.
ethylnorepinephrine (bronchodilator)

ENEM, enem.
enema

ENG
electroneurography
electronystagmogram
electronystagmograph
electronystagmography

ENI
elective neck irradiation

ENIAC
electronic numerical integrator and
    computer

ENK
enkephalin

ENL
erythema nodosum leprosum
erythema nodosum leprosy
erythema nodosum leproticum

enl.
enlarge
enlarged
enlargement

ENO1
enolase-1 (re: genetics)

ENO2
enolase-2 (re: genetics)

Eno
enolase

ENQ
enquiry character (re: computers/data
    processing)

ENR
eosinophilic nonallergic rhinitis
extrathyroidal neck radioactivity

ENS
enteric nervous system

E.N.S.
ethylnorsuprarenin
    (ethylnorepinephrine—a broncho-
    dilator)

ENT
extranodal tissue
extranodular tissue

ENT, E.N.T.
ear(s), nose, and throat

Entom, entom.
entomology

ENU
N-ethyl-N-nitrosourea (mutagen;
    ethylating agent)

environ.
environment
environmental

enz.
enzymatic
enzyme

EO
effect of opening (of eyes—re: EEG)
elbow orthosis
eosinophilia
ethylene oxide
eyes open

EO, eo.
eosinophil (leukocyte)

E_O
electric affinity
skin dose (re: radiation therapy)

$E_o{}^+$
oxidation-reduction potential

ϵ_O
permittivity of free space
permittivity of vacuum (ratio of electric
   displacement to electric field strength
   when no polarization is present)

EOA
effective orifice area
end of address (code—re: computers/
   data processing)
erosive osteoarthritis
esophageal obturator airway
examination, opinion, and advice

EOB
emergency observation bed
end of block (code—re: computers/data
   processing)

EOD
electric organ discharge
entry on duty

EOD, eod, e.o.d.
every other day

EOE
ethiodized oil emulsion (re: CT contrast)

EOF
end of file (re: computers)

EOG
electro-oculography
electro-olfactogram

EOG, eog.
electro-oculogram

EOJ
end of job (re: computers)
extrahepatic obstructive jaundice

EOL
end of life

EOM
end of message (code—re: computers/
   data processing)
equal ocular movements
error of measurement (re: statistics)
external otitis media
extraocular motion
extraocular movement(s)
extraocular muscles

EOM F & Conj
extraocular movements full and
   conjugate

EOMI
extraocular muscles intact

EOP
efficiency of plating
emergency outpatient

EOR
exclusive OR (re: binary logic)

EOS, Eos, eos.
eosinophils

Eosins, eosins
eosinophils

EOT
effective oxygen transport
end of tape (marker—re: computers/
   data processing)
end of text (re: computers)
end of transmission (character—re:
   computers/data processing)

EOU
epidemic observation unit

EP
ectopic pregnancy
edible portion (re: food)
electrophoresis
electrophysiologic
electroprecipitin
emergency physician
endogenous pyrogen
endoperoxide
endpoint
enteropeptidase
enzyme product
eosinophilic pneumonitis
ependymal (cell)
epicardial
epithelioid
erythrocyte protoporphyrin
erythrophagocytosis
erythropoietic porphyria
esophageal pressure
evoked potential (re: EEG)
extreme pressure

EP, Ep
erythropoietin (erythropoiesis
   stimulating factor)

EP, ep.
epithelial
epithelium

EPA
eicosapentaenoic acid (5,8,11,14,17-
eicosapentaenoic acid—re:
prostaglandin biosynthesis, marine
food chain)
erect posterior-anterior
ethylphenacemide (anticonvulsant)
exact posteroanterior (position)
exophthalmos-producing activity
extrinsic plasminogen activator

Epa antigen
alloantigens specific to epidermal cells
(mouse—re: genetics)

EPAP
expiratory airway pressure

EPAQ
Extended Personal Attributes
Questionnaire

EPB
extensor pollicis brevis

EPC
end-plate current
epilepsia partialis continua
external pneumatic compression

EPCA
external pressure circulatory
assist(ance)

Ep cells, ep. cells
epithelial cells

EPCG
endoscopic pancreatocholangiography

EPD
effective pressor dose

EPDML
epidemiological
epidemiologist
epidemiology

EPE
erythropoietin-producing enzyme

EPEA
expense per equivalent admission

EPEC
enteropathogenic (strains of)
Escherichia coli

EPF
early pregnancy factor
endocarditis parietalis fibroplastica
endothelial proliferating factor
exophthalmos-producing factor

EPG
eggs per gram (re: parasitology)
electropneumogram
electropneumograph

EPH
edema, proteinuria, hypertension
extensor proprius hallucis

ephed.
ephedrine

EPH gestosis
edema, proteinuria, hypertension
gestosis (re: OB)

EPI
Emotions Profile Index
epileptic
epithelial
epithelium
epitympanic
evoked potential index
extrapyramidal involvement
Eysenck Personality Inventory

EPI, Epi, epi.
epinephrine

Epi
epicardium
epiglottis

epid.
epidemic

epig.
epigastric

epigast.
epigastrium

Epil
epilepsy
epileptic

epineph.
epinephrine

epiph.
epiphysis

epis.
episiotomy
episode(s)
episodic
epistaxis

epistom.
epistomium (a stopper on mouth of a
bottle)

epith.
epithelial
epithelial (cells)
epithelium

EPL
effective patient life
essential phospholipids
extensor pollicis longus
external plexiform layer

EPM
Elderfield pyrimidine mustard
electron probe microanalysis
energy-protein malnutrition

EPN
O-ethyl *O*-*p*-nitrophenyl
phenylphosphonothioate (insecticide;
acaricide)

EPO
erythropoietin
expiratory port occlusion

EPP
equal pressure point
erythropoietic protoporphyria

EPP, e.p.p.
end-plate potential

EPPB
end-positive pressure breathing

EPPS
Edwards Personal Preference Schedule
(re: psychological testing)

EPQ
Eysenck Personality Questionnaire

EPR
electron paramagnetic resonance
electrophrenic respiration
estradiol production rate
extraparenchymal resistance

EPROM
erasable programmable read-only
memory (re: computers)

EPS
elastosis performans serpiginosa
electrophysiologic studies
enzymatic pancreatic secretion
exophthalmos-producing substance (of
anterior pituitary)
expressed prostatic secretion
extrapyramidal side effect (syndrome)
extrapyramidal symptomatology (re:
Neuro)
extrapyramidal symptoms
extrapyramidal syndrome

ep's
epithelial cells

EPSD
E-point to septal distance (re: Cardio)

EPSDT
Early and Periodic Screening,
Diagnosis, and Treatment

EPSE
extrapyramidal side effects

EPSP
excitatory postsynaptic potential (re:
Neuro)

EPSS
E-point septal separation (re: Cardio)

EPT
early pregnancy test
Eidetic Parents Test (re: Psychol)
endoscopic papillotomy

EPTC
S-ethyl dipropylthiocarbamate
(herbicide)

EPTE
existed prior to enlistment

EPTS
existed prior to service

EPXMA
electron probe x-ray microanalyzer

EQ
education quotient
educational quotient
encephalization quotient
energy quotient
equilibrium

EQ, eq.
equation

Eq, eq.
equivalent

eq.
equal

EQA
external quality assessment

eqn.
equation

eqpt.
equipment

EQU
(gram-) equivalent

equilib.
equilibrium

equip.
equipment

equiv.
equivalent
equivocal

ER
early reticulocyte
efficacy ratio
ejection rate
electroresection
endoplasmic reticulum
enhancement ratio
environmental resistance
epigastric region
equine rhinopneumonia
equivalent roentgen (unit)
erythrocyte receptor
esophageal rupture
estradiol receptor
estrogen receptor
evoked response
expiratory reserve
extended release (tablet)
external resistance
external rotation
extraction ratio
eye research

ER, E.R.
Emergency Room

ER +
increased estrogen receptors

ER −
decreased estrogen receptors

E & R
equal and reactive (re: reflexes)
examination and report

Er
erbium (element)

Er, er.
erythrocyte

169Er
radioactive isotope of erbium

171Er
radioactive isotope of erbium

ERA
electric response activity
electrical response activity
electrical response audiometry
electroencephalic (evoked) response
    audiometry
estradiol receptor assay
evoked response audiometry

ERB
ethnic relational behavior (re: Psychol)

ERBF
effective renal blood flow

ERC
ECHO (enterocytopathogenic human
    orphan)-rhino-coryza (viruses)
endoscopic retrograde cholangiography

(pupils) equal, regular, contract (re:
    Ophth)
erythropoietin-responsive cell

ERCP
endoscopic retrograde cannulation of
    the pancreatic (duct)
endoscopic retrograde
    cholangiopancreatography
endoscopic retrograde
    choledochopancreatography

ERD
evoked response detector

ERE
external rotation in extension

ERF
external rotation in flexion

erf
error function

ERFC
erythrocyte rosette-forming cells

ERG
electron radiography

ERG, erg.
electroretinogram
electroretinograph

ERH
egg-laying release hormone

ERHD
exposure-related hypothermia death

ERI
Environmental Response Inventory (re:
    psychological testing)
E (erythrocyte) rosette inhibitor

ERIA
electroradio-immunoassay

ERM
electrochemical relaxation methods
extended radical mastectomy

ERP
early receptor potential
effective refractory period
endoscopic retrograde pancreatography
equine rhinopneumonitis
estrogen receptor protein
event-related (brain) potential

ERPF
effective renal plasma flow

ERPLV
effective refractory period of the left
    ventricle

ERS
endoscopic retrograde sphincterotomy

ERSP
event-related slow-brain potential

ERT
esophageal radionuclide transit
estrogen replacement therapy
external radiation therapy

eruct.
eructation

ERV
equine rhinopneumonitis virus
expiratory reserve volume

ERY
erysipelas

ERY, Ery
Erysipelothrix (genus)
erythrocyte(s)

eryth.
erythema
erythrocyte(s)

ES
Ego Strength (test—re: Psychol)
ejection sound
elastic suspensor
electrical stimulation
electrical stimulus
electroshock
elopement status (re: Psychol)
Emergency Service
emission spectrometry
endoscopic sclerosis
endoscopic sphincterotomy
end to side (anastomosis)
enema saponis (L. soap enema)
enzyme substrate
esophageal scintigraphy
esophagus
esophoria
estimated standard (normal value)
Expectation Score
experimental study
exsmoker
exterior surface
extrasystole

E11S
ECHO 11 (virus) sensitivity

Es
einsteinium (element)

E$_s$
estriol

ESA-4
esterase A4

ESB
electrical stimulation to brain

ESC
electromechanical slope computer
end-systolic count
erythropoietin-sensitive stem cells

ESCA
electron spectroscopy for chemical
analysis

ESCC
electrolyte steroid cardiopathy by
calcification
epidural spinal cord compression

ESCH
electrolyte steroid-produced
cardiopathy (characterized by)
hyalinization

ESCH, Esch
Escherichia (genus)

ESCN
electrolyte and steroid-produced
cardiopathy (characterized by)
necrosis

ESCS
Early Social Communication Scale (re:
Psychol)

ESD
electron-stimulated desorption
electronic summation device
emission spectrometric detector
end-systolic dimension
environmental sex determination
esophagus, stomach, and duodenum
exoskeletal device
external symbol dictionary (re:
computers)

ESD, EsD
esterase D

ESDIAD
electron-stimulated desorption ion
angular distribution

ESE
electrostatische Einheit (Ger.
electrostatic unit)

ESEP
elbow sensory potential

ESF
electrosurgical filter
erythropoiesis-stimulating factor

ESF, E.S.F.
erythropoietic-stimulating factor

ESFL
end-systolic force—length
  (relationship—re: Cardio)

ESG
estrogen

ESI
Ego State Inventory
enzyme substrate inhibitor
epidural steroid injection
extent of skin involvement

ES-IMV
expiration-synchronized intermittent
  mandatory ventilation

ESL
end-systolic (segment) length (re:
  Cardio)
English as a second language

ESM
ejection systolic murmur
endothelial specular microscope

ESN
educationally subnormal
estrogen-stimulated neurophysine

ESO, eso.
esophagoscopy
esophagus

esoph.
esophageal
esophagoscopy
esophagus

esoph. steth.
esophageal stethoscope

ESP
early systolic paradox
effective sensory projection
effective systolic pressure
end-systolic pressure
eosinophil stimulation promotor
epidermal soluble protein
evoked synaptic potential (re: Neuro)
extrasensory perception

esp.
especial (Brit)
especially (Brit)

ESPA
electrical stimulation-produced
  analgesia

espec.
especial (Brit)
especially (Brit)

ESPQ
Early School Personality Questionnaire

ESR
electric skin resistance (re: physiatry)
erythrocyte sedimentation rate

ESR, e.s.r.
electron spin resonance

ESRD
end-stage renal disease

ESRF
end-stage renal failure

ESRS
Extrapyramidal Symptom Rating Scale
  (re: Neuro)

ESS
erythrocyte sensitizing substance
excited skin syndrome

ess.
essence
essential
essentially

Ess Hyper
essential hypertension

Ess Hyper T
essential hypertension

ess. neg.
essentially negative

EST
electroshock therapy
electroshock threshold
endodermal sinus tumor
esterase
exercise stress test

est.
estimate
estimated

esth.
esthetic

est. wgt.
estimated weight

est. wt.
estimated weight

ESU, esu, e.s.u.
electrostatic unit

E sub.
excitor substance

ESV
end-systolic ventricular volume
end-systolic volume
esophageal valve

ESVI
end-systolic volume index

ESVS
epiurethral suprapubic vaginal
  suspension

ESWL
extracorporeal shock-wave lithotripsy

ESWS
end-systolic wall stress

ET
edge thickness
educational therapy
effective temperature
ejection time
embryo transfer
endotracheal
endotracheal (intubation)
endotracheal tube
endurance time
epithelial tumor
esotropia (re: Ophth)
esotropia (for distance—re: Ophth)
essential thrombocythemia
eustachian tube
exchange transfusion
exercise training
exercise treadmill
expiration time
extracellular tachyzoite
extraterrestrial

ET, Et, et
ethyl (group)

ET, et.
etiology

ET'
esotropia for near (re: Ophth)

E/T
effector-to-target ratio

E(T)
intermittent esotropia (re: Ophth)

ET₁
esotropia at near (re: Ophth)

ETA
electron-transfer agent
endotracheal airway
ethionamide (antibacterial;
  tuberculostatic)

ETAB
extrathoracic-assisted breathing

et al.
et alibi (L. and elsewhere)
et alii (L. and others)

ETB
end-of-transmission block (character—
  re: computers/ data processing)

ETC
estimated time of conception

etc.
et cetera (L. and others; and so forth)

ETD
eustachian tube dysfunction

ETEC
enterotoxic *Escherichia coli*
enterotoxigenic *Escherichia coli*
enterotoxins of *Escherichia coli*

ETF
electron-transferring flavoprotein
eustachian tube function

ETH
elixir terpin hydrate
ethionamide (antibacterial;
  tuberculostatic)
ethmoid

eth.
ether

ETH-C, ETH/C
elixir terpin hydrate with codeine

eths
ethmoids

ETIO
etiocholanolone (re: pyogen for
  experimental fevers)

etiol.
etiology

etiol. undet.
etiology undetermined

etiol. unk.
etiology unknown

ETK
erythrocyte transketolase

ETKM
every test known (to) man

ETKTM
every test known to man

ETL
expiratory threshold load

ETM
erythromycin (re: culture and sensitivity
  reports)

ETO
estimated time of ovulation

Et₂O
ether ($C_4H_{10}O$—ethyl ether)

ETOH, EtOH
ethyl alcohol

ETOX
ethylene oxide

ETP
electron transfer particle
electron transport particle
entire treatment period
ephedrine, theophylline, phenobarbital
eustachian tube pressure

ETR
effective thyroxin(e) ratio
estimated thyroid ratio

ETS
Educational Testing Service (re:
    psychological testing)
electrical transcranial stimulation

et seq.
et sequens (L. and the following)
et sequentes (L. and those that follow)

ETT
endotracheal tube
epinephrine tolerance test
exercise tolerance test
exercise treadmill test
extrathyroidal thyroxin(e)

ETTN
ethyltrimethyloltrimethane trinitrate
    (Ettriol trinitrate—coronary
    vasodilator)

ETU
Emergency and Trauma Unit
Emergency Treatment Unit

ETV
educational television

ETX
end of text (character—re: computers/
    data processing)

EU
Ehrlich units (re: bilirubin assays)
emergency unit
endotoxin unit
entropy unit
enzyme unit(s)
esterase unit
expected utility (re: Psychol)

E.U.
etiology unknown

Eu
Euler number (re: fluid dynamics)
European
europium (element)

^{154}Eu
radioactive isotope of europium

^{155}Eu
radioactive isotope of europium

EUA
examination under anesthesia
examination under anesthetic

EUCD
emotionally unstable character disorder

EUL
expected upper limit

EUM
external urethral meatus

E unit
unit of x-ray intensity equivalent to
    about one roentgen per second (now
    obsolete)

EUP
extrauterine pregnancy

EUS
external urethral sphincter

eust.
eustachian

eutroph.
eutrophia
eutrophic

EUV
extreme ultraviolet laser

EV
enterovirus
epidermodysplasia verruciformis
evoked response
excessive ventilation
extravascular

EV, ev.
eversion

eV, ev
electron volt

EVA
ethyl violet azide (broth)

evac.
evacuate(d)

eval.
evaluate
evaluation

evap.
evaporate
evaporated

evapn.
evaporation

EVD
external ventricular drainage

ever.
eversion

EVF
ethanol volume fraction

EVG
electroventriculogram

EVI
endocardial, vascular, interstitial
endocardial, vascular, intestinal

evid.
evidence
evidenced by
evident

EVLW
extravascular lung water

EVM
electronic voltmeter
extravascular mass

evol.
evolution

EVP
evoked visual potential

EVR
endocardial viability ratio
evoked visual response

EVS
endoscopic variceal sclerosis

EVTV
extravascular thermal volume

EW
Emergency Ward

ew.
elsewhere

E wave
expectancy wave

EWB
estrogen withdrawal bleeding

EWHO
elbow-wrist-hand orthosis

EWI
Experiential World Inventory (re:
psychological testing)

EWL
egg-white lysozyme
evaporative water loss

E-W nucleus
Edinger-Westphal nucleus (re: Neuro,
NIII)

Ex, ex.
examination

ex.
exacerbate(d)
exacerbation
exaggerate(d)
examined
examiner
example
excision
exercise
exophthalmos
exposure
extraction

exac.
exacerbate(d)
exacerbation

ex aff.
ex affinibus (L. of the neighboring
[affinity])

EXAFS
extended x-ray absorption fine structure
(spectroscopy)

exag.
exaggerate(d)
exaggeration

exam.
examination
examine
examiner

EXBF
exercise hyperemia blood flow

exc.
excel
excellent
except
excepted
excision

exc. bx.
excisional biopsy

exch.
exchange

excis.
excise
excision

excr.
excrete(d)
excretion

EXD
ethylxanthic disulfide (topical
parasiticide)

EXEC
execute (statement—re: computers)
executive (system—re: computers)

exec.
executive

EXELFS
extended electron-loss fine structure

exer.
exercise

ex gr.
ex grupa (of the group of)

exh.
exhibit
exhibition

exhib.
exhibeatur (L. let it be displayed
  [shown])
exhibit
exhibition

exist.
existing

EXO
exonuclease
exophoria

exog.
exogenous

exoph.
exophthalmia

exos.
exostosis

EXP, Exp, exp.
expired

exp.
expansion
expected
expecting
expectorant
expectorated
experience
experiment
experimental
expiration (die)
expiration (re: respirations)
expiratory
expire
exponent
expose
exposure

expec.
expectorant

expect.
expectoratium (L. expectorant)

exper.
experience
experiment
experimental

ExPGN
extracapillary proliferative glomerular
  nephritis

expir.
expiration
expirator
expiratory

expl.
explain
exploration
exploratory
explore

exp. lap.
exploratory laparotomy

expn.
expression

exp. = sat.
expansion equal and satisfactory (re:
  chest)

expt.
expected
expectorant
expectorate
experimental

exptl.
experimental

EXREM
external radiation-emission-man
  (radiation dose)

EXS
externally supported
extrinsically supported

exsicc.
exsiccatus (L. dried out)

Ext, ext.
extraction (re: Dent)

ext.
extend
extendere (L. to spread; to extend)
extension
extensive
extensor
exterior
external
extern(e)
extract
extracted
extractum (L. extract)
extreme
extremities
extremity

ext. aud.
external auditory

extd.
extended
extracted

extens.
extension
extensor

extentab
extended action tablet

ext. fl.
fluid extract

extr.
extremity

extrap.
extrapolate

extrav.
extravasation

extrem.
extremity

ext. rot.
external rotation (re: Ortho)

↑ **ext. rot.**
increased external rotation (re: Ortho)

↓ **ext. rot.**
decreased external rotation (re: Ortho)

extub.
extubate
extubated
extubation

EXU
excretory urogram

exud.
exudate
exuded

exx
examples

EY
egg yolk
epidemiology year

EYA
egg yolk (pyruvate-tellurite-glycine) agar

Ez
eczema

F

F
bioavailability
coefficient of inbreeding (re: consanguinity measurement)
coupling factors (re: cell mitochondria)
facies
factor
failed
failure
fair
false
family
Faraday constant
far advanced
fascia
fasting (test)
fat
fats
fecal
feces
Fellow
feminine
fermentative
fermi (SI unit of distance equal to 10^{-15}m)
fertility (factor)
fetal
figural (contents—re: Psychol; Aptitudes Research Project testing within structure of intellect model)
filament
Filaria (former genus of nematodes)
filial generation
fine
finger
finger dexterity (re: Psychol; General Aptitude Test Battery)
flexed
flow (of blood)
fluorine (element)
flux
foil (re: Dent)
fontanel(le)
foramen
force
form response
fornix
fossa
fractional concentration (when followed by subscripts indicating location and chemical species)
fragment of an antibody
Francisella (genus)
free

free energy
Freon (a gas refrigerant)
Froude number (re: fluid dynamics)
function
Fusarium (genus)
Fusiformis (an obsolete generic name)
fusion
Fusobacterium (genus)
gas concentration (fractional)
gilbert (unit of magnetomotive force)
Helmholtz free energy
hydrocortisone (compound F)
phenylalanine (a protein amino acid)
ratio of variances
reactional concentration in dry gas stage (primary symbol)
vectorcardiography electrode (left foot)
Wright's inbreeding coefficient (re: genetics)

F, F.
Fahrenheit

F, F., f
field of vision
formula
French (scale for measurement of outside diameter of catheters and sounds)

F, f
farad (practical and SI unit of capacitance)
father
female
fiat (L. let it be made)
fibrous (re: proteins)
fluid
focal length (when followed by a number)
forma (L. form, figure, shape)
formulary
fractional (re: fractional composition of gases)
fracture
frequency
frequency (respiratory)
frontal
full (re: diet)
fundus

F′
secondary focal point (of lens—re: Ophth)

F⁺
good form response

F⁻
fluoride
poor form response

°F
Fahrenheit

F₁
first filial generation (re: genetics)

F₂
second filial generation (produced by
    intercrossed F₁'s —re: genetics)
zinc oxide-eugenol cement (eugenol—a
    dental anaesthetic)

F₃
TFT—trifluorothymidine (antiviral—re:
    Ophth)

F-12
Freon 12

F-18, ¹⁸F
fluorine 18

f
atomic orbital with angular momentum
    quantum number 3
breathing frequency
fac (L. make)
femto- (one quadrillionth [10^{-15}])
fiant (L. let them be made)
fingerbreadth
fission
five
flexion
focal
following (after numeral)
foot
fors (proposed name [1956] for force
    represented by 1 gram weight)
fraction
from

f
general function

FA
false aneurysm
Fanconi anemia
far advanced
fatty acid
febrile antigens
femoral artery
fibrinolytic activity
fibroadenoma
fibrosing alveolitis
field ambulance
filterable agent
filterable air
filtered air
first aid
fluorescein angiography

fluorescent antibody
fluorescent assay
3-fluoro-D-alanine (antibacterial)
folic acid
forearm
formamide (methanamide; industrial
    chemical)
fortified aqueous (re: solutions)
free acid
Freund's adjuvant
functional activities

F/A
fetus active

FAA
folic acid antagonist

2-FAA
N-2-fluorenylacetamide

FAA sol.
formalin, acetic, alcohol solution (a
    fixative)

FAB
fast atom bombardment
formalin ammonium bromide
fragment antigen binding
French-American-British (re:
    morphologic classification)
functional arm brace

FAB, Fab
fragment (of IgG immunoglobulin
    involved in) antigen binding

F(ab')₂
fragment (of IgG immunoglobulin) after
    digestion with the enzyme pepsin

Fabc
fragment, antigen and complement
    binding

FABER
flexion (in) abduction and external
    rotation (re: Ortho)

Fabere
flexion, abduction, external rotation, and
    extension (re: Ortho)

FABF
femoral artery blood flow

FAB/MS
fast atom bombardment mass
    spectrometry

FABP
fatty acid-binding protein
folic acid-binding protein

FAC
5-fluorouracil, Adriamycin (doxorubicin),
    and cyclophosphamide (Cytoxan) (re:
    chemotherapy)

fractional area change
free available chlorine

Fac
factor

fac.
facere (L. to make; to form; construct;
    create)

facil.
facilitate
facilitation
facilitory

FAC-LEV
5-fluorouracil, Adriamycin (doxorubicin),
    cyclophosphamide (Cytoxan), and
    levamisole (re: chemotherapy)

FACP
ftorafur, Adriamycin (doxorubicin),
    cyclophosphamide (Cytoxan), and
    Platinol (cisplatin) (re: chemotherapy)

FACS
fluorescence-activated cell sorter (re:
    cytogenetics)

FACT
Flanagan Aptitude Classification Tests

FAD
familial autonomic dysfunction
fetal activity-acceleration determination
flavin adenine dinucleotide

FADF
fluorescent antibody dark field

FADH₂
flavin adenine dinucleotide, reduced
    form w/hydrogen

FADIR
flexion (in) adduction and internal
    rotation (re: Ortho)

Fadire
flexion, adduction, internal rotation, and
    extension (re: Ortho)

FADN
flavin adenine dinucleotide

FADU
fluorometric analysis of DNA unwinding

FAF
fatty acid free
fibroblast-activating factor

FAHR, Fahr
Fahrenheit

FAI
functional aerobic impairment

FAJ
fused apophyseal joints

FALG
fowl antimouse lymphocyte globulin

FALP
fluoro-assisted lumbar puncture

FAM
5-fluorouracil, Adriamycin (doxorubicin),
    and mitomycin C (re: chemotherapy)

Fam, fam.
family

FAMA
fluorescent antibody to membrane
    antigen (test)

fam. doc.
family doctor

FAME
fatty acid methyl ester
5-fluorouracil, Adriamycin (doxorubicin),
    and MeCCNU (semustine) (re:
    chemotherapy)

fam. hist.
family history

FAMMe
5-fluorouracil, Adriamycin, mitomycin C,
    semustine (re: chemotherapy)

FAMMM
familial atypical mole malignant
    melanoma
familial atypical multiple mole
    melanoma

Fam per. par.
familial periodic paralysis

Fam phys., fam. phys.
family physician

FAM-S
5-fluorouracil, Adriamycin, mitomycin C,
    streptozotocin (re: chemotherapy)

FAN
fuchsin, amido black, and naphthol
    yellow

FANA
fluorescent antinuclear antibodies

FANCAP
fluids, aeration, nutrition,
    communication, activity, and pain (re:
    nursing)

FANCAS
fluids, aeration, nutrition,
    communication, activity, and
    stimulation (re: nursing)

FANPT
Freeman Anxiety Neurosis and
   Psychosomatic Test

FANSS & M
fundus anterior, normal size and shape,
   and mobile

FAP
familial amyloid polyneuropathy
fatty acid poor
fatty acids polyunsaturated
femoral artery pressure
fixed action pattern
frozen animal procedure

FAQ
Family Attitudes Questionnaire (re:
   Psychol)

FAR
Flight Aptitude Rating
fractional albuminuria rate

FAR
immediate good function followed by
   accelerated rejection

far.
farad
faradic

FAS
fetal alcohol syndrome

FASC
free-standing ambulatory surgical
   center

fasc.
fasciculation
fasciculus (L. small bundle)

fasci.
fasciculation

FASF
Factor Analyzed Short Form

FAST
Filtered Audiometer Speech Test
fluorescent antibody staining technique

FAT
family attitudes test
fast axoplasmic transport
fluorescent antibody test

F.A.T.S.A.
Flowers Auditory Test of Selective
   Attention (re: Psychol)

FAV
feline ataxia virus

FAX
facsimile (re: computers/data
   processing)

FAZ
Fanconi-Albertini-Zellweger (syndrome)
foveal avascular zone

FB
fasting blood (sugar)
feedback
fiberoptic bronchoscopy
foreign body

FB, Fb
fingerbreadth(s)

FBA
fecal bile acid

FBC
fully-buffered channel (re: computers)

FBCOD
foreign body, cornea, oculus dexter
   (L. right eye)

FBCOS
foreign body, cornea, oculus sinister
   (L. left eye)

FBD
functional bowel disorder

FBE
full blood examination

FBEC
fetal bovine endothelial cell

FBF
forearm blood flow

FBG
fasting blood glucose
fibrinogen

FBHH
familial benign hypocalciuric
   hypercalcemia

FBI
flossing, brushing, and irrigation (re:
   Dent)

FBM
fetal breathing movement

FBP
femoral blood pressure
fibrin breakdown products
fibrinogen breakdown products

FBR
Frischblut reaction (Ger. fresh-blood
   reaction—re: syphilis)

FBRCM
fingerbreadth below right costal margin

FBS
fasting blood sugar
feedback signal

feedback system
fetal bovine serum

FC
fasciculus cuneatus
fat component (of an axon)
febrile convulsion
fecal coli (broth)
fibrocystic
fibrocyte
finger clubbing
finger counting (re: Ophth/Neuro)
flucytosine (5-fluorocytosine—
    antifungal)
Foley catheter
font change (character—re: computers/
    data processing)
form response determined by color
foster care
free cholesterol
frontal cortex
functional class

F/C
flare and cell (re: Ophth)

F + C
flare and cell (re: Ophth)

5-FC
5-fluorocytosine (antifungal)

Fc, F$_c$
fragment, crystallizable (of Ig)

Fc'
fragment produced in addition to Fc
    fragments following papain digestion
    of Ig molecules
shade response to light gray area

fc
foot-candle (former unit of illumination,
    replaced by lumen)

FCA
ferritin-conjugated antibodies
fracture, complete, angulated
Freund's complete adjuvant

F. cath.
Foley catheter

FCC
follicular center cells
fracture, complete, compound
fracture, compound, comminuted

FCCC
fracture, complete, compound,
    comminuted

FCD
fecal collection device
fibrocystic dysplasia
focal cytoplasmic degradation
fracture, complete, deviated

F$^+$ cell
bacterial cell that serves as a genetic
    donor (re: genetics)

F$^-$ cell
bacterial cell lacking an F plasmid (re:
    genetics)

FCF
fetal cardiac frequency
fibroblast chemotactic factor

FCFC
fibroblast colony-forming cells

FCHL
familial combined hyperlipidemia

FCI
fixed-cell immunofluorescence
food-chemical intolerance

fcly
face lying

FCM
flow cytometry (re: cell cycle)

FCP
final common pathway (re: Neuro)
5-fluorouracil, cyclophosphamide, and
    prednisone (re: chemotherapy)
Functional Communication Profile (of
    aphasic adults— re: Psychol)

FCR
flexor carpi radialis
fractional catabolic rate

FCRA
fecal collection receptacle assembly

F$_c$ receptor
cell surface component which binds
    crystallizable fragment (F$_c$) portion of
    Ig to certain cells in nonantigen-
    specific manner (re: genetics)

FCS
fecal containment system
feedback control system
fetal calf serum

FCT
food composition table

fct.
function

FCU
flexor carpi ulnaris
fraud control unit

FCVD
fracture, complete, varus deformity

FCx
frontal cortex

FD
familial dysautonomia
family doctor
fan douche
fetal danger
fibrinogen derivative
field desorption
Filatov-Dukes (disease)
fluorescence depolarization
Folin-Denis (assay)
freedom from distractibility
freeze-dried
frequency deviation (re: statistics)

FD, F.D.
fatal dose
focal distance
foot drape
forceps delivery

FD$_{50}$
median fatal dose (that fatal to 50% of
test subjects)

Fd
ferredoxin
fundus
heavy chain portion of an Fab
(fragment, antigen binding)

fd
frequency times deviation (re: statistics)

FDA
Food and Drug Administration

FDA, F.D.A.
frontodextra anterior (position of fetus)

FDBL
fecal daily blood loss

FDC
frequency dependence of compliance
perfluorodecalin (blood substitute)

FDC Act
Food, Drug and Cosmetic Act

FDCT
Franck Drawing Completion Test (re:
Psychol)

FDDC
ferric dimethyldithiocarbonate
(ferbam—fungicide)

FDDQ
Freedom from Distractibility Deviation
Quotient

FDDS
Family Drawing Depression Scale

FDE
female day equivalent
final drug evaluation

FDF
fast death factor
further differentiated fibroblast

fdg.
feeding

FDGF
fibroblast-derived growth factor

FDH
familial dysalbuminemic
hyperthyroxinemia

FDI
first dorsal interosseus

F distribution
the probability distribution of the
statistic F

FDIU
fetal death in utero

FDL
flexor digitorum longus

FDLMP
first day of last menstrual period

FDM
fetus of diabetic mother
frequency division multiplex (re:
computers)

FDNB
1-fluoro-2,4-dinitrobenzene
(fluorodinitrobenzene— Sanger's
reagent)

F donor
cell that donates F factor in bacterial
conjugation

FDP
fibrin/fibrinogen degradation product
flexor digitorum profundus
fructose diphosphate (fructose-1,6-
diphosphate)

FDP, F.D.P.
frontodextra posterior (position of fetus)

FDPALD
fructose diphosphate aldolase

FDPase
fructose diphosphatase

fdp/Fdp
fibrin-fibrinogen degradation products

FDQB
flexor digiti quinti brevis

FDR
fractional disappearance rate
frequency dependence of resistance

FDS
flexor digitorum sublimis
flexor digitorum superficialis

FDT, F.D.T.
frontodextra transversa (position of
   fetus)

F$_3$dTMP
trifluorothymidylate

F-duction
the transfer of an F′ plasmid from an F
   donor cell to an F recipient cell (re:
   bacteriology)

FdUMP
5-fluoro-2′-deoxyuridylate

FDV
Friend disease virus

FDX
full duplex (re: computers)

FDZ
fetal danger zone

FE
fatty ester
fecal emesis
fetal erythroblastosis
fetal erythrocyte
fluid extract
fluorescing erythrocyte
forced expiratory
formalin and ethanol
format effector (character—re:
   computers)
freely eating

Fe
ferrum (L. iron [an element])

Fe, fe.
female

Fe^{2+}, Fe(II)
ferrous

Fe^{3+}, Fe(III)
ferric

^{52}Fe
radioactive iron isotope (re: iron
   metabolism)

^{55}Fe
radioactive iron isotope (re: iron
   metabolism)

^{59}Fe
radioactive iron isotope (re: iron
   metabolism)

feb.
febrile
febris (L. fever)

feb. agglut.
febrile agglutinin

feb. dur.
febre durante (L. while the fever lasts)
febris durantibus (L. while the fevers
   last)

FEBP
fetoneonatal estrogen-binding protein

FEC
forced expiratory capacity
free erythrocyte coproporphyrin
Friend's erythroleukemia cell

FECG
fetal electrocardiogram

FeCl$_3$
ferric chloride (catalyst, purifier,
   manufacturing chemical)

F$_{ECO_2}$
fractional concentration of carbon
   dioxide in a sample of expired gas

FECP
free erythrocyte coproporphyria
free erythrocyte coproporphyrin

FECT
factor eight (VIII) correctional time
fibro-elastic connective tissue

FeD
iron (ferrum) deficiency

Fed
federal
federation

Fe def.
iron (ferrum) deficiency anemia

Fed spec.
federal specifications

FEE
forced equilibrating expiration

FEEG
fetal electroencephalogram

FEF
Family Evaluation Form
forced expiratory flow (re: Resp)

FEF$_{25}$
forced expiratory flow after 25% of vital
   capacity has been expelled (re:
   Resp)

FEFO
first-ended, first-out (re: computers/data
   processing)

FEFV
forced expiratory flow volume

FEIBA
factor eight (VIII) inhibitor bypassing
  activity

FEKG
fetal electrokardiogram
  (electrocardiogram)

FEL
familial erythrophagocytic
  lymphohistiocytosis

Fel
Fellow

FELC
Friend erythroleukemia cell

FeLV, FeIV
feline leukemia virus

FEM
femoris (L. of the thigh)
finite element method
fluid-electrolyte malnutrition

fem.
female
feminine
femoral
femur

Fem intern., fem. intern.
femoribus internus (L. at the inner side
  of the thighs)

FENa
excreted fraction of (filtered) sodium
  (natrium)

Fe_{O_2}
the fractional concentration of oxygen in
  a sample of expired gas

FEP
fluorinated ethylene-propylene polymer
free erythrocyte protoporphyrin

FEPB
functional electronic peroneal brace

FEPP
free erythrocyte protoporphyrin

FER
flexion, extension, and rotation
fractional esterification rate

Fer
ferrum (L. iron)

fertd., fert'd
fertilized

ferv.
fervens (L. boiling)

FES
Family Environment Scale (re: Psychol)

fat embolism syndrome
flame emission spectroscopy
forced expiratory spirogram (re: Resp)
functional electrical stimulation
further examples see

FESA
finite element stress analysis

fest.
festination

FeSV
feline sarcoma virus

FET
field effect transistor (voltage amplifier)
forced expiratory time (re: Resp)

fet.
fetus

fetal h.
fetal hemoglobin

FETE
far eastern tick-borne encephalitis

Fe/TIBC
iron (ferrum) saturation of serum
  transferrin

FETS
forced expiratory time in seconds (re:
  Resp)

FEUO
for external use only

FEV
forced expiratory volume (re: Resp)

FEV_1
forced expiratory volume in one second
  (re: Resp)

FEVB
frequency ectopic ventricular beat

FEV-1 sec.
forced expiratory volume in the first
  second after the start of expiration
  (re: Resp)

FEV_1/VC
forced expiratory volume (in one
  second) vital capacity (re: Resp)

FEXE
formalin, ethanol, xylol, ethanol

FeZ
iron zone

FF
fat free (diet)
father factor
fear of failure
fecal frequency

fertility factor
fields of Forel (re: Neuro)
filtration factor
filtration fraction
fine fiber
fine fraction
finger flexion
finger to finger (re: Neuro)
fixing fluid
flat feet
flip-flop (re: electronic logic circuitry)
fluorescent foci
forearm flow
form feed (character—re: computers/
    data processing)
foster father
Fox-Fordyce (disease)
free fraction
fresh frozen
further flexion (re: PM&R)

FF, ff
force fluid(s)
forward flexion

fF
ultrafine fiber
ultrafine fraction

ff
following (after numeral—also f)

f.f.
fundus firm

f→f
finger to finger

FFA, F.F.A.
free fatty acids

F factor
fertility factor

FFAP
free fatty acid phase

FFB
fast feedback
flexible fiberoptic bronchoscopy

FFC
fixed flexion contracture (re: Ortho)
free from chlorine

FFCS
forearm flexion control strap (re: Ortho/
    physiatry)

FFD
focal film distance (re: radiology)
focus film distance (re: radiology)
focus to film distance (re: radiology)

FFDW
fat-free dry weight

FFE
fecal fat excretion

FFEM
freeze fracture electron microscopy

FFF
field-flow fractionation
flicker fusion frequency (test—re:
    Ophth)

f→f & f→n
finger to finger and finger to nose (tests)

FFFT
forward flexion fingertips to _____

FFI
free from infection
fundamental frequency indicator

FFIT
fluorescent focus inhibition test

FFM
fat-free mass

FFMTP
fatigue fracture of the medial tibial
    plateau

FFP
fresh frozen plasma

FFR
frequency-following response

FFROM
full, free range of motion

FFS
failure of fixation suppression
fat-free solid
fat-free supper
fee for service

FFT
fast Fourier transform (re: computers)
flicker fusion test

FFT, F.F.T.
flicker fusion threshold

FFU
focus-forming unit

FFW
fat-free weight

FFWC
fractional free water clearance

FFWW
fat-free wet weight

FG
fasciculus gracilis (re: muscles)
fast glycolytic (re: muscle fiber)
fibrinogen

field gain
French gauge

FG, F-G
Feeley-Gorman (agar)

fg
femtogram (10^{-15} grams—1
quadrillionth)

FGAR
formylglycinamide ribonucleotide

FGB
fully granulated basophil

FGC
fibrinogen gel chromatography

FGD
fatal granulomatous disease

FGDS
fibrogastroduodenoscope

FGF
father's grandfather
fibroblast growth factor
fresh gas flow

FGG
focal global glomerulosclerosis
fowl gamma globulin

FGL
fasting gastrin level

FGM
father's grandmother

FGN
focal glomerulonephritis

FGS
fibrogastroscope
focal glomerulosclerosis

FGT
female genital tract (re: cytologic
smear)
fluorescent gonorrhea test

FGU
French gauge, urodynamic

FH
familial hypercholesterolemia
family history
Fanconi-Hegglin (syndrome)
fasting hyperbilirubinemia
favorable histology
fetal head
fetal heart
fibromuscular hyperplasia
floating hospital
follicular hyperplasia
Frankfort horizontal (plane of skull)

fumarate hydratase (re: tricarboxylic
acid cycle)

f.h.
fiat haustus (L. let a draught be made)

FHA
familial hypoplastic anemia
filamentous hemagglutinin
filterable hemolytic anemia
fimbrial hemagglutinin
fulminant hepatic failure

FHC
familial hypercholesterolemia
family health center

FHD
family history of diabetes

FHF
fetal heart frequency
fulminant hepatic failure

FHH
familial hypocalciuric hypercalcemia
family history of hirsutism
fetal heart heard

FHL
flexor hallucis longus
functional hearing loss

FHLDL
familial hypercholesterolemia (low
density lipoprotein)

FH-M
fumarate hydratase, mitochondrial

FHN
family history negative

FHNH
fetal heart not heard

FHP
family history positive

FHR
familial hypophosphatemic rickets
fetal heart rate
fetal heart rhythm

FHRDC
family history, research diagnostic
criteria

FHR-NST
fetal heart rate nonstress test

FHS
fetal heart sounds
fetal hydantoin syndrome

FH-S
fumurate hydratase, soluble

FHT, f.h.t.
fetal heart tone(s)

FHTG
familial hypertriglyceridemia

FHVP
free hepatic vein pressure

F Hx, FH$_x$
family history

FI
congenital limb absence—fibula,
    complete
fasciculus interfascicularis
fever caused by infection
fibrinogen
fixed internal (reinforcement—re:
    Psychol)
fixed interval (schedule)
flame ionization
forced inspiration
fronto-iliacus
functional inquiry

fi
congenital limb absence—fibula,
    incomplete

FIA
fluorescent immuno-assay
Freund's incomplete adjuvant

FIB
fibrin
fibrositis

FIB, fib.
fibrinogen
fibula

Fib, fib.
fibrillation

fib.
fiber
fibrous

fibr.
fibrillation

fibrill.
fibrillation

fibrin.
fibrinogen

FI$_{co}$
inspirated concentrations (re: Resp)

FICO$_2$
forced inspiratory carbon dioxide
    (concentration of carbon dioxide in
    inspired gas)

FID
flame ionization detector

free induction decay
fungal immunodiffusion

FIF
feedback inhibition factor
(human) fibroblast interferon
    (antineoplastic; antiviral)
forced inspiratory flow (re: Resp)
formaldehyde-induced fluorescence

FIFN
(human) fibroblast interferon
    (antineoplastic; antiviral)

FIFO
first in, first out (re: computer data)

FIFR
fasting intestinal flow rate

fig.
figuratively
figure

FIGLU
formiminoglutamic acid (re: histidine
    catabolism or conversion, folic acid
    deficiency, liver disease)

FIGO
International Federation of Gynecology
    and Obstetrics (re: classification of
    tumor staging)

FIH
fat-induced hyperglycemia

FIL
father-in-law

fil.
filament
filamentous
filial

filt.
filter
filtered
filtra (L. filter [imperative form])

FIM
field ion microscope
field ion microscopy

FIME
5-fluorouracil, ICRF-159 (razoxane), and
    MeCCNU (methyl-CCNU—
    semustine) (re: chemotherapy)

FIN
fine intestinal needle

F insulin, F-insulin
fibrous insulin

FIO$_2$
forced inspiratory oxygen (re: Resp)

fraction of inspired oxygen
fractional % of oxygen in inspired gas

Fior c̄ Cod
Fiorinal with codeine

FIP
feline infectious peritonitis

FIPAPA
Flame Ionization-Pulse Aerosol Particle
  Analyzer

FIQ
full-scale intelligence quotient

FIR
far infrared
fold increase in resistance

FIRDA
frontal irregular rhythmic delta activity
  (re: EEG)

FIRO-B
Fundamental Interpersonal Relations
  Orientation—Behavior

FIRO-F
Fundamental Interpersonal Relations
  Orientation— Feelings

FIS
forced inspiratory spirogram

Fish conc.
Fishberg concentration

Fish dil.
Fishberg dilution

FISS
Flint Infant Security Scale (re: Psychol)

Fiss, fiss.
fissure

fist.
fistula

FIT
Flanagan Industrial Tests (re: Psychol)
fluorescein isothiocyanate (fluorescent
  label—re: histology)
fusion-inferred threshold test

FITC
fluorescein isothiocyanate (fluorescent
  label—re: histology)

FIUO
for internal use only

FIV$_1$
forced inspiratory volume in one second

FIVC
forced inspiratory vital capacity

F-J
Fisher-John (melting point method)

FJN
familial juvenile nephrophthisis

FJRM
full joint range of movement

FJROM
full joint range of motion

FJS
finger joint size

FK
Feil-Klippel (syndrome)
Foster Kennedy (syndrome)
functioning kasai (Belgian Congo
  anemia)

FL
factor level
fatty liver
fibers of Luschka
fibroblast-like
Fiessinger-Leroy (syndrome)
filtration leukapheresis
fluorescence
fluorescent
Friend (erythro)leukemia
frontal lobe (re: Neuro)
functional length

FL, F/L
full liquid (diet)

FL, Fl
fluorescein
focal length

FL, Fl, fl.
fluid

Fl
florentium (former name for
  promethium)
flow

Fl, f.l.
filtered load

fL, fl.
femtoliter (1 quadrillionth or 10^{-15})

fl
foot lambert (unit of brightness)

fl.
flank
flexion
fluidus (L. fluid)
flutter

FLA
fluorescent-labeled antibody

FLA, F.L.A.
frontolaeva anterior (position of fetus)

f.l.a.
fiat lege artis (L. let it be done according
to rule of the art)

flac.
flaccid

flash pt.
flash point

flav.
flavus (L. yellow)

FLB
funny-looking beat (re: EKG)

FLC
fatty liver cell
fetal liver cell
Friend leukemia cells
funny-looking child (re: Ped)

FLD
fibrotic lung disease

FLD, Fld, fld.
fluid

fldext.
fluidum extractum (L. fluidextract)
fluidius extractus (L. fluidextract)

fl. dr.
fluid drachm (dram)

fl. drs.
fluff dressing

fld. ext.
fluidextract

fldxt.
fluidum extractum (L. fluidextract)
fluidius extractus (L. fluidextract)

FLES
Fairview Language Evaluation Scale
(re: mentally retarded)

flex.
flex
flexed
flexion
flexor

flex-ext inj.
flexion-extension injury

fl. ext.
fluidextract

FLK
funny-looking kid (re: Ped)

FLKS
fatty liver and kidney syndrome

FLM
fasciculus longitudinalis medialis

flocc.
flocculation

flor.
flores (L. flowers)

FL OZ, fl. oz.
fluid ounce

FLP, F.L.P.
frontolaeva posterior (position of fetus)

FLR
Fiessinger-Leroy-Reiter (syndrome)

FLS
fibrous long spacing (collagen)
flow-limiting segment
Functional Life Scale

FLSA
follicular lymphosarcoma

FLSP
fluorescein-labeled serum protein

FLT, F.L.T.
frontolaeva transversa (position of
fetus)

FLTAC
Fisher-Logemann Test of Articulation
Competence (re: Psychol)

fluid.
fluidus (L. fluid [adj.])

fluor.
fluorescent
fluorometry
fluoroscopy

fluores.
fluorescence
fluorescent

fluoro.
fluoroscopy

Fl up, fl. up
flare up
follow up

FLV
feline leukemia virus
Friend leukemia virus

flx.
flexion

F + ly
fair plus lying

FM
face mask
fathom

feedback mechanism
fetal movement
fibromuscular
filtered mass
flavin mononucleotide
flowmeter
fluid movement
foramen magnum
forensic medicine
formerly married
foster mother
Friend-Moloney
full mouth (re: dental x rays)
functional movement
fusobacteria microorganisms

FM, fm
frequency modulation

F.M., f.m.
fiat mistura (L. let a mixture be made)

Fm
fermium (element)

fm
femtometer
from

FMAC
fetal movement acceleration test

FMB
full maternal behavior

FMD
family medical doctor
fibromuscular disease
fibromuscular dysplasia
foot-and-mouth disease (virus)

FMDV
foot-and-mouth disease virus

FME
full-mouth extraction (re: Dent)

FMEL
Friend murine erythroleukemia

FMEN
familial multiple endocrine neoplasia

FMET
formylmethionine

fMet-tRNA, f-met-tRNA
N-formylmethionine-transfer ribonucleic
  acid (re: protein synthesis)

fMet-tRNA^Met
bound *N*-formylmethionine–transfer
  ribonucleic acid (re: protein
  synthesis)

FMF
familial Mediterranean fever
fetal movement felt

flow microfluorometry
forced mid-expiratory flow

FMFD1
familial multiple factor deficiency 1

FMG
fine mesh gauze
foreign medical graduate

FMH
family medical history
fat-mobilizing hormone
fetomaternal hemorrhage
fibromuscular hyperplasia

FMIR
frustrated multiple internal reflexion

FML
flail mitral leaflet
fluorometholone (anti-inflammatory;
  glucocorticoid)

f-MLP
formyl-methionyleucylphenylalanine

FMN
first malignant neoplasm
flavin mononucleotide

FMNH
flavin mononucleotide (reduced form)

FMNH$_2$
flavin mononucleotide (reduced form)

Fmoc
9-fluorenylmethoxycarbonyl

fmol
femtomole (1 quadrillionth—10^{-15})

FMP
first menstrual period
fructose monophosphate

FMR
Friend-Moloney-Rauscher (mouse
  leukemia virus)

FMR virus
Friend-Moloney-Rauscher (mouse
  leukemia virus)

FMS
fat-mobilizing substances
full-mouth series (re: dental x rays)

FMSTB
Frostig Movement Skills Test Battery
  (re: Psychol)

FMX
full-mouth radiography (re: Dent)

FN
false-negative
fastigii nucleus (re: Neuro)

fibronectin
final nitrogen
flip number (re: righting ability of
　　animals)
fluoride number

FN, F-N
finger to nose (test—re: Neuro)

F→N
finger to nose (test—re: Neuro)

fn
function

FNA
fine needle aspiration

FNAB
fine needle aspiration biopsy

FNC
fatty nutritional cirrhosis

Fneg
false negative

FNF
false-negative fraction
femoral neck fracture
finger-nose-finger (test—re: Neuro)

FNH
focal nodular hyperplasia

fn. p.
fusion point

FNS
functional neuromuscular stimulation

FNT
false (adrenergic) neurochemical
　　transmitter

f-number, f number, f number
focal length (numerical expression of
　　relative aperture of camera lens)

FO
fast oxidative
fiberoptic
foot orthosis
foramen ovale (re: Cardio)
forced oscillation
fronto-occipital (fetal position)

Fo
Fourier number (re: heat transmission)

fo.
fomentation

FOAM
5-FU, Oncovin, Adriamycin,
　　mitomycin C (re: chemotherapy)

FOAVF
failure of all vital forces

FOB
fecal occult blood
feet out of bed
fiberoptic bronchoscope
fiberoptic bronchoscopy
foot of bed

FOB, FO/B
foreign object/body

↗FOB
elevate foot of bed

FOC
Frequency of Contact (scale)
fronto-occipital circumference

FOCAL
formula calculation (re: computer
　　language)

FOCMA
feline oncornavirus-associated cell
　　membrane antigen

FOD
free of disease

FOG
fast-oxidative-glycolytic (re: muscle
　　fiber)

fol.
folia (L. leaves)
folium (L. a leaf)
follow
following

FOMI
5-fluorouracil, Oncovin (vincristine), and
　　mitomycin (re: chemotherapy)

FOOB
feet out of bed

FOP
forensic pathology

FOPR
full outpatient rate

FOR
forensic pathology

for.
foreign

for. body
foreign body

form.
formation
forming
formula

fort.
fortis (L. strong)

FORTRAN
formula translation (re: computer language)

FOS
fissura orbitalis superior
fractional osteoid surface

Found, found.
foundation

FOW
fenestration oval window (re: Oto)

FP
false-positive
family physician
family planning
Family Practice
family practitioner
family product
Fanconi-Petrassi (syndrome)
fibrinolytic potential
fibrinopeptide
filling pressure
filter paper
final pressure
first pass
fixation protein
flat paper
flat plate (re: x-ray film—obsolete term)
flavin phosphate (riboflavin-5′-phosphate)
flavoprotein
flexor profundus
fluorescence polarization
food poisoning
foreperiod
frontoparietal
frozen plasma
full period
fusion point

FP, fp
foot-pound

FP, fp, f.p.
freezing point

FP, f.p.
forearm pronated

F-P
femoral popliteal

F/P
fluorescein to protein (ratio)

F1P, F-1-P
fructose-1-phosphate

F-6-P
fructose-6-phosphate

f.p.
fiat potio (L. let a potion be made)

fiat pulvis (L. let a powder be made)
flexor pollicis (brevis, longus)

FPA
fibrinopeptide A
filter paper activity
fluorophenylalanine

FPB
femoral popliteal bypass
fibrinopeptide B
flexor pollicis brevis

FPC
familial polyposis coli
fish protein concentrate
forced pair copulation

FPCL
fibroblast-populated collagen lattice

FPD
flame photometric detector

FPDD
familial pure depressive disease

FPE
first-pass effect

FPF
false-positive fraction
fibroblast pneumocyte factor

FPG
fasting plasma glucose
fluorescence plus Giemsa
focal proliferative glomerulonephritis

FPGN
focal proliferative glomerulonephritis

FPH$_2$
flavin phosphate, reduced

FPHE
formalin-treated pyruvaldehyde-stabilized human erythrocytes

FPI
femoral pulsatility index
Freiburger Personality Inventory (re: psychological testing)

f. pil.
fiant pilulae (L. let pills be made)
fiat pilula (L. let a pill be made)

f. pil. xi
fac pilulas xi (L. make 11 pills [lower-case letter roman numerals for number of pills])

FPK
fructose-6-phosphokinase

FPL
fasting plasma lipid
flexor pollicis longus

FPLA
fibrin plate lysis area

FPM
filter paper microscopic (test)
full passive movements

fpm
feet per minute

FPN reagent
ferric chloride, perchloric acid, and nitric
    acid reagent

FPO
freezing point osmometer

FPP
free portal pressure

FPPH
familial primary pulmonary hypertension

FPR
fluorescence photobleaching recovery

FPRA
first-pass radionuclide angiogram

FPS
footpad swelling

FPS, fps
foot-pound-second

fps
feet per second
frames per second

FPU
Family Participation Unit

FPV
fowl pest virus
fowl plague virus

FPVB
femoral popliteal vein bypass

FR
failure rate (re: contraception)
Favre-Racouchot (disease)
feedback regulator
fibrinogen related
fixed ratio
flocculation reaction (Sachs-Georgi
    test)
flow rate
fluid restriction
fluid retention
formatio reticularis (L. reticular
    formation)
free radical
Friend (virus)

fructus (L. fruit, enjoyment)
full range
functional residual (capacity)

FR, Fr
French (scale of measurement of
    outside diameter of catheters and
    sounds)

FR, fR
frequency of respiration

F & R
force and rhythm (of pulse)

Fr
francium (element)
franklin (unit charge in electrostatic
    centimeter- gram-second system)

fr.
fried
from

FRA
fibrinogen-related antigen
fluorescent rabies antibody

fra
fragile site (re: cytogenetics)

frac.
fracture

Fract, fract.
fraction
fracture

fract. dos.
fracta dosi (L. in a divided dose)

frag.
fragile
fragility
fragment
fragmented

frag. test
fragility test

FRAP
fluorescence recovery after
    photobleaching

FRAT
free radical assay technique

FRBB, FR BB, Fr BB
fracture of both bones

FRBS
fast red B salt

FRC
frozen red cells
functional reserve capacity (of lungs)
functional residual capacity (of lungs)

FRCD
fixed ratio combination drugs

FRD
flexion-rotation-drawer (re: Ortho)

frem.
fremitus vocalis (L. vocal + roaring,
    murmuring, growling [a thrill caused
    by speaking—on auscultation])

freq.
frequency
frequent

FRF
fasciculus retroflexus
follicle-stimulating hormone-releasing
    factor

FRH
follicle-stimulating hormone-releasing
    hormone

FRh
fetal rhesus kidney

FRHS
fast-repeat high sequence

frict.
friction (rub)

Fried
Friedman's (test for pregnancy)

frig.
frigidus (L. cold)

FRJM
full range joint motion
full range joint movement

FRN
fully resonant nucleus

FRNS
frequently relapsing nephrotic
    syndrome

FROM
full range of motion (re: Ortho)
full range of movement (re: Ortho)

FROS
front routing of signal

FRP
functional refractory period

FRPS
functional resting position splint

FRR
functional recovery routines (re:
    computers/data processing)

FR r, Fr r, fr. r.
friction rub

FRS
ferredoxin-reducing substance
first rank symptoms (Schneider's
    [schneiderian]— re: psychiatry)
furosemide

FRT
Family Relations Test (re: Psychol)
full recovery time

Fru, fru.
fructose

frust.
frustillatim (L. by small pieces)

FS
factor of safety
field stimulation
file separator (character—re:
    computers/data processing)
fine structure
fire setter (re: Psychol)
forearm supinated
Fourier series
fracture, simple
Freeman-Sheldon (syndrome)
full and soft (diet order)
full scale (IQ)
full strength
forequarter shoulder (re: veterinary)
fracture site
function study

FS, f.s.
frozen section

F & S
full and soft

FSA
fetal sulfoglycoprotein antigen

f.s.a.
fiat secundum artem (L. let it be made
    skillfully)

f.s.a.r.
fiat secundum artis regulas (L. let it be
    made according to the rules of the
    art)

FSB
fetal scalp blood

FSBT
Fowler single breath test

FSC
fracture, simple, complete
free secretory component

FSCC
fracture, simple, complete, comminuted

FSD
focal skin distance (re: radiology)
focus skin distance (re: radiology)

focus to skin distance (re: radiology)
fracture, simple, depressed
full-scale deflection

FSDQ
Frost Self-Description Questionnaire
(re: Psychol)

FSE
filtered smoke exposure

FSF
fibrin-stabilizing factor (Factor XIII)

FSG
fasting serum glucose
focal sclerosing glomerulonephritis
focal segmental glomerulosclerosis

FSGN
focal sclerosing glomerulonephritis

FSGO
floating spherical gaussian orbital

FSGS
focal segmental glomerulosclerosis

FSH
fascioscapulohumeral
follicle-stimulating hormone

F sheet
field sheet

FSH/LH-RH
follicle-stimulating hormone and
luteinizing hormone-releasing
hormone

FSHRF, FSH-RF
follicle-stimulating hormone-releasing
factor

FSHRH, FSH-RH
follicle-stimulating hormone-releasing
hormone

FSI
foam stability index
foam stabilizing index
Function Status Index

FSIA
foot shock-induced analgesia

FSIQ
Full-Scale Intelligence Quotient

FSL
fasting serum level
fixed slight light
formal semantics language (re:
computers)

FSM
flying-spot microscope
furosemide

FSP
familial spastic paraplegia
fibrin/fibrinogen-split products
fibrinolytic split products
fine-suspended particulate
free secretory piece

F-SP
forma specialis (re: taxonomy)

FSR
film screen radiography
fragmented sarcoplasmic reticulum
fusiform skin revision

FSS
Fear Survey Schedule (re: Psychol)
French steel sound
front support strap
Functional Systems Scale

FSST
Full-Scale Score Total

FST
file status table (re: computers/data
processing)
foam stability test

F$^+$ strain
donor-behaving *E. coli* during
unidirectional genetic transfer

F$^-$ strain
recipient-behaving *E. coli* during
unidirectional genetic transfer

FSV
feline fibrosarcoma virus

FSW
field service worker

FT
false transmitter
family therapy
fast twitch
ferromagnetic tamponade
fetal tonsil
fibrous tissue
finger tapping
fingertip
follow through (after barium meal—re:
radiology)
formol toxoid (toxin treated with
formaldehyde—destroys toxicity but
retains antigenicity)
Fourier transform
free thyroxin(e)
full term (re: OB)
functional test

FT$_3$
free triiodothyronine

FT$_4$
free (unbound) thyroxin(e)

Ft, ft
feet
foot

F$_t$
ferritin

ft.
fac (L. make)
fiant (L. let them be made)
fiat (L. let it be made)

ft^2
square foot

ft^3
cubic foot

FTA
fluorescein treponema antibody (test)
fluorescent treponemal antibodies
fluorescent treponemal antibody (test)

FTA-AB
fluorescent treponemal antibody
    absorption (test)

FTA-ABS, FTA-Abs
fluorescent treponemal antibody
    absorption (test)

FTAG, F-TAG
fast-binding target-attaching globulin

FTAT
fluorescent treponemal antibody test

FTB
fingertip blood

FTBD
fit to be detained
full term born dead

FTC
frames to come (re: optometry)
frequency threshold curve

ft c, ft-c
foot candle

ft. catapl.
fiat cataplasma (L. let a poultice be
    made)

ft. cataplasm.
fiat cataplasma (L. let a poultice be
    made)

ft. cerat.
fiat ceratum (L. let a cerate be made
    [medicinal topical formulation made
    with wax for ease of spreading
    without liquifying])

ft. chart. vi
fiant chartulae vi (L. let six powders be
    made [use small letter roman
    numerals for number])

ft. collyr.
fiat collyrium (L. let an eyewash be
    made)

FTD
femoral total density

F3TDR
trifluorothymidine (trifluridine—antiviral
    [ophthalmic])

FTE
full-time equivalent

ft. emuls.
fiat emulsio (L. let an emulsion be
    made)

ft. enem.
fiat enema (L. let an enema be made)

FTF
finger to finger (test—re: Neuro)

FTFTN
finger-to-finger-to-nose (test—re:
    Neuro)

FTG
full-thickness graft

ft. garg.
fiat gargarisma (L. let a gargle be made)

FTI
free thyroxin(e) index

FT$_3$I
free triiodothyronine index

FT$_3$ index
free triiodothyronine index

FT$_4$ index
free thyroxin(e) index
    (tetraiodothyronine)

ft. infus.
fiat infusum (L. let an infusion be made)

ft. injec.
fiat injectio (L. let an injection be made)

FTIR
functional terminal innervation ratio

FTKA
failed to keep appointment

ftL, ft L
foot-lambert (unit describing surface
    luminance— obsolete)

FTLB
full term living birth

ft lb, ft-lb
foot pound (unit of work in foot-pound-second system)

ft. linim.
fiat linimentum (L. let a liniment be made)

FTM
fluid thioglycolate medium
fractional test meal

ft. mas.
fiat massa (L. let a mass be made)

ft. mas. div. in pil.
fiat massa dividenda in pilulae (L. let a mass be made and divided into pills)

ft. mass. div. in pil. xiv
fiat massa et divide in pilulae xiv (L. let a mass be made and divide into 14 pills [lower-case roman numerals for number of pills])

ft. mist.
fiat mistura (L. let a mixture be made)

FTN
finger to nose (test—re: Neuro)

FTNB
full-term newborn

FTND
full term normal delivery

FTNS
functional transcutaneous nerve stimulation

FTNSD
full term, normal, spontaneous delivery

FTO
fructose-terminated oligosaccharide

FTPA
perfluorotripropylamine (blood substitute)

ft. pil. xxiv
fiant pilulae xxiv (L. let 24 pills be made [lower-case roman numerals for number of pills])

ft. pulv.
fiat pulvis (L. let a powder be made)

FTR
fractional turnover rate

FTS
Family Tracking System
feminizing testes syndrome
fingertips

FTSG
full-thickness skin graft

ft. sol.
fiat solutio (L. let a solution be made)

ft. solut.
fiat solutio (L. let a solution be made)

ft. suppos.
fiat suppositorium (L. let a suppository be made)

FTT
failure to thrive
fat tolerance test
fingertips to _____(re: amount of forward flexion)
fraternal twins raised together
fructose tolerance test

ft. troch.
fiant trochisci (L. let lozenges be made)

ft. ung.
fiat unguentum (L. let an ointment be made)

FTX
field training exercise

FU
fecal urobilinogen
fluorouracil (antineoplastic)
fractional urinalysis
fundus

FU, F/U, f/u
follow up (when used as a noun)
follow-up (when used as an adjective)

FU, Fu, F u
Finsen unit (re: ultraviolet ray wavelength intensity)

5FU, 5-FU, 5-fu
5-fluoro-2,4(1H,3H)pyrimidinedione (fluorouracil— antineoplastic)

fu
flux unit (re: radioastronomy energy)

FUB
functional uterine bleeding

FUBAR
fouled up beyond all recognition

FUCA
α-L-fucosidase

FUDR, FUdR
5-fluoro-2′-deoxy-β-uridine (floxuridine; fluorodeoxyuridine—antineoplastic; antiviral)

5-FUDR
5-fluoro-2′-deoxyuridine (antimetabolite)

fulg.
fulguration

FUM
5-fluorouracil and methotrexate (re: chemotherapy)
fumarase
fumarate
fumigate
fumigation

FUMP
fluorouridine monophosphate

funct.
function
functional

FUO, F.U.O.
fever of undetermined origin
fever of unknown origin

FUOV
follow-up office visit

fu p
fusion point

FUR
fluorouracil riboside
5-fluorouridine

FURAM
ftorafur, Adriamycin (doxorubicin), and mitomycin C (re: chemotherapy)

fus.
fusion

FUSE
polykaryocytosis promotor (gene marker symbol—re: molecular genetics)

FUT
fibrinogen uptake test

FUTP
fluorouridine triphosphate

FV
Fahr-Volhard (disease)
femoral vein
flow volume
fluid volume
formaldehyde vapors
Friend virus

FVA
Friend virus anemia

FVC
false vocal cord
forced vital capacity (re: Resp)

FVD
fibrovascular tissue on disk

FVE
fibrovascular tissue elsewhere
forced volume, expiratory (re: Resp)

FVFR
filled voiding flow rate

FVL
femoral vein ligation
force, velocity, length

FVM
familial visceral myopathy

FVP
Friend virus polycythemia

FVR
feline viral rhinotracheitis
forearm vascular resistance

f. vs., f.v.s.
fiat venae sectio (L. let there be a cutting of a vein [venisection])

FW
Falconer-Weddell (syndrome)
Felix-Weil (reaction—re: laboratory)
Folin and Wu's (method—re: laboratory)
forced whisper
fracturing wall
fragment wound
Friderichsen-Waterhouse (syndrome)

fw, f.w.
fresh water

F wave
a compound muscle action potential (re: motor neurons)

FWB
full weight bearing

FWHM
full width (of the photopeak measured at) half the maximal ([count]—re: tomography)
full width (of the line-spread function) half-maximum height

FWR
Felix-Weil reaction

FW reaction
Felix-Weil reaction

FX
fluoroscopy
fornix
fractional
frozen section

FX, Fx, fx.
fracture

fx.
friction

Fx BB
fracture of both bones

FXD
four times daily

Fx-dis, fx-dis
fracture-dislocation

FY
fiber year
fiscal year
full year

FY, Fy
alleles in Duffy system blood group

Fy^a
alleles in Duffy system blood group

Fy^b
alleles in Duffy system blood group

FYI
for your information

Fy^x
alleles in Duffy system blood group

FZ
focal zone

G

G
ganglion
Gasterophilus (genus of botfly—re: veterinary)
gastrin
Gastrodiscoides (genus—*Gastrodiscus*)
gauge
gauss (centimeter-gram-second unit of magnetic flux density)
Gemella (genus)
general learning ability (re: Psychol—General Aptitude Test Battery)
geometric efficiency
Giardia (genus)
giga (10^9 or one billion)
giga- (Gr. giant—prefix)
globular (re: proteins)
globule
globulin
Glossina (genus—tsetse flies)
glycine
glycogen
Gnathostoma (genus—nematode worm—re: veterinary; occasionally in man)
goat (re: veterinary medicine)
gold inlay (re: Dent)
gonidial (re: bacterial colonies)
good
good (re: manual muscle evaluation)
Gordius (genus—horsehair worms; re: veterinary; occasionally in man)
Grafenberg spot (re: GYN)
gravida (pregnant)
gravitational constant (newtonian constant)
gravitational unit
Greek
Gross (leukemia antigen—Ludwik Gross, oncologist)
guanidine
guanine
guanosine
guanylic acid
immunoglobulin G

G, *G*
Gibbs free energy

G, g
conductance
gallop (heart sound)
gap (in cell cycle—re: cytogenetics)
gas

gingival
glucose
gravity
unit of acceleration of gravity (standard value)

G, g, g.
gram (unit of mass in centimeter-gram-second system)

G, g.
green (an indicator color)

Γ
Greek capital letter gamma

G+
gram positive

G 1-4
grade 1 through 4 (re: heart murmur)

G1
Grid 1 (re: EEG)

G_1
Gap $_1$ (re: period in cell cycle)

GI, GII, GIII
number of pregnancies (L. gravida—heavy)

G2
Grid 2 (re: EEG)

G_2
Gap $_2$ (re: period in cell cycle)

G130
granulocyte membrane glycoprotein

g.
gender
grain
gramma (L. gram)
group

$\bar{g}$
physical geometry factor

g%
grams per milliliter
gram percent

$(g)^2$
square grade (unit of solid angle)

γ
a carbon separated from the carboxyl
group by two other carbon atoms (re:
nonaromatic organic compounds)
gamma (third letter of Greek alphabet)
gamma ray (re: radioactive isotopes)
heavy chain of IgG
immunoglobulin
measure of development (re:
photography)
microgram (sometimes used; μg
preferred—re: mass)
one of the hemoglobin monomers in
fetal hemoglobin
photon

γ –
gamma-plasma protein fraction
constituent designator, e.g.,
γ-globulin (gamma globulin)

GA
gastric analysis
gastric antrum
general anesthesia
general appearance
gentisic acid
gestational age
Getting Along (re: psychological testing)
gibberellic acid (plant-growth promoter)
glucuronic acid
Golgi apparatus
gramicidin A
granulocyte adherence
granuloma annulare
guessed average
gut-associated

GA, G/A
gingivoaxial (re: Dent)

Ga
gallium (element)
granulocyte agglutination

^{66}Ga
radioactive isotope of gallium

^{67}Ga
radioactive isotope of gallium

^{68}Ga
radioactive isotope of gallium

^{72}Ga
radioactive isotope of gallium

ga.
gauge (measurement of surgical
needles, wire, etc.)

g.a.
ginger ale

GABA
γ-aminobutyric acid (a
neurotransmitter)

GABA-T
γ-aminobutyric acid transaminase

GABHS
group A beta-hemolytic streptococcus

GABOA
γ-amino-β-hydroxybutyric acid
(anticonvulsant)

GABOB
γ-amino-β-hydroxybutyric (acid—
anticonvulsant)

GABS
group A beta-hemolytic streptococci

γAbu
γ-aminobutyric acid (a
neurotransmitter)

G acid
2-naphthol-6,8-disulfonic acid (re:
manufacture of azo dyes)

G-actin
globular actin (a myofibril protein which,
in absence of salt, becomes globular)

GAD
general acyl-CoA dehydrogenase
generalized anxiety disorder (re:
Psychol)
glutamic acid decarboxylase

GADH
gastric alcohol dehydrogenase

GADS
gonococcal arthritis/dermatitis
syndrome

GAF
giant axon formation

GAG
glycoaminoglycan
glycosaminoglycan

GAGs
glycosaminoglycans

GAHS
galactorrhea-amenorrhea
hyperprolactinemia syndrome

GAI
guided affective imagery (re: Psychol)

GAL
galactosyl
gallus adeno-like (virus)

Gal, gal.
galactose

gal
Galileo (unit of acceleration)

gal.
gallon

GALE
UDP-galactose-4-epimerase

GALK
galactokinase

gal/min
gallons per minute

GalNAc
N-acetyl-D-galactosamine

gal-1-P
galactose-1-phosphate

GALT
galactose-1-phosphate uridyltransferase
gut-associated lymphoid tissue

GAL TT
galactose tolerance test

GALV
gibbon ape leukemia virus

GaLV
gibbon ape lymphosarcoma virus

Galv, galv.
galvanic

galv.
galvanism
galvanized

GAMG
goat antimouse immunoglobulin G

GAN
giant axonal neuropathy

GANC
α-glucosidase C, neutral

gang.
ganglion
ganglionic

gangl.
ganglion
ganglionic

gangr.
gangrene

G antigen
gebundenes (Ger. bound—an internal
   antigen)

GAP
Gardner Analysis of Personality Survey
glyceraldehyde phosphate

GAPD
glyceraldehyde-3-phosphate
   dehydrogenase

GAPDH
glyceraldehyde-3-phosphate
   dehydrogenase

G/A quotient
globulin-albumin quotient

GAR
genitoanorectal (syndrome)
goat antirabbit (gamma globulin)

GARG, garg.
gargarisma (L. a gargle)

GARGG
goat antirabbit gamma globulin

GAS
gastric acid secretion
gastroenterology
generalized arteriosclerosis
Global Assessment Scale
group A streptococcus

GAS, G-A-S
generalized adaptation syndrome
   (Selye's term: 1. alarm reaction; 2.
   stage of resistance; 3. exhaustion)

GAs
gibberellins (plant growth hormones)

GASA
growth-adjusted sonographic age

GASH
guanidinium aluminum sulfate
   hexahydrate

GAST
gastrocnemius (muscle)

Gastroc, gastroc.
gastrocnemius (muscle)

GAT
gas antitoxin
gelatin agglutination test
Gerontological Apperception Test (re:
   Psychol)
group adjustment therapy

GATB
General Aptitude Test Battery

gav.
gavage

GAW
airway conductance (reciprocal of
   airway resistance—G is symbol for
   conductance—re: Resp)

GB
Gilbert-Behçet (syndrome
goofball (barbiturate pill)
Gougerot-Blum (syndrome)
Guillain-Barré(syndrome)

GB, G.B.
gallbladder

Gb
gilbert (centimeter-gram-second unit of magnetomotive force)

GBA
ganglionic-blocking agent
gingivobuccoaxial (re: Dent)

G banding
Giemsa banding (stain)

GBCE
Grassi Basic Cognitive Evaluation (re: Psychol)

GBD
gallbladder disease
glassblower's disease
granulomatous bowel disease

G & B days
good and bad days

GBG
gonadal steroid-binding globulin

GBH
gamma benzene hydrochloride (lindane—pediculicide; scabicide; insecticide)
graphite, benzalkonium, heparin

γ-BHC
gamma benzene hexachloride (lindane—pediculicide; scabicide; insecticide)

GBI
globulin-bound insulin

GBIA
Guthrie bacterial inhibition assay

GBL
glomerular basal lamina

GBM
glomerular basement membrane

GBP
galactose-binding protein
gated blood pool

GBPS
gallbladder pigment stones

GBq
gigabequerel (one billion [10^9] bequerels—re: radioactivity)

GBS
gallbladder series
gastric bypass surgery
glycerin-buffered saline

group β (hemolytic) streptococcus (beta hemolytic streptococcus)
Guillain-Barré syndrome

GB series, G.B. series
gallbladder series

GBSS
Gey's balanced salt solution

GC
ganglion cells
gas chromatography
general circulation
general condition
glucocorticoid
goblet cell
Golgi cell
Golgi complex
gonococcal (infection—gonorrhea)
good condition
Gougerot-Carteaud (syndrome)
granular casts
granule cell
granulocyte cytotoxic
granulomatous colitis
granulosa cell

GC, Gc
gonorrhea
group-specific component (re: genetics—parentage, testing)

GC, gc.
gonococcal
gonococcus

Gc
gigacycle (one billion [10^9] cycles)

GCA
gastric cancerous area
giant cell arteritis

Gca, gca
gonorrhea (a hybridism)

g-cal.
gram-calorie (small calorie)

GCB
gonococcal base

GCDFP
gross cystic disease fluid protein

GCDP
gross cystic disease protein

GCFT
gonococcal complement-fixation test
gonorrhea complement-fixation test

GCI
General Cognitive Index (re: Psychol)

GCII
glucose-controlled insulin infusion

GCIIS
glucose-controlled insulin infusion
　　system

g-cm
gram-centimeter

GCMS, GC-MS
gas chromatography-mass
　　spectrometry

GCN
giant cerebral neuron

GCR
glucocorticoid receptor
group conformity rate

GCRC
General Clinical Research Centers

GCS
general clinical service
Generalized Contentment Scale
Glasgow Coma Scale
glucocorticosteroid

GCSA
Gross cell surface antigen (Ludwik
　　Gross, oncologist)

G-CSF
granulocyte colony-stimulating factor

GCT
general care and treatment
giant cell tumor

GC & T
general care and treatment

GC type
guanine, cytosine type (re: pentose
　　nucleic acids)

GCU
gonococcal urethritis

GCV
great cardiac vein

GCVF
great cardiac vein flow

GCW
glomerular capillary wall

GCY
gastroscopy

GD
gastroduodenal
general duties
gestational day
Gianotti disease
gonadal dysgenesis
Graves' disease

GD, G/D
growth and development

G-D
general diagnostics

G and D
growth and development

Gd
gadolinium (element)

^{153}Gd
radioactive isotope of gadolinium

^{159}Gd
radioactive isotope of gadolinium

gd.
good

GDA
germine diacetate

GDB
gas-density balance

GDC
giant dopamine-containing cell

GDG
generation data group (re: computers/
　　data processing)

GDH
glucose dehydrogenase
glutamate dehydrogenase (used
　　interchangeably with glutamic acid
　　although technically glutamate refers
　　to the negatively charged ion)
glutamic acid dehydrogenase (used
　　interchangeably with glutamate in
　　biochemistry although technically
　　different)
glycerophosphate dehydrogenase
gonadotrop(h)ic hormone
growth and differentiation hormone (in
　　insects)

GDID
genetically determined
　　immunodeficiency diseases

GDM
gestational diabetes mellitus

gdn.
guardian

GDP
gastroduodenal pylorus
gel diffusion precipitin
guanosine diphosphate (guanosine 5'-
　　diphosphate)

GDP-D-mannose
guanosine diphosphate-D-mannose

GDS
Gradual Dosage Schedule

GDT
gel development time

GDW
glass-distilled water

GE
gainfully employed
Gänsslen-Erb (syndrome)
gastric emptying
gastroemotional
gastroenteritis
gastroenterology
gastroenterostomy
gastroesophageal
gastrointestinal endoscopy
gel electrophoresis
generalized epilepsy
gentamicin
glandular epithelium
greater than or equal to (re: computers/
data processing)
Gsell-Erdheim (syndrome)

G/E
granulocyte-erythroid ratio

Ge
Gerbich red cell antigen
germanium (element)

68Ge
radioactive isotope of germanium

71Ge
radioactive isotope of germanium

77Ge
radioactive isotope of germanium

g.e., g-e
gravity eliminated

GEC
galactose elimination capacity

GEE
glycine ethyl ester

GEF
glossoepiglottic fold
gonadotrop(h)in enhancing factor

GEFT
Group Embedded Figures Test (re:
Psychol)

GEH
glycerol ester hydrolase

gel.
gelatin
gelatinous

gel. quav.
gelatina quavis (L. in any kind of jelly)

GEM
geminal

gem-
geminate (two substituents on the same
atom)

GEMS
good emergency mother substitute

GEN
gender
generation
genetics
genital

gen.
general
genitalia
genus (L. kind)

Gen cath.
Gensini catheter

genet.
genetics

gen. et sp. nov.
genus et species nova (L. new genus
and species)

genit.
genitalia

gen'l
general

gen. nov.
genus novum (L. new genus)

gen. proc.
general procedure

geom.
geometric

GEP
gastroenteropancreatic (endocrine
system—re: enterochromaffin cells)

GEPG
gastroesophageal pressure gradient

GER
gastroesophageal reflux
granular endoplasmic reticulum

Ger
German

Ger, ger.
geriatrics

GERD
gastroesophageal reflux disease

Geriat
geriatrics

GERL
Golgi-associated endoplasmic reticulum
 lysosomes

Gerontol
gerontologist
gerontology

GES
glucose electrolyte solution
Group Encounter Survey (re: Psychol)
Group Environment Scale (re: Psychol)

GEST
gestation
gestational

GET
gastric emptying time
graded (treadmill) exercise test

GET½
gastric emptying half-time

GEU
gestation, extra-uterine

GeV
giga electron volt (one billion volts [10^9];
 formerly BeV)

GEX
gas exchange

GF
gastric fistula
gastric fluid
glass factor (tissue culture)
globule fibril
glomerular filtrate
glomerular filtration
gluten-free
grandfather
growth factor
growth failure
growth fraction

GF, Gf
germ-free (animal—re: gnotobiology)

G-F
globular-fibrous (re: proteins)

gf
gram-force

GFA
glial fibrillary acidic (protein)
global force applicator

G factor
general factor (the single variance
 common to different intelligence
 tests—re: Psychol)

g factor
ratio of the magnetic moment of a
 particle to the Bohr magneton (re:
 physics)

GFAP
glial fibrillary acidic protein

GFD
gluten-free diet

GFFS
glycogen-and-fat-free solid

GFH
glucose-free Hanks' (solution)

GFI
glucagon-free insulin

GFL
giant follicular lymphoma

G forces, G-forces
acceleration forces

GFP
gamma-fetoprotein
glomerular filtered phosphate

GFR
grunting, flaring, and retracting (re:
 neonate)

GFR, G.F.R.
glomerular filtration rate

G-F-W Battery
Goldman-Fristoe-Woodcock Auditory
 Skills Test Battery

GG
gamma globulin
genioglossus
glyceryl guaiacolate (guaifenesin—
 reduces viscosity of sputum)
glycylglycine
guar gum (re: pharmaceutical jelly
 formulations)

γG
immunoglobulin G

GGA
general gonadotropic activity

GGCS
gamma-glutamyl-cysteine synthetase

GGE
generalized glandular enlargement
gradient gel electrophoresis

GGFC
gamma globulin-free calf (serum)

GGG, G.G.G.
gummi guttae gambiae (gamboge; New
 L. gambogium; cambugium;

217

gambodium—a gum resin obtained from Cambodia used as drastic hydragogue cathartic)

GGM
glucose-galactose malabsorption

GGPNA
γ-glutamyl-*p*-nitroanilide

GGS
glands, goiter, or stiffness

GG or S
glands, goiter, or stiffness

GGT
γ-glutamyltransferase (gamma-glutamyltransferase; gamma-glutamyl transpeptidase)

GGTP
gamma-glutamyl transpeptidase

GGVB
gelatin, glucose, veronal buffer

GH
Gee-Herter (disease)
general health
general hospital
genetic hypertension
geniohyoid
Gilford-Hutchinson (syndrome)
good health
growth hormone (anterior pituitary)

G + H
Gibbs and Helmholtz (equation)

GHAG
General High Altitude Questionnaire

γ-HCD
gamma-heavy chain disease

GHD
growth hormone deficiency

4G X 6H X 10D
four grains times six hours times ten days

GHK
Goldman-Hodgkin-Katz (equation [Goldman equation])

GHQ
General Health Questionnaire (re: Psychol)

GHR
granulomatous hypersensitivity reaction

GHRF, GH-RF
growth hormone-releasing factor

GHRH, GH-RH
growth hormone-releasing hormone

GHRIF, GH-RIF
growth hormone release-inhibiting factor

GHRIH, GH-RIH
growth hormone release-inhibiting hormone
growth hormone release-inhibitory hormone

GHz
gigahertz (one billion [10^9] hertz [SI unit of frequency])

GI
gastrointestinal
gelatin infusion (medium)
Gingival Index
glomerular index
glucose intolerance
growth inhibiting

GI, G.I.
globin insulin

Gi
good impression (re: California Psychological Inventory)

gi.
gill (¼ pint)

GIA
gastrointestinal anastomosis

GIBF
gastrointestinal bacterial flora

GIC
gastric interdigestive contraction

GICA
gastrointestinal cancer
gastrointestinal cancer antigen

GIF
gonadotrop(h)in-inhibitory factor (somatostatin)
growth hormone-inhibiting factor

GIFT
granulocyte immunofluorescence test

GIGO
garbage in, garbage out (re: computers)

GIH
gastrointestinal hemorrhage
gastrointestinal hormone
growth-inhibiting hormone

GII
gastrointestinal infection

GIK
glucose, insulin, and kalium (potassium—solution)

GILCU
gradual increase in length and
complexity of utterance

GIM
gonadotrop(h)in-inhibitory material

GIN
glutamine

ging.
gingiva (L. gum)

g-ion
gram-ion

GIP
gastric inhibitory peptide
gastric inhibitory polypeptide
giant (cell) interstitial pneumonia
glucose-dependent insulin-releasing
    peptide
glucose insulinotropic peptide
gonorrheal invasive peritonitis

GIR
global improvement rating

GIS
gas in stomach
gastrointestinal series
gastrointestinal symptom
gastrointestinal system

GI series
gastrointestinal series

GIT
gastrointestinal tract
glutathione-insulin transhydrogenase

GITS
gastrointestinal therapeutic system

GITT
gastrointestinal transit time
glucose-insulin tolerance test

GiV
giga (electron) volts (one billion volts
    [10^9]; formerly BeV; GeV preferred)

GIX, Gix
DFDT
    (difluorodiphenyltrichloroethane—a
    powerful insecticide)

GJ
gap junctions
gastrojejunostomy

GJP
graphic job processor (re: computers/
    data processing)

GK
galactokinase

Gasser-Karrer (syndrome)
glycerol kinase

Gk
Greek

GKA
guinea pig keratocyte

GL
Gilbert-Lereboullet (syndrome)
glandula (L. gland)
glomerular layer
glycosphingolipoid
granular layer
greatest length (re: fetus)

GL, Gl, gl.
gland

G/L, g/l
grams per liter

Gl
glucinium (obsolete—now called Be,
    beryllium)

Gl, gl
gill

gl.
glandula(e) (L. gland[s])

GLA
α-galactosidase
giant left atrium
gingivolinguoaxial (re: Dent)

Gla
γ-carboxyglutamic acid

glac.
glacial

GLAD
gold-labeled antigen detection
    (technique)

gland.
glandula (L. gland)
glandular

GLAT
glutamic acid, lysine, alanine, and
    tyrosine

glau.
glaucoma

glauc.
glaucoma

GLB1
β-galactosidase-1

GLB2
β-galactosidase-2

GLC
gas-liquid chromatography

GLC, Glc
glucose

GLC, glc.
glaucoma

GlcA
gluconic acid

GLC/MS
gas-liquid chromatography/mass
spectrometry

GlcN
glucosamine

GlcNAc
N-acetylglucosamine (*N*-acetyl-D-
glucosamine)

GlcUA, Glc-UA
glucuronic acid (D-glucuronic acid)

GLD
globoid leukodystrophy
glutamate dehydrogenase

GLH
germinal layer hemorrhage

GLI
glicentin (formerly enteroglucagon)
glucagon-like immunoreactivity

GLIM
generalized linear interactive model

GLL
glabellolambda line (a craniometric
point)

GLM
general linear model

Gln
glutamine
glutaminyl

GLO
glyoxalase I

GLO1, GLO-I
glyoxalase 1 (I)

GLOB, Glob, glob.
globulin

Glob
globular

glos. dev.
glossal deviation

GLP
glycolipoprotein

good laboratory practice
group-living program

GLPP
glucose, postprandial

GLR
graphic level recorder

GLS
guinea (pig) lung strip

GLTN, Gltn
glomerulotubulonephritis

GLTT
glucose-lactate tolerance test

GLU, Glu, glu.
glutamic acid

GLU, glu.
glucose

Glu
glutamine (glutaminic acid)
glutamyl (radical of glutamic acid)

glu.
glutamate (a salt or ester of glutamic
acid)

GluA
glucuronic acid

gluc.
glucose

gluc. tol.
glucose tolerance

glucur.
glucuronide

glu. ox.
glucose oxidase

Glu-1-P
glucose-1-phosphate

Glut
gluteal

glu. tol.
glucose tolerance

GLV
Gross leukemia virus

glv.
galvanic

Glx
glutaminyl and/or glutamyl (indicates
uncertainty between Glu and Gln)

Gly
glycyl

Gly, gly.
glycine

gly.
glycerite
glycerol

glyc.
glycerin
glyceritum (L. glycerite)

Glycerol-3-P
glycerol 3-phosphate

glyco.
glycogen

GM
gastric mucosa
Geiger-Müller
general medical
General Medicine
genetic manipulation
gentamicin
geometric mean
grand mal
grandmother
grand mutiparity
granulocyte-macrophage
groupmark (re: computers)
growth medium
monosialoganglioside (re: genetic
    marker)

Gm
gamma (allotype, marker)
gramma (L. gram)

Gm, gm
gram (former abbreviation—g now
    used)

Gm +
gram-positive (stain)

Gm −
gram-negative (stain)

Gm%, gm%
grams per hundred milliliters

g-m
gram-meter

g/m
gallons per minute

GMA
glyceryl methacrylate
glycol methacrylate (embedding
    medium—re: histology)
gross motor activities

Gm allotype
gamma allotype (an allotype marker
    found on the heavy chains of IgG)

GMB
gastric mucosal barrier
glioblastoma multiforme

GMBF
gastric mucosal blood flow

GMC
general medical clinic
grivet monkey cell (line)

GMC, G.M.C.
General Medical Council

gm cal
gram calorie (small calorie)

gm/cc
grams per cubic centimeter

GMCD
grand mal convulsive disorder

GM-CFU
granulocyte-macrophage colony-
    forming unit

GM counter
Geiger-Müller counter

GM-CSF
granulocyte-macrophage colony-
    stimulating factors

GMCU
gracilis myocutaneous unit

GMD
geometric mean diameter
glycopeptide moiety (modified)
    derivative

GME
graduate medical education

GMEPP
giant miniature end-plate potential

GMH
germinal matrix hemorrhage

GMK
green monkey kidney (cells)

GML
gut mucosal lymphocyte

gm/l
grams per liter

GMM
Goldberg-Maxwell-Morris (syndrome)

gm-m
gram-meter

Gm marker
gamma marker (an allotype marker
    found on the heavy chains of IgG)

g-mol
gram-molecule

GMP
glucose monophosphate
good manufacturing practice
guanosine-5'-phosphate (guanosine
  monophosphate; guanosine 5'-
  monophosphate; guanylic acid)

GM-P
G-myeloma proteins

3':5'-GMP
guanosine 3':5'-cyclic phosphate (cyclic
  guanosine monophosphate)

GMR
gallops, murmurs, or rubs

GMS
glyceryl monostearate (pharmaceutic
  aid)
Gomori's methenamine-silver (stain)

GM&S, GM & S
general medical and surgical
general medicine and surgery

GM seizure
grand mal seizure

GMT
geometric mean titer

GMT, G.M.T.
Greenwich mean time

GMV
gram molecular volume

GMW
gram molecular weight

GN
Gandy-Nanta (disease)
gaze nystagmus
glomerulonephritis
glucagon
gram negative

GN, G/N
glucose:nitrogen (ratio in urine
  examination)

Gn
gonadotrop(h)in

GNA
general nursing assistance

GNB
gram-negative bacilli

GNBM
gram-negative bacillary meningitis

GN broth
gram-negative broth

GNC
general nursing care
glandular neck cell

GNCA
gastric noncancerous area

GND
gram-negative diplococcus

gnd.
ground

GNID
gram-negative intracellular diplococci

G/N r, G/Nr
glucose-to-nitrogen ratio

GnRF
gonadotrop(h)in-releasing factor

GnRH, Gn-RH
gonadotrop(h)in (hormone)-releasing
  hormone

G/NS
glucose in normal saline

GO
gonorrhea
Gordan-Overstreet (syndrome)

GO, g.o.
glucose oxidase

G&O
gas and oxygen

G$_0$
symbol for a period in cell growth cycle

GΩ
gigohm (unit of electrical resistance
  equal to 1 billion ohms [$10^9\Omega$])

Go
Golgi

G°
standard free energy

GOD
generation of diversity
glucose oxidase

GOD/POD
glucose oxidase-perioxidase (method)

GOE
gas, oxygen, ether (gas-oxygen-ether—
  re: anesthesia)

GOK
God only knows

GOL
glabello-opisthion line (re:
  craniometrics)

Gold sol.
colloidal gold curve solution (test)

GOM
God's own medicine

GON
gonococcal ophthalmia neonatorum

Gonio
gonioscopy

G₀ phase
symbol to indicate cells that leave the mitotic cycle to become quiescent

GOQ
glucose oxidation quotient

GOR
gastroesophageal reflux
general operating room

GOT
goals of treatment

GOT, Got
glutamic oxaloacetic transaminase (aspartate aminotransferase)
glutamine oxaloacetic transaminase

GOT1
glutamate-oxaloacetate transaminase

GOT2
glutamate-oxaloacetate transaminase

Gov
governmental

govt.
government

GP
gastroplasty
general paralysis
general paresis
general practice
general practitioner
general proprioception (re: Neuro)
general purpose
genetic prediabetes
geometric progression
globus pallidus (re: Neuro)
glucose phosphate
glucose production
glutathione peroxidase
D-glycerophosphate
glycoprotein
gram positive
guinea pig
gutta-percha (Malay—gum from a tree; a sealant—re: dental cement, orthopaedic fracture splints)

GP, gp.
group

G-1-P
glucose-1-phosphate

G-1,6-P
glucose-1,6-diphosphate

G-3-P
glyceraldehyde 3-phosphate

G6P, G-6-P
glucose-6-phosphate

[G]p
concentration of glucose in plasma

gp.
group (muscle)

GPA
grade-point averages
guinea pig albumin

GPAIS
guinea pig anti-insulin serum

GPB
glossopharyngeal breathing

GPBP
guinea pig myelin basic protein

GPC
gastric parietal cell
gel permeation chromatography
general purpose computer
giant papillary conjunctivitis
glycerophosphorylcholine
granular progenitor cell
guinea-pig complement

GPD
glucose-6-phosphate dehydrogenase
guinea pig dander

G6PD, G-6-PD, G-6-PD
glucose-6-phosphate dehydrogenase

G6PDA, G-6-PD-A
glucose-6-phosphate dehydrogenase (enzyme) variant A

GPDH
glucose phosphate dehydrogenase (glucose-6-)

G6PDH
glucose-6-phosphate dehydrogenase

GPE
guinea-pig embryo

GPF
glomerular plasma flow
granulocytosis-promoting factor

GPGG
guinea pig gamma globulin

G₁phase
presynthetic gap (re: cell cycle)

G₂phase
postsynthetic gap (re: cell cycle)

GPHN
giant pigmented hairy nevus

GPHV
guinea pig herpes virus

GPI
general paresis of the insane (dementia
    paralytica)
Gingival-Periodontal Index (re: Dent)
glucosephosphate isomerase
glucosephosphate isomerase
    (deficiency)
Gordon Personal Inventory
guinea pig ileum

G.P.I.
general paralysis of the insane
    (dementia paralytica)

GPIMH
guinea pig intestinal mucosal
    homogenate

GPIPID
guinea pig intraperitoneal infectious
    dose

GPK
guinea pig kidney (antigen)

GPKA
guinea pig kidney absorption test

GPLV
guinea pig leukemia virus

Gply
gingivoplasty

GPM
general preventive medicine

GPP
Gordon Personal Profile (re: Psychol)

GPR
good partial response

GPRBC
guinea-pig red blood cell

GPS
Goodpasture's syndrome
guinea pig serum
guinea pig spleen

GPT
glutamate-pyruvate transaminase
    (alanine aminotransferase—ALT)
glutamic pyruvic transaminase (now

known as alanine aminotransferase,
    ALT)
guinea pig trachea

GP TH, GpTh, Gp Th
group therapy

GPTSM
guinea pig tracheal smooth muscle

GPU
guinea-pig unit

GPUT
galactose phosphate uridyl transferase

GPX
glutathione peroxidase

GPX1
glutathione peroxidase-1

GR
gamma ray
gastric resection
general research
generalized rash
glucose response
glutathione reductase
good recovery
granulocyte
gravid

GR, Gr, gr, gr.
grain(s) (smallest unit of mass in
    English system)

GR, gr
gamma roentgen

Gr
Grashof number (re: fluid mechanics)

gr.
grade
graft
grana (L. grains)
granum (L. grain)
gravida (L. heavy; pregnant)
gravity
great
greater
grill
grilled
gross
grossly

gr+
gram-positive (bacteria)

gr−
gram-negative (bacteria)

GRA
gated radionuclide angiography
gonadotrop(h)in-releasing agent

GRAD, grad.
gradatim (L. by degrees; gradually)

grad.
gradient
gradual
gradually
graduate
graduated

GRAE
generally recognized as effective
generally regarded as effective

gran.
granular
granulation
granulatus (L. granulated)

Gr antigen
Vw antigen (rare antigen associated
with MNS blood group)

GRAS
generally recognized as safe
generally regarded as safe (re: food
additives)

Gr I AS
grade I arteriosclerotic (cardiovascular
disease)

Grav, grav.
gravida (L. heavy; pregnant)

grav.
gravid
gravity

grav. I
gravida una (L. heavy; pregnant once)
primigravida (L. first heavy; first
pregnancy)

grav. $\dot{\mathrm{I}}$
primigravida (L. first heavy; first
pregnancy)

grav. $\dot{\mathrm{I}}$/Ab. $\dot{\mathrm{I}}$
gravida 1, aborta 1 (L. one pregnancy,
one abortion)

gravid.
gravida (L. heavy; pregnant)

GRD
beta-glucuronidase (β-glucuronidase—
re: determination of blood steroid
conjugants or urinary steroids)
gender role definition

grd.
ground

grds.
grounds

GRE
Graduate Record Examinations
(Aptitude Test—re: Psychol)

GREAT
Graduate Record Examinations
Aptitude Test (re: Psychol)

GRF
gonadotrop(h)in-releasing factor
growth (hormone)-releasing factor

GRH
gonadotrop(h)in-releasing hormone
growth hormone-releasing hormone

GRID
gay-related immunodeficiency

GRIF
growth hormone release-inhibiting
factor

GRIP
graphics interaction with proteins
(system)

GRL
granular layer

gr.m.p.
grosso modo pulverisatum (L. ground in
a coarse way)

GRN
granules

Grn
glycerone

gros.
grossus (L. coarse)

GRP
gastrin-releasing peptide

GrP
gram-positive

grp.
group

$Gr_1P_0AB_1$
one pregnancy, no births, one abortion

GRPS
glucose-Ringer-phosphate solution

GRS
β-glucuronidase (re: urinary steroids or
blood steroid conjugants
determination)

GRTP
guanosine triphosphate

Gr Tr
graphite treatment

GRW
giant ragweed (test)

GR WT, gr. wt.
gross weight

GS
gallstone
Gardner syndrome
gastric shield
gastrocnemius soleus
general surgery
Gilbert's syndrome
Glanzmann-Saland (syndrome)
glomerular sclerosis (re: Uro)
glucagon secretion
glutamine synthetase
goat serum
graft survival
granulocyte substance
Groenblad-Strandberg (syndrome)
Guérin-Stern (syndrome)

GS, gs
group specific

G/S
glucose and saline

Gs
gauss (centimeter-gram-second unit of
    magnetic flux density)

g/s
gallons per second

GSA
general somatic afferent (nerve)
Gross virus antigen (Ludwik Gross,
    oncologist)
group-specific antigen

G salt
sodium salt of G acid (2-naphthol-6,8-
    aminobutyric acid)

GSAS
glutamate-γ-semialdehyde synthetase

GSB
graduated spinal block

GSBG
gonadal steroid-binding globulin

GSC
gas-solid chromatography
gravity settling culture (plate)

G-SC
guanosine-coupled spleen cell

g scale
(force of) gravity scale

GSCN
giant serotonin-containing neuron

GSD
genetically significant dose (of
    mutagenic radiation)
glutathione synthetase deficiency
glycogen storage disease

GSE
general somatic efferent (nerve)
gluten-sensitive enteropathy (celiac
    sprue)

GSF
galactosemic fibroblasts

GSH
γ-glutamylcysteinylglycine
    (glutathione—reduced form)
glomerular stimulating hormone
golden Syrian hamster

G_1, S, G_2, M
cell cycle phases (G_1 = presynthetic
    gap, S = a DNA synthetic period, G_2
    = postsynthetic gap, and M = a brief
    mitotic period)

GSN
giant serotonin neuron

GSP
galvanic skin potential

GSR
galvanic skin response
generalized Shwartzman reaction
    (phenomenon)
glutathione reductase

GSS
gamete-shedding substance

GSSG
glutathione (oxidized form)

GSSG-R
glutathione reductase

GSSI
Global Sexual Satisfaction Index

GSSR
generalized Sanarelli-Shwartzman
    reaction

GST
gold salt therapy
graphic stress telethermometry
graphic stress thermography

GSW
gunshot wound

GSWA
gunshot wound to the abdomen

G syndrome
first letter of surname of first person
    reported with syndrome:

characteristic facies associated with
hypospadias, ventral penile curvature,
dysphagia

GT
gait training
gastrostomy
Gee-Thaysen (disease)
generation time
genetic therapy
gingiva, treatment of
glucose therapy
glucose tolerance
glucose transport
glutamyl transpeptidase
great toe
greater trochanter
group therapy

G & T
gowns and towels

GT1
glycogenosis type 1

γ-T
γ-tocopherol

gt.
gutta (L. drop)

g/t
granulation time
granulation tissue

GTD
gestational trophoblastic disease

GTF
glucose tolerance factor

GTH
gonadotrop(h)ic hormone

GTM
grade, location (anatomical site), (lymph
node involvement) and metastases
(re: Surgical Staging System for bone
sarcomas)

GTN
gestational trophoblastic neoplasia
gestational trophoblastic neoplasms
glomerulotubulonephritis
glyceryl trinitrate (nitroglycerin—re:
coronary vasodilator)

GTO
Golgi tendon organ

GTP
glutamyl transpeptidase
guanosine triphosphate (guanosine 5'-
triphosphate)

GTR
galvanic tetanus ratio

generalized time reflex
granulocyte turnover rate

GTS
glucose transport system

GTSTD
Grid Test of Schizophrenic Thought
Disorder

GTT
glucose tolerance test

gtt.
guttae (L. drops)

GTT agar
gelatin-tellurite-taurocholate agar

gtts.
guttae (L. drops)

GU
gastric ulcer
glucose uptake
glycogenic unit
gonococcal urethritis
gravitational ulcer

GU, G-U
genitourinary

[G]u
concentration of glucose in urine

Gua
guanine

guid.
guidance

GUK1
guanylate kinase-1

GUO, Guo
guanosine (in ribonucleosides)

GUS
genitourinary system

GUSB
β-glucuronidase

gutt.
gutturi (L. to the throat)

guttat.
guttatim (L. drop by drop)

gutt. quibusd.
guttis quibusdam (L. with a few drops)

GV
gastric volume
gentian violet
granulosis virus
griseoviridin (antibiotic substance
obtained from *Streptomyces griseus*)
Gross virus (Ludwik Gross, oncologist)

GVA
general visceral afferent (nerve)

G value
unit used in radiation chemistry

GVB
gelatin-veronal buffer

GVBD
germinal vesicle breakdown

GVE
general visceral efferent (nerve)

GVF
good visual fields

GVG
gamma-vinyl-GABA
(GABA—γ-aminobutyric acid)

GVH, GvH
graft versus host

GVHD
graft-versus-host disease

GVHR, GvHR
graft-versus-host reaction

GVL
graft versus leukemia

Gvty
gingivectomy

GW
gigawatt (one billion watts)
glycerin in water
group work

G/W
glucose in water

G & W, G&W
glycerin and water

GWBS
global ward behavior scale

GWE
glycerin and water enema

GWG
generalized Wegener's granulomatosis

GXT
graded exercise test

Gy
gray (unit of absorbed dose of ionizing
radiation)

GYN, Gyn, gyn.
gynecological
gynecologist
gynecology

gyn.
gynecologic

gyro.
gyroscope

GZ
Guilford-Zimmerman personality test

Gz
Graetz number (heat transfer—re:
pipes)

GZAS
Guilford-Zimmerman Aptitude Survey
(re: Psychol)

GZTS
Guilford-Zimmerman Temperament
Survey

H

H
enthalpy
the Fraunhofer line at γ 3968 due to calcium (prominent lines of the solar spectrum)
Haemaphysalis (genus of ticks)
Haemophilus (genus)
Hauch (Ger. haze, bloom [film]— designates flagellate or motile type of microorganism)
heart
heart disease
heavy
heelstick
hemagglutination
hemisphere
henry (practical and SI unit of inductance)
heparin
hernia
heroin
Heterophyes (genus)
Hippelates (genus)
Histoplasma (genus)
Holzknecht unit (unit of roentgen-ray exposure)
homosexual
hormone
horse (re: veterinary medicine)
hospital
hot
Hounsfield unit (re: CT scans)
human
husband
hydrogen (element)
hydrolysis
hygiene
Hymenolepis (genus of tapeworms)
hyoscine (scopolamine)
hyperphoria
hyperplasia
hypothalamus
magnetic field strength
oersted (Oe—magnetic field strength in CGS system)
vectorcardiography electrode (neck)

H, h
haustus (L. a draught; a drink)
height
high
hora (L. hour)
horizontal
hour
hypermetropia

hyperopia
hyperopic
hypodermic

(H)
hip

Ⓗ
hypodermic injection

H+, H$^+$
hydrogen ion (the proton)

(H$^+$)
hydrogen ion concentration

H$_1$
alternative hypothesis (re: statistics)
H1 histone (re: histology)

H$_3$
H3 histone (re: histology)
procaine hydrochloride

H4
H4 histone (re: histology)

^{1}H
protium (light hydrogen)

^{2}H
deuterium (heavy hydrogen, hydrogen-2)

^{3}H
hydrogen-3 (tritium; triterium; T)

$^3_1$H
tritium (triterium; T)

h
hecto (prefix)
heteromorphic regions (re: cytogenetics)
human response
hundred
the secondary constriction of a chromosome

h, *h*
Planck's constant (quantum constant)

HA
halothane anesthesia
H antigen
hearing aid
height age
hemadsorbent

hemadsorption (test, virus)
hemagglutinating activity
hemagglutinating antibody
hemagglutination
hemolytic anemia
hepatic adenoma
hepatic artery
hepatitis A
hepatitis associated (virus)
herpangina
heterophil antibody
Heyden antibiotic
high anxiety
hippuric acid
histamine
histocompatibility antigen
Horton's arteritis
hospital acquired
hospital admission
household activity
hyaluronic acid
hydroxyapatite (durapatite—prosthetic
    aid—bone and teeth)
hyperalimentation
hypersensitivity alveolitis
symbol for "an acid"

HA, H/A
headache

HA, Ha
hyperopia, absolute (re: Ophth)

H/A
head-to-abdomen (ratio)

HA1
hemadsorption (virus, type 1)

HA2
hemadsorption (virus, type 2)

H2A
H2A histone (re: histology)

Ha
hahnium (name and symbol proposed
    for artificially made element 105)
Hartmann number (re: fluid flows in
    transverse magnetic field)

H/a
home with advice

HAA
hearing aid amplifier
hemolytic anemia antigen
hepatitis-associated antigen (Australia
    antigen)
hospital activity analysis

HABA
hydroxybenzeneazobenzoic acid
    (p-hydroxyazobenzene-benzoic acid)

HABF
hepatic artery blood flow

HAb/HAd
horizontal abduction/adduction

habit.
habitat

habt.
habeatur (L. let the patient have)

HAc
acetic acid (CH_3COOH; ethanoic acid—
    re: reagent)

HAChT
high/affinity choline transport

HACS
hyperactive child syndrome

HAD
hemadsorption
hexamethylmelamine, Adriamycin
    (doxorubicin), and cis-
    diamminedichloroplatinum (cisplatin)
    (re: chemotherapy)
hospital administrator
hypophysectomized alloxan diabetic

HAD, HAd
hospital administration

HADH
hydroxyacyl-CoA dehydrogenase

HAE
health appraisal examination
hearing aid evaluation
hepatic artery embolization
hereditary angioedema
hereditary angioneurotic edema

HAF
hepatic arterial flow

HaF
Hageman factor

HAFP
human alpha-fetoprotein

HAG
heat-aggregated globulin

HAGG
hyperimmune antivariola gamma
    globulin

HAHTG
horse antihuman-thymus globulin

HAI
hemagglutination inhibition (procedure)
hemagglutinin inhibition

HAL
haloperidol

HAL, hal.
halothane

Hal
halogen

halluc.
hallucination

HALT
Heroin Antagonist and Learning
   Therapy

HaLV
hamster leukemia virus

HAM
hearing aid microphone
helical axis of motion
hexamethylmelamine, Adriamycin
   (doxorubicin), and melphalan (re:
   chemotherapy)
hexamethylmelamine, Adriamycin,
   methotrexate (re: chemotherapy)
human albumin microsphere
human alveolar macrophage
hypoparathyroidism-Addison's disease-
   mucocutaneous candidiasis

HAMA
Hamilton Anxiety (Scale)
human antimouse antibody

HAMD
Hamilton Depression (Scale)

HAMM
human albumin minimicrosphere

Hams
hamstrings (re: musculoskeletal)

HAN
hyperplastic alveolar nodules

HANA
hemagglutinin neuraminidase

HANDICP
handicapped

HANE
hereditary angioneurotic edema

H antigens
Hauch antigens (Ger. haze, bloom
   [film]—antigens localized in flagella of
   motile bacteria, first seen on film of
   spreading agar)

HAP
held after positioning
heredopathia atactica polyneuritiformis
high amplitude peristalsis
histamine acid phosphate
humoral antibody production
hydrolyzed animal protein
hydroxyapatite (fractionation procedure)

HAPA
hemagglutinating antipenicillin antibody

HAPC
hospital-acquired penetration contact

HAPE
high altitude pulmonary edema

HAR
high altitude retinopathy

Har
homoarginine

HARH
high altitude retinal hemorrhage

HARM
heparin assay rapid (easy) method

harm.
harmonic

HARS
Hamilton Anxiety Rating Scale

HAS
Hamilton Anxiety Scale
highest asymptomatic (dose)
hyperalimentation solution
hypertensive arteriosclerotic

HASCVD
hypertensive arteriosclerotic
   cardiovascular disease

HASHD
hypertensive arteriosclerotic heart
   disease

H&ASHD
hypertension and arteriosclerotic heart
   disease

HAT
Halstead Aphasia Test
head, arms, trunk
heterophil antibody titer
hospital arrival time

HATG
horse antihuman-thymocyte globulin

HATH
Heterosexual Attitudes Toward
   Homosexuality (scale)

HAT medium
hypoxanthine, aminopterin, and
   thymidine (tissue culture)

HAU
hemagglutinating unit
hemagglutination unit

haust.
haustus (L. a draught; a drink)

HAV
hemadsorption virus
hepatitis A virus

HA virus
hemadsorption virus

HAWIC
Hamburg-Wechsler Intelligence Test for
  Children

HB
head backward
heart block
heel to buttock
held backward
hemolysis blocking
hepatitis B
His bundle (re: Cardio)
hold breakfast
housebound
Hutchinson-Boeck (disease)
hyoid body

HB, Hb, Hb., hb
hemoglobin

H2B
H2B histone (re: histology)

H-2^b
strain of mouse cells

HBA
hemoglobin α chain
2-(hexyloxy)benzamide (antifungal)

HbA, Hb A
major component of (normal) adult
  hemoglobin

Hb A°
hemoglobin determination

Hb A$_1$
major component of adult hemoglobin

Hb A$_{1a}$, Hb A$_{1b}$, Hb A$_{1c}$
glycosylated forms of hemoglobin that
  can be separated from the main
  hemoglobin fractions Hb A$_1$ and
  Hb A$_2$

Hb A$_2$
minor fraction of adult hemoglobin

HBAb
hepatitis B antibody

HBAg, HB Ag
hepatitis B antigen

H band
heller band (Ger. lighter—the paler area
  in the center of the A band—re:
  sarcomere)

Hb A-S, Hb As
(heterozygosity for) hemoglobin A and
  hemoglobin S, the sickle cell trait

HBB
hemoglobin β chain
non-α-globin genes

Hb Bart's
Bart's hemoglobin (an abnormal
  hemoglobin)

HbBC
hemoglobin-binding capacity

HB/BW
hold breakfast for blood work

HBC
hepatitis B core

HB$_c$
hepatitis B core (antigen)

Hb C
second most common abnormal
  hemoglobin

HB$_c$Ab
hepatitis B core antibody

HBCAG, HBcAg, HB$_c$Ag
hepatitis B core antigen

HBCG
heat-aggregated bacille Calmette-
  Guérin

HBCO
carbon monoxide hemoglobin

HbCO, Hb CO
carboxyhemoglobin

Hb CS
hemoglobin Constant Spring

HBD
has been drinking
hemoglobin δ chain
α-hydroxybutyrate dehydrogenase
hypophosphatemic bone disease

Hb D
an abnormal hemoglobin variant

HBDH
α-hydroxybutyrate dehydrogenase

HBDT
human basophil degranulation test

HBE
hemoglobin ϵ chain
His bundle electrogram

HBE$_1$
His bundle electrogram, distal

HBE$_2$
His bundle electrogram, proximal

HBe
hepatitis B e antigen

Hb E
third most prevalent abnormal
  hemoglobin

HBeAg, HB_eAg
hepatitis B e antigen

HBF
hand blood flow
hemispheric blood flow
hemoglobinuric bilious fever
hepatic blood flow
hypothalamic blood flow

HbF, Hb F, Hb-F
fetal hemoglobin

HBG1
hemoglobin γ chain A

HBG2
hemoglobin γ chain G

Hbg
hemoglobin

HBGM
home blood glucose monitoring

Hb H
an abnormal hemoglobin (re: alpha
  thalassemia)

Hb-Hp
hemoglobin-haptoglobin complex

HBI
high (serum-)bound iron

HBIG, HBIg
hepatitis B immunoglobulin

Hb Kansas
an abnormal hemoglobin

HBL
hepatoblastoma

HBLA
human B lymphocyte antigen

HBM
hypertonic buffered medium

Hb M
hemoglobin M (associated with
  methemoglobinemia)

Hb M$_M$
hemoglobin mobility, Milwaukee

HB M$_{Milwaukee}$
hemoglobin mobility, Milwaukee

Hb M$_S$
hemoglobin mobility, Saskatoon

HB M$_{Saskatoon}$
hemoglobin mobility, Saskatoon

HBO
hyperbaric oxygen (therapy)

HBO, HbO
oxygenated hemoglobin

HbO$_2$
oxyhemoglobin (oxygenated
  hemoglobin)

HBOT
hyperbaric oxygen treatment

HBP
hepatic-binding protein
high blood pressure

HbP
primitive (fetal) hemoglobin

HBr
hydrobromic acid

HbR
methemoglobin reductase

HBS
hepatitis B surface
hyperkinetic behavior syndrome

HbS, Hb S
sickle cell hemoglobin

HB$_s$A
hepatitis B surface associated

HBSAG, HB$_s$Ag, HB$_s$AG, HB$_s$Ag
hepatitis B surface antigen

HBSC
hemopoietic blood stem cell

HbSC
sickle cell hemoglobin C

HBSS
Hanks' balanced salt solution

HbSS
homozygosity for hemoglobin S

HBSSG
Hanks' balanced salt solution plus
  glucose

HBT
human breast tumor

HBV
hepatitis B virus

HBW
high birth weight

H/BW
heart-to-body weight (ratio)

HBZ
hemoglobin ζ chain

HC
hair cell
hairy cell
handicapped
head check
head circumference
head compression
heart cycle
heat conservation
heavy chain
heel cord
hemoglobin concentration
hemorrhage, cerebral
heparin cofactor
hepatic catalase
hepatocellular cancer
hereditary coproporphyria
high calorie
hippocampus (re: Neuro)
histamine challenge
histochemistry
home call
home care
hospital corps
hospitalized controls
house call
Huntington's chorea
hyaline casts
hydranencephaly
hydraulic concussion
hydrocarbon
hydrocortisone
hydroxycorticoid
hyoid cornu
hypercholesterolemia (with
   xanthomatosis)
hypertrophic cardiomyopathy

H & C
hot and cold

HCA
heart cell aggregate
hepatocellular adenoma
hydrocortisone acetate

HCAP
handicapped

H-CAP
hexamethylmelamine,
   cyclophosphamide, Adriamycin,
   Platinol (re: chemotherapy)

HCC
heat conservation center
hepatitis contagiosa canis (virus)
hepatocellular carcinoma
hepatoma carcinoma cell
hexachlorocyclohexane (lindane—
   pediculi-, scabicide)
history of chief complaint
hydroxycholecalciferol (vitamin D)

25-HCC
25-hydroxycholecalciferol (calcium
   regulator)

HCD
health care delivery
heavy chain disease (protein)
high caloric density
high carbohydrate diet
homologous canine distemper
   (antiserum)

HCF
hereditary capillary fragility
highest common factor
hypocaloric carbohydrate feeding

HCFSH
human chorionic follicle-stimulating
   hormone

HCFU
1-(*n*-hexylcarbamoyl)-5-fluorouracil
   (carmofur—antineoplastic)

HCG, hCG
human chorionic gonadotrop(h)in

hCG-α subunit
human chorionic gonadotrop(h)in-alpha
   subunit

hCG-β subunit
human chorionic gonadotrop(h)in-beta
   subunit

HCH
1,2,3,4,5,6-hexachlorocyclohexane
   (lindane; also γ-HCH; benzene
   hexachloride—insecticide, pediculi-,
   scabicide)

HCH, Hch
hemochromatosis

HCHO
formaldehyde, gas

HcImp
hydrocolloid impression (re: Dent)

HCL
hairy cell leukemia
hard contact lens
hemacytology index (unproven method
   for diagnosis/ treatment of cancer)
human cultured lymphoblastoid (cells)

HCl
hydrochloric acid
hydrogen chloride

HCLF
high carbohydrate, low fiber (diet)

HCM
health care maintenance
hypertrophic cardiomyopathy

HCMV
human cytomegalovirus

HCN
hydrocyanic acid
hydrogen cyanide (prussic acid—
  compressed gas and insect and
  rodent exterminator on ships)

HCO$_3$, HCO$_3$ $^-$
bicarbonate

H colony
Hauch colony (Ger. bloom, haze [film]—
  a colony of motile organisms forming
  a thin film of growth)

HCP
handicapped
hepatocatalase peroxidase
hereditary coproporphyria
hexachlorophene
high cell passage

HCR
heme-controlled repressor
human controlled represssor
hysterical conversion reaction (re:
  psychiatry)

H'crit
hematocrit

HCS
hourglass contraction of stomach
human cord serum

HCS, hCS
human chorionic somatomammotropin
  (human placental lactogen)

17-HCS
17-hydroxycorticosteroids

HCSM, hCSM
human chorionic somatomammotropin
  (human placental lactogen)

HCT
Health Check Test
heart-circulation training
homocytotrophic
human chorionic (placental)
  thyrotrophin
hydrochlorothiazide

HCT, Hct, hct.
hematocrit

HCT, hCT
human calcitonin

hct, hct.
hundred count

HCTD
hepatic computed tomography density

high cholesterol and tocopherol
  deficient

HCTS
high cholesterol and tocopherol
  supplemented

HCTU
home cervical traction unit

HCTZ, Hctz
hydrochlorothiazide

HCU
homocystinuria
hyperplasia cystica uteri

HCV
human coronary viruses

HCVD
hypertensive cardiovascular disease

HCVR
hypercapnic ventilatory response

HCVS
human corona virus sensitivity

Hcy
hemocyanin(s)
homocysteine

HD
Haab-Dimmer (syndrome)
Hajna-Damon (broth)
Hansen's disease (leprosy)
hearing disease
hearing distance
heart disease
helium dilution
heloma durum (L. hard corn—re:
  podiatry)
hemidiaphragm
hemodialysis
hemolytic disease
hemolyzing dose
herniated disc
high density
high dosage
high dose
hip disarticulation
Hirschsprung's disease
Hodgkin's disease
hormone dependent
hospital day
house dust
Huntington's disease
hydatid disease
hypnotic dosage

HD$_{50}$
50 percent hemolyzing dose of
  complement

hd.
head

h.d.
hora decubitus (L. at bedtime)

HDBH
α-hydroxybutyrate dehydrogenase

HDC
histidine decarboxylase
human diploid cell

HDCS
human diploid cell strain

H and D curve
Hurter and Driffield curve (re: radiology)

HDCV
human diploid cell (rabies) vaccine

HDD
high dose depth

HDF
high dry field (re: laboratory tests)
host defensive factor
human diploid fibroblasts

HDFL
human development and family life

HDG
high-dose group

HDH
heart disease history
Hostility and Direction of Hostility
(questionnaire)

HDHQ
Hostility and Direction of Hostility
Questionnaire

HDI
hemorrhagic disease of infants

H disease
Hartnup disease (congenital metabolic
disorder)

HDL
high-density lipoprotein

HDLC
high-density lipoprotein cholesterol

HDL-c
high-density lipoprotein-cell surface
(receptor)

HDLP
high-density lipoprotein

HDLW
hearing distance, left, watch

HDMP
high-dose methylprednisolone (re:
chemotherapy)

HDMTX
high-dose methotrexate (re:
chemotherapy)

HDMTX-CF
high-dose methotrexate-citrovorum
factor (re: chemotherapy)

HDMTX/LV
high-dose methotrexate and leucovorin
(re: chemotherapy)

HDN
hemolytic disease of the newborn

hDNA
deoxyribonucleic acid, histone

HDP
hexose diphosphate
high density polyethylene

HDRS
Hamilton Depression Rating Scale

HDRV
human diploid rabies vaccine

HDRW
hearing distance, right, watch

HDS
health delivery system
herniated disc syndrome

HDU
head-drop unit (curare standard)
hemodialysis unit

HDW
hearing distance (with) watch

HDZ
hydralazine

HE
hard exudate
hemagglutinating encephalomyelitis
hemoglobin electrophoresis
hepatic encephalopathy
hereditary elliptocytosis
high explosive
hollow enzyme
human enteric (viruses)
hypogonadotrophic eunuchoidism
hypophysectomy

H and E, H&E
hematoxylin and eosin (stain)
hemorrhage and exudate
heredity and environment

H + E
hematoxylin and eosin (stain)
heredity and environment

He
Hedstrom number (non-dimensional
    parameter—re: non-newtonian fluids)
helium (element)

³He
helium-3

⁴He
helium-4

he.
head

HEA
hexone-extracted acetone
human erythrocyte antigen

He antigen
MNS blood group antigen

HEART
Health Evaluation and Risk Tabulation

HEAT
human erythrocyte agglutination test

HEB
hematoencephalic barrier (blood brain
    barrier)

HEBDOM, hebdom.
hebdomada (re: first week of life; Gr. the
    seventh day—considered a critical
    period)

HEC
hamster embryo cell
human endothelial cell
hydroxyergocalciferol

HED
hydrotropic electron donor

HED, H.E.D.
Haut-Einheits-Dosis (Ger. unit skin
    dose—re: radiology)
Haut-Erythem-Dosis (Ger. skin
    erythema dose—re: radiology)

HeD
helper determinant

HEDSPA
⁹⁹ᵐTc etidronate (ethane-1-hydroxyl-1,1-
    diphosphonate —re: bone-imaging
    agent)

HEENT
head, eyes, ears, nose, and throat

HEF
hamster embryo fibroblast

HEG
hemorrhagic erosive gastritis

HEHR
highest equivalent heart rate

HEI
high-energy intermediate
homogeneous enzyme immunoassay

HE inj.
hyperextension injury

HEIR
health effects of ionizing radiation
high-energy ionizing radiation

HEIS
high-energy ion scattering

HEK
human embryo kidney
human embryonic kidney (cells)

HEL
hen's egg-white lysozyme
human embryo lung (cell culture)
human embryonic lung
human erythroleukemia

HeLa cells
a continuously cultured carcinoma cell
    line used for tissue cultures (named
    for patient, Henrietta Lacks)

HELF
human embryonic lung fibroblasts

HELLP
hemolysis, elevated liver enzymes, and
    low platelet (count)

HELP
Hawaii Early Learning Profile
heat escape lessening posture

Hem
hematology

Hem, hem.
hemolysis (re: blood fragility test)
hemolytic

hem.
hematuria
hemorrhage
hemorrhoid

HEMAT, hemat.
hematology

hemat.
hematocrit

hematem.
hematemesis

Hematol, hematol.
hematologist
hematology

Hemi
hemisphere

hemi.
hemiparalysis
hemiplegia

hemo.
hemoglobin
hemophilia

hemocyt.
hemocytometer

hemo. F
hemoglobin free

hemop.
hemoptysis

hemorr.
hemorrhage
hemorrhagic

hemorrh.
hemorrhage

HEMPAS
hereditary erythroblastic multinuclearity
  associated with a positive acidified
  serum

HEOD
1,2,3,4,10,10-hexachloro-6,7-epoxy-
  1,4,4a,5,6,7,8,8a- octahydroendo,exo-
  1,4:5,8-dimethanonaphthalene
  (dieldrin; compound 497—formerly
  used as insecticide; manufacture has
  been discontinued in the U.S.)

HEP
hemolysis end point
hepatic
hepatoerythropoietic porphyria
high egg passage (strain of virus)
high energy phosphate
human epithelial cells

HEPA
high efficiency particulate air (filter)

Hep/Clav
hepatoclavicular

HEPM
human embryonic palatal mesenchymal
  (cells)

HER
hemorrhagic encephalopathy of rats

her.
hernia

herb. recent.
herbarium recentium (L. of fresh herbs)

hered.
hereditary
heredity

hern.
hernia
herniated
herniation

HES
hematoxylin-eosin stain
human embryonic skin
human embryonic spleen
hydroxyethyl starch (cryoprotective
  agent)
hypereosinophilic syndrome

H and E staining
hematoxylin and eosin staining

HET
helium equilibration time
heterozygous

Het
heterophil (antibody)

HETE
hydroxyeicosatetraenoic (acid)

5-HETE
5-hydroxy-6,8,11,14-eicosatetraenoic
  (acid)

HETP
height equivalent to a theoretical plate
  (re: gas chromatography)

HEV
health and environment
hemagglutination encephalomyelitis
  virus
hepato-encephalomyelitis virus
human enteric virus

HE virus
human enteric virus

HEW
Health, Education, and Welfare

HEXA, Hex A
hexosaminidase A (α-subunit)

HexaCAF, Hexa-CAF
hexamethylmelamine,
  cyclophosphamide, methotrexate,
  5-fluorouracil (re: chemotherapy)

HEXB, Hex B
hexosaminidase B (β-subunit)

HF
Hageman factor (Factor XII)
haplotype frequency
hard feces
hard filled (capsules)
harvest fluid
hay fever
head of fetus
head forward
heart failure

helper factor
hemofiltration
hemorrhagic factor
hemorrhagic fever
hepatocyte function
Hertz frequency
high fat (diet)
high flow
high frequency
hot fomentation
house formula
human fibroblasts
hydrogen fluoride (catalyst)

HF, hf.
half

H/F
HeLa/fibroblast (hybrid)

H of F
height of fundus

Hf
hafnium (element)

175Hf
radioactive isotope of hafnium

181Hf
radioactive isotope of hafnium

HFAK
hollow fiber artificial kidney

HFC
hard filled capsules
high frequency current
histamine-forming capacity

HFCS
high-fructose corn syrup

HFCWC
high-frequency chest wall compression

HFD
hemorrhagic fever of deer
high fiber diet
high forceps delivery
Human Figure Drawing (Techniques—
   re: psychological testing)

HFDK
human fetal diploid kidney (cells)

HFDL
human fetal diploid lung (cells)

HFEC
human foreskin epithelial cell

HFF
human foreskin fibroblast

HFI
hereditary fructose intolerance
human fibroblast interferon

HFIF
human fibroblast interferon

HF inj.
hyperflexion injury

HFJV
high-frequency jet ventilation

HFL
human fetal lung

HFM
hemifacial microsomia

HFO
hard food orientation
high-frequency oscillation

HFOV
high-frequency oscillatory ventilation

HFP
hypofibrinogenic plasma

HFPPV
high-frequency positive pressure
   ventilation

HFR
heart frequency

HFR, Hfr
high frequency (of) recombination (re:
   genetics)

Hfr
high frequency

Hfr mutant
high-frequency recombination mutant
   (re: genetics)

HFRS
hemorrhagic fever with renal syndrome

Hfr strain
high frequency (of) recombination (an
   E. coli strain— re: genetics)

HFS
hemifacial spasm

HFSH, hFSH
human follicle-stimulating hormone

HFST
hearing-for-speech test

HFT
high-frequency transduction
high-frequency transfer

HFUPR
hourly fetal urine production rate

HFV
high-frequency ventilation

HG
handgrip (exercise)
herpes gestationis
Herter-Gee (syndrome)
Heschl's gyri (re: Neuro)
high glucose
human gonadotrop(h)in
human growth factor
Hutchinson-Gilford (syndrome)
hypoglycemia

HG, Hg, hG, hg.
hemoglobin

Hg
hydrargyrum (New Latin from Gr.
   hydrarguros—silver water [the
   element, mercury])

197Hg
radioactive isotope of mercury
   (hydrargyrum)

203Hg
radioactive isotope of mercury
   (hydrargyrum)

hg, hg.
hectogram (100 grams)

HGA
homogentisate (homogentisic acid
   oxidase)
homogentisic acid (an alkapton body—
   in urine)

HGB, Hgb, hGB, hgb.
hemoglobin

Hgb & Hct
hemoglobin and hematocrit

H gene
gene that produces a fucosal
   transferase (H = one of its alleles)

HGF
hyperglycemic-glycogenolytic factor
   (glucagon)

Hg-F
fetal hemoglobin

HGG
herpetic geniculate ganglionitis

HGG, hGG
human gamma globulin

HGH
high growth hormone

HGH, hGH
human (pituitary) growth hormone

Hg-Hg Cl
calomel half cells (one electrode +

surrounding solution [calomel;
   mercurous chloride; HgCl])

HGM
hog gastric mucin
human glucose monitoring

HGMCR
human genetic mutant cell repository

HGO
hepatic glucose output
human glucose output

HgO
mercuric oxide

HGP
hepatic glucose production
hyperglobulinemia purpura

HGPRT
hypoxanthine-guanine
   phosphoribosyltransferase

HGPRT'ase
hypoxanthine-guanine
   phosphoribosyltransferase

HGSHS
Harvard Group Scale of Hypnotic
   Susceptibility

Hgt
height

HH
halothane hepatitis
hard of hearing
Head-Holms (syndrome)
Henderson and Haggard (inhaler)
hiatal hernia
hiatus hernia
holistic health
Hunter-Hurler (syndrome)
hydroxyhexamide
hypergastrinemic hyperchlorhydria

H & H, H&H
hemoglobin and hematocrit

Hh
hemopoietic histocompatibility

HHA
hereditary hemolytic anemia
home health agency
hypothalamic-hypophyseal-adrenal

HHAA
hypothalamo-hypophyseal-adrenal axis

HHB, HHb
un-ionized hemoglobin

HHb
reduced hemoglobin

HHC
home health care

HHD
high heparin dose
hypertensive heart disease

HHDN
1,2,3,4,10,10-hexachloro-1,4,4a,5,8,8a-
hexahydro-1,4:5,8-
dimethanonaphthalene (aldrin—
insecticide; manufacture and use
discontinued in U.S.)

HHE
health hazard evaluation
hemiconvulsions, hemiplegia, epilepsy

HHG
hypertrophic hypersecretory
gastropathy

HHH
hyperornithinemia type I (characterized
by) hyperammonemia and
homocitrullinemia

HHHO
hypotonia-hypomentia-hypogonadism-
obesity (Prader- Willi syndrome)

HHM
hemohydrometry

H & Hm, H and Hm
compound hypermetropic astigmatism

H + Hm, H + Hm
compound hypermetropic astigmatism

HHNK
hyperglycemic hyperosmolar nonketotic
(coma)

HHNKS
hyperglycemic hyperosmolar nonketotic
syndrome

HHPC
hyperoxic-hypercapnic

HHRH
hypothalamic hypophysiotropic-
releasing hormone

HHS
Hearing Handicap Scale

HHT
head halter traction
hereditary hemorrhagic telangiectasia
heterotopic heart transplantation
12-L-hydroxy-5,8,10-heptadecatrienoic
(acid)

HHTA
hypothalamo-hypophyseal-thyroidal
axis

HHTx
head halter traction

HI
hearing impaired
heart infusion
heat inactivated
heat input
hemagglutination inhibition
hepatobiliary imaging
high impulsiveness
hormone independent
hormone insensitive
hospital induced
hospital insurance
humoral immunity
hydriodic acid
hydrogen iodide
hydroxyindole
hyperglycemic index
hypothermic ischemia

HI, Hi
histidine

HIA
heat infusion agar
hemagglutination inhibition antibody
hemagglutination inhibitory antibody

HIAA
5-hydroxyindoleacetic acid

5-HIAA
5-hydroxyindoleacetic acid

HIB
Haemophilus influenzae type B
hemolytic immune body

H-ICDA
International Classification of Diseases,
Adopted Code for Hospitals

Hi CHO
high carbohydrate (diet)

HiCN
cyanmethemoglobin (also called
hemiglobincyanide— re: hemoglobin
assay)

HID
headache, insomnia, depression
(syndrome)
herniated intervertebral disc
human infectious dose
hyperkinetic impulse disorder

HIE
human intestinal epithelial (cell)
hyperimmunoglobulin E

HIF
higher intellectual function (re: Psychol)
histoplasma tissue inhibitory factor
Historical Information Form

HIFBS
heat-inactivated fetal bovine serum

HIFC
hog intrinsic factor concentrate

HIFCS
heat-inactivated fetal calf serum

HIg
human immunoglobulin

HIHA
high impulsiveness, high anxiety

HiHb
hemiglobin

HII
hemagglutination inhibition
    immunoassay

HILA
high impulsiveness, low anxiety

HIM
hemopoietic inductive
    microenvironment
hepatitis-infectious mononucleosis
hexosephosphate isomerase
Hill Interaction Matrix (re: psychological
    testing)

HIMC
hepatic intramitochondrial crystalloid

HIMP
high-dose intravenous
    methylprednisolone (re: chemo-
    therapy)

HIMT
hemagglutination inhibition morphine
    test

Hind II, III
restriction endonucleases from
    Haemophilus influenzae

H inf.
hypodermoclysis infusion

HINT, Hint
Hinton (flocculation test for syphilis)

Hint test
Hinton test (flocculation test for syphilis)

HIO
hypoiodism
hypoiodite (salt of hypoiodous acid)

HIO₃
iodic acid (astringent, disinfectant)

HIP
hydrostatic indifference point

HiPIP
high potential iron protein

Hi Prot
high protein

HIR
high irradiance response

HIS
Haptic Intelligence Scale
Health Information System (re: medical
    records)
Health Interview Survey
hospital information systems
hyperimmune serum
hyperimmunized suppressed

HIS, His, his.
histidine

His
histidyl

HISG
human immune serum globulin

HISMS
How I See Myself Scale (re:
    psychological testing)

Hist
histamine
histidinemia
history

hist.
histologist
histology

Histol
histology

histo spots
chorioretinal scars (of ocular
    histoplasmosis)

HIT
hemagglutination inhibition test (for
    pregnancy)
histamine inhalation test
histamine ion transfer
Holtzman Inkblot Technique (re:
    psychological testing)
hypertrophic infiltrative tendinitis
hypertrophied inferior turbinate

HITB
Haemophilus influenzae type B
    (meningitis)

HITES
hydrocortisone, insulin, transferrin,
    estradiol, selenium

HIU
hyperplasia interstitialis uteri

HJ
Howell-Jolly (bodies)

HJB
Howell-Jolly bodies

HJR
hepatojugular reflux (formerly reflex)

HJ reflux
hepatojugular reflux (formerly reflex)

HK
heat-killed
Hefnerkerze (absolute unit of luminous
    intensity)
hexokinase
Hoffa-Kastert (syndrome)
human kidney (cells)

HK, H-K
hand to knee (test)
heel to knee (test)

H→K
hand to knee (coordination)

HK1
hexokinase-1

HKAFO
hip-knee-ankle-foot orthosis

HKAO
hip-knee-ankle orthosis

HKC
human kidney cell

HK cells
human kidney cells

HKH
hyperkinetic heart syndrome

HKLM
heat-killed *Listeria monocytogenes*

HL
hairline
half-life (of radioactive element)
harelip
hearing level
hemolysis
heparin lock
histiocytic lymphoma
histocompatibility locus
Hodgkin's lymphoma
human leukocyte
hyperlipidemia
hyperlipoproteinemia (familial type of
    triglyceridemia)
hypertrichosis lanuginosa
lateral habenular (nucleus—re: Neuro)

HL, Hl
latent hypermetropia (hyperopia—re:
    Ophth)

HL, h.l.
hearing loss

H/L
hydrophil/lipophil (number)

H & L, H&L
heart and lungs

hl
hectoliter (Gr. one hundred [liters])

HLA
histocompatibility locus antigen
homologous leukocyte antibodies
homologous leukocytic antibodies
human lymphocyte antibody
human lymphocyte (histocompatibility)
    antigen (system)

HLA, HL-A
human leukocyte antigen (system)

HLAA, HLA-A
human leukocyte antigen A

HLA-A
human lymphocyte (histocompatibility)
    antigen, locus A

HL-A antigen
original designation for human
    lymphocyte (histocompatibility) locus
    A (now HLA-A—re: genetics)

HLAB, HLA-B
human leukocyte antigen (locus) B (re:
    genetics)
human lymphocyte antigen (locus) B
    (re: genetics)

HLAC
human leukocyte antigen (locus) C (re:
    genetics)

HLA-C
human lymphocyte antigen (locus) C
    (re: genetics)

HLAD, HLA-D
human leukocyte antigen (locus) D (re:
    genetics)

HLA-D
human lymphocyte antigen (locus) D
    (re: genetics)

HLA-DR
human leukocyte antigen (locus) DR
    (re: genetics)

HLA-L
human leukocyte antigen (locus) L (re:
    genetics)

HLALD
horse liver alcohol dehydrogenase

HL-A-LD
human lymphocyte-antigen-lymphocyte
  defined

H,L,A negative
heart, lungs, and abdomen negative

$$\left.\begin{array}{l} H \\ L \\ A \end{array}\right\} 0$$

heart, lungs, and abdomen negative

HL-A-SD
human lymphocyte-antigen-
  serologically defined

HLB
hydrophil-lipophil balance (re:
  surfactants)
hypotonic lysis buffer

HLBI
human lymphoblastoid interferon

HLC
heat loss center

HLCL
human lymphoblastoid cell line

HLD
hepatolenticular degeneration
herniated lumbar disc
hypersensitivity lung disease
von Hippel-Lindau disease

HLDH
heat (stable) lactic dehydrogenase

HLE
human leukocyte elastase

HLEG
hydrolysate lactalbumin Earle's glucose

HLF
heat-labile factor
human lung field

HLFCB
horizontal laminar flow clean benches

HLH
hypoplastic left heart

HLH, hLH
human luteinizing hormone

HLI
hemolysis inhibition
human leukocyte interferon
human lymphocyte interferon

HLK, H-L-K
heart, liver, kidney(s)

HLN
hilar lymph node

human Lesch-Nyhan (cell)
hyperplastic liver nodules

HL number
hydrophil-lipophil number

H & L OK
heart and lungs normal (OK)

HLP
hepatic lipoperoxidation
hind leg paralysis (re: veterinary
  medicine)
hyperlipoproteinemia

HLR
heart-lung resuscitation
heart-lung resuscitator

HLT
human lipotropin

HLT, hLT
human lymphocyte transformation

hlth.
health

HLV
herpes-like virus

HM
hand motion
hand movements
harmonic mean
health maintenance
heart murmur
hepatic metabolism
heavily muscled
Heine-Medin (disease)
heloma molle (L. soft corn—re:
  podiatry)
Holter monitoring (re: Cardio)
human milk
hydatidiform mole (re: OB)
hyperimmune mice
hypoxic-metabolic
median habenular (nucleus—re: Neuro)

HM, Hm
hyperopia, manifest (hypermetropia—
  re: Ophth)

hm
hectometer (Gr. hecto-; one hundred)

HMAS
hyperimmune mice ascitic (fluid)

HMB
homatropine methylbromide
  (anticholinergic)
Horton-Magath-Brown (disease)

HMBA
hexamethylenebisacetamide

HMC
hand mirror cell
health maintenance cooperative
heroin, morphine, cocaine
hyoscine-morphine-codeine

3-HMC
3-hydroxymethyl-β-carboline (re: study
    of benzodiazepine receptors)

HMCCMP
human mammary carcinoma cell
    membrane proteinase

HMD
hyaline membrane disease
α-hydrazino-α-methyl-β-(3,4-
    dihydroxyphenylpropionic acid
    monohydrate (for parkinsonism in
    combination with levodopa—
    carbidopa)

HME
heat, massage, exercise
heat and moisture exchanger
9-hydroxy-2-methylellipticinium acetate
    (antineoplastic)

H-meromyosin
heavy meromyosin (a product of tryptic
    digestion of myosin)

HMF
5-(hydroxymethyl)-2-furaldehyde
hydroxymethylfurfural (re: synthesis of
    glycols, ethers, dialdehydes)

HMG
high mobility group
human menopausal gonadotrop(h)in
3-hydroxy-3-methylglutaric acid
    (meglutol—antihyper-
    lipoproteinemic)
hydroxymethylglutaryl (3-hydroxy-3-
    methylglutaric acid—
    antihyperlipoproteinemic)

HMGA
3-hydroxy-3-methylglutaric acid
    (meglutol—antihyper-
    lipoproteinemic)

HMG CoA, HMG-CoA
3-hydroxy-3-methylglutaryl coenzyme A

HMI
healed myocardial infarction

HML
human milk lysozyme

HMM
heavy meromyosin (of muscle)
hexamethylmelamine (altretamine—
    antineoplastic)
hexamethylomelamine (investigational
    chemotherapeutic agent)

HMMA
4-hydroxy-3-methoxymandelic acid
    (misnamed vanillylmandelic acid)

HMO
health maintenance organization
heart minute output
hypothetical mean organism

HMP
hexamethylphosphoramide
hexose monophosphate (pathway)
hot moist packs
human menopausal
hydromotive pressure

HMPA
hexamethylphosphoramide (hempa—
    solvent; chemosterilant; mutagen)

HMPG
(4-hydroxy-3-methoxyphenyl)ethylene
    glycol (hydroxymethoxy-
    phenylglycol—re: neuropsychiatry)

HMPS
hexose monophosphate shunt

HMPT
hexamethylphosphoric triamide
    (hempa—solvent; chemosterilant;
    mutagen)

HMR
histiocytic medullary reticulosis

H-mRNA
H-chain messenger ribonucleic acid

HMRTE
human milk reverse transcriptase
    enzyme

HMS
hexose monophosphate shunt
hydroxymesterone (glucocorticoid)
hypermobility score
hypermobility syndrome
hypothetical mean strain

HMSAS
hypertrophic muscular subaortic
    stenosis

HMSN
hereditary motor and sensory
    neuropathy

HMT
hematocrit
hexamethylenetetramine
    (methenamine—antibacterial;
    veterinary—urinary antiseptic)

HMTA
chexamethylenetetramine
    (methenamine—antibacterial;
    veterinary—urinary antiseptic)

HMW
high molecular weight

HMWC
high molecular weight component

HM, WM
heavily muscled, white male

HMX
heat-massage-exercise

HN
head and neck
Heller-Nelson (syndrome)
hemagglutinin neuraminidase
hematemesis neonatorum
hemorrhage of newborn
hereditary nephritis
hilar node
histamine-containing neuron
human nutrition
hypertrophic neuropathy

H & N, H&N
head and neck

HN2
nitrogen mustard (a gas warfare agent;
  Mustargen hydrochloride or
  mechlorethamine hydrochloride—
  antineoplastic)

h.n.
hoc nocte (L. tonight)

HNA
heparin-neutralizing activity

HNB
human neuroblastoma

HNC
hypernephroma cell
hyperosmolar nonketotic coma
hyperoxic normocapnic
hypothalamic-neurohypophyseal
  complex

HNKDS
hyperosmolar nonketotic diabetic state

HNLN
hospitalization no longer necessary
hospitalization no longer needed

H & N mot.
head and neck motion

HNP
herniated nucleus pulposus

hnRNA
heterogeneous nuclear ribonucleic acid

HNS
head, neck, and shaft (of a bone)
head and neck surgery

HNSHA
hereditary nonspherocytic hemolytic
  anemia

HNTD
highest nontoxic dose

HNTLA
Hiskey-Nebraska Test of Learning
  Aptitude

HNV
has not voided

HO
hand orthosis
heterotopic ossification
high oxygen
hip orthosis
Holt-Oram (syndrome)
House Officer
hyperbaric oxygen

H/O, h/o
history of

H_2O
water

H_2O_2
hydrogen peroxide

Ho
holmium (element)

Ho, H_o
null hypothesis (re: statistics)

^{166}Ho
radioactive isotope of holmium

HOA
hip osteoarthritis
hypertrophic osteoarthritis

HOADH
β-hydroxyacyl-CoA dehydrogenase (an
  enzyme of the fatty acid oxidation
  cycle)

Ho antigen
low frequency blood group antigen
  found only in members of very few
  families

HOAP-BLEO
hydroxydaunomycin (doxorubicin),
  Oncovin (vincristine), ara-C
  (cytarabine), prednisone, and
  bleomycin (re: chemotherapy)

HoaRhLG
horse anti-rhesus lymphocyte globulin

HoaTTG
horse anti-tetanus toxoid globulin

HOB
head of bed

HOB UPSOB
head of bed up for shortness of breath

HOC
human ovarian cancer
hydroxycorticoid

HOCM
hypertrophic obstructive
  cardiomyopathy

hoc vesp.
hoc vespere (L. this evening)

HOD
hereditary opalescent dentin (re: Dent)
Hoffer-Osmond Diagnostic (re:
  psychiatry)
hospital day
hyperbaric oxygen drenching

HOF
hepatic outflow

Hoff
Hoffmann's (reflex)

Hoff refl.
Hoffmann's reflex

Hoff resp.
Hoffmann's reponse

HOGA
hyperornithinemia type II (characterized
  by) gyrate atrophy

HOH
hard of hearing

HOI
hospital onset of infection
hypoiodous acid (oxidizing agent)

Holg
horse immunoglobulin

HOM
highest occupied molecular (orbital)

homatrop.
homatropine

HOME
Home Observation for Measurement of
  the Environment
Home Oriented Maternity Experience

Homeo
homeopathy

HOMO
highest occupied molecular orbital

Homo, homo.
homosexual

Homolat, homolat.
homolateral

HON
δ-hydroxy-γ-oxo-L-norvaline

HOOD
hereditary osteo-onychodysplasia

HOOI
Hall Occupational Orientation Inventory
  (re: psychological testing)

HOP
high oxygen pressure
hydroxydaunomycin (doxorubicin),
  Oncovin (vincristine), and prednisone
  (re: chemotherapy)

HOPE
Healthcare Options Plan Entitlement
health-oriented physician education

HOPI
History of Present Illness

HOPP
hepatic occluded portal pressure

hor.
horizontal

hor. decu.
hora decubitus (L. at bedtime)

hor. decub.
hora decubitus (L. at bedtime)

hor. interm.
hora intermedia (L. at the intermediate
  hour)
horis intermediis (L. at the intermediate
  hours)

horiz.
horizontal

hor. som.
hora somni (L. at the hour of sleep; at
  bedtime)

hor. 1 spat.
horae unius spatio (L. one hour's time)

hor. un. spatio
horae unius spatio (L. one hour's time)

HOS
human osteosarcoma

HoS
horse serum

Hosp, hosp.
hospital

hosp.
hospitalization
hospitalize

Hosp Ins
hospital insurance

HOST
hypo-osmotic shock treatment

HOT
human old tuberculin
hyperbaric oxygen therapy

5-HOT
5-hydroxytryptamine

HP
Haemophilus pleuropneumonia
handicapped person
hard palate
Harvard pump
hastening phenomenon
health professional
heater probe
heat production
heel to patella
hemipelvectomy
hemoperfusion
heparin
high potency
high power
high pressure
high protein
highly purified
Hodgen and Pearson (re: Ortho)
hot pad
House Physician
human pituitary
hybridoma product
hydrophobic protein
hydrostatic pressure
hyperparathyroidism
hyperphoria
hypersensitivity pneumonitis
hypertension plus proteinuria
hypoparathyroid

HP, H.P.
hot pack (pad)

HP, Hp, hp.
haptoglobin

HP, hp
horsepower

H→P
heel to patella

H & P, H&P
history and physical
Hodgen and Pearson (re: Ortho)

Hp
hematoporphyrin
hemiplegia

Hp¹
allelic autosomal genes (re:
    haptoglobin)

Hp²
allelic autosomal genes (re:
    haptoglobin)

hp.
heaping

HPA
α-haptoglobin
hemagglutinating penicillin antibody
Hereford Parental Attitude (Survey)
hypothalamic-pituitary-adrenal (axis)
hypothalamic-pituitary-adrenocortical

HPAA
hydroxyphenylacetic acid (urinary
    antiseptic)

HPBC
hyperpolarizing bipolar cell

HPBF
hepatotrop(h)ic portal blood factor

HPBL
human peripheral blood leukocyte

HPC
hemangiopericytoma
hippocampal pyramidal cell
history of present complaint
history of present condition
3-hydroxy-2-phenylcinchoninic acid
    (oxycinchopen—antidiuretic;
    uricosuric)

HPD
high protein diet
highly probably drunk
home peritoneal dialysis

HPD, Hpd
hematoporphyrin derivative

HPE
hepatic portoenterostomy
high permeability edema
history and physical examination
hydrostatic pulmonary edema

5-HPETE
5-hydroperoxy-6,8,11,14-
    eicosatetraenoic acid

HPF
heparin-precipitable fraction
hepatic plasma flow
high pass filter
hypocaloric protein feeding

HPF, hpf, h.p.f.
high-power field

/HPF, /hpf
per high-power field

HPFH
hereditary persistence of fetal
  hemoglobin

HPFSH, hPFSH
human pituitary follicle-stimulating
  hormone

HPG
hypothalamic-pituitary-gonadal

HPG, hPG
human pituitary gonadotrop(h)in

HPH
halothane-percent-hour

HPI
hepatic perfusion index
Heston Personality Inventory (Test)
History of Present Illness (re: a medical
  record)

HPL
human parotid lysozyme
human peripheral lymphocyte

HPL, hPL
human placental lactogen

HPLA
hydroxyphenyllactic acid (re:
  tyrosinemia; ascorbic acid deficiency)

HPLAC
high-pressure liquid affinity
  chromatography

HPLC
high-performance liquid
  chromatography
high-pressure liquid chromatography

HPLE
hereditary polymorphic light eruption

HPM
Harding-Passey melanoma

HPMC
human peripheral mononuclear cell

HPMF
dihydro-3,4-bis[(3-
  hydroxyphenyl)methyl]-2(3H)-
  furanone

HPN
home parenteral nutrition

HPN, hpn.
hypertension

HPO
high-pressure oxygen
hypertrophic pulmonary osteoarthritis
hypertrophic pulmonary
  osteoarthropathy

HPP
hereditary pyropoikilocytosis
history of presenting problems
hydroxyphenylpyruvate (re: tyrosinemia;
  ascorbic acid deficiency)
4-hydroxypyrazolo[3,4-d]pyrimidine
  (allopurinol—a xanthine oxidase
  inhibitor)

HPP, hPP
human pancreatic polypeptide

2 HPP
two hours postprandial

HPPA
hydroxyphenylpyruvic acid (re:
  tyrosinemia; ascorbic acid deficiency)

HPPH
hydroxyphenyl-phenylhydantoin

HPPO
high partial pressure of oxygen

HPr
human prolactin

hPRL
human prolactin

HPRP
human platelet-rich plasma

HPRT
hot plate reaction time
hypoxanthine
  phosphoribosyltransferase
  (hypoxanthine guanine
  phosphoribosyltransferase)

HPS
hematoxylin, phloxine, saffron
Hermansky-Pudlak syndrome
high protein supplement
His-Purkinje system (re: Cardio)
human platelet suspension
hypertrophic pyloric stenosis

H & P susp. trx
Hodgen-Pearson suspension traction

HPT
histamine provocation test
hot plate test
human placenta thyrotrop(h)in
hyperparathyroidism
hypothalamic-pituitary-thyroid

Hpt
haptoglobin

HPTH
hyperparathyroid hormone

HPTIN
human pancreatic trypsin inhibitor

HPV
Haemophilus pertussis vaccine
hepatic portal vein
human papillomaviral infection
human papilloma virus
hypoxic pulmonary vasoconstriction

HPVD
hypertensive pulmonary vascular
   disease

HPV-DE
high-passage virus—duck embryo

HPV-DK
high-passage virus—dog kidney

HPVG
hepatic portal venous gas

HPX
hypophysectomized
partial hepatectomy

Hpx
hemopexin (a serum protein)

HPZ
high pressure zone

HQNO
2-heptyl-4-hydroxyquinoline *N*-oxide
   (specialized electron transfer
   inhibitor)

HR
Hamman-Rich (syndrome)
hemirectococcygeus
hemorrhagic retinopathy
heterosexual relations (scale)
higher rate
high resolution
high resolving
hormone responsive
hospital record
hospital report
Howship-Romberg (syndrome)
O-(β-hydroxyethyl)rutinosides
   (mixture— troxerutin; re: treatment of
   venous disorders)
hypoxic responder

HR, H/R
heart rate

H & R, H&R
hysterectomy and radiation

hr, hr.
hour

HRA
high right atrium
histamine-releasing activity

HRAE
high right atrium electrogram

H ray
hydrogen nuclei stream (protons)

HRB
histamine release (from) basophils

HRBC
horse red blood cells

HRC
help-rejecting complainer (re: Psychol)
high resolution chromatography
horse red cells

HRE
high resolution electrocardiogram
high resolution electrocardiography
hormone-receptor enzyme

HREC
hepatic reticuloendothelial cell

H reflex
Hoffmann's reflex

HREH
high renin essential hypertension

HREM
high resolution electron microscope

H response
Hoffmann's response

HRH
hypothalamic-releasing hormone

HRIG, HRIg
human rabies immune globulin

HRL
head rotated left

HRLA
human reovirus-like agent

hRNA
heterogeneous ribonucleic acid

HRP
high-risk pregnancy
histidine-rich protein
horseradish peroxidase

HRR
head rotated right
heart rate range

HRS
Hamilton Rating Scale
hepatorenal syndrome
hormone receptor site
humeroradial synostosis

hrs
hours

HRT
half relaxation time

heart rate
hormone replacement therapy

HRTE
human reverse transcriptase enzyme

HRTEM
high resolution transmission electron
  microscopy

HRV
heart rate variability
human rotavirus

HRVL
human reovirus-like

HS
half strength
Hallervorden-Spatz (syndrome)
hamstring
hand surgery
Hartman's solution (re: Dent)
head signs
head sling
healthy subject
heart sounds
heat stable
heavy smoker
heme synthetase
Henoch-Schönlein (syndrome)
heparin sulfate
hereditary spherocytosis
herpes simplex
hidradenitis suppurativa
Holländer-Simons (syndrome)
homologous serum
Hopelessness Scale
horizontally selective (re: visual cell)
horse serum
hospital stay
human serum
Hurler's syndrome
hypersensitivity
hypertonic saline

HS, H.S.
house surgeon (House Surgeon)

HS, h.s.
hora somni (L. hour of sleep; at
  bedtime)
hour of sleep

H/S
helper/suppressor
hemorrhage and shock
homestyle

H&S
hemorrhage and shock
hysterectomy and sterilization

H→S, h→s
heel-to-shin (maneuver)

H₂S
Hering's law—EOM innervation, both
  (2) eyes; Sherrington's law—EOM
  innervation, one eye

Hs
hypochondriasis

HSA
Hazardous Substances Act
health service area
health systems agency
horse serum albumin
human serum albumin
hypersomnia-sleep apnea (syndrome)

HSAG
HEPES (hydroxyethylpiperazine
  ethanesulfonic acid) saline-albumin-
  gelatin

HSAP
heat-stable alkaline phosphatase

HSAS
hypertrophic subaortic stenosis

HSC
Hand-Schüller-Christian (syndrome)
health sciences center
health screening center
hemopoietic stem cell
horizontal semicircular canal (re: ENT)
human skin collagenase

HSCD
Hand-Schüller-Christian disease
  (syndrome)

HSCL
Hopkins Symptom Check List

HSD
Honest Significance Difference
hydroxysteroid

HSDA
high single dose alternate day

HSE
herpes simplex encephalitis
human serum esterase

Hse
homoserine

HSF
heated soybean flour
histamine-induced suppressor factor
histamine-sensitizing factor
hypothalamic secretory factor

HSG
herpes simplex genitalis
hysterosalpingogram
hysterosalpingography

hSGF
human skeletal growth factor

HSGP
human sialoglycoprotein

HSHC
hemisuccinate of hydrocortisone

HSI
heat stress index
human seminal (plasma) inhibitor

hskpg.
housekeeping

HSL
herpes simplex labialis

HSLC
high-speed liquid chromatography

HSM
hepatosplenomegaly
high-speed memory (re: computers)
holosystolic murmur (re: Cardio)

HSN
hereditary sensory neuropathy

h. som.
hora somni (L. hour of sleep; bedtime)

HSP
Henoch-Schönlein purpura
high-speed printer (re: computers)
human serum prealbumin
human serum protein

H spike
His bundle electrogram deflection (re:
    Cardio)

HSPM
hippocampal synaptic plasma
    membrane (re: Neuro)

HSPQ
High School Personality Questionnaire
    (re: psychological testing)

HSR
Harleco synthetic resin
high-speed reader (re: computers)
homogeneous staining region (re:
    chromosomes)

HSRD
hypertension secondary to renal
    disease

HSRS
Health-Sickness Rating Scale
Hess School Readiness Scale (re:
    psychological testing)

HSS
Hallervorden-Spatz syndrome

hepatic stimulator substance
high-speed supernatant
hypertrophic subaortic stenosis

HST
Hemoccult slide test
horseshoe tear

HSTF
human serum thymus factor

H substance
a glycolipid on cell membranes or a
    glycoprotein in secretions, etc (re: A,B
    antigen production in ABO group)

HSV
herpes simplex virus
high selective vagotomy
hyperviscosity syndrome

HSV-1
herpes simplex virus 1

HSV-2
herpes simplex virus 2

HSVE
herpes simplex virus encephalitis

HSVtk
herpes simplex virus thymidine kinase

HSyn
heme synthase

HT
Hand Test (re: psychological testing)
Hashimoto's thyroiditis
hearing test
hearing threshold
heart transplant
hemagglutination titer
high temperature
home treatment
horizontal tabulation (character—re:
    computers/data processing)
hospital treatment
Hubbard tank (re: physical therapy)
Huhner test (re: OB-GYN)
human thrombin
hydrocortisone test
hydrotherapy
hydroxytryptamine (serotonin)
hypertension
hyperthyroidism
hypertransfusion
hypertropia

HT, Ht
hyperopia, total (hypermetropia)
hypothalamus

HT, Ht, ht.
heart

HT, h.t.
heart tone(s)
high tension
hypodermic tablet

H&T
hospitalization and treatment

3-HT
3-hydroxytyramine (dopamine)

5HT, 5-HT
5-hydroxytryptamine (serotonin)

Ht
heterozygote

ht.
haustus (L. a draught; a drink)
heat
height

HTA
heterophil transplantation antigen
human thymocyte antigen
hydroxytryptamine (serotonin)
hypophysiotropic area (of
　hypothalamus—re: Neuro)

HTACS
human thyroid adenyl-cyclase
　stimulator

HTB
hot tub bath

HTC
hepatoma cells
hepatoma tissue culture
homozygous typing cells

HTCA
human tumor colony assay

HTCVD
hypertensive cardiovascular disease

HTD
human therapeutic dose

HTF
heterothyrotrop(h)ic factors
house tube feeding

HTG
hypertriglyceridemia

HTH
homeostatic thymus hormone

Hth
hypothalamus

HTHD
hypertensive heart disease

HTI
hemisphere thrombotic infarction

HTIG
homologous tetanus immune globulin

hTIg
human tetanus immunoglobulin

HTK
heel to knee

HTL
hamster tumor line
hearing threshold level
human T-cell leukemia
human T-cell lymphoma

HTLA
high-titer, low acidity
human T lymphocyte antigen

HTLV
human T-cell leukemia virus
human T-cell lymphoma virus

HTLV-III
human T-cell leukemia/lymphoma virus
　(re: AIDS)

HTN
hypertension
hypertensive
hypertensive nephropathy

HTO
hospital transfer order

HTP
hypothromboplastinemia

HTP, H-T-P
House-Tree-Person (Projective
　Technique—re: psychological testing)
hydroxytryptophan

5-HTP
5-hydroxytryptophan

HTPN
home total parenteral nutrition

HTS
head traumatic syndrome
heel-to-shin (test—re: Neuro)
human thyroid stimulator

hTSAb
human thyroid-stimulating antibody

HTSCA
human tumor stem cell assay

HTSH, H-TSH, hTSH
human thyroid-stimulating hormone

HTST
high temperature-short time
　(pasteurization)

HTT
hand thrust test

HTV
herpes-type virus

HTVD
hypertensive vascular disease

HU
heat unit
hemagglutinating unit
hemagglutinin unit
hemolytic unit
Hounsfield unit
hydroxyurea
hyperemia unit

Hu
human

Hu antigen
rare antigen of MNS blood group

HUC
hypouricemia

HUI
Headache Unit Index

HUIS
high-dose urea in invert sugar

HUM
hematourimetry

hum.
humerus

H unit
Holzknecht unit (⅕ erythema dose—re:
   roerɪtgen-ray exposure)

HUP
Hospital Utilization Program (re:
   medical records)

HURT
hospital utilization review team

HUS
hemolytic uremic syndrome
hyaluronidase unit for serum

HuSA
human serum albumin

husb.
husband

HUTHAS
human thymus antiserum

HUV
human umbilical vein

HV
hallux valgus
heart volume
hepatic vein
hepatic venous
herpesvirus

high voltage
high volume
hospital visit
hyperventilation

H & V
hemigastrectomy and vagotomy

H$_v$, *hv*
energy of a photon (h = Planck's
   constant, v = frequency of radiation)

h.v.
hoc vespere (L. this evening)

HVA
homovanillic acid

HVD
hydroxyethylvinyldeuteroporphyrin
hypertensive vascular disease
hypoxic ventilatory drive

HVE
hepatic venous effluence
high-voltage electrophoresis

HVFP
hepatic vein free pressure

HVG
hematoxylin and van Gieson (stain)
host versus graft (response)

HVGS
high voltage galvanic stimulator (re:
   physical therapy)

HVH
herpesvirus hominis

HVHMA
herpesvirus hominis membrane antigen

HVID
horizontal visible iris diameter

HVJ
hemagglutinating virus of Japan

HVL, hvl
half-value layer

HVLP
high volume, low pressure

HVM
high-velocity missile
hypothalamic ventromedial (nucleus)

HVPE
high-voltage paper electrophoresis

HVPG
hepatic venous pressure gradient

HVR
hypoxic ventilatory response

HVS
herpesvirus sensitivity
hyperventilation syndrome

HV1S
herpes simplex virus type 1 sensitivity

HVS-2
herpesvirus, type 2

H vs A
home versus (against) advice

HVSD
hydrogen-detected ventricular septal
  defect

hv sites
hypervariable sites

HVT
half-value thickness
herpesvirus of turkeys

HVTEM
high-voltage transmission electron
  microscopy

HW
Hayrem-Widal (syndrome)
healing well
heart weight
hemisphere width
Hertwig-Weyers (syndrome)
His-Werner (disease)

HW, H/W, h.w.
housewife

HWB, h.w.b.
hot water bottle

HWE
hot water extract

HWOK
heel walking OK

HWP
hot wet pack
Hutchinson-Weber-Peutz (syndrome)

HWRS
Habits of Work and Recreation Survey

HWS
hot water soluble

HWY
hundred woman years (of exposure)

HX
histocytosis X
hydrogen exchange
hypophysectomized

HX, Hx, hx
history

Hx, Hx
hypoxanthine

2-HxG
di(hydroxyethyl)glycine (chelating
  agent)

HXIS
hard x-ray imaging spectrometer

HXM
hexamethylomelamine (former name for
  trimethylomelamine—an
  antineoplastic)

HXR
hypoxanthine riboside

HY
hypophysis (re: Neuro)

HY, Hy
hypermetropia
hyperopia

HY, hy.
hysteria

Hy
history
hypothenar

HYD
hydralazine
hydrated
hydroxyurea

Hyd
hydrocortisone
hydrostatics

hyd.
hydration
Hydrogenomonas (genus)
hydrostatic

hydr.
hydraulic

hydrarg.
hydrargyrum (New Latin from Gr.
  hydrarguros—silver water [the
  element, mercury])

Hydro, hydro.
hydrotherapy

hydrox.
hydroxyline

hyd. and tur.
hydration and turgor

Hyg, hyg.
hygiene

HYL, Hyl
hydroxylysine

Hyl
hyroxylysyl

HYP, Hyp
hydroxyproline (4-hydroxy-L-proline)
hypnosis

Hyp
symbol for the radicals of hypoxanthine
and hydroxyproline

HYP, Hyp, hyp.
hyperresonance
hypertrophy

hyp.
hypalgesia

hyper A
hyperactive

hyperact.
hyperactive

hyperal.
hyperalimentation

hypersens.
hypersensitive

hyperten.
hypertension

hypertens.
hypertensive

hypervent.
hyperventilation

hypes.
hypesthesia

Hypn, hypn.
hypertension

hypno.
hypnosis

hypnotism
hypnotist

hypnot.
hypnotic
hypnotism

HYPO, Hypo, hypo.
hypodermic (injection)

hypo.
hypochromasia
hypochromia

hypo A
hypoactive

hypoact.
hypoactive

Hypox
hypophysectomized

HypRF
hypothalamic-releasing factor

Hypro
hydroxyproline (4-hydroxy-L-proline)

HYS, hys.
hysteria
hysterical

hys.
hysterectomy

HYST, hyst.
hysterectomy

Hyv
hydroxyisovaleric acid

HZ, Hz
herpes zoster

Hz
hertz (one cycle/sec—SI unit of
frequency)

HZV
herpes zoster virus

I

I
electric current
I blood group (designation for)
implantation
implications (products—re: Psychol;
Aptitudes Research Project within
structures of intellect model)
incisivus (L. cut into)
incisor (permanent)
independent
index
indicated
induction
inhalation
inhibition
inhibitor
inosine
inspiration
inspired gas (when used as a
subscript—secondary symbol)
insulin
intake
intensity of electrical current
intensity of magnetism
intensity of radiation
intercalary (re: congenital limb absence)
internal medicine
internist
Iodamoeba (genus)
iodine (element)
ionic strength
isotope
Ixodes (genus of ticks)
luminous intensity
moment of inertia
roman numeral one
vector cardiography electrode (right
midaxillary line)

I, i.
insoluble

I-
iso-

I_1, I_2, I_3, etc.
first, second, third, etc., generations
obtained by inbreeding

^{125}I
radioactive isotope of iodine

^{130}I
radioactive isotope of iodine

^{131}I
radioactive isotope of iodine

^{132}I
radioactive isotope of iodine (clinical
use supplanted by ^{123}I and ^{131}I)

i
isochromosome (re: cytogenetics)

i.
incisor (deciduous)
optically inactive (re: chemicals)

i-
meso- (archaic term—re: chemistry)
optically inactive by internal
compensation

ι
iota (the ninth letter of the Greek
alphabet)

IA
immune adherence
immunobiologic activity
impedance angle
inactive alcoholic
incidental appendectomy
indolaminergic-accumulating (cells)
indolic acids
indulin agar
infected area
inferior angle
inhibitory antigen
internal auditory
intra-alveolar
intra-amniotic
intra-aortic
intra-atrial
intra-auricular

IA, i.a.
intraarterial (intra-arterial)
intraarticular (intra-articular)

I.A.
intrinsic activity

I & A
irrigation and aspiration

Ia
immune (region) associated antigen

IAA
indole-3-acetic acid (indoleacetic acid—
   re: regulation of plant growth)
infectious agent, arthritis
iodoacetic acid

IAAR
imidazoleacetic acid ribonucleotide

IAB
intra-abdominal
intra-aorta balloon

IABA
intra-aortic balloon assistance

IABC
intra-aortic balloon counterpulsation

IABCP
intra-aortic balloon counterpulsation

IABP
intra-aortic balloon pump
intra-aortic balloon pumping

IABPA
intra-aortic balloon pumping assistance

IAC
internal auditory canal
intra-arterial chemotherapy
Inventory of Anger Communications

IACD
intra-atrial conduction defect

IACP
intra-aortic counterpulsation

IAD
inactivating dose
inhibiting antibiotic dose
internal absorbed dose

IADH
inappropriate antidiuretic hormone

IADHS
inappropriate antidiuretic hormone
   syndrome

IADS
immunoadsorbent

IAE
intra-atrial electrocardiogram

IAFI
infantile amaurotic familial idiocy

IAH
idiopathic adrenal hyperplasia
implantable artificial heart

IAHA
idiopathic autoimmune hemolytic
   anemia
immune adherence hemagglutination

IAHD
idiopathic acquired hemolytic disease

IAM
internal auditory meatus

i amniot.
intra-amniotic

IAN
idiopathic aseptic necrosis
intern admit note

IANC
International Anatomical Nomenclature
   Committee

IAO
immediately after onset
intermittent aortic occlusion

IAP
immunosuppressive acidic protein
innervated antral pouch
inosinic acid pyrophosphorylase
intermittent acute porphyria
islet-activating protein

IAR
immediate asthmatic reaction
inhibitory anal reflex
instruction address register (re:
   computers)
iodine-azide reaction

IARF
ischemic acute renal failure

IARSA
idiopathic acquired refractory
   sideroblastic anemia

i arter.
intra-arterial

IAS
immunosuppressive acidic substance
interatrial septum
interatrial shunting
internal anal sphincter
intra-amniotic saline (infusion)

IASD
interatrial septal defect
interauricular septal defect

IASH
isolated asymmetric septal hypertrophy

IAT
immunoaugmentative therapy
   (unproven method for diagnosis/
   treatment of cancer)
instillation abortion time
invasive activity test
iodine azide test

IAV
intermittent assisted ventilation
intra-arterial vasopressin

IAVM
intramedullary arteriovenous
  malformation

IB
birth instrument
Ibrahim-Beck (disease)
immune balance
immune body
inclusion body
index of (body) build
infectious bronchitis (chickens)

I-B
interbody (vertebral)

ib.
ibidem (L. in the same place)

I band
isotropic band (disk—re: striated
  muscle fiber)

IBB
intestinal brush border

IBBBB
incomplete bilateral bundle branch
  block

IBC
iodine-binding capacity
iron-binding capacity
isobutyl cyanoacrylate (surgical tissue
  adhesive)

IBCA
isobutyl cyanoacrylate (surgical tissue
  adhesive)

IBD
inflammatory bowel disease

IBF
immature brown fat (cells)
immunoglobulin-binding factor

IBG
insoluble bone gelatin

IBI
intermittent bladder irrigation
ischemic brain infarction

ibid.
ibidem (L. in the same place)

IBK
infectious bovine keratoconjunctivitis

IBL
immunoblastic lymphadenopathy

IBM
inclusion body myositis
isotonic-isometric brief maximum

IBP
iron-binding protein

IBPMS
indirect blood pressure measuring
  system

IBQ
Illness Behavior Questionnaire

IBR
infectious bovine rhinotracheitis (virus)

IBRV
infective bovine rhinotracheitis virus

IBS
Interpersonal Behavior Survey
irritable bowel syndrome
isobaric solution

IBSA
iodinated bovine serum albumin

iBSA
immunoreactive bovine serum albumin

IBT
ink blot test

IBU
ibuprofen (anti-inflammatory)
international benzoate unit

IBV
infectious bronchitis vaccine
infectious bronchitis virus

IBW
ideal body weight

IC
icteric
immune complex
immune cytotoxicity
immunocytochemistry
impedance cardiogram
incomplete (diagnosis)
indirect calorimetry
individual counseling
inferior colliculus
inhibiting concentration
inorganic carbon
inspiratory capacity
inspiratory center
instruction counter (re: computers)
integrated circuit
intensive care
intercostal
intermediate care
intermittent claudication
internal capsule
internal carotid

internal cerebral
internal cholecystectomy
internal conjugate
interstitial cells
intracardiac
intracarotid
intracavitary
intracellular
intracellular concentration
intracerebral
intracisternal
intracranial
intracutaneous
intrapleural catheter
irritable colon
islet cells (of pancreas)
isovolumic contraction

I/C
invalid chair

I c̄
independent with (equipment)

i.c.
inter cibos (L. between meals)

ICA
internal carotid artery
intracranial aneurysm
islet cell antibodies

iCa
calicum, ionized

ICAb
islet cell antibody

ICAF
internal carotid artery flow

ICAO
internal carotid artery occlusion

ICAP
intracisternal A particle

i card.
intracardial

ICAV
intracavity

ICBF
inner cortical blood flow

ICBP
intercellular binding proteins
intracellular binding proteins

ICC
immunocompetent cells
immunocytochemistry
Indian childhood cirrhosis
intensive coronary care
interchromosomal crossing-over
intermediate cell column

internal conversion coefficient (re:
    radiology)
item characteristic curve (re: statistics)

ICCE
intracapsular cataract extraction

ICCE c̄ PI
intracapsular cataract extraction with
    peripheral iridectomy

ICCM
idiopathic congestive cardiomyopathy

ICCU
intensive coronary care unit
intermediate coronary care unit

ICD
I-cell disease (inclusion cells)
immune complex disease
induced circular dichroism
intercanthal distance
internal cervical device
International Classification of Diseases
    (of World Health Organization)
intracervical device
intrauterine contraceptive device
ischemic coronary disease
isocitrate dehydrogenase (isocitric
    [acid] dehydrogenase)

ICDA
International Classification of Diseases,
    Adapted (for use in the United States)

ICDCD
International Classification of Diseases
    and Causes of Death

ICDH
isocitric dehydrogenase

ICD-O
International Classification of Diseases
    for Oncology

ICDS
Integrated Child Development Scheme

ICE
ice, compression, elevation
Individual Career Exploration (re:
    Psychol)

I cell disease
inclusion cell disease (mucolipidosis II)

ICET
(Forty-Eight) Item Counseling
    Evaluation Test

ICF
indirect centrifugal flotation
intensive care facility
intercellular fluorescence
interciliary fluid
intermediate care facility

intracellular fluid
intravascular coagulation and
  fibrinolysis (syndrome)

ICFA
incomplete Freund's adjuvant
induced complement-fixing antigen

IC fx
intracapsular fracture

ICG
indocyanine green (Cardio-Green™)

ICGN
immune complex-mediated
  glomerulonephritis

ICH
infectious canine hepatitis
intracerebral hemorrhage
intracerebral hypertension
intracranial hemorrhage
intracranial hypertension

ICHPPC
International Classification of Health
  Problems in Primary Care

ICI
Interpersonal Communication Inventory
intracardiac injection
intracisternal

ICIDH
International Classification of
  Impairments, Disabilities, and
  Handicaps

ICLH arthroplasty
Imperial College, London Hospital
  arthroplasty

ICM
inner cell mass
intercostal margin
intracytoplasmic membrane
ion conductance modulator
ipsilateral competing message

ICN
Intensive Care Nursery
Intermediate Care Nursery

ICNC
intracerebellar nuclear cell

ICO
impedance cardiac output
initial check out (only)

i coch.
intracochlear

ICP
incubation period
inductively coupled plasma
infectious cell protein

intermittent catheterization protocol
intracranial pressure
intracytoplasmic

↑ ICP
increased intracranial pressure

ICPMM, I,C,PM,M; I, C, PM, M
incisors, canines, premolars, molars (re:
  Dent)

ICP monitor
intracranial pressure monitor

ICPS
Interpersonal Cognitive Problem-
  Solving

ICR
intermittent catheter routine
international calibrated ratio
intracardiac catheter recording
intracranial reinforcement
ion cyclotron resonance

ICRS
Index Chemicus Registry System

ICRU
International Commission on
  Radiological Units

ICS
ileocecal sphincter
impulse-conducting system
Intensive Care, Surgical
intercellular space
intercostal space
intracranial stimulation

ICSA
islet cell surface antibody

ICSC
idiopathic central serous
  chorioretinopathy

ICSH
interstitial cell-stimulating hormone
  (luteinizing hormone)

ICSS
intracranial self-stimulation

ICT
icteric
immunoglobulin consumption test
indirect Coombs' test
indirect Coombs' titer
insulin convulsive therapy
intensive conventional therapy
intermittent cervical traction
interstitial cell tumor
intracardial thrombus (intracardiac)
intracranial tumor
intradermal cancer test (unproven

method for diagnosis/ treatment of cancer)
intra-oral cariogenicity test
isovolumic contraction time

ICT, I.C.T.
inflammation of connective tissue
insulin coma therapy

ICT, ict.
icterus

iCT
immunoreactive calcitonin
immunoreactive (human) calcitonin

ict. ind.
icteric index
icterus index

ICTS
idiopathic carpal tunnel syndrome

ICTX
intermittent cervical traction

ICU
infant care unit
intensive care unit
intermediate care unit

i cut.
intracutaneous

ICV
intracellular volume

ICV, icv
intracerebroventricular

i.c.v.
into cerebral ventricles

ICW
intact canal wall
intensive care ward
intracellular water

ICX
immune complex

ID
identification
identifier (re: computers/data processing)
iditol dehydrogenase
ill-defined
immunodeficiency
immunodiffusion (test)
immunoglobulin deficiency
inappropriate disability
inclusion disease
index of discrimination
individual dose
induction delivery
infant deaths
infectious disease
inhibitory dose

inhomogeneous deposition
initial diagnosis
initial dose
injected dose
inner diameter
inside diameter
insufficient data
interdigitating (cells)
internal diameter
interstitial disease
intradermally
intraduodenal

ID, I.D.
infective dose

ID, id.
intradermal

I & D, I&D
incised and drained
incision and drainage

ID$_\infty$
infective dose

ID$_{50}$
median infective dose

Id
idiotypic

id.
idem (L. the same)

i.d.
in diem (L. during the day)

IDA
image display and analysis
iminodiacetic acid
insulin-degrading activity
iron-deficiency anemia

id. ac
idem ac (L. the same as)

IDBS
infantile diffuse brain sclerosis

IDC
idiopathic dilated cardiomyopathy
interdigitilating cell

IDCI
intradiplochromatid interchange

I-D curve
intensity-duration curve (re: physiatry)

IDD
insulin-dependent diabetes

IDDF
investigational drug data form

IDDM
insulin-dependent diabetes mellitus

IDDS
investigational drug data sheet

IDDT
immuno-double diffusion test

IDE
inner dental epithelium

IDEM effect
ischemic, drug, electrolyte, metabolic
effect

i derm.
intradermal

IDG
intermediate-dose group

IDH
isocitric dehydrogenase

IDH1
isocitrate dehydrogenase, soluble

IDH2
isocitrate dehydrogenase, mitochondrial

IDH-M
isocitrate dehydrogenase, mitochondrial

IDH-S
isocitrate dehydrogenase, soluble

IDI
immunologically detectable insulin
induction-delivery interval

I disk
isotropic disk (I band—re: striated
muscle fibers)

IDK
internal derangement of knee (joint)

IDL
difference limen for intensity
intermediary density lipoprotein
intermediate density lipoprotein

IDM
idiopathic disease of the myocardium
immune defense mechanism
indirect method
infant of diabetic mother
intermediate-dose methotrexate

IDMC
interdigestive motility complex
interdigestive motor complex

IDMEC
interdigestive myoelectric complex

IDMS, ID-MS
isotope dilution-mass spectrometry

IDNA
intercalary deoxyribonucleic acid

idon. vehic.
idoneo vehiculo (L. in a suitable vehicle)

IDP
immunodiffusion procedures
initial dose period
inosine diphosphate (inosine
5′-diphosphate)
instantaneous diastolic pressure

IDPH
idiopathic pulmonary hemosiderosis

IDR
intradermal reaction

IDS
immunity deficiency state
inhibitor of DNA synthesis
intraduodenal stimulation
investigational drug service

IDT
immune diffusion test
instillation delivery time
interdivision time
intradermal typhoid (and paratyphoid
vaccine)

IDU
idoxuridine (5-iodo-2-deoxyuridine—
antiviral—re: Ophth)
Ivy dog unit

IdUA
iduronic acid (found in proteoglycans
such as heparin)

IDUR
idoxuridine (5-iodo-2-deoxyuridine—
antiviral—re: Ophth)

IDV, I.D.V.
intermittent demand ventilation

IDVC
indwelling venous catheter

IdX
cross-reactive idiotype

IE
immunoelectrophoresis
infective endocarditis
inner ear
intake energy
internal ear
internal elastica
intra-epithelial
Introversion-Extroversion (scale)

IE, I.E.
immunitäts Einheit (Ger. immunizing
unit)

I/E
inspiratory-expiratory ratio

I & E
internal and external

i.e.
id est (L. that is)

IEA
immediate early antigen
immunoelectroadsorption (immuno-
    electro-adsorption)
immuno-electrophoretic analysis
    (immunoelectrophoretic)
infectious equine anemia
intravascular erythrocyte aggregation

IEC
injection electrode catheter
International Electrotechnical
    Commission
intra-epithelial carcinoma
ion exchange chromatography

IE Ca cx
intra-epithelial carcinoma of the cervix

IEE
inner enamel epithelium

IEF
isoelectric focusing

IEI
isoelectric interval

IEL
internal elastic lamina
intimal elastic lamina
intra-epithelial lymphocytes

IEM
immunoelectron microscopy
inborn error of metabolism

IEMG
integrated electromyogram

IEOP
immunoelectro-osmophoresis

IEP
immunoelectrophoresis
individual education plan
isoelectric point

IER test
Institute of Educational Research
    (intelligence) test

IES
ingressive-egressive sequence

I-E Scale
internal versus external (control of
    reinforcement) scale (Rotter—re:
    Psychol)

IF
idiopathic fibroplasia

immersion foot
immunofluorescence
inferior facet
infrared
inhibiting factor
initiation factor
interferon
intermediate factor
intermediate filament
intermediate frequency
internal friction
interstitial fluid
intracellular fluid
intrinsic factor (Castle's—vitamin B_{12}
    utilization)
involved field (re: radiotherapy)

IF, I.F.
internal fixation

IF1
interferon-1

IF2
interferon-2

IF3
interferon-3 (fibroblast)

IF-1, IF-2, IF-3
prokaryote initiation factors (re: protein
    synthesis)

IFA
immunofluorescent antibody
immunofluorescent assay
incomplete Freund's adjuvant
indirect fluorescence assay
indirect fluorescent antibody

IFAT
indirect fluorescent antibody test

IFC
inspiratory flow cartridge
intrinsic factor concentrate

IFCL
intermittent flow centrifugation
    leukapheresis

IFCS
inactivated fetal calf serum

IFE
interfollicular epidermis

IFF
inner fracture face

IFGS
interstitial fluids and ground substance

IFI
Institutional Functioning Inventory (re:
    psychological testing)

IFL
immunofluorescence

IFLrA, IFL-rA
recombinant human leukocyte
   interferon A

IFM
internal fetal monitor
intrafusal muscle

IFN
immunoreactive fibronectin
interferon (antineoplastic; antiviral)

IFN-α
(leukocyte) interferon (antineoplastic;
   antiviral)

IFN-β
(human) fibroblast interferon
   (antineoplastic; antiviral)

If nec.
if necessary

IFP
insulin, hydrocortisone (Kendall's
   compound F), prolactin
intermediate filament protein
intrapatellar fat pad

IFR
infrared
inspiratory flow rate

IFRA
indirect fluorescent rabies antibody
   (test)

IFRC
interferon receptor-21

IFS
interstitial fluid space

IFT
immunofluorescence technique
immunofluorescence test
International Frequency Tables

IFU
interferon unit

IFV
interstitial fluid volume
intracellular fluid volume

IFVC
instantaneous force-velocity curve

IFX
ifosfamide

IG
immature granule
immune globulin
intragastric

I-G
insulin-glucagon

Ig
immunoglobulin (of any of the five
   classes)

I$_\gamma$
specific gamma-ray emission or specific
   gamma-ray output

iG
immunoreactive human gastrin

i.g.
intragastrically

IGA
infantile genetic agranulocytosis

IgA
immunoglobulin A

IGD
interglobal distance

IgD
immunoglobulin D

IGDM
infant of gestational diabetic mother

IgE
immunoglobulin E

IGF
insulin-like growth factor

IGF-I
insulin-like growth factor I

IGF-II
insulin-like growth factor II

IGFET
insulated gate field-effect transistor

IgG
immunoglobulin G

IgG$_1$, IgG$_2$, IgG$_3$
immune gamma globulins

IGH
idiopathic growth hormone
immunoreactive growth hormone

IGI
Institutional Goals Inventory (re:
   psychological testing)

IGIV
immunoglobulin, intravenous

IgM
immunoglobulin M

IGP
intestinal glycoprotein

IGR
immediate generalized reaction
integrated gastrin response

IGS
inappropriate gonadotrop(h)in secretion

IgSC
immunoglobulin-secreting cell

IGT
impaired glucose tolerance

IgT
hypothetical antigen receptor on T-cell
surfaces

IGTT
intravenous glucose tolerance test

IGV
intrathoracic gas volume

IH
immediate (type) hypersensitivity
incomplete healing
indirect hemagglutination
inguinal hernia
inhibiting hormone
inhibitory hormone
in hospital
inner half
Inpatient Hospital
intermittent heparinization
intracerebral hematoma
iron hematoxylin

IH, I.H.
infectious hepatitis

IHA
idiopathic hyperaldosteronism
indirect hemagglutination antibody

IHBT
incompatible hemolytic blood
transfusion

IHBTD
incompatible hemolytic blood
transfusion disease

IHC
identified hair cell
idiopathic hemochromatosis
idiopathic hypercalciuria
inner hair cells (of cochlea)
intrahepatic cholestasis

IHCA
isocapnic hyperventilation with cold air
(re: Resp)

IHD
in-center hemodialysis
ischemic heart disease

IHG
ichthyosis hystrix gravior

IHGD
isolated human growth deficiency

IHH
idiopathic hypogonadotrop(h)ic
hypogonadism
infectious human hepatitis

IHHS
idiopathic hyperkinetic heart syndrome

IHMS
sodium isonicotinylhydrazide
methanesulfonate (tuberculostatic)

IHO
idiopathic hypertrophic
osteoarthropathy

IHP
idiopathic hypoparathyroidism
idiopathic hypopituitarism
inverted hand position

IHPC
intrahepatic cholestasis

IHPH
intrahepatic portal hypertension

IHR
intrahepatic resistance
intrinsic heart rate

IHRA
isocapnic hyperventilation with room air

IHS
inactivated horse serum
infrahyoid strap

IHSA
iodinated human serum albumin (also
^{125}I-HSA, ^{131}I-HSA; normal serum
albumin [human] mildly iodinated with
radioactive ^{131}I)

^{125}I-HSA
iodinated I 125 human serum albumin
(also IHSA)

^{131}I-HSA
iodinated I 131 human serum albumin
(also IHSA)

IHSC
immunoreactive human skin
collagenase

IHSS
idiopathic hypertrophic subaortic
stenosis

IHT
intravenous histamine test
ipsilateral head turning

IHW
inner heel wedge (re: podiatry)

II
image intensifier
irradiated iodine

II, I.I.
icteric index

I or I
illness or injuries

I and i antigens
I blood group antigens

IIC
integrated ion current

IID
insulin-independent diabetes

IIDM
insulin-independent diabetes mellitus

IIE
idiopathic ineffective erythropoiesis

IIF
immune interferon
indirect immunofluorescence
indirect immunofluorescent

IIIVC
infrahepatic interruption of the inferior
vena cava

IIP
idiopathic interstitial pneumonia
idiopathic intestinal pseudo-obstruction
indirect immunoperoxidase
Intra- and Interpersonal (Relations
Scale)

IIS
intensive immunosuppression

IIT
ineffective iron turnover
integrated isometric tension

IJ
intrajejunal

IJ, I-J
internal jugular (vein)

IJD
inflammatory joint disease

IJ line
internal jugular (vein) line

IJP
inhibitory junction potential
internal jugular pressure

IJV
internal jugular vein

IK
immobilized knee
infusoria killing (unit)
interstitial keratitis

IK, I.K.
Immunekörper (Ger. immune bodies)

IKE
ion kinetic energy

IKI, I-KI
iodine potassium iodide (Lugol's
solution)

I₂KI
Lugol's solution (potassium iodide and
iodine in pure water)

IKI catgut
catgut sterilized in a solution of iodine
and potassium, 1:100

IK unit
infusoria-killing unit

IL
ileum
iliolumbar
illustration
incisolingual (re: Dent)
independent laboratory
insensible (weight) loss
inspiratory loading
intensity level
interleukin
intestinal lymphocyte
intralipid
intralumbal
intralumbar

I-L
intensity-latency

IL 1, IL-1
interleukin 1

IL 2, IL-2
interleukin 2

Il
illinium (element—former name of
promethium)
illustration

i.l.
intralesional

ILA
insulin-like activity

ILa
incisolabial (re: Dent)

ILB
infant, low birth (weight)

ILBBB
incomplete left bundle branch block

ILBW
infant, low birth weight

ILC
ichthyosis linearis circumflex
incipient lethal concentration

ILD
interstitial lung disease
ischemic leg disease
ischemic limb disease
isolated lactase deficiency

ILDCSI
Individual Learning Disabilities
    Classroom Screening Instrument

ILE, Ile, ile
isoleucine

Ile
isoleucyl (radical of isoleucine)

i lesion
intralesional

ILEU, Ileu, ileu.
isoleucine (abbreviation Ile is preferred)

ILGF
insulin-like growth factor

ILL
intermediate lymphocytic lymphoma

ill.
illusion
illustrating
illustration

illic. lag. obturat.
illico lagena obturatur (L. let the bottle
    be closed at once)

illus.
illustrated
illustration

ILM
insulin-like material
internal limiting membrane

ILo
iodine lotion

ILR
irreversible loss rate

ILS
increase in life span

infrared liver scanner
interrupt level subroutine (re:
    computers)
intralobular sequestration

ILSS
intraluminal somatostatin

IM
immunosuppression method
Index Medicus
indomethacin
infectious mononucleosis
inner membrane
innocent murmur
inspiratory muscle
intermediate megaloblast
internal malleolus
internal mammary (artery)
internal medicine
intestinal mesenchyme
intramedullary
invasive mole

IM, im.
intramuscular (injection site)
intramuscularly

im-
(indicates presence of) =NH group

IMA
inferior mesenteric artery
internal mammary artery (implant)

IMAA
iodinated macroaggregated albumin

IMAI
internal mammary artery implant

IMB
intermenstrual bleeding

IMBC
indirect maximum breathing capacity

IMC
interdigestive migrating complex
interdigestive migrating contraction
interdigestive myoelectric complex
intestinal (mucosal) mast cell

IMCU
Intermediate Medical Care Unit

IMD
immunologically mediated diseases

ImD$_{50}$
immunizing dose to protect 50 percent

IMDC
intramedullary metatarsal
    decompression

IME
independent medical examination
independent medical examiner

IMEM
improved minimum essential medium

IMEM-HS
improved minimum essential medium,
    hormone supplemented

IMET
isometric endurance time

IMF
idiopathic myelofibrosis
intermaxillary fixation
intermediate filament

IMG
inferior mesenteric ganglion
internal medicine group (re: group
    practice)

IMH
idiopathic myocardial hypertrophy

IMHT
indirect microhemagglutination test

IMH test
indirect microhemagglutination test

IMI
imipramine
immunologically measurable insulin
impending myocardial infarction
indirect membrane
    immunofluorescence
inferior myocardial infarction
intermeal interval
intramuscular injection

imit.
imitation
imitative

IML
initial machine load (re: computers/data
    processing)
initial microprogram load (re:
    computers/data processing)
internal mammary lymphoscintigraphy

IMLA
intramural left anterior (descending
    artery)

IMLAD
intramural left anterior descending
    (artery)

ImLy
immune lysis

IMM
inhibitor-containing minimal medium
internal medial malleolus

immat.
immature

immed.
immediate
immediately

immob.
immobile
immobilize

immobil.
immobilize

ImmU
immunizing unit

Immun, immun.
immunity
immunization

immun.
immune
immunize
immunology

Immunol, immunol.
immunology

IMN
internal mammary (lymph) node

IMP
idiopathic myeloid proliferation
incomplete male
    pseudohermaphroditism
inosine-5′-phosphate (inosine
    monophosphate; inosinic acid)
Inpatient Multidimensional Psychiatric
    (scale)
intramembranous particle

imp.
impacted
imperfect
important
impressed
impression
improve
improved
improvement

IMPA
incisal mandibular plane angle

impair.
impaired
impairment

imperf.
imperfect
imperforate

IMPEX
immediate postexercise

IMPL
impulse

impr.
impressed
impression
improve
improved
improvement

impreg.
impregnate
impregnated

IMPRV
improvement

IMPS
Inpatient Multidimensional Psychiatric Scale

impvt.
improvement

Impx
impaction

IMR
infant mortality rate
infectious mononucleosis receptors
institution for the mentally retarded

IMRAD, Imrad
introduction, material, results, and discussion (re: formal structure of a scientific article)
introduction, methods, results, and discussion (re: formal structure of a scientific article)

IMRD
introduction, methods, results, discussion (re: formal structure of a scientific article)

IMS
incurred in military service
industrial methylated spirit
international metric system

IMSS
In-flight Medical Support System

IMT
indomethacin
induced muscular tension

IMU
international milliunit

IMV
inferior mesenteric vein

IMV, I.M.V.
intermittent mandatory ventilation
intermittent mechanical ventilation

IMVC
indole, methyl red, Voges-Proskauer, citrate (re: bacteriology)

IMVCi
indole, methyl red, Voges-Proskauer, and citrate (re: bacteriology)

IMViC, imvic
indole production, methyl red test, Voges-Proskauer, (and the ability to utilize) citrate as a sole source of carbon (i is inserted for euphony—re: *E. coli, Enterobacter aerogenes*, related organisms)
indole, methyl red, Voges-Proskauer, citrate (reactions— re: bacteriology)

IN
icterus neonatorum
impetigo neonatorum
incidence
incompatibility number
infantile nephrotic (syndrome)
infundibular nucleus
initial (dose) insulin
intermedial nucleus (intermediomedial—re: Neuro)
interneuron
interstitial nephritis
intranasal

In
Index
indium (element)
insulin
inulin

^{111}In
radioactive isotope of indium

^{114}In
radioactive isotope of indium

in.
inch
inches

in^3
cubic inches

INA
infectious nucleic acid (re: transfection)
inferior nasal artery

INAA
instrumental neutron activation analysis

inac.
inactive

INAD
infantile neuroaxonal dystrophy
investigational new animal drug

inadeq.
inadequate

INAH
isonicotinic acid hydrazide

INB
ischemic necrosis of bone

INC
inside-the-needle catheter
interstitial nucleus of Cajal (re: Neuro)

INC, inc.
incomplete
inconclusive
incontinent
increase
increased
increasing

INC, Inc, inc.
incorporated

Inc
including

inc.
incision
incisional
increment
incurred

IncB
inclusion body

INCD
infantile nuclear cerebral degeneration

incid.
incide (L. cut)

incl.
include
including
inclusive

incoher.
incoherent

incompat.
incompatible

incompl.
incomplete

incont.
incontinence
incontinent

INCR, Incr, incr.
increase(d)

inc(R), inc (r)
increase (relative)

incr.
increasing
increment

incur.
incurable

IND
indomethacin (analgesic; anti-
  inflammatory)
industrial
investigational new drug
investigative new drug

ind.
independent
index
indicate
indicating
indication
indigent
indigo
indirect
induction

in d.
in die (L. in a day)
in dies (L. daily)

indef.
indefinite

indic.
indicated
indication

indig.
indigestion

INDIV
individual

INDM
infant of nondiabetic mother

Ind.Med.
Index Medicus

Ind-Med
industrial medicine

INDO
indomethacin (analgesic; anti-
  inflammatory)
intermediate neglect of differential
  overlap (method)

INDOR
internuclear double resonance

Ind-Surg
industrial surgery

ind. th.
individual therapy

induct.
induction

indur.
induration

indust.
industrial
industry

INE
infantile necrotizing
  encephalomyelopathy

in extrem.
in extremis (L. in the last [hours of life])

INF
infectious (disease)
infundibulum (of neurohypophysis)

INF, Inf, inf.
infusion

INF, inf.
infant
infantile
infected
infection
inferior
infirmary
infunde (L. pour in)
infusum (L. an infusion)

inf.
infancy
infarct
infarction
infect
infectious
infirmary
information

in f.
in fine (L. finally; at the end)

infarct.
infarction

infec. dis.
infectious disease

infect.
infection
infectious

infer.
inferior

infl.
inflamed
inflammation
influence
influx

inflam.
inflamed
inflammation
inflammatory

inflamm.
inflammation
inflammatory

infl. proc.
inflammatory process

Inf. MI
inferior (wall) myocardial infarction

info.
information

infor.
information

infra.
infrared

inf. turb.
inferior turbinate

infund.
infunde (L. pour in)

ING
isotope nephrogram

Ing, ing.
inguinal

ingest.
ingestion

INH
isonicotinoylhydrazine (isoniazid;
  isonicotinic acid hydrazide;
  isonicotinylhydrazine—
  tuberculostatic)

INH, inh.
inhalation

inhal.
inhalatio (L. inhalation)

inher.
inherent

INH-G
isonicotinoylhydrazone of D-glucuronic
  acid lactone (glyconiazide—
  antitubercular)

inhib.
inhibit
inhibition
inhibitor
inhibitory

INI
intranuclear inclusion (agent)

init.
initial

INJ, inj.
inject

inj.
injectable
injected
injectio (L. an injection)
injection
injured

injurious
injury

inject.
injection

inj. enem.
injiciatur enema (L. let an enema be
   injected)

INK
injury not known

inl.
inlay

in. lb., in-lb
inch-pound

in litt.
in litteris (L. in correspondence)

in loc. cit.
in loco citato (L. in the place cited)

INN
International Nonproprietary Name

innerv.
innervated
innervation

innom.
innominate

INO
infantile nephrotic (syndrome), other
   (types)
internuclear ophthalmoplegia
   (Bielschowsky-Lutz-Cogan
   syndrome)

INO, Ino, ino.
inosine

Ino
inosyl (radical of inosine; rarely used)

INOC, inoc.
inoculate

inoc.
inoculated
inoculation

inor.
inorganic

inorg.
inorganic

in. oz.
inch ounce

INPAV
intermittent negative pressure assisted
   ventilation

INPC
O-isopropyl N-phenyl carbamate
   (herbicide)

INPEA
N-isopropyl-p-nitrophenylethanolamine
   (beta adrenergic blocker)

INPRCNS
information processing in central
   nervous system

INPRONS
information processing in the (central)
   nervous system

in pulm.
in pulmento (L. in gruel)

INPV
intermittent negative pressure
   (assisted) ventilation

INQ
inferior nasal quadrant

INR
international normalized ratio

INREM
internal (radiation dose) roentgen
   equivalent man
internal (radiation dose) roentgen-
   equivalent—man

INS
idiopathic nephrotic syndrome

INS, ins.
insulin

ins
insertion (re: cytogenetics)

ins.
inches
insurance

insid.
insidious

insol.
insoluble

Insp, insp.
inspiration
inspiratory

insp.
inspect
inspection

insp'd
inspected

insp'd & p's'd
inspected and passed

INSPEC
inspection
inspector

Inspir, inspir.
inspiration
inspiratory

Inst, inst.
institute
institution
institutional

inst.
instructions
instrument

instab.
instability

instill.
instillation

Instn
institution

Instr
instruction
instructor

insuf.
insufficient
insufflatio (L. an insufflation)

insuff.
insufficiency
insufficient

INT, Int
intern
internist
internship

INT, Int, int.
intermittent
internal

int.
intact
integral
interest
interesting
intermediates
interval
intestinal
intime (L. to the innermost)

int. cib.
inter cibos (L. between meals)

INTEG
integument

intell.
intelligence
intelligent

intercond.
intercondylar

intermit.
intermittent

intern.
internal

internat.
international

intertroch.
intertrochanteric

intes.
intestinal
intestine

INTEST, intest.
intestinal

intest.
intestine

Int/Ext
internal/external (rotation—re: Ortho)

INTH
intrathecal

Int Hist, int. hist.
interval history

INTL
internal

INTMD
intermediate

IntMed, Int Med, int. med.
internal medicine

int. noct.
inter noctem (L. during the night)

INTOX, intox.
intoxicated
intoxication

INTR
intermittent

intracal.
intracalvarium

INTREX
Information Transfer Experiment

Int rot., int. rot.
internal rotation (re: Ortho)

↑ **int. rot.**
increased internal rotation

↓ **int. rot.**
decreased internal rotation

int. trx
intermittent traction

intub.
intubate
intubation

INV
inferior nasal vein

inv, inv.
inversion (re: cytogenetics)

inv.
invalid
inverse
inverted
investigate
investigation
involuntary

inval.
invalid

inver.
inversion

invest.
investigate
investigation

invet.
inveterate

Inv/Ev
inversion/eversion

invol.
involuntary

involv.
involve (L. roll on [coat])
involvement

IO
incisal opening
inferior oblique (eye muscle)
inferior olive (re: Neuro)
inside-out (vesicle)
internal os (cervix)
intestinal obstruction
intraocular

I/O
input/output (re: computers)

I & O
in and out

I & O, I&O
intake and output

Io
ionium (a radioactive isotope of
    thorium)

IOA
inner optic anlage (Ger. anlage—
    primordium)

IOB
input-output buffer (re: computers)

IOC
in our culture
input-output controller (re: computers)
intern on call

IOCS
input/output control subroutine (re:
    computers)
input-output control system (re:
    computers/data processing)

IOD
injured on duty
integrated optical density (re: Ophth)
interorbital distance (re: Ophth)

IOFB
intraocular foreign body

IOH
idiopathic orthostatic hypotension

IOL
intraocular lens (re: Ophth)

IOL implant
intraocular lens implant (re: Ophth)

ION
ischemic optic neuropathy

IOP
input/output processor (re: computers)
intraocular pressure (re: Ophth)

IOR
information outflow rate
input/output register (re: computers)

IORT
intraoperative radiation therapy

IOT
intraocular tension (re: Ophth)
intraocular transfer (re: Ophth)
ipsilateral optic tectum (re: Neuro)

IOTA
information overload testing aid

IOU
intensive (therapy) observation unit
international opacity unit

IP
icterus praecox
immune precipitate
immunoblastic plasma
immunoperoxidase
implantation test
inactivated pepsin
incisoproximal (re: Dent)
incisopulpal (re: Dent)
incontinentia pigmenti
incubation period

induced protein
induction period
industrial population (re: statistics)
infection prevention (re: testing
  antiseptics)
infundibular process (re:
  neurohypophysis)
infusion pump
initial pressure
inorganic phosphate
inosine phosphorylase
instantaneous pressure
International Pharmacopoeia
interpeduncular nucleus (re: Neuro)
interpharyngeal
interpositus nucleus (re: Neuro)
interpupillary
intestinal pseudo-obstruction
intracellular proteolysis
ionization potential
isoproterenol

IP, I.P.
isoelectric point

IP, I.P., Ip, i.p.
intraperitoneal (injection site)
intraperitoneally

IP, I-P, I/P
interphalangeal (joint)

IP, I/P
inpatient

I$_p$
peak alternating current

[I] p
concentration of insulin in plasma

IPA
incontinentia pigmenti achromians
indole, pyruvic acid
International Phonetic Alphabet
isopropyl alcohol

IPAR
Institute of Personality Assessment and
  Research

I para, I-para
primipara

IPAT
(Cattell's) Institute for Personality and
  Ability Testing (Anxiety Scale)
Iowa Pressure Articulation Test

IPC
industrial process control (re:
  computers)
ion-pair chromatography
isopropyl chlorophenyl
O-isopropyl N-phenyl carbamate (N-
  phenyl isopropyl carbamate; also
  called propham—an herbicide)

IPCS
intrauterine progesterone contraceptive
  system

IPD
immediate pigment darkening
increase in pupillary diameter
incurable problem drinker
inflammatory pelvic disease
intermittent peritoneal dialysis
interpupillary distance
Inventory of Psychosocial Development

IPE
infectious porcine encephalomyelitis
injury pulmonary edema
interstitial pulmonary emphysema

IPEH
intravascular papillary endothelial
  hyperplasia

i periton.
intraperitoneal

IPF
idiopathic pulmonary fibrosis
infection-potentiating factor
International Primary Factors (Test
  Battery—re: Psychol)
interstitial pulmonary fibrosis

IPG
impedance plethysmography
inspiratory phase gas
isopropyl thiogalactoside
  (isopropylthiogalactoside)

IPGE, iPGE
immunoreactive prostaglandin E

IPH
idiopathic pulmonary hemosiderosis
infant passive hand
inflammatory papillary hyperplasia
interphalangeal
intraparenchymal hemorrhage

IPI
Imagined Process Inventory
interphonemic interval
interpulse interval

IPIA
immunoperoxidase infectivity assay

IPK
intractable plantar keratosis (re:
  podiatry)

IPKD
infantile polycystic kidney disease

IPL
initial program load (re: computers)

inner plexiform layer (stratum
   moleculare [retina] or cerebral cortex)
intrapleural

i pleur.
intrapleural

IPM
impulses per minute
inches per minute
infant passive mitt

IPN
intern progress note
interpeduncular nucleus (re: Neuro)
interpenetrating polymer network

IPn
interstitial pneumonitis

IPNA
N-isopropylnoradrenalin(e)
   (isoproterenol—adrenergic
   [bronchodilator])

IPO
improved pregnancy outcome

IPOF
immediate postoperative fitting

IPOP
immediate postoperative prosthesis

IPP
independent practice plan
inorganic pyrophosphate
inosine, pyruvate, (inorganic) phosphate
intermittent positive pressure
intrahepatic portal pressure
intrapleural pressure

IPPA
inspection, palpation, percussion,
   auscultation

IPPB
intermittent positive pressure breathing
   (device)

IPPB/I
intermittent positive pressure breathing/
   inspiratory

IPPB(R,V)
intermittent positive pressure breathing
   (respiration, ventilation)

IPPC
isopropyl *N*-phenyl-carbamate (an
   herbicide)

IPPI
interruption of pregnancy for psychiatric
   indication

IPPO
intermittent positive pressure (inflation)
   with oxygen

IPPR
integrated pancreatic polypeptide
   response
intermittent positive pressure respiration

IPPT
Inter-Person Perception Test (re:
   Psychol)

IPPUAD
immediate postprandial upper
   abdominal distress

IPPV
intermittent positive pressure ventilation

IPQ
Intermediate Personality Questionnaire
   (for Indian Pupils—re: psychological
   testing)
Intimacy Potential Quotient (re:
   psychological testing)

IPR
insulin production rate
interval patency rate
intraparenchymal resistance

I-PR, IPr
isopropyl- (prefix denoting a
   1-methylethyl group)

IPRL
isolated perfused rabbit lung
isolated perfused rat liver

IPRT
Interpersonal Reaction Test

IPS
impulse per second
inches per second (re: computers)
infundibular pulmonary stenosis
initial prognostic score
intermittent photic stimulation (re: EEG)
Interpersonal Perception Scale
intraperitoneal shock

Ips
p-iodophenylsulfonyl (pipsyl)

ips
inches per second

IPSB
intrapartum stillbirth

IPSC
inhibitory postsynaptic current

IPSF
immediate postsurgical fitting (re:
   prostheses)

IPSID
immunoproliferative small intestinal
   disease

IPSP
inhibitory postsynaptic potential

IPT
immunoprecipitation
interpersonal psychotherapy
isoproterenol
   (N-isopropylnoradrenalin[e]—
   adrenergic [bronchodilator])

IPTG
isopropylthiogalactose
isopropylthiogalactoside

iPTH
immunoreactive parathyroid hormone

IPTX
intermittent pelvic traction (re: Ortho)

IPU
inpatient unit

IPV
inactivated poliomyelitis vaccine
inactivated poliomyelitis virus (vaccine)
inactivated polio vaccine
inactivated poliovaccine
inactivated poliovirus vaccine
incompetent perforator vein
infectious pustular vaginitis
infectious pustular vulvovaginitis (of
   cattle)
intrapulmonary vein

IPVD
Index of Pulmonary Vascular Disease

IPW
interphalangeal width

IPZ
insulin-protamine zinc

IQ, I.Q.
intelligence quotient

i.q.
idem quod (L. the same as)

IQ&S
iron, quinine and strychnine

IR
ileal resection
immunization rate
immunological response
immunoreactive
immunoreagent
index of response
individual reaction
inferior rectus (muscle)
information retrieval (re: computers)
infrared

infrared (rays)
inside radius
insoluble residue
inspiratory reserve
inspiratory resistance
insulin receptor
insulin requirement
insulin response
integer ratio
internal resistance
internal rotation
intrarachidian
inversion recovery
inverted repeats (re: genetics)
irritant reaction
isovolumetric relaxation

IR, Ir
immune response

IR, i.r.
intrarectal
intrarenal

I-R
Ito-Reenstierna (test/reaction)

Ir
iridium (element)

192Ir
radioactive isotope of iridium

194Ir
radioactive isotope of iridium

IRA
immunoradioassay
immunoregulatory alpha-globulin

IRB
Institutional Review Board

IRBBB
incomplete right bundle branch block

IRBC
infected red blood cell

iRBC
immature red blood cell

IRC
inspiratory reserve capacity
instantaneous resonance curve

IRCA
intravascular red cell aggregation

IRCS
International Research
   Communications System

IRCU
intensive respiratory care unit

IRD
isorhythmic dissociation

IRDS
idiopathic respiratory distress syndrome
infant respiratory distress syndrome

IRE
internal rotation in extension

IRF
idiopathic retroperitoneal fibrosis
internal rotation in flexion

IRG
immunoreactive gastrin
immunoreactive glucagon

Ir genes
immune response genes

IRGH
immunoreactive growth hormone

IRGI
immunoreactive glucagon

IRH
intraretinal hemorrhage

IRHC
immunoradioassayable human
   chorionic (somatomammotropin)

IRhCS
immunoreactive human chorionic
   somatomammotropin

IRHGH, IR-HGH, IRhGH
immunoreactive human growth
   hormone

IRhPL
immunoreactive human placental
   lactogen

IRI
immunoreactive insulin
insulin radioimmunoassay
iris

IRIA
indirect radioimmunoassay

IRI/G
immunoreactive insulin (to serum or
   plasma) glucose (ratio)

IRIg
insulin reactive immunoglobulin

IRL
information retrieval language (re:
   computers)

IRM
innate releasing mechanism

IRMA
immunoradiometric assay
intraretinal microvascular abnormalities
   (re: Ophth)

iRNA
immune ribonucleic acid

IROS
ipsilateral routing of signal

IRP
immunoreactive plasma
immunoreactive proinsulin
incus replacement prosthesis
inhibitor of radical processes
insulin-releasing polypeptide
International Reference Preparation

IRR
infrared refractometry
intrarenal reflux
irritation

IRR, Irr
irritant

IRR, irr.
irradiation

irreg.
irregular

IRRG
irrigated
irrigation

irrig.
irrigate
irrigation

IRS
immunoreactive secretin
infrared spectrophotometry
insulin receptor species

IRSA
idiopathic refractory sideroblastic
   anemia
iodinated rat serum albumin

IRT
immunoreactive trypsin
interresponse time
item response theory (re: psychological
   testing)

IRTO
immunoreactive trypsin output

IRTU
integrating regulatory transcription unit

IRU
interferon reference unit

IRV
inferior radicular vein
inspiratory reserve volume

IS
ileal segment
immediate sensitivity

immune serum
immunosuppressive
incentive spirometer
index of saponification
index of sexuality
infant size
infrahyoid strap
initial segment
insertion sequence (element—re: DNA)
insulin secretion
intercellular space
intercostal space
interictal spike (re: EEG)
internal standard
interstitial space
intracardial shunt (intracardiac)
intraspinal
intrasplenic
intrastriatal
intraventricular septum
inventory by system
ischemic score
isoproterenol

IS, i.s.
in situ (L. in [original] place)
interspace

I-10-S
invert sugar (10%) in saline

Is, is.
isolation

is.
island
isolate

ISA
intrinsic stimulating activity
intrinsic sympathomimetic activity
iodinated serum albumin
irregular spiking activity (re: EEG)

ISA$_5$
internal surface area of lung at volume
  of five liters

ISADH
inappropriate secretion of antidiuretic
  hormone

ISAM
indexed-sequential access method (re:
  computers)
integrated switching and multiplexing
  (re: computers)

ISC
immunoglobulin-secreting cell
insoluble collagen
intensive supportive care
International Statistical Classification
interstitial cells
intersystem crossing
irreversibly sickled cell

ISCCO
intersternocostoclavicular ossification

ISCF
interstitial cell fluid

ISCN
International System for (Human)
  Cytogenetic Nomenclature

ISCP
infection surveillance and control
  program

ISD
immunosuppressive drug
inhibited sexual desire
interatrial septal defect
interventricular septal defect
isosorbide dinitrate

ISDB
indirect self-destructive behavior (re:
  Psychol)

ISDN
isosorbide dinitrate

ISE
inhibited sexual excitement
integrated square error
ion-selective electrode

ISED
Interview Schedule for Events and
  Difficulties

IS-ELEMENT
insertion sequence element

ISF
interstitial fluid

ISFET
ion-specific field-effect transducer

ISG
immune serum globulin

ISH
icteric serum hepatitis

ISI
infarct size index
initial slope index
injury severity index
International Sensitivity Index
interstimulus interval

ISIH
interspike interval histogram

ISL
inner scapular line
interspinous ligament
isoleucine

ISM
intersegmental muscles

ISO
International Organization for
 Standardization
isoproterenol (adrenergic
 [bronchodilator])

ISO, iso.
isotropic

isoenz.
isoenzymes

Isol
Isolette®

isol.
isolate
isolated
isolation

Is of Lang
islands (islets) of Langerhans

isoln.
isolation

isom.
isometric
isometrophic

IsoPPC
O-isopropyl N-phenyl carbamate
 (propham—herbicide)

IsoRAS
isorenin-angiotensin system

ISP
distance between iliac spines
immunoreactive substance P
interspace
intraspinal

ISPT
interspecies (ovum) penetration test

ISPX
Ionescu-Shiley pericardial xenograft

i.s.q.
in status quo (L. unchanged)

ISR
insulin secretion rate

ISS
Injury Severity Scale
interrupt service subroutine (re:
 computers)
ion-scattering spectroscopy
ion surface scattering

ISSN
international standard serial number

IST
insulin sensitivity test
insulin shock therapy
interstitiospinal tract
ischemic ST (depression)
isometric systolic tension

ISTD
insulin standard

I-sub
inhibitor substance

I substance, I-substance
inhibitor substance

ISW
interstitial water

ISWI
incisional surgical wound infection

ISY
intrasynovial

IT
immunity test
immunotherapy
implantation test
individual therapy
industrial therapy
information technology
inhalation test
insulin treatment
intension tremor
intensive therapy
intermittent traction
internal thoracic
internal transition
interstitial tissue
intertrochanteric
intertuberous (pelvic diameter)
intolerance and toxicity
intracellular tachyzoite
intradermal test
intrathecal
intrathoracic
intratracheal
intratracheal tube
intratumoral
intubercular
ischial tuberosity
isomeric transition (re: radioactive
 isotopes)

IT, I.T.
inhalation therapy

I/T
intensity/time (duration)

ITA
inferior temporal artery
itaconic acid

ital.
italic
italicize

ITC
imidazolyl-thioguanine chemotherapy

ITCVD
ischemic thrombotic cerebrovascular
   disease

ITD
insulin-treated diabetic

ITE
in the ear (hearing aid)
intrapulmonary interstitial emphysema

ITET
isotonic endurance test

ITF
interferon

ITFS
incomplete testicular feminization
   syndrome

ITH, ITh, I Th
intrathecal (intraspinal—re: injections)

i thec.
intrathecal

ITI
intertrial interval

ITLC
instant thin-layer chromatography

ITLC-SG
instant thin-layer chromatography-silica
   gel

ITM
intrathecal methotrexate
Israel turkey meningoencephalitis

ITOU
intensive therapy observation unit

ITP
idiopathic thrombocytopenic purpura
immune thrombocytopenic purpura
inosine 5′-triphoshate
islet (cell) tumor of pancreas

ITPA
Illinois Test of Psycholinguistic Abilities
inosine triphosphatase (gene marker
   symbol— re: genetics)

ITQ
inferior temporal quadrant

ITR
intraocular tension recorder
intratracheal

i trach.
intratracheal

ITSC
It Scale for Children (re: psychological
   testing)

ITSHD
isolated thyroid-stimulating hormone
   deficiency

ITT
identical twins (raised) together
insulin tolerance test
internal tibial torsion

ITU
intensive therapy unit

ITV
inferior temporal vein

ITX
intertriginous xanthoma

ITyr
3-iodotyrosine (monoiodotyrosine)

IU
intrauterine
in utero
5-iodouracil

IU, I.U.
immunizing unit
international unit

[I] U
concentration of insulin in urine

IUB
International Union of Biochemistry (re:
   standardization)

IUC
idiopathic ulcerative colitis

IUCD
intrauterine contraceptive device

IUD
intrauterine death
intrauterine (contraceptive) device

IUDR
5-iododeoxyuridine (idoxuridine; 5-iodo-
   2′-deoxyuridine)

IUFB
intrauterine foreign body

IUFD
intrauterine fetal demise

IUFGR
intrauterine fetal growth retardation

IUG
infusion urogram

intrauterine gestation
intrauterine growth

IUGR
intrauterine growth rate
intrauterine growth retardation

IU/L
international units per liter

IUM
internal urethral meatus
intrauterine (fetally) malnourished
intrauterine malnourishment
intrauterine membrane

IUP
intrauterine pregnancy
intrauterine pressure

IUPAC
International Union of Pure and Applied
Chemistry (re: standardization)

IUPAP
International Union of Pure and Applied
Physics

IUPD
intrauterine pregnancy, delivered

IUP,TBCS
intrauterine pregnancy, term birth,
cesarean section

IUP,TBLC
intrauterine pregnancy, term birth, living
child

IUP,TBLI
intrauterine pregnancy, term birth, living
infant

IUT
intrauterine transfusion

IV
ichthyosis vulgaris
interventricular (heart)
intervertebral
intravascular
intravertebral
invasive
in vitro
in vivo

IV, I-V
intraventricular

IV, iv.
intravenous
intravenously

IV, i.v.
iodine value

IVag
intravaginal

IVAP
in vivo adhesive platelet

IVAR
insulin variable

IVB
intraventricular block
intravitreal blood

IVBAT
intravascular bronchioalveolar tumor

IVC
individually viable cells
inferior vena cava
inspiratory vital capacity
inspired vital capacity
integrated vector control
intravascular coagulation
intravenous cholangiogram
intravenous cholangiography
isovolumic contraction (period)

IVCC
intravascular consumption
coagulopathy

IVCD
intraventricular conduction defect
intraventricular conduction delay

IVCh
intravenous cholangiogram

IVCP
inferior vena cava pressure

IVCT
isovolumic contraction time

IVCV
inferior venacavography

IVD
intervertebral disc

IVF
interventricular foramen
intravascular fluid
intravenous fluids
in vitro fertilization
in vivo fertilization

IVGTT
intravenous glucose tolerance test

IVH
intravenous hyperalimentation
intraventricular hemorrhage

IVJC
intervertebral joint complex

IVM
immediate visual memory
intravascular mass

IVMP
intravenous methylprednisolone

IVN
intravenous nutrition

IVNF
intravitreal neovascular frond (re:
    Ophth)

IVP
intravenous push (dose)
intravenous pyelogram
intraventricular pressure
intravesical pressure

IVPB
intravenous piggypack

IVPD
in vitro protein digestibility

IVPF
isovolume pressure flow (curve)
isovolumic pressure flow

IVR
internal visual reference
intravaginal ring
isolated volume responders
isovolumic relaxation time

IVRD
in vitro rumen digestibility (re:
    veterinary)

IVRT
isovolumic relaxation time

IVS
inappropriate vasopressin secretion
intact ventricular septum
intervening sequence
interventricular septum
intervillous space
intraventricular septum

IVSD
interventricular septal defect

IVSE
interventricular septal excursion

IVT
index of vertical transmission
intravenous transfusion
intraventricular
isovolumic time

IVTTT
intravenous tolbutamide tolerance test

IVU
intravenous urogram
intravenous urography

IVV
influenza virus vaccine
intravenous vasopressin

IV Vol.
intravenous Volutrol

IW
inner wall

I-5-W
invert sugar (5%) in water

IWI
interwave interval

IWL
insensible water loss

IWMI
inferior wall myocardial infarction

IWS
Index of Work Satisfaction

IZ
infarction zone

IZS
insulin zinc suspension

J

J
Jewish
joint
Joule's equivalent
journal
Jurassic (geological time division)
juvenile
juvenile (amaurotic idiocy)

J, J
joule (practical and SI unit of work)

J, j
juice

J
flux density
mechanical equivalent (15° calorie)

J1, J2, J3, etc.; J-1, J-2, J-3, etc.
Jaeger test type number 1, 2, 3, etc. (re:
  Ophth)

j
in prescription writing, used as a roman
  numeral as the equivalent of "i" for
  one, or at the end of a number (EX: j,
  ij, iij, vij, etc.)

JA
juvenile atrophy
juxta-articular

JAI
juvenile amaurotic idiocy

JAS
Jenkins Activity Survey (re:
  pyschological testing)
Job Attitude Scale

jaund.
jaundice

JBC
Jesness Behavior Checklist

JBE
Japanese B encephalitis

JC
Jakob-Creutzfeldt (syndrome)
joint contracture

J/C
joule per coulomb

jc.
juice

JCA
juvenile chronic arthritis

JCAH
Joint Commission on Accreditation of
  Hospitals

JCF
juvenile calcaneal fracture

J chain
a polypeptide chain

JCL
job control language (re: computers)

JCML
juvenile chronic myelocytic leukemia

JCP
juvenile chronic polyarthritis

jct.
junction

JCV
Jamestown Canyon virus

JD
jejunal diverticulitis
juvenile diabetes

JDM
juvenile diabetes mellitus

JE
Japanese encephalitis
junctional escape

JEE
Japanese equine encephalitis

JEJ, Jej, jej.
jejunum

jentac.
jentaculum (L. breakfast)

JEPI
Junior Eysenck Personality Inventory

JEV
Japanese encephalitis virus

JF
jugular foramen
junctional fold

JFET
junction field-effect transistor

JFS
jugular foramen syndrome

JG
June grass (test)
juxtaglomerular

JGA
juxtaglomerular apparatus

JGC
juxtaglomerular cell

j-g complex
juxtaglomerular complex

JGCT
juxtaglomerular cell tumor

JGI
jejunogastric intussusception
juxtaglomerular granulation index
juxtaglomerular index

JGP
juvenile general paralysis

JH
juvenile hormone (of insects)

j_H
heat transfer factor

JHA
juvenile hormone analogue

JHR
Jarisch-Herxheimer reaction

JI
jejunoileal

JIB
jejunoileal bypass

JIH
joint interval histogram

JJ
jaw jerk

Jk
Kidd system blood group (alleles Jk^a,
Jk^b, anti-Jk^a, anti-Jk^b)

JKST
Johnson-Kenney Screening Test (re:
psychological testing of early learning
disability)

JL
Jadassohn-Lewandowski (syndrome)
Jaffe-Lichtenstein (syndrome)

JLP
juvenile laryngeal papilloma

j_M
mass transfer factor (re: heat transfer)

JMS
junior medical student

JNA
Jena Nomina Anatomica (re:
anatomical terminology)

JND
just noticeable difference

jnt.
joint

JOD
juvenile-onset diabetes

JODM
juvenile-onset diabetes mellitus

JOMACI
judgment, orientation, memory,
abstraction, and calculation intact (re:
psychiatry)

Jour, jour.
journal

JP
juvenile periodontitis

JPB
junctional premature beat

JPC
junctional premature contraction

JPD
juvenile plantar dermatosis

JPI
Jackson Personality Inventory

JPS
joint position sense

JR
Jolly's reaction
junctional rhythm

jr.
junior

JRA
juvenile rheumatoid arthritis

J receptor
juxtapulmonary-capillary receptor

jrl.
journal

jrnl.
journal

JS
jejunal segment
junctional slowing
Junkman-Schoeller (unit of
  thyrotrop[h]in)

Js^a antigen
Sutter antigen (Kell system blood
  group)

JSI
Jansky Screening Index (re:
  psychological testing)

JS unit
Junkman-Schoeller unit (of
  thyrotrop[h]in)

JT, jt.
joint

jt. asp.
joint aspiration

jucund.
jucunde (L. pleasantly)

jug.
jugular

jug. comp.
jugular compression (test)

junct.
junction

juv.
juvenile

juve.
juvenile

JUXT, juxt.
juxta (L. near)

JV
jugular vein
jugular venous

JVD
jugular venous distention

JVIS
Jackson Vocational Interest Survey

JVP
jugular vein pulse
jugular venous pressure
jugular venous pulse

JVPT
jugular venous pulse tracing

JW, j.w.
jump walker

JXG
juvenile xanthogranuloma

K

K
absolute zero (temperature)
calyx, calix (Gr. kalyx—cup)
capsular antigen
carrying capacity (re: genetics)
coefficient of scleral rigidity (re: Ophth)
cretaceous
electron capture (re: radioactive isotopes)
electrostatic capacity
equilibrium constant
a gastric tube (i.e., K-10)
gene required for maintenance of kappa in *Paramecium aurelia* (re: genetics)
ionization constant
kalium (from Arabic—qali [potash]—potassium, an element)
kallikrein inhibiting unit (re: enzyme)
kanamycin
kappa (capital tenth letter of Greek alphabet)
Kell blood system
kelvin (SI—fundamental unit of temperature; previously °K)
kidney
killer (cells)
Klebsiella (genus)
knee
lysine
motor coordination (re: General Aptitude Test Battery test)
phylloquinone (or phylloquinone K)
1024 (symbol for the number of bytes in a kilobyte—re: computers)
radius of curvature of flattest meridian of apical cornea (re: fitting of contact lenses)

K, K.
kathode (obsolete for cathode)

K, k
kilogram
one thousand

K
symbol for dissociation constant

°K
previous abbreviation for kelvin (replaced in 1968 by the CGPM with the single word kelvin; K now used)

K-10
gastric tube

17K
17-ketosteroid excretion

17-K
17-ketosteroids

⁴⁰K
potassium-40

⁴²K
potassium-42 (a reactor-produced radionuclide)

⁴³K
potassium-43

k
Boltzmann constant (a fundamental physical constant)
constant
kilo (prefix)
reaction rate constant

k
constant, rate or velocity

κ
kappa (tenth letter of Greek alphabet)
magnetic susceptibility
one of the two immunoglobulin light chains

KA
keratoacanthoma (re: Derma)
ketoacidosis

KA, K-A
King-Armstrong (units)

KA, Ka, ka.
kathodal (obsolete for cathodal)
kathode (obsolete for cathode)

K/A
ketogenic to antiketogenic (ratio)

K/A, K:A
ketogenic-antiketogenic (ratio)

K_a
acid ionization (dissociation) constant

KAAD mixture
kerosene, alcohol, acetic acid, dioxane mixture (re: killing insect larvae)

KAB
knowledge, attitude, behavior

KABC
Kaufman Assessment Battery for
Children

KAF
killer-assisting factor
kinase-activating factor

KAFO
knee-ankle-foot orthosis

$K_a = [H^+][A^-]/[HA]$
acid ionization constant ([ ] denote
concentration, HA = undissociated
acid, H^+ and A^- are its ions)

Kal
kalium (L. potassium; from Arabic—qali
[potash]— an element)

KAP
knowledge, aptitude, and practices (re:
fertility)

K/A ratio
ratio of ketogenic to antiketogenic
substances (re: diets)

KAS
Katz Adjustment Scales (re:
psychological testing)

KAST
Kindergarten Auditory Screening Test

kat
katal (unit of measurement for
catalyzing agents— enzyme unit)

KAU
King-Armstrong unit

KB
Kashin-Bek (disease)
ketone bodies
kilobytes (per second—re: computers)
knee brace

K/B
knee bearing (prosthesis—re: Ortho)

K_b
base ionization constant
dissociation constant of a base

Kb, kb
kilobase (re: nucleic-acid molecules)

kbp
kilobase pair (re: nucleic-acid
molecules)

kb pair
kilobase pair (re: nucleic-acid
molecules)

KBr
potassium bromide

KBS
Klüver-Bucy syndrome

KB splint
knuckle-bender splint

KC
kathodal (cathodal) closing
keratoconus (re: Ophth)
keratoma climacterium
kilo characters (per second—re:
computers)
knees to chest
knuckle cracking
Kupffer cell

kc, kc.
kilocycle

K Cal, Kcal, kcal, kcal.
kilocalorie (1000 calories)

K capture
radioactive decay by electron capture
(involving K-shell electron)

KCC
kathodal (cathodal) closing contraction

KCCT
kaolin-cephalin clotting time

K cell
killer cell

KCG
kinetocardiogram

kCi
kilocurie

KCl
potassium chloride

KCNS
potassium thiocyanate

K complex
slow waves related to sleep arousal (re:
EEG)

kcps, kc.p.s.
kilocycles per second

KCS
keratoconjunctivitis sicca

kc/s
kilocycles per second

KCT
kathodal (cathodal) closing tetanus

KCTe
kathodal (cathodal) closing tetanus

KD
kathodal (cathodal) duration

Kawasaki disease
killed

K_d
dissociation constant
distribution coefficient (re: solute)
partition coefficient (re: solute)

kd
kilodalton

KDA
known drug allergies

KDC
kathodal (cathodal) duration contraction

KDO
2-keto-3-deoxy-octonate

KDS
Kaufman Development Scale (re:
  psychological testing)

kd/sec
kilocycles per second

KDSM
keratinizing desquamative squamous
  metaplasia

KDT
kathodal (cathodal) duration tetanus

KD Te
kathodal (cathodal) duration tetanus

KE
Kendall's compound E (cortisone)
kinetic energy

K_e
exchangeable body potassium

KEC
Klebsiella, Enterobacter, Citrobacter

Kemo Tx
chemical therapy

Kera
keratitis

KERV
Kentucky equine respiratory virus

keto.
17-ketosteroid(s)

keV, kev.
kiloelectron volt(s)

KF
Kenner-fecal medium
Klippel-Feil (syndrome)

kf
symbol indicating flocculation speed in
  antigen- antibody reactions

KFAB
kidney-fixing antibody

K factor
gamma (γ) ray dose (roentgens/hr. at
  1 cm from 1 mCi
  point source of radiation)

KFAO
knee-foot-ankle orthosis

KFD
Kinetic Family Drawings (re:
  psychological testing)
Kyasanur Forest disease (of South
  India)

KFS
Klippel-Feil syndrome

KG-1
Koeffler Golde-1 (cell line)

kG
kilogauss

kg, kg.
kilogram (fundamental unit of mass in
  metric system)

KGC
Keflin, gentamicin, and carbenicillin

Kg-cal, kg cal, kg/cal, kg-cal
kilogram-calorie

KGHT
kidney Goldblatt hypertension

kg-m
kilogram-meter

kgps
kilogram per second

KGS
ketogenic steroid(s)

17-KGS
17-ketogenic steroids

KH
Krebs-Henseleit (cycle)

KHB
Krebs-Henseleit bicarbonate buffer

KHb
potassium hemoglobinate

KHC
kinetic hemolysis curve

KHD
kinky hair disease

KHF
Korean hemorrhagic fever

K hgb.
potassium hemoglobinate

KHN
Knoop hardness number (re: solids)

KHS
Krebs-Henseleit solution

KHZ, kHz
kilohertz

KI
karyopyknotic index (re: squamous cell
index)
Krönig's isthmus (Kroenig's)
potassium iodide

K_I
dissociation of enzyme-inhibitor
complex
inhibition constant

KIA
Kligler iron agar (medium)

KIC
ketoisocaproate (ketoisocaproic acid)

KICB
killed intracellular bacteria

KIDS
Kent Infant Development Scale

kilo
kilogram
kilometer
one thousand

KIMSA
Kirsten murine sarcoma (virus)

KIMSV, Ki-MSV
Kirsten murine sarcoma virus

KIP
key intermediary proteins

KIS
Krankenhaus Informations System

KISS
key integrative social system

KIT
Kahn Intelligence Tests

KIU
kallikrein inactivator units
kallikrein inhibiting unit (re: enzymes)

KJ, kj, k.j.
knee jerk (knee kick)

kJ
kilojoule (unit of energy, work, or heat)

KK, Kk
knee kick (knee jerk)

KL
kidney lobe
Kleine-Levin (syndrome)

Kl, kl, kl.
kiloliter

kl.
Klang (Ger. a compound musical
overtone; a ringing— re: acoustics)

KL bac., K.L. bac.
Klebs-Löffler bacillus (diphtheria
bacillus)

Kleb
Klebsiella (genus)

Klebs
Klebsiella (genus)

K level
lowest level (re: x rays)

KLH
keyhole limpet hemocyanin

KLS
kidneys, liver, spleen

KLST
Kindergarten Language Screening Test

KM
kanamycin
κ-immunoglobulin light chains
Kraepelin-Morel (disease)

Km, K_m
Michaelis-Menten dissociation constant

K_m
Michaelis constant (re: enzyme assays)

km, km.
kilometer

kMc
kilomegacycle

K-MCM
potassium-containing minimal
capacitation medium

kMcps, kMc.p.s.
kilomegacycles per second

KMEF
keratin, myosin, epidermin, fibrin (class
of proteins)

KMnO
potassium permanganate

KMnO₄
potassium permanganate

kmps
kilometers per second

km/s
kilometers per second

KMV
killed measles (virus) vaccine
killed measles virus (vaccine)

KN, Kn, kn.
knee

Kn
Knudsen number (re: low-pressure gas
   flow)

K nail
Küntscher nail (re: Ortho)

knork
KNife and fORK (re: physiatry)

KNRK
normal rat kidney cells transformed by
   Kirsten sarcoma virus

KO
killed organism
knee orthosis

KO, K/O
keep open
knocked out

KO, K/o
keep on (continue)

KOC
kathodal (cathodal) opening contraction

KOH
potassium hydroxide

KOIS
Kuder Occupational Interest Survey (re:
   psychological testing)

KOT
Knowledge of Occupations Test (re:
   psychological testing)

KP
Kaufmann-Peterson (base)
keratic precipitates (punctate keratitis;
   keratitis punctata—re: Ophth)
keratio punctata (Gr. kera—"horn"—
   keratotic patches)
keratitic precipitates (re: Ophth)
kidney protein
kidney punch
killed parenteral (vaccine)
Klebsiella pneumoniae

kPa
kilopascal (unit of pressure)

KPB
ketophenylbutazone (kebuzone—
   antirheumatic)
kalium (potassium) phosphate buffer

KPE
Kelman phacoemulsification (re: Ophth)

KPI
karyopyknotic index

KPR
key pulse rate
Kuder Preference Record

KPR-V
Kuder Preference Record—Vocational
   (re: psychological testing)

KPs
keratic precipitates (keratitic)

KPT
kidney punch test

KPTI
Kunitz pancreatic trypsin inhibitor

KPV
killed parenteral vaccine

KR
knowledge of results

Kr
krypton (element)

79Kr
radioactive isotope of krypton

85Kr
radioactive isotope of krypton

KRA
Klinefelter-Reifenstein-Albright
   (syndrome)

KRBB
Krebs-Ringer bicarbonate buffer

KRBG
Krebs-Ringer bicarbonate buffer
   (containing) glucose

KRBS
Krebs-Ringer bicarbonate solution

KRP
Kolmer (test) with Reiter protein
Krebs-Ringer phosphate

KRPS
Krebs-Ringer phosphate (buffer)
   solution

KRRS
kinetic resonance Raman spectroscopy

KS
Kaposi's sarcoma
Kartagener's syndrome
ketosteroid
Klinefelter's syndrome
Kugel-Stoloff (syndrome)
Kveim-Siltzbach (test)

17-KS
17-ketosteroids

KSA
knowledge, skills, and abilities

KSCN
potassium thiocyanate (broth)

KSK
Kathodenschließungs-Kontraktion
(kathodal [cathodal] closing
contraction)

KS/OI
Kaposi's sarcoma and opportunistic
infections

KSP
kidney-specific protein

K_{sp}
solubility product

KSR
keyboard send-receive (set—re:
computers)

KST
Kathodenschließungs-Tetanus
(kathodal [cathodal] closing tetanus)

K.S.U. Speech Discrimination Test
Kent State University Speech
Discrimination Test

KT
kidney transplant
Klippel-Trenaunay (syndrome)

KTS
kethoxal thiosemicarbazone

KTSA
Kahn Test of Symbol Arrangement

KUB
kidney and upper bladder

KUB, K.U.B.
kidneys, ureters, and bladder

KUS
kidney(s), ureter(s), and spleen

KV
kanamycin-vancomycin
killed vaccine

kV, kv.
kilovolt (unit of electrical potential)

kVA, kVa, kva
kilovolt-ampere

K value
proportion of relatives affected divided
by the birth frequency in the general
population of the same sex (re:
genetics)

KVBA
kanamycin-vancomycin blood agar

KVCP, kVcp, kvcp
kilovolt constant potential

KVE
Kaposi's varicelliform eruption

KVLBA
kanamycin-vancomycin laked blood
agar

KVO
keep vein open

KVO C D5W
keep vein open cum (L. with) dextrose
5% in water

KVP, kVP, kVp, kvp
kilovolt(s) peak (peak kilovoltage)

KW
Kimmelstiel-Wilson (syndrome)
Kugelberg-Welander (disease)

KW, K-W
Keith-Wagener (re: Ophth)

K_w
dissociation constant of water

kW
kilohm (unit of electrical resistance—
formerly k)

kW, kw.
kilowatt (unit of power)

KWB
Keith, Wagener, Barker (classification of
eyeground findings—re: Ophth)

kWh
kilowatt hour

kW-hr, kw hr, kw-hr
kilowatt-hour

KWIC
keyword in context (re: computers)

K wire, K-wire
Kirschner wire (re: Ortho)

KWOC
keyword out of context (re: computers)

KYB
Know Your Body

kyph.
kyphosis

KZ
Kaplan-Zuelzer (syndrome)

L

L
angular momentum
coefficent of induction
heat labile component of protein antigen of vaccinia and variola viruses
inductance (usually measured in henries)
Lactobacillus (genus)
lambert (unit of luminance)
Latin
left eye
Legionella (genus)
Leishmania (genus)
Leptospira (genus)
Leptotrichia (genus)
leucine
Leuconostoc (genus)
lewisite
liber (L. book)
licensed (to practice)
lidocaine
ligament
light (chain of protein molecules)
light sense
lilac (an indicator color)
limen (threshold)
lingual
liquor
Listeria (genus)
liver
lowest
lues (L. plague—syphilis)
lung
lymph
lymphocyte
lymphogranuloma
lysosome
roman numeral 50

L, l.
left
length
lethal (Erlich's symbol for fatal)
longitudinal (re: sections)
lumen

L, l
lesser
libra (L. pound; balance)
licensed
light
limes (boundary—used with subscript, lower-case letter, and/or plus sign as symbol for various doses of toxin)

liter (subsidiary unit of volume in metric system; in US—L sometimes used instead of l to distinguish from number 1, although SI system recommends using lower case "l")
living
low (when followed by another abbreviation; e.g. LBP— low blood pressure)
lower
lumbal
lumbar (re: vertebral formulae)

Ⓛ
left

(L)
left
lunch

L+
limes tod (Ehrlich's symbol for toxin-antitoxin mixture which contains one fatal dose in excess and which will kill the experimental animal—L. limes—boundary lines, threshold + to[xic] d[ose])

L₊
limes tod (L. boundary line, threshold + toxic dose)

L-
a compound structurally related to L-glyceraldehyde
levo- (in configurational sense only), the opposite of D-
a stereodescriptor (re: optically active organic compounds)

LI, LII, LIII
lues, first, second, third stage

L₁, L₂
lumbar nerves
lumbar vertebrae 1 through 5

L/3
lower third (re: long bone)

Λ
kX unit to ångström conversion factor

Λ, λ
lambda (eleventh letter of Greek alphabet)

λ
decay constant
microliter (now obsolete)
one of the two forms of immunoglobulin
    light chain
wavelength

l.
left (eye)
levo
line
long
radioactive constant

l-
levo- (prefix abbreviation for
    counterclockwise or levorotatory; [in
    configurational sense only] opposite
    of *d*—re: chemical formulae)

LA
lactic acid
language age
large amount
late antigen
latex agglutination
Latin American
left angle
left angulation
left arm
left atrial
left atrium
left auricle
leucine aminopeptidase
leukemia antigen
leukoagglutinating
levator ani
lichen amyloidosis
Lightwood-Albright (syndrome)
linguo-axial (re: Dent)
linoleic acid
lobuloalveolar
local anesthesia
long-acting (drug)
long arm (cast)
low anxiety
Ludwig's angina

L & A, L&A
living and active (re: family history)

L & A, L&A, L + A, l&a
light and accommodation

La
labial
lanthanum (element)

140La
radioactive isotope of lanthanum

l.a.
lege artis (L. according to the art)

LAA
left atrial appendage

left auricular appendage
leukemia-associated antigen
leukocyte ascorbic acid

LAAM
l-acetyl-α-methadol (α-*l* form of
    methadyl acetate; levomethadyl
    acetate—analgesic, narcotic)

LAAO
L-amino acid oxidase

LAB
Leisure Activities Blank (re: Psychol)

Lab, lab.
laboratory
a rennet ferment coagulating milk
    (chymosin—Ger. Lab)

lab. proc.
laboratory procedure

LABS
Laboratory Admission Baseline Studies

LABVT
left atrial ball-valve thrombus

LAC
La Crosse (arbovirus)
left atrial contraction
linguo-axiocervical (re: Dent)
long arm cast
low amplitude contraction

LaC
labiocervical (re: Dent)

lac.
laceration(s)
lactate
lactation

lac. & cont.
lacerations and contusions

lacr.
lacrimal

LACT
Lindamood Auditory Conceptualization
    Test (re: Psychol)

lact.
lactate
lactating

lact. (acid)
lactic acid

LAD
lactic acid dehydrogenase
language acquisition device
left anterior descending (coronary
    artery)
left axis deviation
linoleic acid depression

lipoamide dehydrogenase
lymphocyte-activating determinant

LADA
laboratory animal dander allergy
left acromiodorso-anterior (position of
    fetus)

LADCA
left anterior descending coronary artery

LADD
left anterior descending diagonal
    (branch of coronary artery)

LADH
lactic acid dehydrogenase
liver alcohol dehydrogenase

LADME
liberation, absorption, distribution,
    metabolism, excretion

LADP
left acromiodorsoposterior (position of
    fetus)

LADu
lobuloalveolar-ductal

LAE
left atrial enlargement
long above elbow (cast)

LAEI
left atrial emptying index

laev.
laevus (L. left)

LAF
laminar air flow
Latin American female
leukocyte-activating factor
lymphocyte-activating factor
lymphocyte-activation factor

LAFB
left anterior fascicular block

LAFR
laminar air flow room

LAFU
laminar air flow unit

LAG
linguo-axiogingival (re: Dent)
lymphangiogram
lymphangiography

LAG, LaG
labiogingival (re: Dent)

lag.
lagena (L. a flask, bottle)

LAH
lactalbumin hydrolysate

left anterior hemiblock
left atrial hypertrophy
lithium-aluminum hydride (aluminum
    lithium hydride— a reducing agent)

LAHB
left anterior hemiblock

LAHV
leukocyte-associated herpes virus

LAI
latex (particle) agglutination inhibition
leukocyte adherence inhibition (assay)

LAI, LaI
labioincisal (re: Dent)

LAIF
leukocyte adherence inhibition factor

LAIT
latex agglutination inhibition test

LAK
lymphokine-activated killer (cells)

LAL
limulus amebocyte lysate
low air loss

LaL
labiolingual (re: Dent)

L-Ala
L-alanine

LALI
lymphocyte antibody lymphocytolytic
    interaction

LAM
late ambulatory monitoring
Latin American male
left anterior measurement
left atrial myxoma
lymphangioleiomyomatosis

LAM, Lam, lam.
laminectomy

Lam
laminogram

lam. & fus.
laminectomy and fusion

LA-MAX
maximal left atrial (dimension)

lami.
laminotomy

LAMMA
laser microprobe mass analyzer

LAN
long-acting neuroleptic

LANC
long arm navicular cast

LANV
left atrial neovascularization

LAO
left anterior oblique
left atrial overloading

LAP
left arterial pressure
left atrial pressure
leucine aminopeptidase
leukocyte alkaline phosphatase
low atmospheric pressure
lyophilized anterior pituitary (tissue)

LAP, Lap, lap.
laparotomy

lap.
laparoscopy

LAPA
leukocyte alkaline phosphatase activity

lapid.
lapideum (L. stony)

LAPOCA
L-asparaginase, prednisone, Oncovin
    (vincristine), cytarabine, and
    Adriamycin (doxorubicin) (re:
    chemotherapy)

LAP stain
leukocyte alkaline phosphatase stain

LAPW
left atrial posterior wall

LAR
late asthmatic response

LAR, lar.
laryngology

LAR, l.a.r.
left arm, reclining
left arm, recumbent

lar.
larynx

LARC
leukocyte automatic recognition
    computer

LARS
Language-Structured Auditory
    Retention Span (Test—re:
    psychological testing)
leucyl-tRNA synthetase (gene-marker
    symbol—re: genetics)

laryn.
laryngeal

laryngitis
laryngoscopy

Laryng
laryngology

Laryngol
laryngologist
laryngology

LAS
laxative abuse syndrome
left anterior-superior
left arm sitting (re: blood pressure)
linear alkyl sulfonate (a more
    biodegradable detergent—replacing
    alkylbenzene sulfonates)
local adaptation syndrome
long arm splint
lower abdominal surgery

LASER, laser
light amplification by stimulated
    emission of radiation

LASFB
left anterior-superior fascicular block

LASH
left anterior-superior hemiblock (re:
    Cardio)

L-ASP
L-asparaginase

LASS
labile aggregation-stimulating
    substance
Linguistic Analysis of Speech Samples

LAT
latent
latex agglutination test
left anterior thigh

lat.
lateral
latitude

LAT-A
latrunculin A

lat. admov.
lateri admoveatum (L. let it be applied to
    the side)

LAT-B
latrunculin B

lat. bar
latissimus (dorsi) bar (re: Ortho)

lat. bend.
lateral bending

lat. dol.
lateri dolenti (L. to the painful side)

lat. & loc.
lateralizing and localizing

lat. men.
lateral meniscectomy

LATP
left atrial transmural pressure

lat. Rin.
lactated Ringer's

lat. rot.
lateral rotation

LATS
long-acting thyroid stimulator
long-acting transmural stimulator

LATSP, LATS-P
long-acting thyroid stimulator-protector

LATu
lobuloalveolar tumor

LAV
lymphadenopathy-associated virus

LAW
left atrial wall

Lax, lax.
laxative

lax.
laxity

LB
laboratory data
lamellar body
large bowel
lateral bending
Lederer-Brill (syndrome)
left bundle
left buttock
leiomyoblastoma
lipid body
live birth(s)
liver biopsy
Living Bank
loose body
low back
low breakage
lung biopsy

L-B
Liebermann-Burchard (test—re:
   cholesterol)

L&B
left and below

L + B
left and below

lb, lb.
libra (L. pound; balance)

LBA
left basal artery

lb ap.
libra apothecary (L. apothecary pound)

lb av.
libra avoirdupois (L. avoirdupois pound)

LBB
left bundle branch
low back bend
low back bending

LBBB
left bundle branch block

LBBSB, LBBsB
left bundle branch system block

LBBX, LBBx
left breast biopsy examination

LBC
lidocaine blood concentration

LBCD
left border (of) cardiac dullness

LBCF
Laboratory Branch Complement
   Fixation (test)

LBD
large bile duct
left border dullness (of heart to
   percussion)

LBDQ
Leader Behavior Description
   Questionnaire

LBE
long below elbow (cast)

LBF
Lactobacillus bulgaricus factor
   (pantetheine)
limb blood flow
liver blood flow

lb-ft
pound-feet
pound-foot

LBH
length, breadth, height

LBI
low serum-bound iron

LBL
labeled lymphoblast
lymphoblastic lymphoma

LBM
lean body mass
loose bowel movements

LBNP
lower-body negative pressure

LBP
low back pain
low blood pressure

LBRF
louse-borne relapsing fever

LBS
lactobacillus selector (agar)

lbs
librae (L. pounds)

LBSA
lipid-bound sialic acid

LBT
low back tenderness
low back trouble
lupus band test

lb t.
libra troy (L. pound[s] troy)

LBTI
lima bean trypsin inhibitor

LBV
lung blood volume

LBW
lean body weight
low birth weight

LBWI
low-birth-weight infant

LBWR
lung-body weight ratio

LC
Laennec's cirrhosis
lamina cortex
Langerhans' cells
large chromophobe
large cleaved (cell)
late clamped (umbilical cord)
Launois-Cléret (syndrome)
left circumflex
lethal concentration
life care
light chain
light coagulation
linguocervical (re: Dent)
lining cell
lipid cytosomes
liquid chromatography
liquid crystal
lithocolic acid
liver cirrhosis
liver clinic
living children
locus ceruleus
long-chain (triglycerides)

longus capitus
low calorie
lung cancer
lung cell
lymph capillary
lymphocyte count
lymphocytotoxin
lymphoma culture

l.c.
loco citato (L. in the place cited)

λ_c
Compton wavelength of electron

LCA
left circumflex artery
left coronary artery
lymphocyte chemoattractant activity
lymphocytotoxic antibody

LCAO
linear combination of atomic orbitals

LCAO-MO
linear combination of atomic orbital-
molecular orbital

LCAR
late cutaneous anaphylactic reaction

LCAT
lecithin-cholesterol acetyl-transferase
lecithin cholesterol acyl transferase
lecithin cholesterol acyl-transferase
lecithin cholesterol acyltransferase
lecithin-cholesterol acyltransferase
lecithin-cholesterol-acyl tranferase
lecithin-cholesterol-acyltransferase
lecithin-cholesterol-acyltransferase
(deficiency)
lecithin:cholesterol acyltransferase
(ratio)

LCB
left costal border

↑ LCB
elevated left costal border
upper left costal border

↓ LCB
lower left costal border

LCBF
local cerebral blood flow

LCC
lactose coliform count
left common carotid
left coronary cusp
liver cell carcinoma

LCCA
late cortical cerebellar atrophy
left common carotid artery

LCCP
limited channel-capacity processes

LCCS
low cervical cesarean section

LCD
liquid crystal display
liquor carbonis detergens (coal tar
    solution)

LCDD
light chain deposition disease

LCED
liquid chromatography with
    electrochemical detection

LCF
least common factor
left circumflex (coronary artery)
linear correction factor
low-frequency current field
lymphocyte culture fluid

LCFA
long-chain fatty acid

LCFAO
long-chain fatty acid oxidation

LCFC
linear combination of fragment
    configuration

LCFU
leukocyte colony-forming units

LCG
Langerhans' cell granule

LCGU
local cerebral glucose utilization

LCH
lentil agglutinin binding (gene marker
    symbol—re: genetics)

L chain
light chain (polypeptides with low
    molecular weight)

L-chain disease
light chain (polypeptides with low
    molecular weight— re: Bence Jones
    myeloma)

LCI
length complexity index

LCIS
lobular carcinoma in situ

LCL
Levinthal-Coles-Lillie (cytoplasmic
    inclusion bodies)
lower confidence limit
lymphoblastoid cell line

lymphocytic choriomeningitis (virus)
lymphocytic leukemia
lymphocytic lymphosarcoma
lymphoid cell line

LCM
latent cardiomyopathy
left costal margin
leukocyte-conditioned medium
lowest common multiple
lymphatic choriomeningitis
lymphocyte choriomeningitis
lymphocytic choriomeningitis

LCMG
long-chain monoglyceride

LCMV
lymphocytic choriomeningitis virus

LCN
lateral cervical nucleus
left caudate nucleus

LCP
Legg-Calvé-Perthes (disease)
long chain polysaturated (fatty acids)

λ_{cp}
Compton wavelength of proton

LCPD
Legg-Calvé-Perthes disease

LCQG
left caudal quarter ganglion

LCR
leurocristine (vincristine—
    antineoplastic)

LCS
large (capacity) core storage (re:
    computers)
left coronary sinus
liquor cerebrospinalis

LCT
liver cell tumor
long-chain triglyceride
lung capillary time
lymphocytotoxicity test
lymphocytotoxin

LCU
life change unit

LCX, LCx
left circumflex (coronary artery)

LD
labyrinthine defect
lactate dehydrogenase
lactic (acid) dehydrogenase
L-dopa
learning disability
learning disabled
learning disorder

left deltoid
Legionnaires' disease
Leishmania donovani
lethal dose
light-dark
light difference (perception of low
  density)
limited disease
linear dichroism
linguodistal (re: Dent)
lipodystrophy
lithium discontinuation (re: psychiatry)
liver disease
living donor
loading dose
long day (re: plant growth)
longitudinal diameter (of heart)
long (time) dialysis
low density
low dosage
low dose
lung destruction
lymphocyte defined
lymphocyte depletion
lymphocytically determined

LD, L-D
Leishman-Donovan (bodies)

LD, Ld
laboratory data

L/D
light-dark (ratio)

L & D
light and distance (re: Ophth)

L & D, L + D
labor and delivery

LD$_\infty$
lethal dose

LD$_{50}$, LD50
median lethal dose (lethal for 50% of
  test subjects)

LD$_{100}$
completely lethal dose

LDA
laser Doppler anemometry
left dorso-anterior (position of fetus)
linear displacement analysis
lithiodiisopropylamine (re: organic
  synthesis)
lymphocyte-dependent antibody

LDAR
latex direct agglutination reaction

LDB
lamb dysentery bacillus
Legionnaires' disease bacillus

LD (bacillus)
lamb dysentery bacillus (type B toxins
  of *Clostridium perfringens*)

L-D bodies
Leishman-Donovan bodies

LDCT
late distal cortical tubule

LDD
late dedifferentiation
light-dark discrimination

LDDS
local dentist

LDE
lauric diethamide

LDF
limit dilution factor

LDG
lactic dehydrogenase
long-distance group
low-dose group

LDH
lactate dehydrogenase (lactic [acid]
  dehydrogenase)
low-dose heparin

LDHA
lactate dehydrogenase A

LDHB
lactate dehydrogenase B

LDIH
left direct inguinal hernia

LDL
loudness discomfort level
low-density lipoproteins
low-density lymphocyte

LDLC
low density lipoprotein-cholesterol

LDLP
low-density lipoprotein(s)

L-dopa
L-dihydroxyphenylalanine
levodopa (antiparkinsonism,
  anticholinergic)

L doses
limes doses (re: toxin/antitoxin
  combining power)

L+ dose, L₊ dose
alternative for L†, the limes tod dose of
  diphtheria toxin (i.e., smallest dose of
  toxin mixed with 1 unit of antitoxin
  which will kill experimental animal
  within 96 hours)

LDP
left dorsoposterior (position of fetus)
lumbodorsal pain

L. Drom.
Levo-Dromoran (narcotic, analgesic)

LDS
ligating, dividing stapler

LDT
left dorsotransverse (position of fetus)

LDU
long double upright

LDUB
long double upright brace

LDV
lactic dehydrogenase virus
large dense-cored vesicle
laser Doppler velocimetry
lateral distant view (re: Radio)

LE
left ear
left eye
leukocyte elastase
leukoerythrogenetic
live embryo
lupus erythematosus

LE, L/E
lower extremity

Le
Leonard (unit for cathode ray)
Lewis number (diffusivity:diffusion
    coefficient of a fluid)

LEA
language experience approach
lower extremity amputation

Le^a
regarding Lewis blood group

LEADS
Leadership Evaluation and
    Development Scale (re: Psychol)

LEB
lupus erythematosus body

Le^b
regarding Lewis blood group

LEC
leukoencephalitis

LE cell
lupus erythematosus cell

LECP
low-energy charged particle

Lect
lecturer

lect.
lecture

LED
light-emitting diode
lowest effective dose
lupus erythematosus disseminatus

LEED
low-energy electron diffraction

LEEDS
low-energy electron diffraction
    spectroscopy

LEEP
left end-expiratory pressure

LEER
lower extremity equipment related

LEF
leukokinesis-enhancing factor
lupus erythematosus factor

leg.
legal
legally
legislation
legislative

leg. com.
legal commitment
legally committed

LeIF
leukocyte interferon (antineoplastic;
    antiviral)

LEIS
low-energy ion scattering

LEJ
ligation of the esophagogastric junction

LEL
lowest effect level (of toxicity)

LEM
lateral eye movements
leukocyte endogenous mediator
light electron microscope

LEMO
lowest empty molecular orbital

lenit.
leniter (L. gently)

LEOPARD syndrome
lentigines, electrocardiographic
    (conduction abnormalities), ocular
    (hypertelorism), pulmonary
    (stenosis), abnormal (genitalia),
    retardation (of growth), and
    (sensorineural) defects

LEP
lethal effective phase
lipoprotein electrophoresis
low egg passage (strain of virus)
lower esophageal (segment, sphincter, stricture)

LE prep.
lupus erythematosus preparation

Lept
Leptospira (genus)

LER
lysosomal enzyme release

LERG
local electroretinogram

LES
Life Experience Survey
Locke egg serum (medium)
lower esophageal segment
lower esophageal sphincter
lower esophageal stricture
lupus erythematosus, systemic

LES, l.e.s.
local excitatory state

les.
lesion

LESA
liposomally entrapped second antibody

LESP
lower esophageal sphincter pressure

LET
language enrichment therapy
lineal energy transfer
linear energy transfer
low energy transfer

LETD
lowest effective toxic dose

LETS
large, external transformation-sensitive (fibronectin)

LEU
leukocyte equivalent unit

LEU, Leu, leu.
leucine

Leu, leu.
leucine radical

leuko.
leukocytes

lev.
levis (L. light)
levorotatory

levit.
leviter (L. lightly)

LEW
Lewis (rat)

LEX
lactate extraction

L ext., l/ext
lower extremity

LF
labile factor
laryngofissure
latex fixation
lavage fluid
leaflet
left foot
leucine flux
low fat (diet)
low forceps

LF, Lf
limit (of) flocculation

LF, lf
low frequency

Lf, L$_f$
limes flocculation units (dose—of toxin per ml)

LFA
left femoral artery
left forearm
left frontoanterior (position of fetus)
leukotactic factor activity

LFB
lingual-facial-buccal
liver, iron, and B complex

LFC
left frontal craniotomy
low fat and cholesterol

LFD
lactose-free diet
large for date
least fatal dose
low fat diet
low fiber diet
low forceps delivery

LFECT, L-FECT
loose fibroelastic connective tissue

LFER
linear free-energy relationship

L-F f.
Laki-Lorand factor (Factor XIII; fibrin-stabilizing factor)

LFH
left femoral hernia

LFL
left frontolateral

LFN
lactoferrin

LFP
left frontoposterior (position of fetus)

LFR
lymphoid follicular reticulosis

L fraction
labile fraction (membrane potential)

LF-RF
local regional failure

LFS
limbic forebrain structure
liver function series

LFT
latex fixation test
latex flocculation test
left frontotransverse (position of fetus)
liver function tests
low frequency tetanic (stimulation)
low frequency transduction
low frequency transfer

LFTSW
left foot switch

LFU
lipid fluidity unit

LFV
Lassa-fever virus
low frequency ventilation

L fx
linear fracture

LG
lactoglobulin
lamellar granule
laryngectomy
left gluteal
left gluteus
linguogingival (re: Dent)
lipoglycopeptide
liver graft
low glucose
lymph glands

Lg, lg.
large
leg

Lg
prefix (re: asymmetric atoms)

lg.
long

LGA
large for gestational age (re: OB)
left gastric artery

LGB
Landry-Guillain-Barré (syndrome)
lateral geniculate body

LGC
left giant cell

LGD
Leaderless Group Discussion (re:
    Psychol; situational test)

LGd
dorsal lateral geniculate (nucleus)

lge.
large

LGF
lateral giant fiber

LGH
lactogenic hormone
little growth hormone

LGI
large glucagon immunoreactivity

LGL
large granular leukocytes
large granular lymphocyte
Lown-Ganong-Levine (syndrome)

LGMD
limb-girdle muscular dystrophy

LGN
lateral geniculate nucleus (re: Neuro)
lobular glomerulonephritis

LGT
late generalized tuberculosis

Lgt
ligamentum

lgt.
ligament

lgts.
ligaments

LGV
large granular vesicle
lymphogranuloma venereum

LH
late healed
lateral hypothalamus
left hand
left hemisphere
left hyperphoria
liver homogenate
lower half
lues hereditaria (hereditary syphilis)

lung homogenate
luteinizing hormone
luteotrop(h)ic hormone

LHA
lateral hypothalamic area
left hepatic artery

LHb
lateral habenular

LHBV
left heart blood volume

LHC
left heart catheterization
left hypochondrium

LHCG
luteinizing hormone-chorionic
  gonadotrop(h)in (hormone)

LHF
left heart failure
ligament of the head of the femur

LHFA
lung Hageman factor activator

LH/FSH-RF
luteinizing hormone/follicle-stimulating
  hormone- releasing factor

LHG
left hand grip
localized hemolysis in gel

LHI
lipid hydrocarbon inclusions

LHL
left hepatic lobe

LHM
lisuride hydrogen maleate

LHN
lateral hypothalamic nucleus (re: Neuro)

LHPZ
lower (esophageal) high-pressure zone

LHR
leukocyte histamine release (test)
liquid holding recovery

l hr, l-hr
lumen hour (a unit quantity of light)

LHRF
luteotrop(h)in hormone-releasing factor

LHRF, LH-RF
luteinizing hormone-releasing factor

LHRH, LH-RH
luteinizing hormone-releasing hormone

LHS
left hand side
left heart strain
lymphatic and hematopoietic system

LHT
left hypertropia

L-5HTP
5-hydroxy-L and D-tryptophan
  (antidepressant; anti-epileptic)

LI
labeling index (re: cell cycle)
lactose intolerance
lamellar ichthyosis
large intestine
learning impaired
left injured
left involved
Leptospirosis icterohaemorrhagiae
  (now *L. interrogans*)
life island
linguoincisal (re: Dent)
lithogenic index
low impulsiveness

L & I
liver and iron

Li
lithium (element)

li.
links

LIA
leukemia-associated inhibitory activity
leukemia cell-derived inhibitory activity
lock-in amplifier
lymphocyte-induced angiogenesis
  (factor)
lysine-iron agar

LIAC
light-induced absorbance change

LIAF
lymphocyte-induced angiogenesis
  factor

LIAFI
late infantile amaurotic familial idiocy

lib.
libra (L. balance; "pound" [about 12 troy
  ounces])

LIBC
latent iron-binding capacity

LiBr
lithium bromide

LIC
left internal carotid
limiting isorrheic concentration

LICA
left internal carotid artery

LICC
lectin-induced cellular cytotoxicity

LICD
lower intestinal Crohn's disease

LICM
left intercostal margin

Li₂CO₃
lithium carbonate

LICS
left intercostal space

LID
late immunoglobulin deficiency
late-onset immunoglobulin deficiency
lymphocytic infiltrative disease

LIDC
low intensity direct current

LIDO
lidocaine

LIF
laser-induced fluorescence
left iliac fossa
left index finger
leukocyte infiltration factor
leukocyte inhibitory factor
leukocytosis-inducing factor

LIFE
Longitudinal Interval Follow-up
   Evaluation

LIFO
last in, first out (re: computer data)

LIFT
lymphocyte immunofluorescence test

Lig, lig.
ligament
ligamentum

lig.
ligate
ligature

ligg.
ligamenta
ligaments
ligature

ligs.
ligaments

LIH
left inguinal hernia

LIHA
low impulsiveness, high anxiety

LII
Leisure Interest Inventory (re: Psychol)

LILA
low impulsiveness, low anxiety

LIM
limes (L. boundary)

lim.
limit
limitation

LIMA
left internal mammary artery

lin.
linear
linimentum (L. a liniment)

LINAC
linear accelerator

ling.
lingual
lingular

linim.
liniment

Linn
Linnaeus, Linnaean, Linnean (re:
   taxonomic classification and
   nomenclature originated by Carolus
   Linnaeus)

LIO
left inferior oblique (muscle)

Li₂O
lithium oxide

LiOH
lithium hydroxide

LIP
lithium-induced polydipsia

LIP, L.I.P
lymphocytic interstitial pneumonia

Lip
lipoate (lipoic acid)

LIPA
lysosomal acid lipase A

LIPB
lysosomal acid lipase B

LIPHE
Life Interpersonal History Enquiry (re:
   Psychol)

LIPS
Leiter International Performance Scale

LIQ
lower inner quadrant

LIQ, Liq, liq.
liquid
liquor

liq.
liquor (L. a liquor; a solution)

LIR
left iliac region
left inferior rectus

LIRBM
liver, iron, red bone marrow

LIS
lateral intercellular space
left intercostal space
lobular in situ (carcinoma)
low ionic strength

LISP
List Processing Language (re:
    computers)

LISS
low ionic-strength solution (a medium
    test)

lit.
literal
literally

LIV
law of initial value (Joseph Wilder)
left innominate vein
liver (battery test—re: Dent)
living

LIV-BP
leucine, isoleucine, valine-binding
    protein

LIVC
left inferior vena cava

LIVIM
lethal intestinal virus of infant mice

LJ
Larsen-Johansson (syndrome)

LJM
Löwenstein-Jensen medium

LK
Landry-Kussmaul (syndrome)
left kidney
lichenoid keratosis
Löhr-Kindberg (syndrome)

LK+
low potassium ion

LKM
liver-kidney microsomal

LKP
lamellar keratoplasty

LKS
liver, kidneys, spleen

LKSB
liver, kidneys, spleen, bladder

LKS non. pal.
liver, kidneys, spleen not palpable

liver, kidneys, and spleen negative

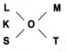

liver, kidneys, and spleen negative, no
    masses or tenderness

LKV
laked kanamycin vancomycin (agar)

LL
large local
large lymphocytes
lateral lemniscus (re: Neuro)
left lateral
left leg
left lower
left lung
lepromatous leprosy
Lewandowski-Lutz (syndrome)
lines
lingual lipase
lipoprotein lipase
long leg
loudness level
lower lid
lower lobe
lung length
lymphocytic lymphoma
lymphoid leukemia
lysolecithin

LL, l.l.
lid lag

LLA
limulus lysate assay

L lam.
lumbar laminectomy

LLB
left lateral bending
left lateral border
long leg brace
lower lobe bronchus

LLBCD
left lower border of cardiac dullness

LLBP
long leg brace with pelvic (band)

l.l. brace
long leg brace

LLC
Lewis lung carcinoma
long leg cast
lymphocytic leukemia, chronic

LL cast
long leg cast

LLCC
long leg cylinder cast

LLD
left lateral decubitus
leg length discrepancy
liquid liquid distribution
long-lasting depolarization
long leg discrepancy

LLD factor
Lactobacillus lactis Dorner factor
(vitamin B_{12})

LL discrep.
leg length discrepancy

LLE
left lower extremity

LLF
Laki-Lorand factor (fibrinase, fibrin-
stabilizing factor—Factor XIII)
left lateral femoral (site of injection)
left lateral flexion

LLL
left liver lobe
left lower leg
left lower (eye)lid
left lower lobe
left lower lung

LLL, L.L.L.
left lower lobe (of lung)

L LL brace
left long leg brace

LLLE
left lower lid, eye
lower lid left eye (lower lid, left eye)

LLLNR
left lower lobe, no rales

LLM
localized leukocyte mobilization

LLO
legionella-like organism(s)

LLOD
lower lid, oculus dexter (right eye)

LLOS
lower lid, oculus sinister (left eye)

LLP
late luteal phase
long-lasting potentiation

LLQ
left lower quadrant

LLR
large local reaction
left lateral rectus (re: Ophth)
left lumbar region

LLRE
lower lid, right eye

LLS
lateral loop suspensor
long leg splint

LLSB
left lower scapular border
left lower sternal border

LLT
left lateral thigh
lysolecithin

LLV
lymphatic leukemia virus
lymphoid leukosis virus

LLV-F
Friend virus-associated lymphatic
leukemia virus

LLW
low-level waste

LLWC
long leg walking cast

LLX
left lower extremity

LM
lactose malabsorption
laryngeal muscle
lateral malleolus
left main
left median
legal medicine
lemniscus medialis
light microscope
light microscopy
light minimum
lincomycin
linguomesial (re: Dent)
lipid mobilizing (hormone)
liquid membrane
Listeria monocytogenes
longitudinal muscle
Looser-Milkman (syndrome)
lower motor (neuron)

5 L/M
five liters per minute

lm
lumen (SI unit of luminous energy flow
    in terms of its visual effect)

LMA
left mentoanterior (position of fetus)
limbic midbrain area
liver membrane antibody
liver membrane autoantibody

LMB
Lawrence-Moon-Biedl (syndrome)
leiomyoblastoma

LMBBS
Lawrence-Moon-Bardet-Biedl syndrome
    (Lawrence-Moon- Biedl-Bardet)

LMC
large motile cells
lateral motor column
left main coronary
left middle cerebral (artery)
lymphocyte-mediated cytolysis
lymphocyte-mediated cytotoxicity
lymphomyeloid complex

LMCA
left main coronary artery
left middle cerebral artery

LMCAD
left main coronary artery disease

LMCAT
left middle cerebral artery thrombosis

LMCL
left midclavicular line

LMCT
ligand-to-metal charge transfer

LMD
left main disease (re: Cardio)
lipid-moiety modified derivative
local medical doctor
low molecular (weight) dextran

LMDF
lupus miliaris disseminatus faciei

LMDX
low molecular (weight) dextran

LME
left mediolateral episiotomy
leukocyte migration enhancement

L-meromyosin
light (molecular weight) meromyosin
    (re: muscle [myosin] activity)

LMF
left middle finger

Leukeran (chlorambucil), methotrexate,
    and 5-fluorouracil (re: chemotherapy)
leukocyte mitogenic factor
lymphocyte mitogenic factor

LMFBR
liquid metal fast-breeder reactor

LMG
lethal midline granuloma
low mobility group

LMH
lipid mobilizing hormone

LM hormone
lipid mobilizing hormone

LMI
leukocyte migration inhibition (assay)

LMIF
leukocyte migration inhibition factor

L/min.
liters per minute

L/min/m²
liters per minute per square meter

LMIR
leukocyte migration inhibition reaction

LMIT
leukocyte migration inhibition test

LML
large and medium lymphocytes
left mediolateral (episiotomy)
left middle lobe
lower midline

LML scar s̄ h
lower midline scar without hernia

LML scar w/h
lower midline scar with hernia

LMM
lactobacillus maintenance medium
lentigo maligna melanoma
light molecular (weight) meromyosin
    (re: muscle [myosin] activity)

LMN
lower motor neuron

LMNL
lower motor neuron lesion

LMO
localized molecular orbital

LMP
lumbar puncture

LMP, L.M.P.
last menstrual period
left mentoposterior (position of fetus)

LMR
left medial rectus (re: Ophth)
linguomandibular reflex
log magnitude ratio

LMS
leiomyosarcoma

LMSV
left maximal spatial voltage

LMT
left mentotransverse (position of fetus)
leukocyte migration technique
luteomammotrophic hormone

LMTA
Language Modalities Test for Aphasia

lmtd.
limited

L-3-MTO
L-3-methoxy-4-hydroxyphenylalanine

LMW
low molecular weight

LMWD
low molecular weight dextran

LN
later (onset) nephrotic (syndrome)
Lesch-Nyhan (syndrome)
lipoid nephrosis
lupus nephritis
lymph node

L/N
letter-numerical (system)

ln
logarithm, natural

LNAA
large neutral amino acid

LNC
lymph node cells

LNG
liquified natural gas

LNH
large number hypothesis

LNI
log(arithm) neutralization index

LNL
lower normal limit

LNMP
last normal menstrual period

LNNB
Luria-Nebraska Neuropsychological
Battery

LNP
large neuronal polypeptide

LNPF
lymph node permeability factor

LNS
lateral nuclear stratum
Lesch-Nyhan syndrome
lymph node seeking (equivalent)

LO
linguo-occlusal (re: Dent)
love object
low

L_0
limes nul (Ehrlich's symbol for a
    neutralized mixture of a toxin-antitoxin
    and thus will not kill an animal)

LOA
leave of absence
Leber optic atrophy
left occipito-anterior (position of fetus)

LOC
laxative of choice
level of consciousness
liquid organic compound
Locus of Control (re: Psychol)
loss of consciousness

loc.
local
localized
location

LoCa
low calcium

lo. cal.
low calorie (diet)

lo. calc.
low calcium (diet)

LOC-C
Locus of Control-Chance (re: Psychol)

loc. cit.
loco citato (L. in the place cited)

Lo CHO
low carbohydrates

lo. chol.
low cholesterol

loc. dol.
loco dolenti (L. to the painful spot)

LOC-E
Locus of Control-External (re: Psychol)

LOC-I
Locus of Control-Internal (re: Psychol)

LOC-PO
Locus of Control-Powerful Others (re: Psychol)

LOD
line of duty

lo. fat
low fat

log
base 10 logarithm (Briggsian logarithms)
logarithm

log₁₀
logarithm to the base 10 (Briggsian logarithms)

logₑ
logarithm to the base e

LOH
loop of Henle

LOI
level of incompetence
Leyton Obsessive Inventory

LOI, l.o.i.
limit of impurities

LOIH
left oblique inguinal hernia

LoK
low kalium (potassium)

LOL
left occipitolateral (position of fetus)

LOM
left otitis media
limitation of motion
limitation of movement
loss of motion
loss of movement

LOMPT
Lincoln-Oseretsky Motor Performance Test

LOMSA
left otitis media, suppurative, acute

LOMSC
left otitis media, suppurative, chronic

LOMSCh
left otitis media, suppurative, chronic

LoNa
low sodium

long.
longitude
longitudinal
longus (L. long)

LOP
leave on pass
left occiput posterior (position of fetus)

LOPS
length of patient stay

LOQ
Leadership Opinion Questionnaire (re: Psychol)
lower outer quadrant

LOR
lorazepam

lord.
lordosis
lordotic

LOS
length of stay
loss of site
low output syndrome

lo. salt
low salt

LOT
lateral olfactory tract
left occiput transverse (position of fetus)
lengthened off time

lot.
lotio (L. a lotion)

LOV
large opaque vesicle

LOWBI
low birth weight infant

lox
liquid oxygen

LP
labile peptide
labile protein
laboratory procedure(s)
lactoperoxidase
lamina propria
laryngeal-pharyngeal
latency period
latent period
lateral plantar
lateral pylorus
(nucleus) lateralis posterior (re: thalamus)
latex particle
leading pole
Legionella pneumophila
leukocyte-poor
levator palati
lichen planus
ligamentum patella
light perception
lightly padded
linear programming (re: computers)

linguopulpal (re: Dent)
lipoprotein
lost privileges
low potency
low power (microscopy)
low pressure
low protein
lumbar puncture
lumboperitoneal
lung parenchyma
lymphocyte predominant
lymphoid plasma
lymphoid predominance

L/P
lactate/pyruvate (ratio)
liver to plasma (concentration ratio)
lymphocyte/polymorph (ratio)
lymph-plasma (ratio)

LPA
larval photoreceptor axon
latex particle agglutination
left pulmonary artery

LPAM, L-PAM
L-phenylalanine mustard (melphalan—
    antineoplastic)

LPB
lipoprotein B
low profile bioprosthesis

LPBP
low profile bioprosthesis

LPC
late positive component
lysophosphatidyl choline (deacylated
    derivative of plasmalogens)

LPc̄P
light perception with projection (re:
    Ophth)

LPCT
late proximal cortical tubule

LPD
luteal phase defect

LPE
lipoprotein electrophoresis

LPerc
light perception

LPF
leukocyte-promoting factor
leukopenia factor
lipopolysaccharide factor
localized plaque formation
lymphocyte-promoting factor

LPF, L.P.F.
leukocytosis-promoting factor

LPF, l.p.f.
low-power field (microscopy)

LPFB
left posterior fascicular block

LPFN
low pass filtered noise

LPFS
low pass filtered signal

LPG
liquified petroleum gas

LPH
left posterior hemiblock
lipotrop(h)ic hormone
lipotrop(h)ic pituitary hormone
lipotrop(h)in

LPHB
left posterior hemiblock

LPI
left posterior-inferior
long process of incus (re: Oto)

LPIFB
left posterior-inferior fascicular block

LPIH
left posterior-inferior hemiblock

LPK
liver pyruvate kinase

LPL
lamina propria lymphocytes
lichen planus-like lesion
lipoprotein lipase

LPLA
lipoprotein lipase activity

LPM
lateral pterygoid muscle
left posterior measurement
lines per minute (re: computers)
liver plasma membrane
localized pretibial myxedema

LPM, lpm
liters per minute

LPO
left posterior oblique
light perception only
lobus parolfactorius

LPOA
lateral preoptic area

LpOH
lysopine dehydrogenase

LPP
lateral pterygoid plate

LP & P, LP + P
light perception and projection

LPPH
late postpartum hemorrhage

LPR
lactate-pyruvate ratio
late phase response

L/P ratio
lactate-pyruvate ratio

LProj, L Proj
light projection

LPS
levator palpebrae superioris (muscle)
linear profile scan
lipase
lipopolysaccharide (complex
    [endotoxin])
London Psychogeriatric Scale

LP$\overline{s}$
light perception without (projection—re:
    Ophth)

lps
liters per second

LPSR
lipopolysaccharide receptor

LPT
lipotrop(h)in

LPV
left portal view
left pulmonary veins
lymphopathia venereum

LPW
lateral pharyngeal wall

lpw
lumens per watt

LP-X
lipoprotein-X

LQ
longevity quotient
lordosis quotient
lower quadrant
lowest quadrant

l.q.
lege quaeso (L. I ask by law)

LR
labeled release (experiment)
laboratory references
laboratory report
labor room
lactated Ringer's (solution)
large reticulocyte
latency reaction

latency relaxation
lateral rectus (muscle)
left rotation
ligand receptor
light reaction
light reflex
lymphocyte recruitment

L & R
left and right

L/R
left to right (ratio)

L>R
left greater than right

L<R
left less than right

L→R
left to right

Lr
lawrencium (element—formerly Lw)

Lr, L$_r$
limes reacting (dose—L. boundary; the
    smallest amount of toxin-antitoxin to
    yield a minimum positive reaction in a
    laboratory animal)

LRA
low right atrium

LRC
locomotor-respiratory coupling
longitudinal redundancy check
    (character—re: computers)
lower rib cage

LRD
living related donor

LRDT
live related donor transplant

LRE
leukemic reticuloendotheliosis
lymphoreticuloendothelial
lymphosarcoma reticuloendothelial

LREH
low renin essential hypertension

LRF
latex and resorcinol formaldehyde
liver residual factor
liver residue factor
luteinizing (hormone)-releasing factor

LRH
luteinizing (hormone)-releasing
    hormone

LRI
lower respiratory illness

lower respiratory infection
lymphocyte reactivity index

LRM
left radical mastectomy

LRMP
last regular menstrual period

LRN
lateral reticular nucleus

LRNA
low renin, normal aldosterone

LROP
lower radicular obstetrical paralysis

LRP
lichen ruber planus

LRQ
lower right quadrant

LRQG
left rostral quarter ganglion

LRR
labyrinthine righting reflex (re: Oto/
Neuro)
lymphatic return rate

LRS
lactated Ringer's solution

LRSF
lactating rat serum factor
liver regenerating serum factor

LR-SH
left-right shunt

LR$_6$(SO$_4$)^3
lateral rectus (innervated by) sixth
cranial nerve; superior oblique by
fourth cranial nerve; rest of EOMs
(extraocular muscles) by third cranial
nerve (a mnemonic)

LRSP
long-range systems planning

LRT
lower respiratory tract

LRTI
lower respiratory tract illness
lower respiratory tract infection

LS
lateral septal
lateral suspensor
left sacrum
left septum
left side
legally separated
leiomyosarcoma
length of stay

lesser sac
Letterer-Siwe (disease)
Libman-Sacks (disease)
light sleep
liminal sensitivity (liminial)
linear scleroderma
lipid synthesis
liver and spleen
low sodium (diet)
lower segment
lumbar spine
lumbosacral
lung strip
lymphosarcoma

L-S
lipid-saccharide

L/S
lactase/sucrase (ratio)
lecithin/sphingomyelin (ratio)

L & S, L + S
liver and spleen

L5-S1
lumbar fifth vertebra to sacral first
vertebra

L$_s$
prefix (re: asymmetric atoms)

LSA
left sacro-anterior (position of fetus)
left subclavian artery
leukocyte specific activity
lichen sclerosis et atrophicus (re:
Derma)
lipid-bound sialic acid
lymphosarcoma

LS&A
lichen sclerosis et atrophicus (re:
Derma)

LSA/RCS
lymphosarcoma-reticulum cell sarcoma

LSB
least significant bit (re: binary numbers)
left scapular border
left sternal border

LSC
late systolic click
least significant character (re:
computers)
left-sided colon (cancer)
lichen simplex chronicus (re: Derma)
liquid scintillation counting
liquid-solid chromatography

LSCA, LScA
left scapuloanterior (position of fetus)

LSCL
lymphosarcoma cell leukemia

LSCP, LScP
left scapuloposterior (position of fetus)

LSCS
lower segment caesarean section
(cesarean)

LSD
least significant difference
least significant digit (re: computers)
low salt diet
low sodium diet
D-lysergic acid diethylamide
(lysergide—psychomimetic)

LSD-25
D-lysergic acid diethylamide
(lysergide—psychomimetic)

LSEP
left somatosensory evoked potential

LSF
lymphocyte-stimulating factor

LSH
lutein-stimulating hormone
lymphocyte-stimulating hormone
(factor)

LSI
large scale integrated (circuit)
large scale integration (re: computers)
Life Satisfaction Index
light scattering index

LSK
liver, spleen, kidneys

LSKM
liver-spleen-kidney megalia

LSL
left sacrolateral (position of fetus)
lymphosarcoma (cell) leukemia

L SL brace
left short leg brace

LSM
late systolic murmur
lymphocyte separation medium

LSN
left substantia nigra
left sympathetic nerve

LSO
left salpingo-oophorectomy
left superior oblique
left superior olive (of brain)
lumbosacral orthosis

LSP
left sacroposterior (position of fetus)
life space
liver specific protein

LSp, L sp.
life span

L sp., L-sp
lumbar spine

LSQ
least square

LSR
lanthanide shift reagent (re: nuclear
magnetic resonance imaging)
left superior rectus

LSRA
low septal right atrium

L-S ratio, L/S ratio
lecithin to sphingomyelin ratio

LSS
Life Span Study
Life Study Sample
life support station

LSSA
lipid-soluble secondary anti-oxidant

LST
lateral spinothalamic tract
left sacrotransverse (position of fetus)
local sojourn time

LSTC
laparoscopic tubal cautery

LSTL
laparoscopic tubal ligation

LST tract
lateral spinothalamic tract

LSU
lactose-saccharose-urea (agar)
life support unit

LSV
lateral sacral vein
left subclavian vein

LSVC
left superior vena cava

LSWA
large-amplitude, slow-wave activity (re:
EEG)

LT
heat-labile enterotoxin
laminar tomography
left thigh
lethal time
leukotriene
Levin tube
levothyroxine
long term
low temperature
lues test (L. plague—re: syphilis)

lymphocyte transformation
lymphocyte transitional
lymphocytotoxin
lymphotoxin

LT, lt.
left
light

lt.
low tension

LTA
leukotriene A (5-*trans*-5,6-oxido-7,9-
   trans-11,14-*cis*-eicosatetraenoic acid;
   LTA$_4$)
lipoate transacetylase (lipoate
   acetyltransferase)
lipoteichoic acid
local tracheal anesthesia
lymphocyte-transforming activity

LTA$_4$
leukotriene A (5-*trans*-5,6-oxido-7,9-
   trans-11,14-*cis*-eicosatetraenoic acid)

LTAF
local tissue-advancement flap

LTAS
lead tetra-acetate Schiff

LTB
laryngotracheal bronchitis
laryngotracheobronchitis
leukotriene B (5,12-dihydroxy-6,8,10,14-
   eicosatetraenoic acid; LTB$_4$)

LTB$_4$
leukotriene B (5,12-dihydroxy-6,8,10,14-
   eicosatetraenoic acid)

LTC
large transformed cell
leukotriene C (5-hydroxy-6-glutathionyl-
   7,9-*trans*-11,14-*cis*-eicosatetraenoic
   acid; LTC$_4$)
lidocaine tissue concentration
long-term care
lysed tumor cell

LTC$_4$
leukotriene C$_4$ (5-hydroxy-6-
   glutathionyl-7,9- *trans*-11,14-*cis*-
   eicosatetraenoic acid)

LTCF
long-term care facility

LTCS
low transverse cervical (cesarean)
   section

LTD
leukotriene D (5-hydroxy-6-cysteinyl-
   glycine-7,9-*trans*-11,14-*cis*-
   eicosatetraenoic acid; LTD$_4$)
long-term disability

LTD$_4$
leukotriene D$_4$ (5-hydroxy-6-cysteinyl-
   glycine-7,9- *trans*-11,14-*cis*-
   eicosatetraenoic acid)

ltd.
limited

LTE
laryngotracheoesophageal
leukotriene E (6-[(2-amino-2-
   carboxyethyl)thio]-5-hydroxy-
   7,9,11,14-eicosatetraenoic acid; LTE$_4$)

LTE$_4$
leukotriene E$_4$ (6-[(2-amino-2-
   carboxyethyl)thio]-5- hydroxy-
   7,9,11,14-eicosatetraenoic acid)

LTF
lipotrop(h)ic factor (or hormone)
lymphocyte-transforming factor

LTH
lactogenic hormone
local tumor hyperthermia
low-temperature holding
   (pasteurization)
luteotrop(h)ic hormone

LTI
low temperature isotropic
lupus-type inclusion

lt. lat.
left lateral

LTM
long-term memory

LTP
leukocyte thromboplastin
long-term potentiation
L-tryptophan

LTPP
lipothiamide pyrophosphate (earlier
   name for lipoic acid; thiotic acid—re:
   treatment, liver disease; *Amanita*
   poisoning)

LTR
long terminal repeats (re: virology;
   genetics)
lymphocyte transfer reaction

L-Trp
L-tryptophan (antidepressant; nutrient)

LTS
long-term storage
long-term surviving
long tract sign (re: Neuro)

LTs
leukotrienes

LTT
lactose tolerance test
leucine tolerance test
limited treadmill testing
lymphoblastic transformation test
lymphocyte transformation test

LTV
lung thermal volume

lt. vent. BBB
left ventricular bundle branch block

lt. vent. BBB occl. assoc. c̄ SOB
left ventricular bundle branch block
  occasionally associated with
  shortness of breath

LTW
Leydig cell tumor of Wistar rats

LTX
lophotoxin (neuromuscular toxin)

LU
left uninjured
left uninvolved
left upper
logical unit (re: computers/data
  processing)
loudness unit (replaced by sone)
lytic unit

LU, Lu
lung (specific lobe of lung is
  subscripted)

L & U
lower and upper

Lu
lutetium (element)

177Lu
radioactive isotope of lutetium

LUA
left upper arm

Lu antigen
re: Lutheran blood group

luc. prim.
luce prima (L. at first light [daybreak])

LUE
left upper extremity

LUIS
low dose urea in invert sugar

LUL
left upper (eye)lid
left upper limb
left upper lung

LUL, L.U.L.
left upper lobe (of lung)

Lumb, lumb.
lumbar

LUMO
lowest unoccupied molecular orbital

LUO
left ureteral orifice

LUOB
left upper outer buttock

LUOQ
left upper outer quadrant

LUP
left ureteropelvic (junction)

LUQ
left upper quadrant

LUSB
left upper scapular border
left upper sternal border

lut.
luteum (L. yellow)

LUTT
lower urinary tract tumor

LUV
large unilamellar vesicles (type of
  liposome)

lux
luminous flux density (SI unit of
  illuminance)

LV
lacto-ovo-vegetarian
laryngeal vestibule
lateral ventricle (re: Neuro)
left ventricle
leucovorin
leukemia virus
live vaccine
live virus
low volume
lumbar vertebra
lung volume

LV, Lv.
Lactobacillus viridescens

Lv, lv.
leave

LVA
left ventricular aneurysm
left ventricular aneurysmectomy
left vertebral artery
low vision aids

LVAD
left ventricular assist device

LVAS
left ventricular assist system

LVBP
left ventricle bypass pump

LVCS
low vertical cesarean section

LVD
left ventricular dysfunction

LV$_D$
left ventricular end-diastolic (pressure)

LVDP
left ventricular diastolic pressure

LVDT
linear variable differential transformer

LVDV
left ventricular diastolic volume

LVE
left ventricular ejection
left ventricular enlargement

LVED
left ventricular end diastolic

LVEDC
left ventricular end-diastolic
circumference

LVEDD
left ventricular end-diastolic dimension

LVEDP
left ventricular end-diastolic pressure

LVEDV
left ventricular end-diastolic volume

LVEF
left ventricular ejection fraction

LVEP
left ventricular end-diastolic pressure

LVESD
left ventricular end-systolic dimension

LVESV
left ventricular end-systolic volume

LVET
left ventricular ejection time

LVETI
left ventricular ejection time index

LVF
left ventricular failure
left ventricular function
left visual field

low voltage fast
low voltage foci

LVFP
left ventricular filling pressure

LVG
left ventral gluteus

LVH
large vessel hematocrit

LVH, L.V.H.
left ventricular hypertrophy

LVI
left ventricular insufficiency
left ventricular ischemia

LVID
left ventricular internal diastolic
left ventricular internal dimension

LVIDd
left ventricular internal dimension
diastole

LVIDP
left ventricular initial diastolic pressure

LVIDs
left ventricular internal dimension
systole

LVIV
left ventricular infarct volume

LVLG
left ventrolateral gluteal (site of
injection)

LVM
lateral ventromedial (nucleus)
left ventricular mass

LVMF
left ventricular minute flow

LVN
lateral ventricular nerve
limiting viscosity number (re:
suspensions)

LVOT
left ventricular outflow tract

LVP
large volume parenteral (solution)
left ventricular pressure
levator veli palatini (muscle)
lysine-vasopressin (vasopressin
8-lysine—re: antidiuretic;
vasopressor)

LVPEP
left ventricular pre-ejection period

LVPSP
left ventricular peak systolic pressure

LVPW
left ventricular posterior wall

LVPWT
left ventricular posterior wall thickness

LVR
limb vascular resistance

L$_1$VR, L$_2$VR
first lumbar ventral (nerve) root; second
    ventral (nerve) root, etc.

LVS
left ventricular strain

LVs
(mean) left ventricular systolic
    (pressure)

LVSEMI
left ventricular subendocardial
    myocardial ischemia

LVSI
left ventricular systolic index

LVSO
left ventricular systolic output

LVSP
left ventricular systolic pressure

LVST
lateral vestibulospinal tract (cells)

LVSV
left ventricular stroke volume

LVSW
left ventricular stroke work

LVSWI
left ventricular stroke work index

LVT
left ventricular tension

LVV
left ventricular volume
live varicella vaccine

LVW
lateral ventricular width
left ventricular wall
left ventricular work

LVWI
left ventricular work index

LVWM
left ventricular wall motion

LVWMA
left ventricular wall motion abnormality

LVWMI
left ventricular wall motion index

LVWT
left ventricular wall thickness

LW
lacerating wound
lateral wall
Lee-White (blood-clotting method)
Léri-Weill (syndrome)
lung width

L/W
living and well

L & W, L&W
living and well

L-10-W
levulose (10%) in water

Lw
lawrencium (former symbol; Lr now
    used)

LWCT
Lee-White clotting time

LWD
living with disease

LWK
large white kidney

LWP
lateral wall pressure

LX
local irradiation

Lx
latex

lx
lux (SI unit of illumination = 1 lumen/
    M^2)

lx.
larynx
lower extremity

LXT
left exotropia

LY
lymphocyte
lyophilization

ly
langley (unit of sun's heat—replaced by
    pyron)

ly.
lying

LYDMA
lymphocyte-detected membrane
    antigen

LYEL
lost years of expected life

LYG
lymphomatoid granulomatosis

LYM
lymph

lym.
lymphocyte

lymph.
lymphocyte

lymphos
lymphocytes

lymphs
lymphocytes

LyNeF
lytic nephritic factor

LYP
lactose, yeast, peptone (agar)
lower yield point

Lyp
lymphosarcoma

LYS
lysosome

LYS, Lys, lys.
lysine (or its radicals in peptides)

lytes
electrolytes

LZM, Lzm, lzm.
lysozyme

M

M
Macaca (genus of monkeys used in research)
macerare (L. to soften)
magnetization
malignant (re: tumors)
Mansonia (genus of mosquitoes)
manual
manual dexterity (re: General Aptitude Test Battery)
maternally contributing (re: genetics)
matrix
matt (dull, slightly granular—re: bacterial colonies)
maximal
maximum
meatus
mediator (chemical, released in the tissues)
medical
medicine
mega (10^6—one million)
mega-(Gr. great, huge [prefix])
membrana
mentum (L. chin)
meridies (L. noon)
mesial
metabolite
metal
metastasis
methionine (a lipotropic)
method in use at National Institutes of Health
methotrexate
Microbacterium (genus)
Micrococcus (genus)
Microsporum (genus)
midvertebral line (vectorcardiography electrode)
mille (L. thousand)
misce (L. mix)
mist
mistura (L. a mixture)
mitochondria
mitosis (cell division)
mitte (L. send)
molar (solution)
molar (tooth, permanent)
mole
molecular weight
Monday
monkey
monocyte
month

Moraxella (genus)
morbus (L. disease, sickness)
morgan (unit of gene separation)
mors (L. death)
mortuus (L. dead)
mother
motile (re: bacteria)
movement response to human figure
Mucor (genus)
mucous (adjective)
mucus (noun)
Multiceps (genus of tapeworm)
multipara (L. many labors—births)
Musca (genus—fly)
muscle
musculus
mutitas (L. dumbness)
Mycobacterium (genus)
Mycoplasma (genus)
myopia (re: Ophth)
myopic
myosin
semantic (contents—re: Psychol; Aptitudes Research Project testing within structure of intellect model)
strength of pole (should be given in terms of dynes when placed in a field of strength H, as there is no name for a pole-strength unit in the centimeter-gram-second unit system)
symbol for a blood factor (re: MNS blood group)
thousand

M, *M*, м
moles per liter

M, m
mean, sample (re: statistics)
meter (fundamental unit of length in metric system)
minim (a unit of fluid measure, from L. minimus—least)
mix
mixture

M, m.
male
manipulus (L. handful)
married
masculine
mass
massage
mature
media (laboratory)

median
medium
membrane
memory (associative)
morphine
mucoid (re: bacterial colonies)
murmur (heart)

M, m, m.
milli- (L. one thousand)

M-1, M₁
mitral first sound, slight dullness

M₁
myeloblast

M₁, M₂, M₃
slight, marked, and absolute dullness
    (auscultation—re: mitral heart
    sounds)

M₂
mitral second sound, marked dullness
promyelocyte (second stage in
    granulocytic maturation)

M²
dose per square meter of body surface
square meters

M/3
middle third (long bones)

M₃
mitral third sound, absolute dullness
myelocyte

M₄
myelocyte

M₅
metamyelocyte

M₆
band form

M₇
polymorphonuclear neutrophil

M130
external membrane protein-130

M195
external membrane protein-195

m
melts at (when followed by a figure
    denoting temperature)
metastable isomer (when given after
    mass number)
micro (Gr. mikros—prefix for small)
minute
molality (number of moles of solute per
    unit mass of solvent)
molar (tooth, deciduous)

m.
by mouth
mane (L. in the morning)
minimum (L. least)
modulus

(m)
by mouth
murmur

μ
chemical potential
dynamic viscosity
heavy chain of IgM
ionic strength (re: intensity of electrical
    field existing in a solution)
linear attenuation coefficient
magnetic moment
mean
micro-(prefix—10^{-6}—one one-millionth)
micrometer (formerly micron—one one-
    millionth of a meter)
micron (former term for micrometer,
    10^{-6}m)
mu (twelfth letter of Greek alphabet,
    lower case)
permeability

m-
mesoposition (prefix)

m-, *m-*
meta

m²
square meter

m³
cubic meter

MA
mandelic acid
manifest achievement
Martin-Albright (syndrome)
masseter
maternal aunt
mean arterial (blood pressure)
medical audit
medical authorization
megaloblastic anemia
membrane antigen
menstrual age
mentum anterior (position of fetus)
Mexican American
microagglutination
microaneurysm
Miller-Abbott (tube)
mitochondrial antibody
mitogen activation
mitotic apparatus
moderately advanced
monoamine
monoclonal antibody
multiple action
muscle activity

mutagenic activity
myelinated axon

MA, M.A.
mental age (re: Psychol)

MA, M.A., ma.
meter angle (meter-angle)

MA, mA, ma
milliamperage (re: radiology)
milliampere

M.A.
metatarsus adductus

M/A
mood and/or affect

Ma
mach number (re: aerodynamics)
masurium (technetium)

μA
microampere

ma.
macera (L. soften)

MAA
macroaggregated albumin
macroaggregates of albumin
melanoma-associated antigen
monarticular arthritis

MAAAP
macroaggregated albumin arterial
perfusion

MAACL
Multiple Affect Adjective Check List (re:
psychological testing)

MABI
Mother's Assessment of the Behavior of
Her Infant

MABOP
Mustargen (nitrogen mustard),
Adriamycin, bleomycin, Oncovin,
prednisone (re: chemotherapy)

MABP
mean arterial blood pressure

MAC
MacConkey (agar)
MacIntosh (blade)
malignancy associated changes
maximal allowable cost
maximum acid concentration
maximum allowable cost
membrane attack complex
methotrexate, actinomycin D,
cyclophosphamide (re:
chemotherapy)
mid-arm circumference
minimal antibiotic concentration

minimum alveolar (anesthetic)
concentration
mitomycin C, Adriamycin (doxorubicin),
and cyclophosphamide (re:
chemotherapy)
mitral anular calcium
modulator of adenylate cyclase
multidimensional actuarial classification

MAC, M.A.C.
maximal allowable concentration
maximum allowable concentration

Mac
macula (re: Ophth)

mac.
macera (L. soften)
macerare (L. to soften)
macerated
maceration

MAC AWAKE
minimal alveolar (anesthetic)
concentration (patient recovering
from general anesthesia able to
respond to instructions)

MACC
methotrexate, Adriamycin (doxorubicin),
cyclophosphamide, and CCNU
(lomustine) (re: chemotherapy)

m. accur.
misce accuratissme (L. mix very
accurately)

MACR
mean axillary count rate

macro.
macroscopic

MAD
maximum allowable dose
MeCCNU (semustine) and Adriamycin
(doxorubicin) (re: chemotherapy)
methandriol (anabolic)
methylandrostenediol (methandriol—a
metabolic)
mind-altering drug
minimum average dose (dosis curativa
minima)

MADRS
Montgomery and Asberg Depression
Rating Scale

MADU
5-(methylamino)-2′-deoxyuridine
(antiviral)

MAE
Multilingual Aphasia Examination

MAF
macrophage-activating factor

macrophage-activation factor
macrophage-agglutinating factor
minimum audible field
mouse amniotic fluid
movement aftereffect

MAFA
mid-arm fat area

MAFH
macroaggregated ferrous hydroxide

MAG
myelin-associated glycoprotein

Mag
magnesium

mag.
magnification
magnify
magnus (L. large)

mag. cit.
magnesium citrate (laxative)

MAGE
mean amplitude of glycerin excursion

MAGF
male accessory gland fluid

MAgF
macrophage-aggregation factor

MAggF
macrophage-agglutination factor

Magic
microprobe analysis generalized
   intensity corrections

magn.
magnus (L. large)

magnif.
magnification

MAGS
Multidimensional Assessment of Gains
   in School (re: psychological testing)

MAHA
microangiopathic hemolytic anemia

MAI
Morbid Anxiety Inventory

MAII
Milwaukee Academic Interest Inventory
   (re: psychological testing)

MAIS
Mycobacterium avium,
   (Mycobacterium) intracellulare,
   (Mycobacterium) scrofulaceum

MAIS complex
isolates possessing characteristics

intermediate between
   Mycobacterium avium and
   Mycobacterium scrofulaceum

MAIS intermediates
Mycobacterium avium,
   (Mycobacterium) intracellulare,
   (Mycobacterium) scrofulaceum

maj.
major
majority

MAKA
major karyotypic abnormality

MAL
malfunction
midaxillary line

Mal
malate

mal.
malanando (L. by blistering)
malandria (L. blisters)
malignant

malad.
maladjusted

Mal-BSA
maleated bovine serum albumin

MALG
Minnesota antilymphoblast globulin

malig.
malignancy
malignant

MALIMET
Master List of Medical (Indexing) Terms
   (EMBASE thesaurus)

maloccl.
malocclusion

MALT
mucosa-associated lymphoid tissue

MAM
methylazomethanol (active component
   of cycasin—a carcinogen)

MAM, MaM, mam
milliampere minute

M + AM, M + Am, M + Am
compound myopic astigmatism

MAMA
midarm muscle area
monoclonal anti-malignin antibody

MAMC
mean arm muscle circumference
mid-arm muscle circumference

MAmg
medial amygdaloid (nucleus)

MA min., ma-min
milliampere-minute

m-AMSA
4'-(9-acridinylamino)methanesulfon-m-anisidide (amsacrine—antineoplastic)

MAN
magnocellular nucleus (of anterior neostratum)

MAN, Man
mannose (or its radicals in polysaccharides)

Man
manipulation

man.
mane (L. morning, in the morning)
manipulate
manipulus (L. a handful)

MANA
α-D-mannosidase A, cytoplasmic

MANB
α-D-mannosidase B, lysosomal

mand.
mandible
mandibular

manif.
manifest
manifestation
manifested

manifest.
manifestation

MANIP, manip.
manipulation
manipulus (L. a handful)

manip. ↓ anesthesia
manipulation under anesthesia

MANOVA
multivariate analysis of variance

Man-6-P
mannose-6-phosphate

man. pr.
mane primo (L. first thing in the morning)

man. prim.
mane primo (L. first thing in the morning)

M antigen
re: β-hemolytic streptococci, *Streptococcus pneumoniae*, and blood group A

M_1, M_2 antigens
MNS blood group antigens

manu.
manufacture

manuf.
manufacture

MAO
maximal acid output
monoamine oxidase

MAOA
monoamine oxidase A

MAOI
monoamine oxidase inhibitor

MAP
maximal aerobic power
mean aortic pressure
mean arterial pressure
megaloblastic anemia of pregnancy
mercapturic acid pathway
methyl acceptor protein
6-α-methyl-17α-acetoxyprogesterone (medroxyprogesterone— progestin)
microlithiasis alveolarum pulmonum
microtubule-associated protein
minimum audible pressure
monophasic action potential
mouse antibody production (test)
muscle-action potential
Musical Aptitude Profile (re: psychological testing)

MAPA
muscle adenosine phosphoric acid

MAPC
migrating action potential complex

MAPE
Multidimensional Assessment of Philosophy of Education (re: psychological testing)

MAPF
microatomized protein food

MAPI
microbial alkaline protease inhibitor

MAPO
methyl aphoxide (metepa— chemosterilant)

MAPS
Make A Picture Story (re: Psychol)
measurement of air pollution from satellites

MAR
Main Admitting Room
marasmus
margin
marrow

maximal aggregation ratio
medication administration record
memory address register (re:
   computers)
microanalytical reagent
minimal angle resolution
mixed antiglobulin reaction

mar
marker chromosome (re: cytogenetics)

MARG
(acute) marginal (branch of the left
   circumflex artery)

marg.
margin
marginal

MARS
Mathematics Anxiety Rating Scale
mouse antirat serum

MARS-A
Mathematics Anxiety Rating Scale—
   Adolescents

marsup.
marsupialization

MARTI
mobile advanced real-time image

MAS
Management Appraisal Survey (re:
   psychological testing)
Manifest Anxiety Scale (Taylor)
Maternal Attitude Scale
meconium aspiration syndrome
milk alkali syndrome
minor axis shortening (of left ventricle)
mobile arm support
Morgagni-Adams-Stokes (syndrome)
motion analysis system

MAS, MaS, mA-s, mas.
milliampere second

mas.
masculine
massa (L. a mass)

masc.
masculine
mass concentration

MASER
microwave amplification by stimulated
   emission of radiation

MASH
Mobile Army Surgical Hospital
multiple automated sample harvester

MASP
microaerophilous stationary phase

mas. pil.
massa pilularum (L. pill mass)

mass.
massa (L. a mass)
massage
massive

MAST
Military Anti-Shock Trousers (used by
   emergency personnel for
   management of hypovolemia)

mAST
mitochondrial aspartate
   aminotransferase

mast.
mastectomy
mastoid

MAT
Manipulative Aptitude Test (re: Psychol)
manual arts therapy
mature
maturity
mean absorption time
medication administration team
Metropolitan Achievement Tests (re:
   Psychol)
microagglutination test
Miller Analogies Test (re: Psychol)
Motivation Analysis Test
multifocal atrial tachycardia
multiple agent (chemo)therapy

Mat
maternity

mat
maternal origin (re: cytogenetics)

mat.
material

MATE
Marital Attitudes Evaluation (re:
   Psychol)

mat. gf.
maternal grandfather

mat. gm.
maternal grandmother

math, math.
mathematical
mathematics

MATSA
Marek's associated tumor-specific
   antigen

MA tube
Miller-Abbott tube

matut.
matutinus (L. in the morning)

MAU
Meyenburg-Altherr-Uehlinger
(syndrome)

MAV
mechanical auxiliary ventricle
minimum apparent viscosity
movement arm vector

MAVA
multiple abstract variance analysis

MAVR
mitral and aortic valve replacement

MAX, Max, max, max.
maximum

max.
maxilla
maxillary
maximal

MaxEP
maximum esophageal pressure

MB
buccal margin
the isoenzyme of creatine kinase that
    contains one M and one B subunit
Mallory body
mamillary body (re: Neuro)
Marie-Bamberger (syndrome)
Marsh-Bendall (factor—an ATP inhibitor
    in muscle tissue; relaxing factor)
maximum breathing
megabytes (per second—re:
    computers)
mercury bougie
mesiobuccal (re: Dent)
methyl bromide
methylene blue
microbiological (assay)
muscle balance
myocardial band

6MB
six-meal bland (diet)

Mb
mandible body
myoglobin

μ·B
magnetic moment of electron (Bohr
    magneton)

mb
millibar (unit of pressure)

m.b.
misce bene (L. mix well)

μb
microbar (unit of pressure)

MBA
methylbenzyl alcohol

methylbis(β-chloroethyl)amine
    (mechlorethamine—gas warfare
    agent base; hydrochloride form as
    antineoplastic)
methylbovine albumin

M-BACOD
methotrexate/citrovorum factor,
    bleomycin, Adriamycin (doxorubicin),
    cyclophosphamide (Cytoxan),
    Oncovin (vincristine), and
    dexamethasone (re: chemotherapy)

M band
monoclonal band (re: paraprotein)

MBAR
myocardial beta-adrenergic receptor

mbar
millibar (unit of pressure)

μbar, μ-bar
microbar (unit of pressure)

MBAS
methylene blue active substance

MBB
modified barbital buffer

MBC
male breast cancer
maximal breathing capacity
maximum bladder capacity
maximum breathing capacity
methyl 2-benzimidazolecarbamate
    (fungicide)
methylthymol blue complex
microcrystalline bovine collagen
minimal bactericidal concentration
minimum bactericidal concentration

MbCO
myoglobin and its combination with
    carbon monoxide

MBCU
metallic bead-chain urethrocystograph

MBD
Mental Deterioration Battery
methotrexate, bleomycin,
    diamminedichloroplatinum
    (cisplatin—re: chemotherapy)
methylene blue dye
minimal brain damage
minimal brain dysfunction
Morquio-Brailsford disease

MBE
medium below elbow (cast)

MBF
medullary blood flow
muscle blood flow
myocardial blood flow

MB factor
Marsh-Bendall factor

MBFLB
monaural bifrequency loudness balance

MBG
mean blood glucose

MBH
maximum benefit from hospitalization
medial basal hypothalamus
mediobasal hypothalamic
methylene blue reduced

MBH$_2$
methylene blue reduced

MBHI
Millon Behavioral Health Inventory

MBK
methyl butyl ketone (2-hexanone)

MBL
menstrual blood loss
minimal bactericidal level

MBLA
mouse-specific bone marrow-derived
   lymphocyte antigen

MBM
mineral basal medium

MBO
mesiobucco-occlusal (re: Dent)

MbO$_2$
hemoglobin and its combination with
   oxygen
oxymyoglobin

MBP
major basic protein
maltose-binding protein
mean blood pressure
melitensis, bovine, porcine (antigen
   from *Brucella melitensis, Brucella
   bovis*, and *Brucella suis*)
mesiobuccopulpal (re: Dent)
myelin basic protein

MBPS
multigated (cardiac) blood pool
   scanning

MBq
megabecquerel (unit of radioactivity)

MBR
memory buffer register (re: computers)
methylene blue reduced

MBRT
methylene blue reduction time

MBSA
methylated bovine serum albumin

MBSD
maple bark stripper disease

MBT
2-mercaptobenzothiazole (zinc or
   sodium salts used as fungicide)
mixed bacterial toxin

MBTI
Myers-Briggs Type Indicator (re:
   psychological testing)

MC
mass casualty
mast cell
maximum concentration
medium-chain (triglycerides)
medullary cavity
medullary cystic (disease)
megacharacters (per second—re:
   computers)
melanoma cell
meningeal carcinomatosis
Merkel cell (meniscus tactus)
mesenteric collateral
mesiocervical
mesocaval (shunt)
metacarpal
methylcellulose
microcephaly
microciliary clearance
microcirculation
midcapillary
midcarpal
Minkowski-Chauffard (syndrome)
mitochondrial complementation
mitomycin C
mitotic cycle
mitral commissurotomy
mixed cellularity
mixed cryoglobulinemia
monkey cells
mononuclear cell
mouth care
mycelial phase (re: fungi)
myocarditis

MC, Mc, mc
megacurie (MCi is preferred)
megacycle (now called megahertz—
   MHz)

MC, M-C
mineralocorticoid (re: adrenal cortical
   hormones)

M-C
Magovern-Cromie (prosthesis)

M & C, M&C
morphine and cocaine

M + C
morphine and cocaine

3-MC
3-methylcholanthrene (re: cancer
   research)

Mc
mandible coronoid

mC
millicoulomb (a unit of charge—re:
   electricity)

mc, mc.
millicurie (former abbreviation—now
   mCi)

μC
microcoulomb (a unit of charge—re:
   electricity)

MCA
major coronary arteries
medical care administration
methylcholanthrene (3-MECA, 3-MC—
   experimental drug—re: cancer
   research)
middle cerebral artery
monochloroacetic acid (herbicide)
monoclonal antibody
motorcycle accident
multichannel analyzer
Multiple Classification Analysis
multiple congenital abnormality
multiple congenital anomaly

Mᶜ antigen
MNS blood group antigen

MCAR
mixed cell agglutination reaction

MCAS
middle cerebral artery syndrome

MCAT
middle cerebral artery thrombosis

m. caute
misce caute (L. mix cautiously)

MCB
membranous cytoplasmic bodies (body)

McB
McBurney's (point)

MCBM
muscle capillary basement membrane

MCBMT
muscle capillary basement membrane
   thickening

MCBP
melphalan, cyclophosphamide, BCNU,
   prednisone (re: chemotherapy)

McB pt.
McBurney's point

MCBR
minimum concentration of bilirubin

MCC
marked cocontraction
mean corpuscular (hemoglobin)
   concentration
medial cell column
metacerebral cell
metastatic cord compression
microcrystalline collagen
minimum complete-killing concentration
mucocutaneous candidiasis

McC
McCarthy (panendoscope)
McCoy (antibodies)

MCCD
minimum cumulative cardiotoxic dose

MCCNU
methyl-CCNU (semustine—re:
   chemotherapy)

MCCU
mobile coronary care unit

MCD
magnetic circular dichroism
margin crease distance (re: Ophth)
mast-cell degranulating (peptide)
mean cell diameter
mean corpuscular diameter
mean of consecutive differences
median control death
medullary collecting duct
medullary cystic disease
metabolic coronary dilation
metacarpal cortical density
minimal cerebral dysfunction
minimal changes disease
multiple carboxylase deficiency
muscle carnitine deficiency

mcD, mcd
millicuries-destroyed (re: radioactivity)

MCDI
Minnesota Child Development
   Inventory

MCDP
mast cell degranulating peptide

MCDT
multiple choice discrimination test

MCE
medical care evaluation

MCES
multiple cholesterol emboli syndrome

MCF
macrophage chemotactic factor
medium corpuscular fragility
microcomplement fixation
monocyte (leukotactic) factor
mononuclear cell factor
most comfortable frequency
myocardial contractile force

MCFA
medium-chain fatty acid
miniature centrifugal fast analyzer

MCFP
mean circulating filling pressure

MCG
magnetocardiogram
membrane coating granule
mesencephalic central gray
Minkowski-Chauffard-Gänsslen
   (syndrome)

mcg.
microgram

MCGC
metacerebral giant cell

MCGF
mast cell growth factor

mcgm.
microgram

MCGN
mesangiocapillary glomerulonephritis
mixed cryoglobulinemia associated with
   glomerulonephritis

MCH
Maternal and Child Health
mean cell hemoglobin
mean corpuscular hemoglobin

mch, mc h, mc-h, mc.h.
millicurie-hour

μc.h.
microcurie-hour

MCHC
maternal and child health care
mean cell hemoglobin concentration
mean corpuscular hemoglobin
   concentration

MCHg
mean corpuscular hemoglobin

MC Hgb
mean corpuscular hemoglobin

mchr, mc-hr
millicurie-hour

μC hr.
microcurie-hour

MCI
mean cardiac index
methicillin

MCi
megacurie

mCi
millicurie

μCi
microcurie

mCid
millicuries destroyed

mCi-hr
millicurie-hour

μCi-hr
microcurie-hour

MCKD
multicystic kidney disease

MCL
maximum comfort level
maximum containment laboratory
medial collateral ligament
midclavian line
midclavicular line
midcostal line
minimal change lesion
mixed culture, leukocyte
modified chest lead
most comfortable listening (level)
most comfortable loudness (level—re:
   Audio)

MCLL
most comfortable listening level
most comfortable loudness level (re:
   Audio)

MCLS
mucocutaneous lymph node syndrome

MCM
Monte Carlo method (re: computers)

MCMI
Millon Clinical Multiaxial Inventory (re:
   Psychol)

MCMN
1-methyl-2-[(carbamoyloxy)methyl]-5-
   nitroimidazole (ronidazole—
   antimicrobial)

MCMV
mouse cytomegalovirus
murine cytomegalovirus

MCN
minimal change nephropathy

MC-N
mixed cell nodular (lymphoma)

MCNS
minimal change nephrotic syndrome

MCO
medical care organization

M colony
mucoid colony

M component
M protein seen in myeloma or
  macroglobulinemia and other plasma
  cell dyscrasias

mcoul
millicoulomb

μcoul
microcoulomb

MCP
master control program (re: computers)
maximal closure pressure
melanosis circumscripta precancerosa
melphalan, cyclophosphamide,
  prednisone (re: chemotherapy)
metacarpal phalangeal
metacarpophalangeal
methyl-accepting chemotaxis protein
2-methyl-4-chlorophenoxyacetic acid
  (weed killer)
mitotic-control protein

MCPA
(4-chloro-2-methylphenoxy)acetic acid
  (weed killer)

MCPH
metacarpal phalangeal
metacarpophalangeal

MCPS
Missouri Children's Picture Series (re:
  psychological testing)

Mcps, Mc.p.s., mcps, mc p s
megacycles per second

MCP test
mucin clot-prevention test

MCQ
multiple choice question

MCR
message competition ratio
metabolic clearance rate (re: steroid[s])

MCS
malignant carcinoid syndrome
Marlow-Crowne (Social Desirability)
  Scale
mesocaval shunt
methylcholanthrene (-induced) sarcoma
moisture control system
multiple combined sclerosis
myocardial contractile state

mc/s
megacycles per second

MCSA
Moloney cell surface antigen

M-CSF
macrophage colony-stimulating factor

MCT
manual cervical traction
mean cell thickness
mean cell threshold
mean circulation time
mean corpuscular thickness
medium-chain triglyceride
medullary cancer, thyroid
medullary carcinoma of thyroid
microtoxicity test
multiple compressed tablet

MCTC
metrizamide computed tomography
  cisternography

MCTD
mixed connective tissue disease

MCTF
mononuclear cell tissue factor

MCT oil
medium-chain triglyceride oil

MCU
maximum care unit
millicurie (mCi now used)

mcU
microunit

MCV
mean cell volume
mean clinical value
mean corpuscular volume
median cell volume
motor conduction velocity (re: Neuro)

MD
macula densa (re: nephron)
magnesium deficiency
main duct
maintenance dose
malate dehydrogenase (malic acid
  dehydrogenase)
malrotation of the duodenum
manic depressive
Marek's disease (avian lymphomatosis)
maternal deprivation
maximal dose
maximum dose
mean deviation
mean diastolic
measurable disease
Meckel's diverticulum
(nucleus) medialis dorsalis (thalamus—
  re: Neuro)

mediastinal disease
Medical Department
medical doctor (Medicinae Doctor,
    Doctor of Medicine)
mediodorsal
medium dosage
mental deficiencies
mentally deficient
mesiodistal (re: Dent)
Minamata disease
minimum dosage
mitral disease
mixed diet
moderate disability
monocular deprivation
movement disorder
multiple deficiencies
muscular dystrophy
myeloproliferative disease
myocardial damage
myocardial disease

M^D
molecular rotation

Md
mendelevium (element)

md.
median

MDA
malondialdehyde
manual dilation of the anus
mentodextra anterior (position of fetus)
3,4-methylenedioxyamphetamine
multivariant discriminant analysis

MDA, M.D.A.
motor discriminative acuity

MDAP
Machover Draw-A-Person (Test—re:
    Psychol)

MDBK
Madin-Darby bovine kidney (cells)

MDC
minimum detectable concentration

MDCK
Madin-Darby canine kidney (cell line)

MDD
major depressive disorder
mean daily dose
mean day of death

MDDA
Minnesota Differential Diagnosis of
    Aphasia

MDDD
Merrill-Demos DD (drug abuse and
    delinquent behavior scale—formerly
    called the TPSC Scale)

MDE
major depressive episode

MDEBP
mean daily erect blood pressure

M-Det
N,N-diethyl-3-methylbenzamide (deet—
    insect repellent)

***m*-DETA**
N,N-diethyl-*m*-toluamide (deet—insect
    repellent)

MDF
mean dominant frequency
myocardial depressant factor

MDGF
macrophage-derived growth factor

MDH
malate dehydrogenase (malic acid
    dehydrogenase)
medullary dorsal horn

MDH1
malate dehydrogenase, soluble

MDH2
malate dehydrogenase, mitochondrial

MDHM
malate dehydrogenase, mitochondrial

MDHR
maximum determined heart rate

MDHS
malate dehydrogenase, soluble

MDHV
Marek's disease herpesvirus

MDI
manic-depressive illness
metered dose inhaler
Multiscore Depression Inventory

m. dict.
more dicto (L. in the manner directed)

MDIT
mean disintegration time

MDM
mid-diastolic murmur
minor determinant mixture

MDMH
monomethyloldimethylhydantoin
    (preservative)

mdn.
median

MDNB
mean daily nitrogen balance

MDOPA
methyldopa (alpha-methyldopa)

MDP
mandibular dysostosis and peromelia
manic-depressive psychosis
maximum deliverable pressure
mentodextra posterior (position of fetus)
^{99m}Tc medronate methylene
　diphosphonate (re: bone imaging
　agent)
muramyldipeptide

MDPI
maximum daily permissible intake

MDQ
memory deviation quotient
minimum detectable quantity

MDR
median duration of response
memory data register (re: computers)
minimum daily requirement
multichannel data recorder (re:
　computers)

MDRH
multidisciplinary rehabilitation hospital

MDS
medical data screen
medical data system
milk drinker syndrome
multidimensional scaling
multiple deficiency syndrome

M.D.S.
misce, da, signa (L. mix, give, label)

MDSBP
mean daily supine blood pressure

MDSO
mentally disordered sex offender

MDT
mast (cell) degeneration test
mean dissolution time
median detection threshold
mentodextra transversa (position of
　fetus)
multidisciplinary team

MDTR
mean diameter-thickness ratio

MDUO
myocardial disease of unknown origin

MDV
Marek's disease virus
mucosal disease virus
multiple dose vial

MDY
month, date, year

ME
macular edema
magnitude estimation
male equivalent
malic enzyme
manic episode
maximum effort
medial eminence
median eminence (of hypothalamus)
medical education
medical examination
medical examiner
member employee
meningoencephalitis
mercaptoethanol
metabolizable energy
metamyelocyte
microembolization
middle ear
mouse epithelial (cells)
muscle examination
myoepithelial (cells)

ME, M.E.
Mache Einheit (Ger. unit—re: radiation
　emanation— now obsolete)

ME-
methyl-

M/E
myeloid-erythroid (ratio)

M:E
myeloid-to-erythroid (precursors in
　bone marrow) ratio

ME1
malic enzyme, soluble

ME$_{50}$
50 percent maximal effect

2 ME, 2ME
2-mercaptoethanol

Me
acetone (Me$_2$CO)
methyl (CH$_3$—)
methyl alcohol (MeOH)

MEA
β-mercaptoethylamine (cysteamine—
　antidote to acetaminophen poisoning)
monoethanolamine (surfactant)
multiple endocrine adenomas
multiple endocrine adenomatosis

MEA I
multiple endocrine adenoma
　(syndrome), type I
multiple endocrine adenomatosis, type I

meas.
measure
measured

measurement
measuring

MEAT
Minnesota Engineering Analogies Test
(re: psychological testing)

MEB, MeB
methylene blue

ME-BH
medial eminence, basal hypothalamus

MeBSA
methylated bovine serum albumin

MEC
median effective concentration
middle ear canals
minimal effective concentration
minimum effective concentration

mec.
meconium

3-MECA
3-methylcholanthrene (re: cancer
research)

Mecano, mechano.
mechanotherapy

Mec Asp
meconium aspiration (re: OB)

Me-CCNU
methyl-CCNU (semustine) (re:
chemotherapy)

mech.
mechanical
mechanism

MECT
maximum extrapolated clotting time

MECTA
mobile electroconvulsive therapy
apparatus

MECY
methotrexate, cyclophosphamide (re:
chemotherapy)

MED
median erythrocyte diameter
Meekeren-Ehlers-Danlos (syndrome)
minimum effective dosage
minimum effective dose

MED, M.E.D.
minimal effective dose
minimal erythema dose

MED, med.
median
medical
medicine

med.
medial
medicamentum (L. a medicine)
medication
medicinal
medium (re: bacteriology)

MEDAAC
Medical Data (System for) Analysis (of)
Clinical (Information)

MEDAC syndrome
multiple endocrine deficiency—
Addison's disease—candidiasis

med. elig.
medical eligibility

MEDEM
medical emergency (stat report)

MEDLARS
Medical Literature Analysis and
Retrieval System (the National
Library of Medicine's computerized
index system)

MEDLINE
telehone linkage between MEDLARS
and various medical libraries in the
U.S.

med. men.
medial meniscectomy
medial meniscus

MEDPRO
Medical Education (Resources)
Program

MEDS, meds.
medications
medicines

MedSurg
medicine and surgery

Med Tech, med. tech.
medical technology

MEE
methylethyl ether (methoxyethane)
middle ear effusion

MEF
maximal expiratory flow (re: Resp)
middle ear fluid
midexpiratory flow
migration enhancement factor
mouse embryo fibroblasts
mouse embryonic fibroblasts

MEF$_{50}$
mean maximum expiratory flow

MEFR
maximal expiratory flow rate (re: Resp)
maximum expiratory flow rate (re: Resp)

MEFSR
maximum expiratory flow-static recoil
(curve)

MEFV
maximal expiratory flow-volume (curve)
(re: Resp)
maximum expiratory flow volume (re:
Resp)

MEFVC
maximum expiratory flow volume curve
mechanical expiratory flow volume
curve

MEG
magnetoencephalogram
magnetoencephalograph

MEG, meg
megacycle

MEG, meg.
megakaryocytes

meg.
megaloblastic

MEGA-DATS
(Indiana) Medical Genetics Acquisition
and Data Transmission System

mEGF
mouse epidermal growth factor

MEK
methyl ethyl ketone

MEL
metabolic equivalent level
mouse erythroleukemia
murine erythroleukemia

mel.
melena

MELC
murine erythroleukemia cell

MELI
met-enkephalin-like immunoreactivity

MEM
macrophage electrophoretic migration
macrophage electrophoretic mobility
(test)
minimal essential medium
minimum essential medium

MEm
mitochondrial malic enzyme

mem.
member

memb.
membrane

MEMPHIS
Memphis Educational Model Providing
Handicapped Infant Services (re:
psychological testing)

MEN
multiple endocrine neoplasia

MEN I
multiple endocrine neoplasia, type I
(Wermer syndrome)

MEN II
multiple endocrine neoplasia, type II
(Sipple syndrome)

MEN III
multiple endocrine neoplasia, type III (or
IIb—mucosal neuroma syndrome)

men.
meningeal
meninges
meningitis

mening.
meningeal
meninges
meningitis

menst.
menstrual
menstruate
menstruating

menstru.
menstrual
menstruate
menstruation

MEN syndrome
multiple endocrine neoplasia

ment.
mental
mentation

MEO
malignant external otitis

MeOH
methyl alcohol

MEOS
microsomal ethanol oxidizing system

MEP
maximal expiratory pressure
mean effective pressure
motor end plate (re: Neuro)

MEP, mep.
meperidine (Demerol)

MEPC
miniature end-plate current

MEPP
miniature end-plate potential

MePr
methylprednisolone

MEPS
Means-Ends Problem-Solving
　(Procedure—re: Psychol)

MEq, mEq., meq.
milliequivalent

mEq/L
milliequivalents per liter

MER
mean ejection rate
methanol-extruded residue
molar esterification rate
multimodality evoked response

M/E ratio
myeloid-erythroid ratio

MERB
met-enkephalin receptor binding

MERG
macular electroretinogram

MES
maintenance electrolyte solution
maximal electroshock
maximal electroshock seizure
muscles in elongated state
myoelectric signal

Mes
mesencephalic
mesencephalon

Mesc
mescaline

MESGN
mesangial glomerulonephritis

MESH
Medical Subject Headings (re:
　MEDLARS)

MET
metabolic (equivalent; energy
　expended while in a resting state)
metabolic equivalent of the task
midexpiratory time
multistage exercise testing

MET, Met, met.
methionine (or its radicals in peptides—
　lipotrophic)

MET, met.
metastasis

met.
metabolic

metabolism
metabolites
metal
metallic (re: chest sounds)
metallic (re: foreign body)
metastatic

meta.
metahead (re: podiatry)
metatarsal (re: podiatry)

metab.
metabolic
metabolism
metabolites

metaph.
metaphysics
metaphysis

metas.
metastasis
metastasize
metastasizing
metastatic

M et f. pil.
misce et fiant pilulae (L. mix and let pills
　be made)

M et f. pulv.
misce et fiat pulvis (L. mix and let a
　powder be made)

METH
methicillin

Meth
methedrine (methylamphetamine
　hydrochloride)

meth.
method
methyl

MetHb, metHb
methemoglobin

methyl-GAG
methylglyoxyl bis(guanylhydrazone)
　(mitoguazone dihydrochloride—an
　antineoplastic)

metMb
metmyoglobin

m. et n.
mane et nocte (L. morning and night)

METS
metabolic equivalents

Mets
metastases

met. series
metastatic series

M et sig., m. et sig.
misce et signa (L. mix and label)

METT
maximum exercise tolerance test

Met-tRNA
methionine-transfer RNA (re: eukaryote
  protein synthesis initiator)

MEV
maximal exercise ventilation
murine erythroblastosis virus

MeV
mega electron volt

Mev, mev.
million electron volts (10^6 eV)

MF
mass fragmentography
meat free
medium frequency
megafarad
microfibrile
microfilament
microfilia
microflocculation
microscopic factor
mid-forceps
Miller Fisher (syndrome)
Millipore filter
mitochondrial fragments
mitogenic factor
mitomycin, 5-fluorouracil (re:
  chemotherapy)
mitotic figure
mossy fiber
mucosal fluid
multifactorial
multiplying factor
mutation frequency
mutton fat (keratic precipitates,
  granulomatous type— re: Ophth)
mycosis fungoides
myelin figure(s)
myelofibrosis
myocardial fibrosis
myofibrillar

M-F
masculinity-femininity

M/F, M:F
male to female (ratio)

M & F
mother and father

Mf
masculine-feminine

Mf, mf.
microfilaria

mF, mf
millifarad (mF preferred)

μF, μf
microfarad

MFA
monofluoroacetamide (insecti-,
  rodenticide)
multifunctional acrylic
multiple factor analysis

MFAT
multifocal atrial tachycardia

MFB
medial forebrain bundle
metallic foreign body

MFC
mean frequency of compensation
minimal fungicidal concentration

m-FC
membrane fecal coli (broth)

MFD
mandibulofacial dysostosis
Memory-For-Designs (Test—re:
  Psychol)
midforceps delivery
milk-free diet

MFD, M.F.D.
minimum fatal dose

MFG
modified (heat degraded) gelatin (a
  plasma extender)

mfg.
manufactured
manufacturing

MFH
malignant fibrohistiocytoma
malignant fibrous histiocytoma

MFID
multielectrode flame ionization detector

M flac, m. flac.
membrana flaccida (L. flaccid
  membrane [pars flaccida membrana
  tympani]—Shrapnell's membrane)

MFM
Millipore filter method

MF method
membrane filter method (re:
  bacteriology)
Millipore filter method

MFO
mixed-function oxidase

MFP
melphalan, 5-fluorouracil,
　medroxyprogesterone acetate (re:
　chemotherapy)
monofluorophosphate
myofascial pain

m.f. pil.
misce, fiant pilulae (L. mix, let pills be
　made)

MFR
mean flow rate
median flow rate
mucus flow rate

mfr.
manufacture
manufacturer

MFRL
maximum force at rest length

MFS
medical fee schedule

MF sol.
merthiolate-formaldehyde (stock)
　solution

MF/SS
mycosis fungoides/Sézary's syndrome

MFT
multifocal atrial tachycardia
muscle function test

m. ft.
mistura fiat (L. let a mixture be made)

MFU
medical follow up

MFW
multiple fragment wounds

MG
Marcus Gunn (pupil—Gunn pupil;
　relative afferent pupillary defect)
margin
medial gastrocnemius
membranous glomerulonephritis
menopausal gonoadotrop(h)in
mesiogingival (re: Dent)
methylglucoside (α-methylglucoside—
　an industrial chemical)
methylglyoxal (pyruvaldehyde)
Michaelis-Gutmann (bodies)
Millard-Gubler (syndrome)
minigastrin
monoclonal gammopathy
monoglyceride
mucigen granule
mucous granule
muscle group
myasthenia gravis

Mycoplasma gallisepticum
myoglobin

Mg
magnesium (element)

^{28}Mg
radioactive isotope of magnesium

mg, mg.
milligram

mg%
milligram(s) percent
milligrams per deciliter
milligrams per hundred milliliters

mγ
micromilligram (nanogram)
milligamma (nanogram)
millimicrogram (nanogram)
nanogram

μg
microgram

$\mu\gamma$
microgamma (picogram)
micromicrogram (picogram)
picogram

MGA
medical gas analyzer
melengestrol acetate (a progestin)

M^g antigens
MNS blood group antigens

MGB
medial geniculate body

MGBG
methylglyoxal bis(guanylhydrazone)

MGC
minimal glomerular change
　(nephrology)

MgCl$_2$
magnesium chloride

MGD
mixed gonadal dysgenesis

mgd
million gallons per day

MG-EL, mg. el., mg-el
milligram-element (radioactive)

MGES
multiple gated equilibrium scintigraphy

MGF
macrophage growth factor
maternal grandfather
mother's grandfather

MGG
May-Grünwald-Giemsa (stain)
molecular and general genetics
mouse gamma globulin

MGGH
methylglyoxal bis(guanylhydrazone)
(mitoguazone— an antineoplastic
agent)

MGH, mgh, mg h
milligram-hour (milligramage—re:
radioactivity)

mg-hr
milligram-hour (milligramage—re:
radioactivity)

mg/hr
milligrams per hour

MGI
macrophage- and granulocyte-inducing
(proteins)

mg/kg
milligrams per kilogram

MGM
maternal grandmother
mother's grandmother

mgm
milligram

mgm/100 ml
milligrams per 100 milliliters

mgmt.
management

MGN
medial geniculate nucleus (re: Neuro)
membranous glomerulonephritis

MgO
magnesium oxide

MGP
marginal granulocyte pool
membranous glomerulopathy
mucin glycoprotein
mucous glycoprotein

MGR
modified gain ratio
multiple gas rebreathing

mgr.
manager

MGSA
melanoma growth-stimulating activity

MgSO₄
magnesium sulfate (Epsom salt)

mgt.
management

mgtis
meningitis

MGUS
monoclonal gammopathy of
undetermined significance

MGW
magnesium sulfate, glycerin, water
(enema)

MH
maleic hydrazide (plant growth inhibitor)
malignant histiocytosis
malignant hyperpyrexia
malignant hyperthermia
mammotrophic hormone (prolactin)
marital history
medial hypothalamus
medical history
melanophore hormone
menstrual history
mental health
mid-half (re: expiratory flow)
military history
moist heat
murine hepatitis
mutant hybrid
myohyoid

M.H.
mercuri-hematoporphyrin disodium salt
(merphyrin— antineoplastic)

M-H
Mueller-Hinton (agar)

Mh
mandible head

mH, mh
millihenry

μH
microhenry

MHA
2-hydroxy-4-(methylthio)butyric acid
(calcium salt in poultry feed)
methemalbumin
microangiopathic hemolytic anemia
microhemagglutination (test for syphilis)
middle hepatic artery
mixed hemiadsorption
Mueller-Hinton agar

MHATP, MHA-TP
microhemagglutination-*Treponema
pallidum*

MHB
maximum hospital benefit
Mueller-Hinton base (a medium)

MHb
medial habenula

methemoglobin
myohemoglobin

MHBSS
modified Hank's balanced salt solution

MHC
major histocompatibility complex
mental health clinic
multiphasic health checkup

μ-HCD
μ (mu) heavy-chain disease

mhcp
mean horizontal candle power

MHD
magnetohydrodynamics
maintenance hemodialysis
mean hemolytic dose
Metahydrin
minimum hemolytic dilution

MHD, M.H.D.
minimum hemolytic dose

MHDPS
Mental Health Demographic Profile
System

MHEC
Multiphasic Health Examination Clinic

mHg
millimeters of mercury

MHI
malignant histiocytosis of the intestine

MHIP
1-(3-methylphenoxy)-2-hydroxy-3-
isopropylaminopropane (toliprolol—
β-adrenergic blocker)

MHLC
Multidimensional Health Locus of
Control (diagnostic scale)

MHLS
metabolic heart load simulator

MHMA
3-methoxy-4-hydroxymandelic acid
(misnamed vanillylmandelic acid)

MHN
massive hepatic necrosis
morbus haemolyticus neonatorum

MHNTG
multiheteronodular toxic goiter

MHO
microsomal heme oxygenase

mho
reverse ohm; reciprocal of impedance;
siemens unit

MHP
maternal health program
mercurihydroxypropane (1-mercuri-2-
hydroxypropane)

MHPA
mild hyperphenylalaninemia
Minnesota-Hartford Personality Assay

MHPG
3-methoxy-4-hydroxyphenylglycol
(biochemical tool)

MHR
major histocompatibility region
maternal heart rate
maximal heart rate
maximum heart rate
methemoglobin reductase

MHRI
Mental Health Research Institute

MHS
major histocompatibility system
malignant hyperthermia susceptible
(patients)

MHSA
microaggregated human serum albumin

MHT
multiphasic health testing

MHTI
minor hypertensive infant

MHV
magnetic heart vector
minimal height velocity
mouse hepatitis virus
murine hepatitis virus

MH virus
murine hepatitis virus

MHW
medial heel wedge (re: podiatry)
mental health worker

M Hx
medical history

MHz
megahertz

MI
massa intermedia (adhesio
interthalamica)
maturation index
medical inspection
melanophore index
menstrual induction
mental illness
mesio–incisal (re: Dent)
metabolic index
migration index
migration inhibition

mild irritant
mitotic index (re: cell cycle)
mitral incompetence
mitral insufficiency
mononucleosis infectiosa
morphology index
motility index
myocardial ischemia
myo-inositol

MI, M.I.
myocardial infarction

Mi
mitomycin

MIA
medically indigent adult

MIAN
Medicine intern admit note

MIAP
modified innervated antral pouch

MIBK
methyl isobutyl ketone (solvent)

MIC
major immunogene complex
maternal and infant care
maternity and infant care
medical intensive care
methacholine inhalation challenge
    (response)
minimal inhibitory concentration
minimal isorrheic concentration
minimum inhibition concentration
minimum inhibitory concentration (re:
    lab tests)
model immune complex

MIC, mic.
microscopic
microscopic (findings in centrifuged
    urinary sediment)
microscopy

MiC
minocycline (antibacterial)

MICC
mitogen-induced cellular cytotoxicity

MICG
macromolecular insoluble cold globulin

mic. pan.
mica panis (L. bread crumb)

MICR
magnetic ink character recognition (re:
    computers)
methacholine inhalation challenge
    response

micro.
microscopic

microscopic (findings)
microscopy

Microbiol, microbiol.
microbiology

microbiol.
microbiological

microcryst.
microcrystalline

MICU
medical intensive care unit
mobile intensive care unit

MID
maximum inhibiting dilution
mesioincisodistal (re: Dent)
minimal inhibiting dose
minimal inhibitory dose
minimum inhibitory dilution
minimum irradiation dose
multi-infarct dementia
multiple ion detection

MID, M.I.D.
minimal infecting dose
minimum infective dose

mid.
middle

mid. sag.
midsagittal

MIF
macrophage-inhibiting factor
macrophage inhibitory factor
maximal inspiratory flow (rate)
melanocyte inhibitory factor
melanocyte (-stimulating hormone)-
    inhibiting factor
melanocyte (-stimulating hormone
    release-) inhibiting factor
melanotrop(h)ic-inhibiting factor
    (melanostatin)
merthiolate-iodine-formaldehyde
    (technique for fecal examination)
microimmunofluorescence
midinspiratory flow
migration inhibition factor
migration inhibitory factor (for
    macrophages)
migratory-inhibiting factor
mixed immunofluorescence
müllerian-inhibiting factor

MIFA
mitomycin C, 5-fluorouracil, and
    Adriamycin (doxorubicin) (re:
    chemotherapy)

MIFR
maximal inspiratory flow rate (re: Resp)
maximum inspiratory flow rate (re:
    Resp)

343

MIF tech.
merthiolate iodine formaldehyde
   technique

MIFV
Maferr Inventory of Feminine Values

MIG
measles immune globulin

MIg
malaria immunoglobulin
measles immunoglobulin
membrane immunoglobulin

MIGW
maximum increment in growth and
   weight

MIH
MSH (melanocyte-stimulating
   hormone)-inhibitory hormone
minimal intermittent (dosage of) heparin

MIKA
minor karyotypic abnormalities

MIKE
mass-analyzed ion kinetic energy

MIL
mother-in-law

mil.
military
milliliter

millihg
millimeters of mercury (pressure)

millisec.
millisecond

MILP
mitogen-induced lymphocyte
   proliferation

mil. TB
miliary tuberculosis

MIME
mean indices of meal excursions

MIMR
minimal inhibitor mole ratio

MIMV
Maferr Inventory of Masculine Values
   (re: Psychol)

MIN
medial interlaminar nucleus

MIN, min.
minim
minimal
minimum (L. minimum)
minute

min.
mineral
minor

/min.
per minute

MINA
monoisonitrosoacetone
   (isonitrosoacetone)

MINDO
modified intermediate neglect of
   differential overlap (method)

MINIA
monkey intranuclear inclusion agent
   (virus)

Mini-COAP
cyclophosphamide, Oncovin
   (vincristine), ara-C (cytarabine), and
   prednisone (re: chemotherapy)

MIO
motility indole ornithine (medium)

MIO, M.I.O.
minimal identifiable odor
minimum identifiable odor

MIP
maximum inspiratory pressure
mean incubation period
mean intravascular pressure
metacarpointerphalangeal (joint)
middle interphalangeal (joint—re:
   podiatry)
minimal inspiratory pressure

MIPN
Medicine intern progress note

MIQ
Minnesota Importance Questionnaire
   (re: Psychol)

MIR
multiple isomorphous replacement
   (method)

MIRD
Medical Internal Radiation Dose

MIRF
macrophage immunogenic (antigen)
   recruitment factor

MIRU
Myocardial Infarction Research Unit

MIS
management information system (re:
   computers/data processing)
medical information system (re:
   computers)
meiosis-inducing substance
müllerian-inhibiting substance

Mi S
mitral stenosis

Mis Astig
mixed astigmatism (L. miscere—to mix
one thing with another)

misc.
miscarriage
miscellaneous

MISG
modified immune serum globulin

MISS
Modified Injury Severity Scale

MISSGP
mercury in Silastic strain gauge
plethysmography

mist.
mistura (L. a mixture)

MIT
Male Impotence Test
marrow iron turnover
melodic intonation therapy
metabolism inhibition test
miracidial immobilization test
mitomycin
monoiodotyrosine (3-iodotyrosine; ITyr)

mit.
mitte (L. let go)

mit. insuf.
mitral insufficiency

MITO C
mitomycin C

mitt.
mitte (L. let go)

mitte sang.
mitte sanguinem (L. let go the blood
[blood letting procedure])

mitt. tal.
mitte tales (L. send such)

mitt. x tal.
mitte decem tales (L. send ten like this)

mIU
milli-international unit

μIU
micro-international unit

mixt.
mixtura (L. mixture)

MJ
marijuana
megajoule

MJA
mechanical joint apparatus

MJDQ
Minnesota Job Description
Questionnaire (re: psychological
testing)

MK
main kitchen
menaquinone (menadione—vitamin K_2)
monkey kidney
Morel-Kraepelin (disease)
Mounier-Kuhn (syndrome)

MK-6
menaquinone-6 (vitamin K_2)

MK-7
menaquinone-6 with a 3-heptaprenyl
side-chain (vitamin K_2)

MKB
megakaryoblast

MKC
monkey kidney cell

mkd.
marked

mkdly.
markedly

MKG, mkg
meter kilogram

MKS, M.K.S., mks
meter kilogram second (system)

MKTC
monkey kidney tissue culture

MKV
killed measles vaccine

ML
lingual margin
malignant lymphoma
Marie-Léri (syndrome)
maximal left
maximum (cardiac bulge) to left
medial lemniscus (re: Neuro)
meningeal leukemia
mesiolingual (re: Dent)
middle lobe (of lung)
molecular layer
motor latency
muscular layer
myeloid leukemia

ML, m.l.
marked latency
midline

M/L
monocyte to lymphocyte (ratio)
mother-in-law

M:L
monocyte-lymphocyte (ratio)

ML I
mucolipidosis I (isolate neuraminidase deficiency)

ML II
mucolipidosis II (I-cell disease)

ML III
mucolipidosis III (mild form of ML II)

ML IV
mucolipidosis IV (marked by corneal clouding and psychomotor retardation)

mL
millilambert

ml, ml.
milliliter (1/1000 of a liter)

μl
microliter

MLA
medium long-acting
mentolaeva anterior (position of fetus)
monocytic leukemia, acute
multilanguage aphasia

MLA, MLa
mesiolabial (re: Dent)

MLAI, MLaI
mesiolabio-incisal (re: Dent)

MLAP
mean left atrial pressure

MLaP
mesiolabiopulpal (re: Dent)

MLB
monaural loudness balance

MLb
macrolymphoblast

MLBP
mechanical low back pain

MLC
Marginal Line Calculus (Index)
minimal lethal concentration (re: Bact)
minimum lethal concentration
mixed leukocyte culture
mixed ligand chelate
mixed lymphocyte concentration
mixed lymphocyte culture
morphine-like compound
multilamellar cytosome
myelomonocytic leukemia, chronic

MLCK
myosin light chain kinase

MLCP
myosin light chain phosphatase

MLCR
mixed lymphocyte culture reaction

MLCT
metal-to-ligand charge transfer

MLCW
mixed lymphocyte culture, weak

MLD
marginal limbal distance (re: Ophth)
masking level difference
mesencephalicus lateralis dorsalis
metachromatic leukodystrophy
minimal lethal dose

MLD, M.L.D.
median lethal dose
minimum lethal dose

MLD 50, MLD50, MLD$_{50}$, mld$_{50}$
median lethal dose

MLF
medial longitudinal fasciculus (re: oculomotor and vestibular systems)
morphine-like factor

MLG
mitochondria lipid glucogen

ML-H
malignant lymphoma, histiocytic

MLI
mesiolinguo-incisal (re: Dent)
mixed lymphocyte interaction
motilin-like immunoreactivity

M line
M band (mesophragma—re: myofibrils)

MLL
malignant lymphoma, lymphoblastic

ML method
maximum likelihood method

ml/min/m^2
milliliters per minute per square meter

MLN
mesenteric lymph node

MLNS
mucocutaneous lymph node syndrome

MLO
mesiolinguo-occlusal (re: Dent)

MLP
mentolaeva posterior (position of fetus)
mesiolinguopulpal (re: Dent)
microsomal lipoprotein

ML-PDL
malignant lymphoma, poorly
    differentiated lymphocytic

MLR
mean length of response
middle latency response
mixed lymphocyte reaction
mixed lymphocyte response
mixed lymphocytic reaction

M/L ratio
monocyte-lymphocyte ratio

MLS
mean life span
median life span
median longitudinal section
middle lobe syndrome
mouse leukemia virus
mucolipidoses
myelomonocytic leukemia, subacute

MLT
mean latency time
median lethal time (radiation)
mentolaeva transversa (position of
    fetus)

MLTC
mixed leukocyte-trophoblast culture
mixed lymphocyte tumor cells

MLTI
mixed lymphocyte target interaction

MLU
mean length of utterance

MLV
Moloney's leukemogenic virus
monitored live voice
mouse leukemia virus
multilaminar large vesicles (type of
    liposome)
multilaminar vesicles
murine leukemia virus

MLVSS
mixed liquor volatile suspended solids

MM
the isoenzyme of creatinine kinase that
    contains two M subunits
macromolecule
malignant melanoma
manubrium of the malleus
Marshall-Marchetti (procedure—re:
    urinary incontinence)
megamitochondria
meningococcic meningitis
methadone maintenance
middle molecule
minimal medium
missmatch
morbidity, mortality
multiple myeloma

muscularis mucosae
myeloid metaplasia

MM, M.M., mm, m.m.
mucous membrane(s)

MM, mm.
medial malleolus
muscles

M & M
milk and molasses
morbidity and mortality

Mm
mandible mentum

mM.
millimolar
millimole

mm
methylmalonyl (-CoA mutase)
millimeter

mµ
millimicron (one one-millionth of a
    meter; one one-thousandth of a
    micron [10^{-3}]; nanometer is preferred
    term)

µm
micrometer (formerly micron—one-
    millionth of a meter)

µµ
micromicro (one trillionth or 10^{-12}; pico-
    is preferred)
micromicron

mm^2
square millimeter

mm^3
cubic millimeter

MMA
methylmalonic acid
multiple module access

MMAD
mass median aerodynamic diameter

MMATP
methadone maintenance and aftercare
    treatment program

MMC
migrating motor complex
migrating myoelectric complexes
minimal medullary concentration
minimum medullary concentration
mitomycin C (antineoplastic)

mµc.
millimicrocurie (nanocurie)

μμc.
micromicrocurie (picocurie)

MMD
mass median diameter (of particles)
minimal morbidostatic dose
minimum morbidostatic dose
myotonic muscular dystrophy

MME
M-mode echocardiography
mouse mammary epithelium

MMECT
multiple monitored electroconvulsive
   treatment

MMEF
maximal midexpiratory flow
maximum midexpiratory flow

MMEFR
maximal midexpiratory flow rate
maximum midexpiratory flow rate

M & M enema
milk and molasses enema

MMF
magnetomotive force
maximal midexpiratory flow
maximum midexpiratory flow (rate)
mean maximum flow

μμF
micromicrofarad

MMFG
mouse milk fat globule

MMFR
maximal midexpiratory flow rate
maximal midflow rate
maximum midexpiratory flow rate
maximum midflow rate

MMFV
maximum midexpiratory flow volume

MMG
mean maternal glucose

mμg.
millimicrogram (nanogram)

μmg.
micromilligram

μμg.
micromicrogram (picogram)

MMH
monomethylhydrazine (re: chemical
   syntheses)

mmHg
millimeters of mercury (Hg =
   hydrargyrum)

MMI
macrophage migration index
methylmercaptoimidazole
   (methimazole—re: thyroid inhibitor)
myelomonocytic leukemia

MMK
Marshall-Marchetti-Krantz procedure
   (re: stress incontinence)

MML
myelomonocytic leukemia

mM/L, mM/l
millimol(e)s per liter

MMLV
Moloney murine leukemia virus

MMM
microsome-mediated mutagenesis
myelofibrosis (myelosclerosis) and
   myeloid metaplasia (syndrome)

μmm.
micromillimeter

MMMF
man-made mineral fiber

MMMS
Merck molecular modeling system

MMN
morbus maculosus neonatorum

MMNC
marrow mononuclear cell

MMOA
maxillary mandibular odontectomy
   alveolectomy

M-mode
motion mode (TM-mode—re: diagnostic
   ultrasound)

M-mode u.
motion mode unit (re: ultrasonography)

mmol
millimol(e) (one-thousandth of a gram
   molecule [10^{-3}])

μmol
micromol(e)

mmole
millimol(e) (one-thousandth of a gram
   molecule [10^{-3}])

4 MMPD
4-methoxy-m-phenylenediamine (also
   called 2,4-DAA)

MMPI
Minnesota Multiphasic Personality
   Inventory (test)

mmpp, mm.p.p.
millimeters partial pressure

MMR
mass miniature radiography
maternal mortality rate
measles, mumps, rubella
mobile mass x ray
myocardial metabolic rate

MMS
methyl methanesulfonate (mutagen)

MMSC
methylmethioninesulfonium chloride
  (vitamin U—re: gastric disorders)

MMSE
mini-mental state examination

mm/sec
millimeters per second

MMSEL
mini-mental state examination,
  language

mm st, mmst.
muscle strength

mm str.
muscle strength

MMT
manual muscle test(-ing—re: PM&R)
mouse mammary tumor

MMTP
Methadone Maintenance Treatment
  Program

MMTV
mouse mammary tumor virus

mmu
millimass units

MMuLv
Moloney murine leukemia virus

MMY
Mental Measurements Yearbook (re:
  psychological testing)

MN
malignant nephrosclerosis
melena neonatorum
membranous nephropathy
mesenteric node
metanephrine
MN blood group (MNS blood group)
mononuclear (leukocyte)
motor neuron
mucosal neurolysis
multinodular
myoneural

MN, M/N, mn.
midnight

M-N
motility nitrate (medium)

M & N
morning and night

Mn
manganese (element)

^{52}**Mn**
radioactive isotope of manganese

^{53}**Mn**
radioactive isotope of manganese

^{54}**Mn**
radioactive isotope of manganese

^{56}**Mn**
radioactive isotope of manganese

mN
millinormal

μ**N**
magnetic moment of proton (proton
  magneton)
nuclear magneton

MNA
maximum noise area

MNAP
mixed nerve action potential

MNB
murine neuroblastoma

MNC
mononuclear cell

MNCV
motor nerve conduction velocity

MND
minimal necrosing dose
minimum necrosing dose
modified neck dissection
motor neuron disease

MNG
N-methyl-N'-nitroso-N-nitroguanidine
  (carcinogen; mutagen)

mng.
morning

MNJ
myoneural junction

MNL
maximum number of lamellae
mononuclear leukocytes

MNMK
maximum number of microbes killed

MNNG
N-methyl-N'-nitro-N-nitrosoguanidine
(carcinogen; mutagen)

MNP
mononuclear phagocyte

MNPA
d-2-(6-methoxy-2-naphthyl)propionic
acid (naproxen—anti-inflammatory;
analgesic; antipyretic)

MNSER
mean normalized systolic ejection rate

MNWLT
Modified New World Learning Test

MO
manually operated
Medical Officer
mesio-occlusal (re: Dent)
metastases, zero
mineral oil
Minor-Oppenheim (syndrome)
minute output (re: heart)
molecular orbit (contour)
molecular orbital
mono-oxygenase
morbidly obese

MO, mo.
month

MΩ
megohm (formerly M)

μΩ
microhm

MO$_2$
myocardial oxygen (consumption)

Mo
mode
Moloney (strain)
molybdenum (element)

^{99}Mo
molybdenum-99

mo
morgan (unit of relative distance—re:
genetics)

μo
permeability of free space (rationalized)

MOA
mechanism of action

MOAB
(murine) monoclonal antibodies

MOB
4-methoxy-2-hydroxybenzophenone
(oxybenzone—ultraviolet screen)

(nitrogen) mustard, Oncovin, bleomycin
(re: chemotherapy)

MOB-III
mitomycin C, Oncovin (vincristine),
bleomycin, and cisplatin (re:
chemotherapy)

mob.
mobile
mobility
mobilization

mobil.
mobility

MOC
maximum oxygen consumption

MOCA
4,4'-methylenebis[2-chloroaniline] (also
called DACPM— curing agent)

MoCM
molybdenum-conditioned medium

MOD
maturity onset diabetes
mesio-occlusodistal (re: Dent)

MOD, mod.
moderate

mod.
moderately
modicus (L. moderate-sized)
modified
modulation
modulus (L. a little measure)

MODEM, modem
modulator/demodulator (re: computers)

MODM
mature-onset diabetes mellitus

mod. praesc.
modo praescripto (L. in the manner
prescribed)

MODS
Medically Oriented Data System

MODY
maturity onset diabetes of the young

MOF
marine oxidation/fermentation (medium)
MeCCNU (semustine), Oncovin
(vincristine), and 5-fluorouracil (re:
chemotherapy)
methoxyflurane (an anesthetic)
multiple organ failure

MOF-STREP, MOF-Strep
MeCCNU (semustine), Oncovin
(vincristine), 5-fluorouracil, and
streptozocin (re: chemotherapy)

mohm
mobile ohm (unit of mechanical
  mobility)

MOI
maximum oxygen intake
multiplicity of infection

MOJAC
mood, orientation, judgment, affect,
  content (re: Psychol)

MOL
machine-oriented language (re:
  computers)
molecular layer

mol
mole (unit of quantity of matter—
  elementary entities must be specified
  when mol is used)

mol.
molecular
molecule

molc
molar concentration

moll.
mollis (L. soft)

mol/l
molecules per liter

mol. wgt.
molecular weight

MOL WT, Mol wt., mol wt, mol. wt.
molecular weight

MOM
milk of magnesia
mucoid otitis media

MOMA
methoxyhydroxymandelic acid
  (4-hydroxy-3-methoxymandelic
  acid; misnamed vanillylmandelic
  acid)

MO-MOM
mineral oil and milk of magnesia

MO & MOM
mineral oil and milk of magnesia

MOMP
mechlorethamine, Oncovin (vincristine),
  methotrexate, and prednisone (re:
  chemotherapy)

MON, Mon
Monday

mon.
monocyte
month

Mono
(infectious) mononucleosis

mono.
monocyte

Monos
monocytes

MOP
major organ profile
medical outpatient
Mustargen (nitrogen mustard), Oncovin,
  prednisone (re: chemotherapy)

5-MOP
5-methoxypsoralen (re: psoriasis)

8-MOP
8-methoxypsoralen (pigmentation
  agent)

MOP-BAP
mechlorethamine (nitrogen mustard),
  Oncovin (vincristine), procarbazine,
  bleomycin, Adriamycin (doxorubicin),
  and prednisone (re: chemotherapy)

MOPP
mechlorethamine (nitrogen mustard),
  Oncovin (vincristine), procarbazine,
  and prednisone (re: chemotherapy)
Mustargen hydrochloride
  (mechlorethamine hydrochloride),
  Oncovin (vincristine), procarbazine,
  and prednisone (re: chemotherapy)
Mustine hydrochloride
  (mechlorethamine hydrochloride),
  Oncovin (vincristine), procarbazine,
  and prednisone (re: chemotherapy)

MOPP/ABV hybrid
(nitrogen) mustard, Oncovin,
  procarbazine, prednisone,
  Adriamycin, bleomycin, vinblastine
  (re: chemotherapy)

MOPP-BLEO, MOPP-Bleo
mechlorethamine (nitrogen mustard),
  Oncovin (vincristine), procarbazine,
  prednisone, and bleomycin (re:
  chemotherapy)

MOPPHDB
(nitrogen) mustard, Oncovin,
  procarbazine, prednisone, and high-
  dose bleomycin (re: chemotherapy)

MOPPLDB
(nitrogen) mustard, Oncovin,
  procarbazine, prednisone, and low-
  dose bleomycin (re: chemotherapy)

MOPr
(nitrogen) mustard, Oncovin,
  procarbazine (re: chemotherapy)

MOPV
monovalent oral poliovirus vaccine

MOR
morphine

MORA
mandibular orthopaedic repositioning
appliance

MORD
magnetic optical rotatory dispersion (re:
chemistry)

mor. dict.
more dicto (L. in the manner directed)

morph.
morphine
morphological
morphology

mor. sol.
more solito (L. in the usual way, manner,
as accustomed)

mort.
mortality

mortal.
mortality

MOS
medial orbital sulcus
metal oxide semiconductor (re:
computers)
myelofibrosis osteosclerosis

mOs
milliosmolal
milliosmolar
milliosmole

mos
mosaic (re: cytogenetics)

mos.
months

MOSFET, MOS-FET
metal oxide semiconductor field effect
transistor

MOsm, mOsm, mosm
milliosmolar
milliosmole

m osmole
milliosmole

MOT
mini-object test
mouse ovarian tumor

MOTT
mycobacteria other than tubercle
(bacilli)

MotV
motor nucleus of the trigeminal V (fifth)
nerve

MOUS
multiple occurrences of unexplained
symptoms

MOVC
membranous obstruction of vena cava

MOVE
medically oriented vocational education

MOX
moxalactam (an anti-infective)

MP
macrophage
matrix protein
mean pressure
medial plantar
medical payment
melphalan and prednisone (re:
chemotherapy)
membrane potential
menstrual period
mentum posterior (position of fetus)
mercaptopurine (an antineoplastic
agent)
Merzbacher-Pelizaeus (disease)
mesiopulpal (re: Dent)
metacarpophalangeal
metaphalangeal
metatarsophalangeal
methylprednisolone (a glucocorticoid)
methylprednisolone (sodium
succinate—a glucocorticoid)
middle phalanx
modulator protein
moist pack
monophosphate
motor power
mouthpiece
mouth pressure
mucopolysaccharide
multipara
multiparous
muscle potential
mycoplasmal pneumonia
myenteric plexus

MP, mp.
melting point (melts; melting at—when
followed by a figure denoting
temperature)

MP, m.p.
modo praescripto (L. in the manner
prescribed)

6 MP, 6MP, 6-MP
6-mercaptopurine (antineoplastic
agent)

8-MP
8-methoxypsoralen (pigmentation agent)

MPA
main pulmonary artery
medial preoptic area
medroxyprogesterone acetate (a progestin)
methylprednisolone acetate (a glucocorticoid)
minor physical anomaly

MPa
megapascal

MPAP
mean pulmonary arterial pressure
mean pulmonary artery pressure

MPB
male pattern baldness
menadione dimethylpyrimidinol bisulfite (veterinary— vitamin)
meprobamate

MPC
marine protein concentrate
maximum permissible concentration
mean plasma concentration
meperidine, promethazine, chlorpromazine
(minimum) mycoplasmacidal concentration
minimum protozoacidal concentration

MPCD
minimum perceptible color difference

MPCL
Mooney Problem Check List (re: Psychol)

MPCN
microscopically positive, culturally negative

MPCU
maximum permissible concentration of unidentified (radionucleotides in water)

MPCUR
maximum permissible concentration of unidentified radionuclides

MPD
main pancreatic duct
mean population doubling
membrane potential difference
minimal papular dose
minimal phototoxic dose
minimum perceptible difference
minimum port diameter
Minnesota Percepto-Diagnostic (re: Psychol)
multiplanar display

myeloproliferative disorder
myofascial pain dysfunction

MPD, M.P.D.
maximal permissible dose
maximal pyrogene dosis
maximum permissible dose

MPDS
myofascial pain dysfunction syndrome

MPDT
Minnesota Percepto-Diagnostic Test (re: Psychol)

MPDW
mean percent desirable weight

MPE
maximal possible effect
maximum possible error

MPEC
monopolar electrocoagulation

MPED
minimal phototoxic erythema dose

MPEH
methylphenylethylhydantoin

M period
mitotic period (re: cell growth cycle)

MPF
maturation promoting factor

MPFM
mini-Wright peak flow meter

MPG
magnetopneumography
methyl green pyronin

MPGM
monophosphoglycerate mutase

MPGN
membrane proliferative glomerulonephritis
membranoproliferative glomerulonephritis
membranous proliferative glomerulonephritis
mesangioproliferative glomerulonephritis

MPH
male pseudohermaphroditism
milk protein hydrolysate

mph
miles per hour

M phase
the phase of mitosis (re: cell growth cycle)

MPI
mannosephosphate isomerase
Master Patient Index (re: medical
    records)
Maudsley Personality Inventory
maximal permitted intake
maximum point of impulse
Motor Problems Inventory
Multiphasic Personality Inventory
Multivariate Personality Inventory
myocardial perfusion imaging

MPJ
metacarpophalangeal joint
    (articulationes
    metacarpophalangeae)
metatarsophalangeal joint
    (articulationes metatarsophalangeae)

MP joint
metacarpophalangeal joint
    (articulationes
    metacarpophalangeae)
metatarsophalangeal joint
    (articulationes metatarsophalangeae)

MP Jt
metacarpophalangeal joint
metatarsophalangeal joint

MPL
maximum permissible level
melphalan
mesiopulpolingual

MPLA, MPLa
mesiopulpolabial

MPM
malignant papillary mesothelioma
medial pterygoid muscle
multiple primary malignancy
multipurpose meal
Murphy (kidney) punch maneuver

MPMP
(N-methyl-3-
    piperidyl)methylphenothiazine
    (mepazine—tranquilizer)

MPMT
Murphy punch maneuver test (re:
    kidneys)

MPMV, M-PMV
Mason-Pfizer monkey virus

MPN
most probable number

MPO
maximum power output
myeloperoxidase

MPOA
medial preoptic area (re: Neuro)

MPOD
myeloperoxidase deficiency

MPP
massive periretinal proliferation
maximum perfusion pressure
medial pterygoid plate

MPPG
microphotoelectric plethysmography

MPPT
methylprednisolone pulse therapy

MPQ
McGill Pain Questionnaire

MPR
marrow production rate
massive preretinal retraction
maximum pulse rate

MPRE
minimum pure radium equivalent

M protein
M component (homogeneous protein
    seen in plasma cell dyscrasias, such
    as myeloma and macroglobulinemia)
monoclonal protein

MPS
Managerial Philosophies Scale (re:
    psychological testing)
mononuclear phagocyte system
movement produced stimuli
mucopolysaccharide
mucopolysaccharidosis
multiphasic screening
myocardial perfusion scintigraphy

MPS II
mucopolysaccharidosis II (Hunter)

MPS IIIA
mucopolysaccharidosis IIIA, IIIB
    (Sanfilippo)

MPS IIIB
mucopolysaccharidosis IIIA, IIIB
    (Sanfilippo)

MPS IVA, IVB
mucopolysaccharidosis IVA, IVB
    (Morquio)

MPS VI
mucopolysaccharidosis VI (Maroteaux-
    Lamy)

MPS VII
mucopolysaccharidosis VII (Sly)

MPSI
Mental Process Short Inventory

MPS IH, MPS I-H
mucopolysaccharidosis I (Hurler)

MPS IHS
mucopolysaccharidosis IHS (Hurler-Scheie)

MPS IS, MPS I-S
mucopolysaccharidosis IS (Scheie)

MPSRT
matched pairs signed rank test

MPT
maximum predicted phonation time

MPTAH
Mallory's phosphotungstic acid hematoxylin

MPV
mean platelet volume
metatarsus primus varus (re: podiatry)

MPX
multiplex (re: computers)
multiplexer (re: computers)

MQ
memory quotient

MQC
microbiologic quality control

MQR
multiplier-quotient register (re: computers)

MR
Maddox rod
magneresistant
mandibular reflex
mannose-resistant
maximal right
maximum (cardiac bulge) to right
measles-rubella
medial rectus (muscle)
median raphe
medical record
medical rehabilitation
medical release
medication responder
medicine radiation
medicine reaction
medium range
Melkersson-Rosenthal (syndrome)
menstrual regulation
mental retardation
mentally retarded
mesencephalic raphe
metabolic rate
methemoglobin reductase
methyl red (an indicator)
milk ring (test—re: brucellosis)
mitral reflux
mitral regurgitation
modulation rate
mortality rate
mortality ratio
multicentric reticulohistiocytosis

multiplication rate
multiplicity reactivation
muscle receptor
muscle relaxant
myotactic reflex

MR, M/R, m.r.
may repeat

M R
maintenance and repair

M & R
measure and record

Mr
mandible ramus

M_r
molecular (weight) ratio

mR, mr, mr.
milliroentgen

μR, μr
microroentgen

MRA
main renal artery
marrow repopulating activity
melody, rhythm, accent
mid-right atrium
multivariate regression analysis

mrad
millirad

MRAN
medical resident admitting note
Medicine resident admit note

MRAP
maximal resting anal pressure
mean right atrial pressure

MRAS
main renal artery stenosis

MRBC
monkey red blood cell (receptor)
monkey red blood cells
mouse red blood cell

MRBF
mean renal blood flow

MRC
methylrosaniline chloride (gentian violet, crystal violet)
Müller-Ribbing-Clément (syndrome)

MRD
margin reflex distance (re: Ophth)
maximum rate of depolarization
Medical Record Department
method of rapid determination
minimal reacting dose
minimal renal disease

minimal residual disease
minimum reaction dose

MRD, M.R.D.
minimum reacting dose

MRD$_2$
marginal reflex distance 2

mrd
millirutherford (unit of radioactivity)

MRE
manual resistive exercise (re: physical
  therapy)
maximal respiratory effectiveness
minimum risk estimate

MR-E
methemoglobin reductase

MREI
mean rate ejection index

mrem
millirem
milliroentgen equivalent man
milliroentgen equivalent, man
milliroentgen equivalent—man
milliroentgen-equivalent-man

mrep
milliroentgen equivalent physical
milliroentgen equivalent, physical
milliroentgen equivalent—physical
milliroentgen-equivalent-physical

MRF
medical record form
melanocyte-stimulating hormone-
  releasing factor
mesencephalic reticular formation
midbrain reticular formation
mitral regurgitant flow
moderate renal failure
müllerian regression factor

MRF, mRF
monoclonal rheumatoid factor

MRFC
mouse rosette-forming cells

MRFIT
multiple risk factor intervention trial

MRFT
modified rapid fermentation test

MRH
MSH (melanocyte-stimulating
  hormone)-releasing hormone

MRHA
mannose-resistant hemagglutination

mrhm
milliroentgen per hour at one meter

MRHT
modified rhyme hearing test

MRI
magnetic resonance imaging
moderate renal insufficiency

MRIF
MRH (melanocyte-stimulating hormone)
  release-inhibiting factor

MRIH
melanocyte (stimulating hormone)
  release-inhibiting hormone

M&R I&O
measure and record intake and output

MRK syndrome
Mayer-Rokitansky-Kuester syndrome

MRM
modified radical mastectomy

MRN
malignant renal neoplasm

mRNA
messenger RNA (ribonucleic acid)

MRO
muscle receptor organ
no masses or rebound

MR θ
no masses or rebound

MRP
maximum reimbursement point
mean resting potential

MRPAH
mixed reverse passive antiglobulin
  hemagglutination

MRR
marrow release rate
maximal relaxation rate
maximum rate of rise

MRS
mania rating scale
median range score

MRSA, MR-SA
methicillin-resistant *Staphylococcus*
  aureus

MRT
major role therapy
mean residence time
median reaction time
median recognition threshold
median relapse time
medical records technology
Metropolitan Readiness Tests (re:
  psychological testing)
milk-ring test (abortus-Bang-ring test)

modified rhyme test
muscle response test

MR test
milk ring test (abortus-Bang-ring)

MRU
mass radiography unit
measure of resource use
minimal reproductive units (re:
  bacteriology)

MRUS
maximum rate of urea synthesis

MRV
minute respiratory volume
mixed respiratory vaccine

MRVP
mean right ventricular pressure
methyl red, Voges-Proskauer (test)

M.R. X 1
may repeat one time

MS
Marie-Sée (syndrome)
Marie-Strümpell (disease)
mass spectrometry
mechanical stimulation
mediastinal shift
medical supplies
mental status
(activating) metal (ion) substrate
  (complex)
microscope slide
mitral sounds
modal sensitivity
molar solution
Mongolian spot
Morquio-Silfverskiöld (syndrome)
motile sperm
mucosubstance
multiple sclerosis
muscle shortening
muscle strength
muscular strength
musculoactive substance
musculoskeletal

MS, M.S.
morphine sulfate

MS, m.s.
mitral stenosis

M/S
meters per second

MS-1
strain of hepatitis virus A

MS-2
strain of hepatitis virus B

MS III
third-year medical student

MS IV
fourth-year medical student

MS-222
tricaine methanesulfonate (tricaine; 3-
  aminobenzoic acid ethyl ester
  methanesulfonate—re: veterinary
  medicine)

Ms
murmurs
muscles

Ms, ms
manuscript

M/s^2, m/s^2
meters per second squared

ms
millisecond

ms-
meso- (internally compensated—re:
  chemistry)

μs
microsecond

MSA
major serologic antigen
male specific antigen
mannitol salt agar (plate)
Marriage Skills Analysis
medical short appointment
membrane-stabilizing action
membrane-stabilizing activity
mine safety appliance
mouse serum albumin
multichannel signed averager
Multidimensional Scalogram Analysis
multiplication-stimulation activity

MSAA
multiple sclerosis-associated agent

MSAP
mean systemic arterial pressure

MSAS
Mandel Social Adjustment Scale

MSAT
Minnesota Scholastic Aptitude Test

MSB
mid-small bowel
most significant bit (re: binary numbers)

MSBLA
mouse-specific B lymphocyte antigen

MSBOS
maximum surgical blood order schedule

MSC
most significant character (re: computers)
multiple sib case

MSCA
McCarthy Scales of Children's Abilities

MSCLC
mouse stem cell-like cell

MSCP, mscp
mean spherical candle power

MSCU
medical special care unit

MSD
mean-square deviation
mild sickle (cell) disease
most significant digit (re: binary numbers)
multiple sulfatase deficiency

MSDI
Martin S-D (suicide-depression) Inventory

MSE
medical support equipment
mental status examination

mse
mean square error

msec.
millisecond

μsec, μsec.
microsecond

MSER
mean systolic ejection rate
Mental Status Examination Record

MSES
medical school environmental stress

MSF
macrophage-slowing factor
macrophage-spreading factor
Mediterranean spotted fever
melanocyte-stimulating factor
migration-stimulating factor
modified sham feeding

MSG
monosodium glutamate

MSH
medical self-help
melanocyte-stimulating hormone
melanophore-stimulating hormone (intermedin)

MSHA
mannose-sensitive hemagglutination

MSHIF, MSH-IF
melanocyte-stimulating hormone-inhibiting factor

MSHRF
melanocyte-stimulating hormone-releasing factor

MSIS
Multi-State Information System (re: medical records)

MSK
medullary sponge kidney

MSL
midsternal line
multiple symmetric lipomatosis

MSLA
mouse-specific lymphocyte antigen

MSLR
mixed skin (cell-) leukocyte reaction

MSM
mineral salts medium

MSMA
monosodium methanearsonate (herbicide)

MSN
main sensory nucleus (re: Neuro)
mildly subnormal

MSO
medial superior olive (of brain)

Msp, m. sp.
muscle spasm

MSPGN
mesangial proliferative glomerulonephritis

MSPS
myocardial stress perfusion scintigraphy

MSQ
Managerial Style Questionnaire (re: psychological testing)
Mental Status Questionnaire
Minnesota Satisfaction Questionnaire (re: psychological testing)

MSR
monosynaptic reflex

MSRPP
multidimensional scale for rating psychiatric patients

MSRT
Minnesota Spatial Relations Test

MSS
mental status schedule

Minnesota Satisfactoriness Scales (re: Psychol)
minor surgery suite
motion sickness susceptibility
mucus-stimulating substance
multiple sclerosis susceptibility
muscular subaortic stenosis

MSS, mss
massage

Mss
manuscripts

MSSG
multiple sclerosis susceptibility gene

MSSST
Meeting Street School Screening Test (re: Psychol)

MST
mean survival time
mean swell time (botulism test)
median survival time

MSTh
mesothorium

MSTI
multiple soft tissue injuries

M stim.
muscle stimulation

M str.
muscle strength

MSU
maple syrup urine
Maximum Security Unit
memory for symbolic units (re: psychological testing)
midstream specimen of urine
monosodium urate
myocardial substrate uptake

MSUD
maple syrup urine disease

MSV
Mauriceau-Smellie-Veit (maneuver—re: OB)
maximal sustained (level of) ventilation
mean scale value
Moloney's sarcoma virus
murine sarcoma virus

MSVC
maximal sustained ventilatory capacity

MSVL
maximal spatial vector to the left

MSW
multiple stab wounds

M.S.W.D.
married, single, widowed, divorced

MSWYE
modified sea water yeast extract (agar)

MT
empty
malaria therapy
malignant teratoma
mammary tumor
mammilothalamic tract (re: Neuro)
manual traction
mastoid tip
maximal therapy
medial thalamus
medial thickness
medical treatment
melatonin
membrane thickness
mesangial thickening
methoxytryptamine (hypnotic, sedative potentiator)
methyltyrosine (metyrosine—antihypertensive—re: pheochromocytoma; tyrosine hydroxylase inhibitor)
microtherm
microtome
microtubule
midtrachea
minimum threshold
mitotic time
muscle test
muscles and tendons
music therapy

MT, M.T.
membrana tympana

MT, Mt
metatarsal

M-T
macroglobulin-trypsin (complex)

M/T
(no) masses or tenderness
myringotomy with tubes (inserted)

M & T
Monilia and *Trichomonas*
myringotomy and tubes

MTA
malignant teratoma anaplastic
mammary tumor agent
Management Transactions Audit (re: psychological testing)
metatarsus adductus (re: podiatry)
myoclonic twitch activity

MTAC
mass transfer-area coefficient

MTAD
membrana tympana auris dextrae (L.
  tympanic membrane of the left ear)

MTAI
Minnesota Teacher Attitude Inventory
  (re: psychological testing)

MTAL
medullary thick ascending limb

MTAS
membrana tympana auris sinistrae (L.
  tympanic membrane of the left ear)

MTAU
membranae tympani aures unitae (L.
  tympanic membranes of both ears)

MTB
methylthymol blue
Mycobacterium tuberculosis

MT bar
metatarsal bar (re: podiatry)

MTBE
methyl *tert*-butyl ether

MTBF
mean time between failures (re:
  computers)

MTC
mass transfer coefficient
maximum tolerated concentration
maximum toxic concentration
medullary thyroid carcinoma
mitomycin C (an antineoplastic)

99mTc
technetium-99m

MTD
maximally tolerated dose
maximum tolerated dose
metastatic trophoblastic disease
Monroe tidal drainage (re: urinary
  bladder)
multiple tic disorder

m.t.d.
mitte tales doses (L. send such doses)

MTDDA
Minnesota Test for the Differential
  Diagnosis of Aphasia

mtDNA
mitochondrial DNA (deoxyribonucleic
  acid)

MTDT
modified tone decay test

MTE
medical toxic environment

MTET
modified treadmill exercise testing

MTF
maximum terminal flow
modulation transfer factor
modulation transfer function

MTF(f)
modulation transfer function frequency
  (re: scintillating camera or CT
  scanner)

MTg
mouse thyroglobulin

MTH
mithramycin (an antineoplastic)

MTI
malignant teratoma, intermediate
minimum time interval
moving target indicator

MTLP
metabolic toxemia of late pregnancy

MTM
modified Thayer-Martin medium

mt mRNA
mitochondrial messenger RNA
  (ribonucleic acid)

MTOC
microtubule organizing center
mitotic organizing center

MTP
maximum tolerated pressure
medial tibial plateau
median time to progression
metatarsophalangeal
microtubule protein

MTPJ
metatarsophalangeal joint

MTQ
metolquizolone (methaqualone—
  hypnotic; sedative)

MTR
Meinicke turbidity reaction

MTRG, MTR/G
masses, tenderness, rebound, or
  guarding

MTR-O
no masses, tenderness, or rebound

M
T } 0
R

no masses, tenderness, or rebound

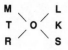

no masses, tenderness, or rebound,
and liver, kidneys,and spleen not
palpable

mt rRNA
mitochondrial ribosomal RNA
(ribonucleic acid)

MTS
multicellular tumor spheroid

MTST
maximal treadmill stress test

MTT
malignant teratoma, trophoblastic
maximal treadmill testing
mean transit time

mt tRNA
mitochondrial transfer RNA (ribonucleic
acid)

MTU
malignant teratoma, undifferentiated
Medical Therapy Unit
methylthiouracil (thyroid inhibitor)

M tuberc.
Mycobacterium tuberculosis

MTV
mammary tumor virus
metatarsus varus (re: podiatry)

MTX
methotrexate (antimetabolite;
antineoplastic)

MU
map unit
mate killers (*Paramecium aurelia*
carrying mu particles— re: genetics)
maternal uncle
Montevideo unit
motor unit (re: muscles)

MU, Mu, M.u.
mache unit (Mache Einheit—Dr.
Heinrich Mache—re: radium
emanations)

MU, mu, m.u.
mouse unit (re: gonadotrophins)

4-MU
4-methylumbelliferone (choleretic;
antispasmodic)

mU.
milliunit

mu
micron

μU, μU.
microunit

MUA
middle uterine artery
multiple unit activity

MUAP, M U A P
motor unit action potential (re:
physiatry)

MUC
maximum urinary concentration
mucosal ulcerative colitis

MUC, muc.
mucilago (L. mucilage)

muc.
mucoid
mucous (adjective)
mucus (noun)

muco-pur
mucopurulent

MUD
minimal urticarial dose

MUE
motor unit estimated

MUGA
multiple gated (image) acquisition
(analysis)

MUGEx
multigated (blood pool images during)
exercise

MUGR
multigated (blood pool images at) rest

mul. inj.
multiple injuries

mult.
multiple
multiplication

Multip, multip.
multipara

multip.
multiparous

multivits
multivitamins

MuLV
murine leukemia virus

MUMPS
Massachusetts (General Hospital)
Utility Multi-Programming System (a
programming language for complex

data, patient records, etc.—re:
computers)

MuMTV, MuMTv
murine mammary tumor virus

MUO
myocardiopathy of unknown origin

MUP
major urinary protein
maximal urethral pressure
motor unit potential (re: PM&R)

MURC
measurable undesirable respiratory
  contaminants

MurNAc
N-acetylmuramate (*N*-acetyl muramic
  acid)

musc.
muscles
muscular

musc. ligt.
musculoligamentous

mus-lig
musculoligamentous

MUST
medical unit, self-contained,
  transportable

mut.
mutilated
mutilation

MUU
mouse uterine units

MUW
mouse uterine weight

MUWU
mouse uterine weight unit

MV
measles virus
mechanical ventilation
megavolt
meningovascular
microvilli
millivolts
minute ventilation
minute volume
mixed venous
multivesicular
multivessel

MV, m.v.
mitral valve

Mv
mendelevium (former symbol; Md now
  used)

mV, mv.
millivolt

μV, μv.
microvolt

MVA
mechanical ventricular assistance
mitral valve area
motor vehicle accident
moving vehicle accident

MVB
multivesicular body

MVC
maximal voluntary contraction
maximum voluntary contraction
myocardial vascular capacity

MVD
Marburg virus disease
mitral valve disease
mouse vas deferens
multivessel (coronary artery) disease

MVE
mitral valve (leaflet) excursion
Murray Valley encephalitis (virus)

MVE-2
maleic vinyl ether

MV grad.
mitral valve gradient

MVH
massive variceal hemorrhage
massive vitreous hemorrhage

MVI
multivalvular involvement
multi-vitamin infusion

MVII
Minnesota Vocational Interest Inventory

MVL
mitral valve leaflet

MVLS
mandibular vestibulolingual sulcoplasty

MVM
microvillose membrane (microvillous)
minute virus of mice

MVMT
movement

MVN
medial ventromedial nucleus

MVO
maximum venous oxygen (saturation)

MVO$_2$
maximum venous oxygen
  (consumption)

mVO₂
minute venous oxygen consumption

MVOA
mitral valve orifice area

MVOS
mixed venous oxygen saturation

MVP
microvascular pressure
mitral valve prolapse

MVPP
(nitrogen) mustard, vinblastine,
  procarbazine, prednisone (re:
  chemotherapy)

MVPS
mitral valve prolapse syndrome

MVPT
Mertens Visual Perception Test (re:
  Psychol)
Motor-Free Visual Perception Test (re:
  Psychol)

MVR
massive vitreous retraction
microvascular research
mitral valve replacement
multiple valve replacement

MVRI
mixed vaccine respiratory infections

MV-SV
mitral valve-semilunar valve

mvt.
movement

MVV
maximal voluntary ventilation
maximum voluntary ventilation

MVV₁
maximal ventilatory volume

MVVPP
(nitrogen) mustard, vincristine,
  vinblastine, procarbazine, prednisone
  (re: chemotherapy)

MVW
Minot-von Willebrand (syndrome)

MW
Mallory-Weiss (syndrome)
mean weight

MW, M.W.
molecular weight

MW, mw
microwave

mW
milliwatt

μW, μw.
microwatt

M wave
muscle response from motor nerve
  stimulation

m wave
Müller cell activity (re:
  electroretinogram)

MWCB
manufacturer's working cell bank

MWD
microwave diathermy (re: physical
  therapy)
molecular weight distribution

MWLT
Modified Word Learning Test

MWMT
Monotic Word Memory Test

MWPC
multiwire proportional chamber

MWT
myocardial wall thickness

MWt
molecular weight

MX
matrix

Mx
maxwell (centimeter-gram-second unit
  of magnetic flux)

MY
myelocyte

MY, My, my.
myopia

My
myxedematous

my.
mayer (unit of heat capacity)

Myco
Mycobacterium (genus)

Mycol
mycology

MYD
myotonic (muscular) dystrophy

Myel
myelocyte

myel.
myelin
myelinated
myelogram

myelo.
myelocyte

myel. sched.
myelogram scheduled

MyG
myasthenia gravis

Myg
myriagram

Myl
myrialiter

Mym
myriameter

MyMD
myotonic muscular dystrophy

MYO
myoglobin

myo.
myocardial
myocardium

myocard.
myocardial
myocardium

Myop
myopia

MYS
myasthenic syndrome

MYX
myxoma

MZ
mantle zone
mezlocillin
monozygotic
monozygous

MZA
monozygotic twins (raised) apart

MZT
monozygotic twins (raised) together

N

N
antigenic determinant of erythrocytes
asparagine
inherited blood factor—MNS blood
  group
Necator (genus of hookworm)
negative
Negro
Neisseria (genus)
neomycin
nervus (L. nerve)
neural
neurologist
neurology
neuropathy
Neurospora (genus of fungi used in
  genetics and cellular biochemistry)
neutron number
neutrophil
newton (SI unit of force)
nicotinamide
Nitrobacter (genus)
nitrogen (element)
Nocardia (genus)
node
nodules
none
nonmalignant (re: tumors)
Nonne (globulin test)
noon
normality, equivalent/liter
nucleus
number of atoms
number density (number of moles of
  substance per unit of volume)
number of molecules
number of observations (re: statistics)
numerical aptitude (re: General
  Aptitude Test Battery)
population size
size of sample

N, *N*
Avogadro constant or number

N, n
haploid chromosome number (2n
  equals diploid number)
index of refraction (refractive index)
nasal
natus (L. born)
nerve
neuter
neutron dosage (unit of)
normal (re: manual muscle evaluation)

normal (re: solutions: 2N equals twice
  normal, N/2 or 0.5N equals one-half
  normal, etc.; also re: organs, structure
  and function)
number

N
normal (concentration)

N/10
decinormal ($\frac{1}{10}$ of normal solution
  strength)

0.1N
decinormal ($\frac{1}{10}$ of normal solution
  strength)

NI, NII, etc.
cranial nerves No. 1, No. 2, etc.

5′-N
5′-nucleotidase

^{13}N
nitrogen-13 (a cyclotron-produced
  radioisotope of nitrogen)

^{14}N
nitrogen-14 (the common nitrogen
  isotope)

^{15}N
nitrogen-15 (heavy nitrogen, the less
  common stable nitrogen isotope)

n
nano (prefix—one billionth of basic
  number, 10^{-9})
naris (L. nostril)
neutron
night
normal (also re: chemicals)
observed number of random events (re:
  statistics)

n
normal, as *n*-propyl

ν
frequency symbol
kinematic viscosity
lower case form of Greek letter nu
neutrino
number of degrees of freedom (re:
  statistics)

n, 2n, 3n, 4n
haploid, diploid, triploid, tetraploid
(number of chromosomes in cell,
strain, organism—re: genetics)

n̄
mean value of n for a number of
observations (re: statistics)

NA
Native American
neuraminidase
neurologic age
neutralizing antibody
neutrophil antibody
nicotinic acid
Nomina Anatomica
nonadherent
nonalcoholic
nonamnionic (nonamniotic)
noradrenaline
not admitted
not antagonized
not attempted
not available
nuclear antibody
nucleic acid
nucleus accumbens (septi—re: Neuro)
nucleus ambiguus (re: Neuro)
nursing action

NA, N.A.
numeric aperture
numerical aperture

NA, N/A
Negro adult
no abnormalities
not applicable
not available

N & A
normal and active

N_A, Na
Avogadro's number (constant)

Na
natrium (L. sodium—an element)
noise rating number (re: acoustics)

^{22}Na
radioactive isotope of sodium

^{24}Na
radioactive isotope of sodium

NAA
α-naphthaleneacetic acid (1-
naphthaleneacetic acid—re: plant
growth regulation)
neutral amino acid
neutron activation analysis
nicotinic acid amide
no apparent abnormalities

NAACP
neoplasia, allergy, Addison's (disease),
collagen (vascular disease), parasites

NAB
Novarsenobenzene
(neoarsphenamine—re: veterinary
medicine)

NaBr
sodium bromide

NAC
accessory nucleus (Monakow's—re:
Neuro)
N-acetyl-L-cysteine
nitrogen mustard, Adriamycin
(doxorubicin), and CCNU (lomustine)
(re: chemotherapy)
nonadherent cell

NAC-EDTA
N-acetyl-L-cysteine ethylenediaminetetraacetic acid

n-Ach
achievement need (re: Psychol)

NaCl
sodium chloride

NaClO
sodium hypochlorite

NaClO$_3$
sodium chlorate

NAcneu
N-acetylneuraminic acid

Na$_2$CO$_3$
sodium carbonate

Na$_2$C$_2$O$_4$
sodium oxalate

NAD
new antigenic determinant
nicotinamide-adenine dinucleotide
(formerly coenzyme I or DPN)
nicotinic acid dehydrogenase
no abnormal discovery
no abnormality demonstrable
no active disease
no acute distress
no apparent distress
normal axis deviation
nothing abnormal detected

NAD, N.A.D.
no appreciable disease

NAD$^+$
isocitrate dehydrogenase
oxidized form of nicotinamide-adenine
dinucleotide

NADH
reduced form of nicotinamide-adenine
  dinucleotide

NADP
nicotinamide-adenine dinucleotide
  phosphate (formerly called coenzyme
  II or TPN)

NADP$^+$
isocitrate dehydrogenase
oxidized form of nicotinamide-adenine
  dinucleotide phosphate

NADPH
reduced form of nicotinamide-adenine
  dinucleotide phosphate

NAE
net acid excretion

NaE, Na$_e$
exchangeable body sodium (natrium)

NAF
nafcillin
Negro adult female
net acid flux

NaF
sodium fluoride

NAG
narrow angle glaucoma
nonagglutinable (vibrios)
nonagglutinating

NAGA
α-N-acetylgalactosaminidase

NaHCO$_3$
sodium bicarbonate

NAI
net acid input (urinary)
neuraminidase inhibition
no acute inflammation
non-accidental injury
non-adherence index

NaI
sodium iodide

NAIR
non-adrenergic inhibitory response

NaI(T)
thallium-activated sodium iodide
  (sodium iodide crystal)

NaI(TI)
thallium-activated sodium iodide crystal
  (re: gamma-ray detectors)

NaK ATPase
sodium- and potassium-activated
  adenosine triphosphate

NAL
non-adherent leukocyte

NALL
null (cell line of) acute lymphocytic
  leukemia

NALP
neuroadenolysis of the pituitary

NAM
natural actomyosins
Negro adult male

NAMN
nicotinic acid mononucleotide

NAN
N-acetylneuraminic acid

NANA
N-acetylneuraminic acid

NANB
non-A, non-B (hepatitis)

NANBH
non-A, non-B hepatitis

NAND
NOT-AND (result is false only if all
  arguments are true; otherwise, the
  result is true; Cf. AND)

NANM
N-allylnormorphine (nalorphine—
  narcotic antagonist)

N ant/post
anterior and posterior "zones" (nerve
  cell groups— nuclei) of hypothalamus

NaOH
sodium hydroxide

NAP
nasion, point A, pogonion
  (measurement of convexity or
  concavity of facial profile)
nasion pogonion (angle of convexity—
  re: craniometrics)
nerve action potential
neutrophil alkaline phosphatase
nucleic acid phosphate

NAPA
N-acetyl-p-aminophenol
  (paracetamol—re: analgesic,
  antipyretic)
N-acetylprocainamide (a metabolite of
  procainamide—an anti-arrhythmic
  agent)

NAPAP
N-acetyl-p-aminophenol
  (paracetamol—re: analgesic;
  antipyretic)

NaPG
sodium pregnanediol glucuronide

NAPH
naphthyl

NAPQI
N-acetyl-*p*-benzoquinonimine

NAR
nasal airway resistance
no action required

NARC
narcotics (officer)

NARC, narc.
narcotic(s)

Narc
nucleus arcuatus (nucleus
   infundibularis—re: Neuro)

narco.
narcotics (hospital)
narcotics (officer)
narcotics (treatment center)

NAS
neonatal airleak syndrome
neuroallergic syndrome
normalized alignment score

NAS, nas.
nasal

NAS, n.a.s.
no added salt

NAT
N-acetyltransferase
natal
nonaccidental trauma

Nat, nat.
national
native
natural
nature

NATB
Nonreading Aptitude Test Battery

Natr
natrium (L. sodium)

NB
nail bed
Negri bodies (re: rabies virus)
nervus buccalis
neurometric (test) battery
newborn
nitrous oxide-barbiturate
normoblast
northbound (re: motor vehicle accident)
nuclear bag (certain intrafusal muscle

fiber nuclei of a neuromuscular
   spindle)
nutrient broth

NB, n.b.
nota bene (L. note well; take notice)

N/B
neopterin to biopterin (ratio)

Nb
niobium (element)

95Nb
radioactive niobium

NBD
neurologic bladder dysfunction
no brain damage

NBE
northern bean extract

NBEI synd.
non-butanol extractable iodine
   syndrome

NBF
not breast fed

NBI
neutrophil bactericidal index
no bone injury
no bony injury

NBICU
Newborn Intensive Care Unit

NB Int
Newborn Intensive (Care—unit)

nbl.
normoblast

NBM
normal bone marrow
nothing by mouth

NBME
normal bone marrow extract

NBN
narrow band noise

NBO
nonbed occupancy

NBP
needle biopsy of prostate

NBS
National Bureau of Standards
N-bromosuccinimide (catalylst)
Neri-Barré syndrome
no bacteria seen
normal blood serum
normal bowel sounds
normal brain stem

NBT
nitroblue tetrazolium
normal breast tissue

NBTE
nonbacterial thrombotic endocarditis

NBTNF
newborn, term, normal, female

NBTNM
newborn, term, normal, male

NBW
normal birth weight

NC
nabothian cyst
nasal cannula
nasal clearance
natural cytotoxic (cells)
natural cytotoxicity
neck complaints
Negro child
neonatal cholestasis
neural crest
neurologic check
neurologic control
nevus comedonicus
nitrocellulose
no card
no casualty
noise criteria
noncirrhotic
noncontributory
normal control
normocephalic
noseclip
not classified
not cultured
nucleocapsid

NC, N/C
no change
no charge
no complaints

N/C
nerves and circulation
numerical control (re: computers)

N:C
nuclear-cytoplasmic (ratio)

N & C
nerves and circulation

nC, nc, nc.
nanocurie (nCi preferred)

NCA
neurocirculatory asthenia
neutrophil chemotactic activity
nodulocystic acne
noncontractile area
nonspecific cross-reacting antigen
nuclear cerebral angiogram

N-CAM
nerve cell adhesion molecule

NCC
noncoronary cusp

NCCLS
National Committee for Clinical
  Laboratory Standards

NCCU
newborn convalescent care unit

NCD
nitrogen clearance delay
no congenital deformities
normal childhood diseases
normal childhood disorders
not considered disabling

NCDV
Nebraska calf diarrhea virus

NCE
negative contrast echocardiography
new chemical entities
nonconvulsive epilepsy

NCF
(polymorphonuclear) neutrophil
  chemotactic factor
no cold fluids

NCF(C)
neutrophil chemotactic factor
  (complement)

NCGL
nucleus corporis geniculati lateralis (re:
  Neuro)

NCI
National Cancer Institute
nuclear contour index (re: cells)
nucleus colliculi inferioris

nCi
nanocurie (one-billionth of a curie,
  10^{-9})

NCL
neuronal ceroid lipofuscinosis

NCMC
natural cell-mediated cytotoxicity

NCNCA
normochromic normocytic anemia

NCO
no complaints offered

NCP
nonclonogenic proliferating (cells
  [doomed])
noncollagen protein

NCPE
noncardiogenic pulmonary edema

NCR
nuclear-cytoplasmic ratio

NCRP
National Council on Radiation
    Protection (and Measurements)

NCS
neocarcinostatin (zinostatin—
    antineoplastic)
newborn calf serum
noncircumferential stenosis
noncoronary sinus

NCT
neural crest tumor
number connection test

NCV
nerve conduction velocity (study)
no commercial value
noncholera vibrio

NCVS
nerve conduction velocity studies

ND
nasal deformation
nasal deformity
nasolacrimal duct
natural death
neonatal death
neoplastic disease
nervous debility
neurotic depression
neutral density
Newcastle disease (avian influenza—
    transmittable to man)
New Drug
no data
no date
no disease
nondetectable
nondetermined
nondiabetic
nondisabling
normal delivery
normal dose
not detectable
not detected
not determined
not diagnosed
not dictated
nothing done
nucleus of Darkschewitsch
nurse's diagnosis

ND, N/D
not done

N/D
no defects

N&D
nodular and diffuse (lymphoma)

Nd
neodymium (element)
number of dissimilar (matches)

N_d, n_D
refractive index

^{147}Nd
radioactive isotope of neodymium

^{149}Nd
radioactive isotope of neodymium

NDA
New Drug Application
no data available
no demonstrable antibodies
no detectable activity

NDC
nondifferentiated cell
nuclear dehydrogenating clostridia

NDCD
National Drug Code Directory

NDE
near-death experience
nondiabetic extremity

NDEA
N-nitrosodiethylamine (anti-oxidant)

NDELA
N-nitrosodiethanolamine (carcinogen)

NDF
neutral detergent fiber
neutrophil diffraction factor
new dosage form
Nicolas-Durand-Favre (disease)

NDGA
nordihydroguaiaretic acid (anti-oxidant)

NDI
nephrogenic diabetes insipidus

NDIR
nondispersive infrared analyzer

NDMA
nitrosodimethylaniline (re: manufacture
    of organic compounds; industrial
    chemical)

N dm/vm
nucleus dorsomedialis-ventromedialis

NDP
net dietary protein
nucleoside 5'-phosphate

NDR
neonatal death rate

normal detrusor reflex
nucleus dorsalis raphe

NDRO
non-destructive read out (re:
  computers)

NDS
New Drug Submission
normal dog serum

NDT
neurodevelopmental treatment (re:
  physical therapy)
noise detection threshold
non-destructive testing

NDTI
National Disease and Therapeutic
  Index

NDV
Newcastle disease virus

Nd-YAG
neodymium-yttrium aluminum garnet
  (surgical laser)

NE
necrotic enteritis
neomycin (re: C & S reports)
nerve ending
nerve excitability (test)
neural excitation
neuroendocrine
neuroepithelium
neurologic examination
neutrophil elastase
never exposed
new employer
no effect
nonelastic
nonendogenous
norepinephrine
not enlarged
not evaluated
not examined
nutcracker esophagus

Ne
neon (element)

NEA
neoplasm embryonic antigen
no evidence of abnormality

NEB
neuroendocrine body

nebul.
nebula (L. a cloud [as a nebulizer])

NEC
necrotizing enterocolitis
neuroendocrine cell
no essential change
nonesterified cholesterol

not elsewhere classifiable
not elsewhere classified
not elsewhere coded
not enough cells

nec.
necessary

NED
no evidence of disease
no expiration date
normal equivalent deviation

NEEE
near east equine encephalomyelitis

NEEP
negative end-expiratory pressure

NEF
nephritic factor

NEFA
nonesterified fatty acids

NEG
neglect

NEG, neg.
negative (symbol: $-$)

Neg
Negro

NEI
National Eye Institute

NEISS
National Electronic Injury Surveillance
  System

NEJ
neuroeffector junction

NEM
N-ethylmaleimide (re: cancer research)
no evidence of malignancy

nema.
nematode (threadworm)

Nemb, nemb.
Nembutal

NEMD
nonspecific esophageal motor disorder
nonspecific esophageal motor
  dysfunction

neo.
neoarsphenamine (re: veterinary
  medicine)
neonatal

neoars.
neoarsphenamine (re: veterinary
  medicine)

neonat.
neonatal
neonatorum

neopl.
neoplasm

Neo-Syn
Neo-Synephrine hydrochloride
(phenylephrine hydrochloride—
adrenergic)

NEP
negative expiratory pressure
nephrology
no evidence of pathology
noise-equivalent power

NEPD
no evidence of pulmonary disease

neph.
nephritis

NEPHGE
nonequilibrium pH (gradient) gel
electrophoresis

NER
no evidence of recurrence

ner.
nervous
nervousness

NERD
no evidence of recurrent disease

NERO
noninvasive evaluation of radiation
output

nerv.
nervous
nervousness

NES
not elsewhere specified

NESS
national excess sodium syndrome

NET
nasoendotracheal tube
nerve excitability test
norethisterone

n. et m.
nocte et mane (L. night and morning)

ne. tr. s. num.
ne tradas sine nummo (L. deliver not
without the money [do not deliver
unless paid])

neu.
neurilemma

Neuro, neuro.
neurology

neuro.
neurologic

Neurol
neurology

neurol.
neurologic

Neuropath
neuropathologist
neuropathology

Neuro-Surg, neurosurg.
neurosurgeon
neurosurgery

neut.
neuter
neutral
neutralize
neutrophil

NEX
nose to ear to xiphoid

NEY
neomycin egg yolk (agar)

NEYA
neomycin egg yolk agar

NF
nafcillin
National Formulary
nephritic factor
neurofibromatosis
neurofilament
neutral fraction
noise factor
none found
nonfiltered
nonfluent
nonfunction
Nonne-Froin (syndrome)
nonwhite female
normal flow
not found
nylidrin hydrochloride (a
sympathomimetic amine)
nylon fiber

NF, N/F
Negro female

nF
nanofarad (formerly millimicrofarad)

NFB
nonfermenting bacteria

NFC
not favorably considered

NFD
neurofibrillary degeneration
no family doctor

NFE, nfe, nf.e.
non-ferrous extract

NFL
nerve fiber layer (re: Ophth)

NFM
northern fowl mite

NFP
natural family planning
no family physician
19-nortestosterone furylpropionate
(nandrolone—an anabolic)

NFPA
National Fire Protection Association (re:
hazardous chemicals)

NFS
nonfire setter

NFT
neurofibrillary tangle
Nitrazine fern test

NFTD
normal full term delivery

NFTSD
normal, full term, spontaneous delivery

NG
new growth
nitroglycerin
nodose ganglion (nodulous)
no growth
nongenetic
nongroupable

NG, N/G
no good

NG, ng.
nasogastric

ng, ng.
nanogram (millimicrogram)

NGA
nutrient gelatin agar

NGC
nucleus (reticularis) gigantocellularis
(re: medulla oblongata)

N-Ger
neurological geriatrics

NGF
nerve growth factor

NG fdgs
nasogastric feedings

NGGR
nonglucogenic/glucogenic ratio

NGI
nuclear globulin inclusion
nurses' global impressions

ng/ml
nanograms per milliliter

NGR
narrow gauze roll

NGS
normal goat serum

NGSA
nerve growth stimulating activity

NGT
normal glucose tolerance

NG tube
nasogastric tube

NGU
nongonococcal urethritis

NH
natriuretic hormone
neonatal hepatitis
neurologically handicapped
nodular histiocytic
nonhuman
nursing home

NH₃
ammonia

NH₄
ammonium (the radical form, NH_4^+
[NH_3 and H^+])
dilute ammonia water (reflex respiratory
stimulant)

NHA
nonspecific hepatocellular abnormality

NHAIS
Naylor-Harwood Adult Intelligence
Scale

NHC
neighborhood health center
neonatal hypocalcemia
nonhistone chromatin
nonhistone chromosomal (protein)
nursing home care

NH₄Cl
ammonium chloride

NHCP
nonhistone chromosomal protein

NHC protein
nonhistone chromosomal protein

NHDC
neohesperidin dihydrochalcone
 (sweetener)

NHDL
nonhigh-density lipoprotein

NHG
normal human globulin

NHH
neurohypophyseal hormone

NHK
normal human kidney

NHL
nodular histocytic lymphoma
non-Hodgkin's lymphoma

NH₃N
ammonia nitrogen

NHP
nonhemoglobin protein
nonhistone protein
normal human (pooled) plasma
nursing home placement

NHR
net histocompatibility ratio

NHS
normal horse serum
normal human serum

NHWM
normal human white matter

NI
neuraminidase inhibition
neurological improvement
no information
Noise Index
not identified
not isolated
nucleus intercalatus (re: Neuro)

Ni
nickel (element)

63Ni
radioactive isotope of nickel

65Ni
radioactive isotope of nickel

NIA
nephelometric inhibition assay (re:
 immunoassays)
neutrophil-inducing activity
no information available

NIA, nia.
niacin

NIB
non-involved bone

NIBS
nearly ideal binary solvent

NIC
Nomarski interference contrast (re:
 Optics—microscope)
nurse interim care

Nic
nicotinyl

NICU
Neonatal (Newborn) Intensive Care Unit
Neurological Intensive Care Unit
Neurosurgical Intensive Care Unit
nonimmunologic contact urticaria

NIDD
noninsulin-dependent diabetes

NIDDM
noninsulin-dependent diabetes mellitus

NIDS
nonionic detergent soluble

NIF
negative inspiratory force
neutrophil immobilizing factor
nifedipine
nonintestinal fibroblast

nif genes
nitrogen fixation (genes for)

NIg
non-immunoglobulin

nig.
niger (L. black)

NIH
National Institutes of Health

NIHL
noise-induced hearing loss

NIL
noise interference level
nothing in light

nil.
nihil (L. nothing)

NIMH
National Institute of Mental Health

NIP
nipple
no infection present
no inflammation present

NIPS
noninvolved psoriatic skin

NIPTS
noise-induced permanent threshold
 shift

NIR
near infrared

NIRA
nitrite reductase

NIRD
non-immune renal disease

NIS
N-iodosuccinimide
no inflammatory signs
non-immune sheep (serum)

NISM
(bed) nucleus of the stria medullaris

NIST
(bed) nucleus of the stria terminalis

NITD
noninsulin-treated disease

nit. ox.
nitrous oxide

nitro.
nitroglycerin

NITTS
noise-induced temporary threshold shift

NIV
nodule-inducing virus

NJ
nasojejunal

NK
natural killer (cell)
normal killer (cell)

NK, n/k
not known

N/K
(name) not known

NKA
no known allergies

NKC
nonketotic coma

NK cell
natural killer cell(s)

NKDA
no known drug allergies

NKH
nonketotic hyperglycemia

NKHA
nonketotic hyperosmolar acidosis

NKHS
normal Krebs-Henseleit solution

NKR
normal rat kidney

NKTS
natural killer target structure

NL
neural lobe
neutral lipid
nodular lymphoma
normal libido
normolipemic
Nyhan-Lesch (syndrome)

NL, Nl
normal

NL, n.l., n/l
normal limits

N_L
Loschmidt number/Loschmidt constant
(re: molecules in cubic meter of ideal
gas at s.t.p. [standard temperature
and pressure])

nl
nanoliter (millimicroliter)

nl.
non licet (L. it is not permitted; it is not
lawful)
non liquet (L. it is not clear)

NLA
neuroleptanalgesia
neuroleptanesthesia
normal lactase activity

NLAL
nodule-like alveolar lesion

NLB
needle liver biopsy

NLC & C
normal libido, coitus, and climax

NL C/Cl
normal libido, coitus, and climax

NLD
nasolacrimal duct
necrobiosis lipoidica diabeticorum

NLDL
normal low density lipoprotein

Nle
norleucine

NLF
nonlactose fermenting (organism)

NLM
National Library of Medicine
noise level monitor

NLMC
nocturnal leg muscle cramp

NLN
no longer needed

NLP
neurolinguistic programming
nodular liquifying panniculitis
no light perception
normal light perception

NLPD
nodular lymphocytic poorly
    differentiated

NLS
nonlinear least squares (method)
normal lymphocyte supernatant

NLSD
normal life span for dogs

NLT
Names Learning Test (re: Psychol)
normal lymphocyte transfer (test)
not less than
nucleus lateralis tuberis

NLX
naloxone (antinarcotic)

NM
neomycin
neuromedical
neuromedicine
nictitating membrane (L. nictitare—to
    wink)
night and morning
nitrogen mustard
nodular melanoma
nodular mixed
nonmalignant
nonmotile (re: bacteria)
nonwhite male
normetadrenaline
normetanephrine
not measurable
nuclear medicine
nuclear membrane

NM, N/M
Negro male
neuromuscular

NM, n/m
not measured
not mentioned

N & M
nerves and muscles

Nm, n.m., nm.
nux moschata (nutmeg)

N·m
newton-meter

nM
nanomolar (millimicromolar)

nm
nocte et mane (L. night and morning)

nm, nm.
nanometer (one-billionth of a meter,
    10^{-9}m)

n & m
nocte et mane (L. night and morning)

NMA
neurogenic muscular atrophy

NMATWT
New Mexico Attitude Toward Work Test
    (re: Psychol)

NMC
neuromuscular control

NMCD
nephrophthisis-medullary cystic disease

NMCPT
New Mexico Career Planning Testing
    (re: Psychol)

NMF
N-methylformamide
nonmigrating fraction (of spermatozoa)

NMI
no mental illness
no middle initial
normal male infant

NMJ
neuromuscular junction

NMJAPT
New Mexico Job Application
    Procedures Test (re: Psychol)

NMKOT
New Mexico Knowledge of Occupations
    Test

NML
nodular mixed lymphoma

NMM
nodular malignant melanoma
Nonne-Milroy-Meige (syndrome)

NMN
nicotinamide mononucleotide
no middle name
normetanephrine

NMN+
nicotinamide mononucleotide (reduced
    form)

nmol
nanomole (one-billionth of a mole,
    10^{-9}mol)

NMOR
N-nitrosomorpholine (4-
nitrosomorpholine—carcinogen)

NMP
normal menstrual period
nucleoside 5'-monophosphate

NMR
Neill-Mooser reaction
neonatal mortality rate
nictitating membrane response (L.
nictitare—to wink)
nuclear magnetic resonance
(spectroscopy)

NMRI
nuclear magnetic resonance imaging

NMS
neuroleptic malignant syndrome
neuromuscular spindle
normal mouse serum

NMSIDS
near-miss sudden infant death
syndrome

NMT
neuromuscular tension
neuromuscular transmission

NMTD
non-metastatic trophoblastic disease

NMTS
neuromuscular tension state

NMU
neuromuscular unit

NN
normally nourished
nurses' notes

NN, nn
neonatal

N:N
the azo group (nitrogen)

nn.
nervi (L. nerves)
nomen novum (L. new name)

NND
neonatal death
New and Nonofficial Drugs

NNE
neonatal necrotizing enterocolitis
non-neuronal enolase

NNI
noise and number index

NNM
neonatal mortality

N-nitrosomorpholine (4-
nitrosomorpholine—carcinogenic)

NNN
Nicolle-Novy-MacNeal (medium)
Novy-MacNeal-Nicolle (medium)
Novy-Nicolle-MacNeal (medium)

n. nov.
nomen novum (L. new name)

NNP
nerve net pulse

NNR
New and Nonofficial Remedies
not necessary to return

NNT
neonatally tolerant
nuclei nervi trigemini

NO
narcotics officer
nitric oxide
nitrous oxide
nonobese
nursing office

NO, n/o
none obtained

N₂O
nitrous oxide (dinitrogen monoxide)

No
nobelium (element)

No, no.
number

no.
numero (L. to the number of)
numerus (L. number)

nob.
nobis (L. to us [as a new species])

NOBT
nonoperative biopsy technique

noc.
noctis (L. of the night—[nocturnal])
nocturia

NO-CCE
no clubbing, cyanosis, or edema

no compl.
no complaints
no complications

Noct, noct.
nocte (L. night)

noct.
noctis (L. of the night—[nocturnal])
nocturia
nox (L. night)

NOCTI
National Occupation Competency
Testing (Program—re: Psychol)

noct. maneq.
nocte maneque (L. night and morning)

NOD
nodular (melanoma)
nonobese diabetic

NOEL
no observed effect level (of toxin)

no ess. abn.
no essential abnormalities

NOK
next of kin

nom. dub.
nomen dubium (L. a doubtful name)

NOMI
nonocclusive mesenteric infarction

nom. nov.
nomen novum (L. new name)

nom. nud.
nomen nudum (L. a naked name
[without designation])

noncontrib.
noncontributory

NON-REM, non-REM
nonrapid eye movement

non rep.
non repetatur (L. do not repeat—[no
refills])

non repet.
non repetatur (L. do not repeat—[no
refills])

NON REPETAT, non repetat.
non repetatur (L. do not repeat—[no
refills])

nonsegs.
nonsegmented (neutrophils)

nonspec.
nonspecific

nontend.
nontender

NOP
not otherwise provided (for)

NO-PYR
N-nitrosopyrrolidine (carcinogen)

NOR
noradrenaline

nucleolar organizing region (re:
cytogenetics)
result is false if and only if any
argument is true (re: logic; Cf. OR)

nor.
normal

nor-
prefix indicating a parent compound (re:
chemistry)

norleu.
norleucine

norm.
normal

normet.
normetanephrine

normoceph.
normocephalic

NORs
nucleolus organizer regions (re:
cytogenetics)

NOS
not on staff
not otherwise specified

nos.
numbers

NOSAC
nonsteroidal anti-inflammatory
compound

NOSIE
Nurses' Observation Scale for Inpatient
Evaluation (re: Psychol)

NOT
nocturnal oxygen therapy
nucleus of the optic tract

NOTT
nocturnal oxygen therapy trial

nov.
novum (L. new)

nov. n.
novum nomen (L. new name)

nov. sp.
nova species (L. new species)

NOW
negotiable order of withdrawal

NP
nasopharyngeal
nasopharynx
near point (re: Ophth)
nerve palsy
neuritic plaque
neuropathology

neuropsychiatric
neuropsychiatry
new patient
Niemann-Pick (disease)
nitrogen-phosphorus (detector—re: gas
    chromatography)
nitrophenide (veterinary—coccidiostat)
nitroprusside
nonpathologic
nonpaying
nonphagocytic
nonpracticing
nonproducer (cells)
no phone
no progression
normal plasma
normal pressure
not palpable
not perceptible
not performed
not practiced
nucleoplasmic (index)
nucleoprotein
nucleoside phosphorylase
nursing procedure

NP, Np
neurophysin

Np
neper (re: unit for comparing magnitude
    of two powers, usually electrical or
    acoustical—8·686 decibels)
neptunium (element)

^{237}Np
radioactive isotope of neptunium

np
nucleotide pair

n.p.
nomen proprium (L. proper name [label
    with])

NPA
nucleus of pretectal area (re: Neuro)

NPA, npa, n.p.a.
near point accommodation (re: Ophth)
near point of accommodation (re:
    Ophth)

NPa
nail patella

NPA acid
N-[3-(5-
    nitrofurfurylidene)carbazoyl]arsanilic
    acid (re: veterinary—coccidiostat)

Np-AVP
neurophysin associated with
    vasopressin

NPB
nodal premature beat
nonprotein bound

NPBF
nonplacental blood flow

NPC
nasopharyngeal carcinoma
nodal premature contractions
nonparenchymal cell
nonproductive cough
nucleus of posterior commissure (re:
    Neuro)

NPC, npc, n.p.c.
near point of convergence (re: Ophth)

NPCa
nasopharyngeal carcinoma

NP cult.
nasopharyngeal culture

NPD
natriuretic plasma dialysate
Niemann-Pick('s) disease
nitrogen-phosphorus detector (re: gas
    chromatography)
no pathologic diagnosis

NP detector
nitrogen-phosphorus detector (re: gas
    chromatography)

NPDL
nodular, poorly differentiated
    lymphocytes
nodular, poorly differentiated
    lymphocytic (lymphoma)

NPDR
nonproliferative diabetic retinopathy

NPE
neurogenic pulmonary edema
neuropsychologic examination
no palpable enlargement

N periv.
nuclei periventriculares (re:
    neuroendocrine)

NPF
nasopharyngeal fiberscope
no predisposing factor

NPFT
Neurotic Personality Factor Test

NPG
nonpregnant

NPH
neutral protamine Hagedorn (insulin)
normal pressure hydrocephalus

NPHI
neutral protamine Hagedorn insulin

NPI
neuropsychiatric institute
no present illness
nucleoplasmic index

NPJT
nonparoxysmal (AV) junctional
tachycardia

NPL
National Physics Laboratory
neoproteolipid

NPN
nonprotein nitrogen

NPO
preoptic nucleus

NPO, n.p.o.
non per os (L. nothing through the
mouth)

NPO/HS, n.p.o./h.s., npo.hs
nulla per os hora somni (L. nothing
through the mouth at bedtime)

NP polio.
nonparalytic poliomyelitis

NPOW
not prisoner of war

NPP
neuropsychologic performance

4-NPP
4-nitrophenylphosphate

NPPNG
nonpenicillinase-producing *Neisseria
gonorrheae*

NPR
net protein ratio (re: dietary protein)

NPS1
nail-patella syndrome, type 1

Nps
nitrophenylsulfenyl (a radical—re:
peptide synthesis, protein chemistry)

NPSA
normal pilosebaceous apparatus

NPSH
non-protein sulfhydryl (group)

NPT
neoprecipitin test
nocturnal penile tumescence
normal pressure and temperature

NPU
net protein utilization (re: dietary
protein)

NPV
negative pressure ventilation
nuclear polyhidrosis virus

NPV, N pv
nucleus paraventricularis (re:
neuroendocrine)

NPYR
N-nitrosopyrrolidine (carcinogen)

NQA
nursing quality assurance

NR
nerve root
neural retina
neutral red (an indicator)
noise reduction
nonreactive
nonrebreathing
nonreimbursable
no radiation
no reaction
no recurrence
no refill
no rehearsal
no report
no respirations
no response
no results
no return
normal
normal range
normal reaction
normotensive rat
not readable
not recorded
not resolved
nurse
nutritive ratio

NR, N_R
Reynold's number (re: turbulent gas
flow—R_e)

NR, n.r.
non repetatur (L. do not repeat—[no
refills])

N/R
not remarkable

nr.
near

NRA
nitrate reductase
nucleus raphe alatus (re: Neuro)
nucleus retroambigualis (re: Neuro)

NRB
non-rejoining (DNA strand) break

NRBC
normal red blood cell

NRBC, NRbc, Nrbc
nucleated red blood cell (mass)

NRC
National Research Council
noise reduction coefficient
not routine care
Nuclear Regulatory Commission

NRC, N.R.C.
normal retinal correspondence (re:
   Ophth)

NRCL
nonrenal clearance

NRD
nonrenal death

NREH
normal renin essential hypertension

NREM
nonrapid eye movements

NREMS
nonrapid eye movements, sleep

NRF
normal renal function

NRFC
nonrosette-forming cell

NRGC
nucleus reticularis gigantocellularis

NRH
nodular regenerative hyperplasia (liver)

NRI
nerve root involvement
nerve root irritation
neutral regular insulin

NRK
normal rat kidney

NRL
nucleus reticularis lateralis (re: Neuro)

NRM
normal range of motion
normal retinal movement
nucleus raphe magnus (re: Neuro)
nucleus reticularis magnocellularis (re:
   Neuro)

NRN
no return necessary

nRNA
nuclear RNA (ribonucleic acid)

NROM
normal range of motion

NRP
nucleus reticularis parvocellularis (re:
   Neuro)

NRPC
nucleus reticularis pontis caudalis (re:
   Neuro)

NRPG
nucleus reticularis paragigantocellularis
   (re: Neuro)

NRR
net reproductive rate
Noise Reduction Rating

NRS
nonimmunized rabbit serum
normal rabbit serum
normal reference serum
numerical rating scale

NRV
nucleus reticularis ventralis (re: Neuro)

NS
needle shower
nephrosclerosis
nephrotic syndrome
nervous system
neurologic survey
neurosecretory
neurosurgeon
neurosurgery
neurosurgical
neurosyphilis
neurotic score
nodular sclerosis
nonsmoker
nonsnorer
nonspecific
nonstimulation
nonstructural (protein)
nonstutterer
nonsymptomatic
Noonan syndrome
normal smoking
normal sodium (diet)
normal study
Norwegian scabies
no sample
no show
not seen
not specified
not stated
not sufficient
nuclear sclerosis (re: Ophth)

NS, N/S
normal saline
normal serum

NS, n.s.
no sequelae
no specimen

not significant
nylon suture

N-S
Northrupp-Sierra (prosthesis)

Ns
nerves

ns
nanosecond
non sequelae (L. no following
   [consequences])

NSA
normal serum albumin
no serious abnormality

NSA, n.s.a.
no salt added
no significant abnormality (-ties)

NSAD
no signs of acute disease

NSAE
nonsupported arm exercise

NSAIA
nonsteroidal anti-inflammatory agent

NSAID, NSAI(D)
nonsteroid anti-inflammatory drugs
nonsteroidal anti-inflammatory drug

NSAR AN
Neurosurgical assistant resident admit
   note

NSC
neurosecretory cells
nonservice connected
nonspecific suppressor cell
not service connected

NSC, n.s.c.
no significant change

NSCD
nonservice-connected disability

N sch.
nucleus suprachiasmaticus (re:
   neuroendocrine)

nsCHE
nonspecific cholinesterase

NSCJ
new squamocolumnar junction

NSCLC
nonsmall-cell lung cancer

NSD
Nairobi sheep disease
neonatal staphylococcal disease
nominal single dose

nominal standard dose (re:
   radiotherapy)
normal spontaneous delivery
normal standard dose
no significant defect
no significant deficiency
no significant deviation
no significant difference
no significant disease

NSE
neuron-specific enolase
nonspecific esterase
normal saline enema

N S̈E
nausea without emesis

nsec, nsec.
nanosecond

NSFTD
normal spontaneous full-term delivery

NSG
neurosecretory granules

nsg, nsg.
nursing

NSGCT
nonseminomatous germ cell tumor

NSGCTT
nonseminomatous germ cell tumor of
   the testis

NSG HX
nursing history

NSHD
nodular sclerosing Hodgkin's disease

NSI
negative self-image
no signs of infection
no signs of inflammation

NSILA
non-suppressible insulin-like activity

NSILA-S
non-suppressible insulin-like acting
   substance

NSILP
non-suppressible insulin-like protein

NSL
non-salt losers

NSLF
normal sheep lung fibroblast

NSM
neurosecretory material
neurosecretory motoneuron (motor
   neuron)

non-antigenic specific mediator
nonsmoker
nutrient sporulation medium (agar)

NSN
nephrotoxic serum nephritis
nicotine-stimulated neurophysin

NSN, Nsn
number of similar negative (matches)

NSND
nonsymptomatic, nondisabling

NSO
Neosporin ointment
supraoptic nucleus

N so.
nucleus supraopticus (re:
    neuroendocrine)

NSP
neuron specific protein

NSP, Nsp
number of similar positive (matches)

NSPF
not specifically provided for

NSPN
Neurosurgery progress note

NSQ
Neuroticism Scale Questionnaire
not sufficient quantity

NSR
nasal septal reconstruction
nonsystemic reaction
normal sinus rhythm

nSRBC
neuraminidase-treated sheep red blood
    cells (erythrocytes)

NSRN
Neurosurgery resident note

NSS
normal saline solution
normal size and shape
not statistically significant
nutrition support service

NSSL
normal size, shape, and location

NSS & M
normal size, shape, and mobility

NS sol.
normal saline solution

NSST
Northwestern Syntax Screening Test
    (re: Psychol)

NSSTT
nonspecific ST-T (wave—re: EKG)

NST
neospinothalamic tract
non-shivering thermogenesis
nonstress test (fetal monitoring)
nutritional status type

NSU
neurosurgical unit
nonspecific urethritis

NSurg, N Surg
neurosurgery

N surg.
neurosurgeon
neurosurgical

NSV
nonspecific vaginitis

NSVD
normal, spontaneous vaginal delivery

NSVT
nonsustained ventricular tachycardia

NSX
neurosurgical examination

Nsy, nsy
nursery

NT
nasotracheal (tube)
neotetrazolium (histological stain)
neurotensin
neutralization technique
neutralization test
neutralizing
nicotine tartrate
nontender
nontumorous
nontypable
normal temperature
normal tissue
normotensive
nortriptyline
nose and throat
no test
not tested

NT, Nt
niton (obsolete symbol for radon—Rn)

N & T, N + T
nose and throat

5'NT, 5'-NT
5'-nucleotidase

nt
nit (meter-kilogram-second unit of
    luminance)

NTA
natural thymocytotoxic autoantibody
nitrilotriacetic acid (chelating/
sequestering agent)

NTAB
nephrotoxic antibody

NTBR
not to be resuscitated

NTC
neotetrazolium chloride (re: staining)
neuroepithelioma teratoides ciliare

NTCC
National Type Culture Collection

NTD
neural tube defect
nitroblue tetrazolium dye
noise tone difference
5′-nucleotidase

NTDs
neural tube defects

NTE
neurotoxic esterase
nontest ear
nuclear tract emulsion

NTG
nitroglycerin
nontoxic goiter
normal triglyceridemic (subject)

NTGO
nitroglycerin ointment

NTHH
nontumorous hypergastrinemic
hyperchlorhydria

N & thr.
nose and throat

NTI
nonthyroid illness

NTLI
neurotensin-like immunoreactivity

NTM
nontuberculous mycobacteria

NTMI
nontransmural myocardial infarction

NTN
nephrotoxic nephritis

NTO
not thrown out (re: motor vehicle
accident)

NTP
nitroprusside
normal tension and pressure

nucleoside triphosphate (nucleoside
5′-triphosphate)

NTP, N.T.P.
normal temperature and pressure

NT & P
normal temperature and pressure

NTR
negative therapeutic reaction
normalized thyroxin(e) ratio
normotensive rat

NTR, ntr.
nutrition

NTS
nephrotoxic serum
nonturning against the self (re: Psychol)
nucleus tractus solitarii (re: Neuro)

NTT
near total thyroidectomy

NTV
nervous tissue vaccine

nt. wt.
net weight

NTX
naltrexone (narcotic antagonist)

NTZ
normal transformation zone (re:
colposcopy)

NU
name unknown

Nu
nucleolus
nucleus
Nusselt number (or biot—re: fluid
dynamics)

nU
nanounit (one billionth or 10^{-9} of a
standard unit)

Nuc
nucleoside

nuc.
nucleated
nucleus

nucl.
nucleus

NUG
necrotizing ulcerative gingivitis

nullip.
nulliparous (re: OB)

num.
numerator

n unit
neutron dose (unit of)

Nut
nutrition

NUV
near ultraviolet

NV
negative variation
neovascularization
neurovascular
new vessels
next visit
nonvaccinated
nonvegetarian
nonvenereal
nonveteran
normal value
normal volunteers
not verified

NV, Nv
naked vision

NV, nv.
nonvolatile

N/V
nausea and vomiting

N & V, N&V
nausea and vomiting

N or V
nausea or vomiting

NVA
near visual acuity

NVB
neurovascular bundle

NVC
nonvalved conduit

NVD
neck vein distention
neovascularization of the disk (re:
   Ophth)
Newcastle virus disease
new vessels on disk (re: Ophth)
nonvalvular (heart) disease
number of vessels diseased

NVD, N/V/D
nausea, vomiting, diarrhea

NVDC-O, NVDC Ө
no nausea, vomiting, diarrhea, or
   constipation

NVE
neovascularization elsewhere (retina—
   re: Ophth)
new vessels elsewhere (re: Ophth)

NVG
neovascular glaucoma (re: Ophth)
nonventilated group

NVI
neovascularization of the iris (re: Ophth)

NVM
nonvolatile matter

NVS
neurological vital signs
nonvaccine serotype

NVSS
normal variant short stature (children)

NVWSC
nonvolatile whole smoke condensate

NW
naked weight
nasal wash
nonwithdrawn
Norman-Wood (syndrome)
not weighed

NWB
nonweight bearing
no weight bearing

NWF
new working formulation

NWm
multiple (breath) nitrogen washout

NWR
normotensive Wistar rat

NWs
single (breath) nitrogen washout

NWSN
Nocardia water-soluble nitrogen

Nx
naloxone (narcotic antagonist)

NYD, N.Y.D.
not yet diagnosed

NYHA
New York Heart Association (re:
   classification of heart disease)

ny. hor.
nystagmus horizontalis (Gr. nystazein—
   to nod; horizontal nystagmus)

NYP
not yet published

ny. rot.
nystagmus rotatorius (Gr. nystazein—to
   nod; rotatory nystagmus)

nyst.
nystagmus (Gr. nystazein—to nod)

NYU insert
New York University insert (re:
  prostheses)

ny. und.
nystagmus undulans (Gr. nystazein—to
  nod; undulant nystagmus)

ny. vert.
nystagmus verticalis (Gr. nystazein—to
  nod; vertical nystagmus)

NZ
normal zone

NZB
New Zealand black (mouse—an inbred
  strain)

NZO
New Zealand obese (mouse)

NZW
New Zealand white (mouse—an inbred
  strain)

O

O
blood group in ABO system
in vivo physiological test
no special preparation necessary (for
   test)
obese
obesity
objective
objective findings
observation(s)
observed number (in a cell of a
   statistical table)
obstetrics
occipital
occiput
occlusal (re: Dent)
oculus (L. eye)
ohm (Ω—unit of electrical resistance)
old
Onchocerca (genus of nematode
   parasite)
Oncomelania (genus of snails—re:
   schistosomiasis)
opening (re: formulae for electrical
   reactions)
operator
operon (re: genetics)
Opisthorchis (genus of flukes,
   trematodes)
opium
orange (an indicator color)
orderly
Ordovician (geological time age)
Oriental
Ornithonyssus (genus of mites)
osteocyte
other
output
oxidative
oxygen (element)
respirations (re: anesthesia chart)
suture size (zero)
zero
zero—no evidence of contractility (re:
   manual muscle evaluation)

O, *O*
ohne Hauch (Ger. no film—designating
   a nonmotile type of microorganism)

O, (O)
oral
orally

O, o.
octarius (L. pint)
orthopaedic

O
denoting attachment to oxygen

O, O̶
negative
nil
no
none

Ō
pint

Ω
mitochondrial sex locus (yeast cell gene
   on its mitochondrial DNA—re:
   genetics)
ohm (unit of electrical resistance)
omega (twenty-fourth capital letter of
   Greek alphabet)

O2, O₂
both eyes
oxygen (symbol for the diatomic gas)

O₃
ozone

O 15, ¹⁵O
oxygen-15 (a cyclotron-produced
   radionuclide)

¹O₂
singlet oxygen

¹⁶O
oxygen-16 (common oxygen isotope)

¹⁷O
oxygen-17 (rarest of stable oxygen
   isotopes)

¹⁸O
oxygen-18 (heavy oxygen—a stable
   oxygen isotope)

o
Greek lower case letter omicron

ω
angular velocity
Greek lower case letter omega

ō̄
negative
none
without

o-
ortho- (re: chemical formulae)

o-
ortho

'o'
orally

"o"
orders

OA
object assembly (re: Psychol)
obstructive apnea
occipital artery
occipito-anterior (fetal position)
ocular albinism
old age
oleic acid
op amps (re: electronic circuits)
opiate analgesia
opsonic activity
optic atrophy
oral airway
oral alimentation
orotic acid (a uricosuric acid)
osteoarthritis
ovalbumin
overall assessment
oxalic acid

O-A
Objective-Analytic (Anxiety Battery—re: Psychol)

O & A
observation and assessment

O$_2$a
oxygen availability

OAA
old age assistance
oxaloacetic acid

OAAD
ovarian ascorbic acid depletion (test)

OABP
organic anion-binding protein

OAD
obstructive airway disease
occlusive arterial disease
organic anionic dye

OADC
oleic acid, albumin, dextrose, catalase (medium)

OADMT
Oliphant Auditory Discrimination Memory Test (re: Psychol)

OAF
open air factor
osteoclast-activating factor

OAG
open angle glaucoma (re: Ophth)

OAH
ovarian androgenic hyperfunction

OAJ
open apophyseal joint

OALF
organic acid labile fluoride

OALL
ossification of anterior longitudinal ligament

O antigen
low frequency blood group antigen

O antigens, O antigens
antigens occurring in cytoplasm (somatic) and cell walls of bacteria (derived from Ger. ohne Hauch—without film)

OAP
Oncovin (vincristine), ara-C (cytarabine), and prednisone (re: chemotherapy)
ophthalmic artery pressure
osteoarthropathy
oxygen at atmospheric pressure

OAPs
Occupational Ability Patterns (re: psychological testing)

OAR
orientation/alertness remediation
other administrative reasons

OARSA
oxacillin, aminoglycoside-resistant *Staphylococcus aureus*

OAS
osmotically active substance

OASDHI
Old Age, Survivors, Disability and Health Insurance (Program—re: Social Security Act)

OASM units
ohm, ampere, second, and meter units

OASP
organic acid soluble phosphorus

OAST
Oliphant Auditory Synthesizing Test (re: Psychol)

OAT
ornithine aminotransferase

OAV
oculoauriculovertebral (dysplasia)

OAW
oral airway

OB
obese
objective benefit
occult bleeding
occult blood
olfactory bulb

OB, Ob
obstetrical
obstetrician
obstetrics

OB, ob.
obiit (L. he died; she died)

O&B
opium and belladonna

OB∗∗∗
observed (value)

OBB
own bed bath

OBD
organic brain disease

OBE
out-of-body experience (re: Psychol/
Parapsychol)

OBF
organ blood flow

OBG
obstetrician-gynecologist
obstetrics and gynecology

OB-GYN, OB-Gyn.
obstetrics-gynecology

Obj, obj.
objective

obj.
object

OBL, obl.
oblique

obli.
oblique

OBP
ova, blood, and parasites (re: stool
exam)

OBPA
10,10′-oxybis-10*H*-phenoxarsine (used
to protect plastics from fungus and
bacteria)

OBS
obstetrical service
organic brain syndrome

OBS, obs.
observation
obstetrics

Obs
observer

Obs, obs.
observed
obsolete

Obst, obst.
obstetrician
obstetrics

obst.
obstipation
obstruct
obstruction
obstructive

obstet.
obstetric

Obstruct
obstruction
obstructive

OC
occlusocervical (re: Dent)
office call
on call
only child
optic chiasm (re: Neuro)
oral contraceptive(s)
organ culture
original claim
outer canthus
ovarian cancer
oxygen consumed

O & C
onset and course (of a disease)

O + C
onset and course (of a disease)

Oc
ochre (suppressor)

o.c.
opere citato (L. in the work cited)

OCA
oculocutaneous albinism
operant conditioning audiometry
oral contraceptive agent

OCA1
olivopontocerebellar atrophy 1

OCAD
occlusive carotid artery disease

O₂ cap.
oxygen capacity

OCBF
outer cortical blood flow

Occ
occlusion

Occ, occ.
occasional
occasionally

occ.
occipital
occiput
occupation
occurrence

occ△
occipital triangle

occas.
occasional
occasionally

occip.
occipital
occiput

occip. F, occip-F
occipitofrontal

occip-F HA
occipitofrontal headache

occl.
occlusion

OCC Th, OccTh, occ. th.
occupational therapy

Occup, occup.
occupation
occupational

occup.
occupies
occupying

Occup Rx
occupational therapy

OCD
osteochondritis dissecans
ovarian cholesterol depletion (test)

OCG
omnicardiogram
oral cholecystogram
oral cholecystography

OCH
oral contraceptive hormone

OCL
Occupational Check List (re: psychological testing)
operation control language (re: computers/data processing)

OCM
oral contraceptive medication

OCN
oculomotor nucleus

O colony
ohne (Ger. without; growth of nonmotile bacteria, single compact colonies; c.f. Hauch)

OCP
oral contraceptive pills

OCR
ocular counterrolling
ocular countertorsion reflex
optical character reader (re: automated reading of written or printed characters)
optical character recognition (re: computers/data processing)

OCS
open canalicular system (of platelets)
oral contraceptive steroid

11-OCS
11-oxycorticosteroid

OCSP
orthopaedic examination, special

OCT
Object Classification Test
optimal cutting temperature (a medium)
oral contraceptive therapy
ornithine carbamoyltransferase
oxytocin challenge test

Oct HA
octanohydroxamic acid (veterinary—antimicrobial; growth promotant)

octup.
octuplus (L. eight-fold)

OCU
observation care unit

OCV
ordinary conversational voice

OD
occupational dermatitis
occupational disease
once a day
on duty
open drop (anesthesia)
open duct
optical density
optimal dose
organization development
originally derived
out-of-date

OD, O.D.
oculo dextro (L. in the right eye)

oculus dexter (L. right eye)
outside diameter

OD, O.D., O/D
(drug) overdose

O-D
original-derived

o.d.
omni die (L. every day)

ODA, O.D.A.
occipitodextra anterior (position of
fetus)

O-DAP
Oncovin (vincristine),
dianhydrogalactitol, Adriamycin
(doxorubicin), and Platinol (cisplatin)
(re: chemotherapy)

ODAT
one day at a time

ODB
opiate-directed behavior

ODC
orotidylate decarboxylase (orotidine-5'-
phosphate decarboxylase—a lyase
class enzyme)
oxygen dissociation curve

ODD
oculo-dental-digital (syndrome)
oculodentodigital dysplasia

OD'd
(drug) overdosed

ODEPA
N-(3-oxapentamethylene)-N',N''-
diethylenephosphoramide

ODM
ophthalmodynamometry

Odont
odontology

odont.
odontogenic

odoram.
odoramentum (L. a perfume)

odorat.
odoratus (L. odorous, smelling,
perfuming)

ODP
occipitodextra posterior (position of
fetus)
offspring of diabetic parents

ODQ
on direct questioning
opponens digiti quinti (muscle)

ODSG
ophthalmic Doppler sonogram

ODT
occipitodextra transversa (position of
fetus)
oculodynamic test

ODU
optical density unit

OD units
optical density units

OE
on examination
orthopaedic examination
otitis externa

O/E
ratio of observed to expected

O&E
observation and examination

Oe
oersted (centimeter-gram-second unit of
magnetic field strength)

OEE
outer enamel epithelium

OEF
oil emersion field

OEM
open-end marriage (re: Psychol)
opposite ear masked
original equipment manufacturer (re:
computers)

OEMO
one-electron molecular orbital (theory)

OER
osmotic erythrocyte (enrichment)
oxygen enhancement ratio

OES
optical emission spectroscopy
oral esophageal stethoscope

OET
oral esophageal tube

OF
occipital-frontal (diameter of head)
occipitofrontal (re: occiput and
forehead; occipital and frontal lobe of
cerebral cortex)
optic fundi
orbitofrontal
osmotic fragility (test)
osteitis fibrosa
Ostrum-Furst (syndrome)

OF, O-F, O/F
oxidation/fermentation (medium)

OFA
oncofetal antigen

OFBM
oxidation-fermentation basal medium

OFC
occipitofrontal circumference (occipital-frontal circumference)
orbitofacial cleft
osteitis fibrosa cystica

ofc.
office

OFD
object-film distance (re: radiology)
oral-facial-digital (dysostosis)

Off, off.
official

off.
office

O-FHA, OF-HA
occipitofrontal headache

OF PF
optic fundi and peripheral fields

OF rad.
occipitofrontal radiation

OG
Obstetrics-Gynecology (department)
occlusogingival (re: Dent)
oligodendrocyte (re: Neuro)
optic ganglion
orange green (stain)
orogastric
orogastrically

O & G
obstetrics and gynecology

OGA
orogastric gonococcal aspirate

OGF
ovarian growth factor
oxygen gain factor

OGH
ovine growth hormone

OGM
outgrowth medium

OGS
oxogenic steroid

OGTT, OGT(T)
oral glucose tolerance test

OH
a hydroxide
hydroxy (prefix for —OH in chemical compounds)

hydroxycorticosteroids
hydroxyl group
hydroxyl radical
obstructive hypopnea
occipital horn
occupational health
occupational history
on hand
open heart (surgery)
out of hospital
Outpatient Hospital

OH, o.h.
omni hora (L. every hour)

OH$^-$
hydroxide ion

17-OH
17-hydroxycorticosteroids

OHA
oral hypoglycemic agent

3-OHA
3-hydroxyamobarbital

OHB$_{12}$
hydroxocobalamin (vitamin B$_{12}$)

OHC
hydroxycholecalciferol (1α-OH-CC; 1α-hydroxyvitamin D$_3$)
outer hair cells

OH-Cbl
hydroxocobalamin

OHCS, OHCs
hydroxycorticosteroid

17-OHCS
17-hydroxycorticosteroids

OHD
1α-hydroxycholecalciferol (synthetic analog to hormonal form of vitamin D$_3$)
organic heart disease

OH-DOC
hydroxydeoxycorticosterone

OHF
Omsk hemorrhagic fever

OHFA
hydroxy fatty acid

OHFT
overhead frame trapeze

OHI
ocular hypertension indicator
Oral Hygiene Index

OH IAA
hydroxyindoleacetic acid

5 OH IAA
5-hydroxyindoleacetic acid

OHI-S
Simplified Oral Hygiene Index (re: Dent)

ohm-cm
ohm-centimeter

OHP
hydroxyproline (hydroxy = —OH
 radical or group)
oxygen under high pressure

17-OHP
17α-hydroxyprogesterone

OHS
obesity hypoventilation syndrome
open heart surgery
Overcontrolled Hostility Scale (re:
 Psychol)

OHT
ocular hypertensive (glaucoma suspect)

OI
objective improvement
obturator internus
occipito-iliacus
opportunistic infection
opsonic index
orgasmic impairment
Orientation Inventory (re: psychological
 testing)
orthoiodohippurate
osteogenesis imperfecta
otitis interna (L. inflammation of the
 inner ear)
ouabain-insensitive
oxygen income
oxygen intake

O-I
outer-to-inner

OID
optimal immunomodulating dose
organism identification (number)

OIF
oil immersion field

OIH
131I orthoiodohippuric acid
ovulation-inducing hormone

oint.
ointment

OIP
organizing interstitial pneumonia

OIT
(Tien) organic integrity test (re:
 psychiatry)

OJ, o.j.
orange juice

OK
all right
approved
correct

OKN
optokinetic nystagmus ("railroad"
 nystagmus—re: Neuro/Ophth)

OKT
Ollier-Klippel-Trenaunay (syndrome)

OL
other location

OL, O.L., o.l.
oculus laevus (L. left eye)

Ol, ol.
oleum (L. oil)

OLA
occipitolaeva anterior (position of fetus)

OLB
olfactory bulb
open-liver biopsy

OLD
obstructive lung disease

OLH, oLH
ovine lactogenic hormone

OLIB
osmiophilic lamellar inclusion body

OLIDS
open-loop insulin delivery system

OLMAT
Otis-Lennon Mental Ability Test

OL OLIV, ol. oliv.
oleum olivae (L. oil of the olive)
oleum olivarium (L. olive oil)

OLP
occipitolaeva posterior (position of
 fetus)

OLR
Otology, Laryngology, and Rhinology

Ol res, ol. res.
oleoresin (oil and resin compound in
 certain plants)

OLRT
on-line real time (re: computers)

OLSIST
Oral Language Sentence Imitation
 Screening Test

OLT
occipitolaeva transversa (position of fetus)

OM
occipitomental (re: fetal head diameter—occipital protuberance to midpoint of chin)
occupational medicine
oculomotor
Osborn-Mendel (rat)
osteomalacia
osteomyelitis
osteopathic manipulation
otitis media
outer membrane
ovulation method (re: birth control)

o.m.
omni mane (L. every morning)

OMAC
otitis media, acute, catarrhal

OMAD
Oncovin (vincristine), methotrexate (and citrovorum factor), Adriamycin (doxorubicin), and dactinomycin (actinomycin D) (re: chemotherapy)

OMAS
otitis media, acute, suppurating

OMC
open mitral commissurotomy (re: Cardio)

OMCA
otitis media, catarrhal, acute

OMCC
otitis media, catarrhal, chronic

OMChS
otitis media, chronic, suppurating

OMD
ocular muscle dystrophy
organic mental disorder
3-O-methyldopa

OM-dopa
3-O-methyldopa

OME
otitis media with effusion

om. ¼ h.
omni quadranta hora (L. every fifteen minutes)

OMI
old myocardial infarction

OMM
outer mitochondrial membrane

om. mane vel. noc.
omni mane vel nocte (L. every morning or night)

OMN
oculomotor nerve
oculomotor nucleus

omn. bid.
omni bidendis (every two days [hybrid term])

omn. bih.
omni bihora (every two hours [hybrid term])

omn. hor.
omni hora (L. every hour)

omn. 2 hor.
omni secunda hora (L. every second hour)

omn. man.
omni mane (L. every morning)

omn. noct.
omni nocte (L. every night)

omn. quad. hor.
omni quadrante hora (L. every quarter of an hour)

omn. sec. hor.
omni secunda hora (L. every second hour)

OMP
olfactory marker protein
oligo-N-methylmorpholinopropylene oxide (a spreading factor)
outer membrane protein

OMPA
octamethyl pyrophosphoramide (insecticide)
otitis media, purulent, acute

OMPC
otitis media, purulent, chronic

OMPCh
otitis media, purulent, chronic

om. quad. hor
omni quadrante hora (L. every quarter of an hour)

OMS
offshore medical school
otomandibular syndrome

OM&S
Osteopathic Medicine and Surgery

OMSA
otitis media, suppurative, acute

394

OMSC
otitis media, secretory, chronic
otitis media, suppurative, chronic

OMT
O-methyltransferase

OMT, OM/T
osteopathic manipulation treatment

OMVC
open mitral valve commissurotomy

ON
occipitonuchal
optic nerve
osteonecrosis

ON, On, o.n.
omni nocte (L. every night)

O-N
zero to neutral

O→N
zero to neutral

ONB
o-nitrobiphenyl (industrial chemical;
    textile fungicide)

ONC
over-the-needle catheter

oncol.
oncological
oncology

ONCORNA
oncogene RNA (ribonucleic acid)

OND
orbitonasal dislocation
other neurological disorders

ONP
operating nursing procedure
ortho-nitrophenyl

ONPG
ortho-nitrophenyl-beta-D-
    galactopyranoside (o-nitrophenyl-β-
    galactoside)

ONPG-GAL
ortho-nitrophenyl-β-galactosidase

ONTG
oral nitroglycerin

ONTR
orders not to resuscitate

OO
oophorectomized

O-O
outer-to-outer

O & O
off and on

o/o
on account of

OOA
outer optic anlage (Ger. anlage—
    hereditary factor)

OOB
out of bed
out-of-body (experience—re:
    parapsychology)

OOBBRP
out of bed, bathroom privileges

OOC
out of control

OOLR
Ophthalmology, Otology, Laryngology,
    Rhinology

OOP
out of plaster
out on pass

OOR
out of room

OOW
out of wedlock

OP
occipitoparietal
occiput posterior
old patient (previously seen)
olfactory peduncle
opening pressure
operating
operative procedure
ophthalmic
opponens pollicis
original package
oropharynx
orthostatic proteinuria
osmotic pressure
osteoporosis
overproof
ovine prolactin

OP, O/P
outpatient

OP, Op
ophthalmology

OP, op.
operation

OP, op., o.p.
other than psychotic

O & P, O&P
ova and parasites

op.
operative
opposite
opus (L. work)

OPAL
Oncovin (vincristine), prednisone,
L-asparaginase (re: chemotherapy)

OPB
outpatient basis

OPC
Outpatient Clinic

OPCA
olivopontocerebellar atrophy

op. cit.
opus citatum (L. the work cited)

OP code
operation code (re: computers)

OPD
obstetric prediabetes
optical path difference
oto-palato-digital (syndrome)
Outpatient Department
Outpatient Dispensary

o,p′-DDD
2,4′-dichlorodiphenyldichloroethane
(mitotane; Lysodren— antineoplastic)

OpDent
operative dentistry

OPDG
ocular plethysmodynamography

OPE
orbiting primate experiment

oper.
operate
operating
operation
operator

OPG
ocular plethysmography
oculoplethysmograph
oculoplethysmography
ophthalmoplethysmograph
oxypolygelatin (re: plasma volume
extension)

opg.
opening

OPH
obliterative pulmonary hypertension

OPH, Oph, oph.
ophthalmia
ophthalmic
ophthalmology

Oph, oph.
ophthalmoscope
ophthalmoscopic

Ophth, ophth.
ophthalmia
ophthalmic
ophthalmologic
ophthalmologist
ophthalmology
ophthalmoscope

OPI
oculoparalytic illusion
Omnibus Personality Inventory

OPK
optokinetic

OPL
osmotic pressure (of proteins in) lymph
outer plexiform layer
ovine placental lactogen

OPLL
ossification of posterior longitudinal
ligament

OPM
occult primary malignancy
ophthalmoplegic migraine

OPP
Oncovin (vincristine), procarbazine, and
prednisone (re: chemotherapy)
osmotic pressure of plasma (colloids)
ovine pancreatic polypeptide
oxygen partial pressure

opp.
opposed
opposing
opposite
opposition

OPPES
oil-associated pneumoparalytic
eosinophilic syndrome

op. reg.
operative region

oprg.
operating

OPRT
orotate phosphoribosyltransferase

oprtg.
operating

OPS
outpatient service
Outpatient Surgery

OPSA
ovarian papillary serous
(cyst)adenocarcinoma

OPSI
overwhelming post-splenectomy
  infection

OPSR
Office of Professional Standards
  Review

OPSR-BQA
Office of Professional Standards
  Review—Bureau of Quality
  Assurance

OPT
outpatient
outpatient treatment

Opt
optometrist

opt.
optical
optician
optics
optimal
optimum
optimus (L. best)
optional

OPV
oral poliovaccine
oral, (attentuated) poliovirus vaccine

OPWL
opiate withdrawal

OR
oil retention
operations research (re: computers)
optic radiation
oral rehydration
orienting response
orthopaedic
orthopaedic research
orthopaedic (surgeon)
own recognizance
oxidized-reduced

OR, O.R.
operating room

OR, O-R
oxidation-reduction

OR, o.r.
open reduction

O$_R$
rate of outflow
right operator

ORA
occiput right anterior (position of fetus)
opiate receptor agonist

ORAN
Orthopaedic resident admit note

ORANS
Oak Ridge Analytical Systems

ORBC
ox red blood cell

ORC
ox red cell

orch.
orchitis

ORD
optical rotatory dispersion (Cotton
  effect—re: wave length of light)

Ord
orotidine

Ord, ord.
orderly

ord.
order
ordered
ordinate

OR en.
oil-retention enema

OR enema
oil-retention enema

OR & F
open reduction and fixation

org.
organ
organic
organism

organiz.
organization
organizational

ORIF
open reduction (with) internal fixation
  (re: Ortho)

OR c̄ IF
open reduction with internal fixation (re:
  Ortho)

orig.
origin
original
originated

oriT
transfer initiated at the origin (re:
  plasmid transfer)

OrJ, Or J
orange juice

ORL
otorhinolaryngology

ORN
Operating Room Nurse

Orn
ornithine (an intermediate in urea cycle)

ORO
Oropouche (an arbovirus)

OROS
oral osmotic

ORP
occiput right posterior (position of fetus)
oxidation-reduction potential

ORPM
orthorhythmic pacemaker

ORS
oral rehydration salt
oral rehydration solution
oral surgeon
orthopaedic surgeon
orthopaedic surgery

ORT
object relations techniques
oral rehydration therapy

orth.
orthopaedics

Ortho, ortho.
orthopaedics

orthop.
orthopedist

orthot.
orthotonus

or. Xl
oriented to time

or. X2
oriented to time and place

or. X3
oriented to time, place, and person

OS
occipitosacral (position of fetus)
occupational safety
opening snap (heart sound)
operating system (re: computers)
oral surgery
Osgood-Schlatter's (disease)
osteogenic sarcoma
osteoid surface
osteosarcoma
ouabain sensitive
overall survival
oxygen saturation

OS, O.S.
oculo sinistro (L. in the left eye)
oculus sinister (L. left eye)

OS, os.
osteosclerosis

Os
osmium (element)

^{185}Os
radioactive isotope of osmium

^{191}Os
radioactive isotope of osmium

^{193}Os
radioactive isotope of osmium

OSA
obstructive sleep apnea

OSAS
obstructive sleep apnea syndrome

O_2 sat.
oxygen saturation

OSBCL
Ottawa School Behavior Check List (re:
    psychological testing)

osc.
oscillate

OSCE
objective structural clinical examination

OSCJ
original squamocolumnar junction

OSD
outside doctor

OSF
outer spiral fibers (of cochlea)
overgrowth stimulating factor

OSFT
outstretched fingertips

OSIQ
Offer Self-Image Questionnaire (for
    Adolescents)

OSL
Osgood-Schlatter lesion

OSM
ovine submaxillary mucin
oxygen saturation meter

OSM, Osm, osm
osmole (unit of osmolality and
    osmolarity)

osm.
osmotic

osmo.
osmolality

osmol.
osmole

OSN
off-service note

OSRD
Office of Scientific Research and
  Development

OSS
Object Sorting Scales (re: psychological
  testing)
osseous
over-shoulder strap

OST
object-sorting test (re: Psychol)

Osteo
osteopath
osteopathy

Osteo, osteo.
osteomyelitis

osteo.
osteoarthritis
osteopathology

osteoarth.
osteoarthritis

osteocart.
osteocartilaginous

OT
objective test (re: Psychol)
occlusion time
ocular tension
Oesterreicher-Turner (syndrome)
office treatment
old term
old terminology
old tuberculin (Koch's)
olfactory threshold
olfactory tubercle
optic tract
orientation test
ornithine transcarbamylase
orotracheal (tube)
orthopaedic treatment
oxytocin

OT, O.T.
occupational therapy

OT, Ot
otolaryngologist
otolaryngology

OT, ot.
otologist
otology

5-OT
5-oxytryptamine (5-hydroxytryptamine;
  serotonin)

OT***
total oxygen content

OTA
Opinions Toward Adolescents (re:
  psychological testing)

OTAP
Ohio Tests of Articulation and
  Perception (of Sounds)

OTC
ornithine transcarbamylase (also
  transcarbamoylase)
oval target cell
over the counter (re: nonprescription
  drugs)
oxytetracycline

OTD
oral temperature device
organ tolerance dose

OTE
optically transparent electrode

OTF
oral transfer factor

OTH
other

OTI
ovomucoid trypsin inhibitor

OTO, Oto, oto.
otology

Oto, oto.
otolaryngology

Otol, otol.
otologist
otology

otolar.
otolaryngology

OTR
ovarian tumor registry

OTS
occipital temporal sulcus

OTU
olfactory tubercle
operational taxonomic unit

OU
observation unit
Oppenheim-Urbach (syndrome)

OU, O.U.
oculi unitas (L. both eyes together)
oculo utro (L. in each eye)

OU, O.U., o.u.
oculus uterque (L. for each eye; each
  eye [of two])

OURQ
outer upper right quadrant

OV
oculovestibular
office visit
Osler-Vaquez (disease)
osteoid volume
outflow volume
ovalbumin
overventilation (hyperventilation)
ovulating

Ov
ovary

O₂v̂
superoxide

ov.
ovum (L. egg)

OVA
ovalbumin

OVD
occlusal vertical dimension (re: Dent)

OVDQ
Organizational Value Dimensions
Questionnaire (re: psychological
testing)

OVIS
Ohio Vocational Interest Survey (re:
psychological testing)

OVIT
Oral Verbal Intelligence Test (re:
Psychol)

OVLT
organum vasculosum of the lamina
terminalis

OVX
ovariectomized

OW
off work
once weekly
open wedge (osteotomy)
ordinary warfare
out of wedlock
outer wall
oval window

O/W
oil in water (re: emulsions)
oil-water (ratio)

OWA
organics-in-water analyzer

OWR
ovarian wedge resection

OWS
overwear syndrome

o.w.u.
open window unit (unit of sound
absorption)

OWVI
Ohio Work Values Inventory (re:
psychological testing)

OX
optic chiasm
orthopaedic examination
oxacillin

OX, ox.
oxymel (honey, water, and vinegar)

Ox
oxygen

O X 3
oriented times three

OXEA
ox erythrocyte antibody

OXP
oxypressin

OXT
oxytocin

OXY
oxytocin

OXY, oxy.
oxygen

oxy.
oxymel (honey, water, and vinegar)

OYE
old yellow enzyme

oz, oz.
ounce

oz. ap.
apothecary ounce

oz. t.
ounce troy

P

P
blood group designation
form perception (re: General Aptitude
    Test Battery)
gas partial pressure
pain
panmictic index (re: genetics)
Paragonimus (genus of trematode
    parasites)
parent
parental
parous
parte (L. part)
partial performance
partial pressure (frequently with
    subscripts indicating chemical
    species and location)
partial tension
Pasteurella (genus)
pater (L. father)
paternally contributing
patient
penicillin
Penicillium (genus)
Peptococcus (genus)
percentile
perceptual speed
percussion
perforation
permeability
Permian (most recent of Paleozoic
    periods)
peta (prefix for SI unit—a unit equal to
    one- quadrillionth of basic unit—10^{15})
peyote
Pfeifferella (genus)
pharmacopoeia
phenolphthalein (an indicator)
phenylalanine
Phlebotomus (genus of biting flies)
phon (unit of loudness)
phosphate (a group; when combined in
    an abbreviation such as ADP, ATP)
phosphoric residue (re: nucleic acid
    terminology)
phosphorus (element)
Phthirus (genus of lice)
physiology
Physopsis (a subgenus of snails—re:
    schistosomiasis)
pin (re: Dent)
pink (an indicator color)
Pityrosporon (genus of yeastlike fungi—
    re: Derma)

placebo
plan
plasma concentration of substance
    (when followed by a subscript)
Plasmodium (genus—re: malaria)
Pneumocystis (genus)
poise (unit of dynamic viscosity)
poison
polarization
polymyxin
pondere (L. by weight)
pondus (L. weight)
pons
poor (re: manual muscle evaluation)
popular response
population
porcelain
porphyrin
position
positive
posterior
postpartum
power
prednisone
premolar
presbyopia (re: Ophth)
pressure (frequently with subscripts
    indicating chemical species and
    location)
pressure of gas (primary symbol)
primary
primipara (re: OB-GYN)
primitive (re: hemoglobin)
private (patient or room)
probable error (re: statistics)
produces
product
prolactin
proline (an amino acid)
propionate
Propionibacterium (genus)
propionic
protein
Protestant
Proteus (genus)
Providencia (genus)
proximal
proximum (L. near)
Pseudomonas (genus)
psychiatrist
psychiatry
psychosis
Pulex (genus of fleas)
pulmonary

punctum proximum (L. near point [of vision])
P waves (re: EKG)

P, p
concentration by weight (after optical rotations only—re: organic chemistry)
page
para
part
per (L. by; through; excessive)
pint
post (L. after)
probability

P, p.
parity
passive (re: PM&R)
plasma
point
pole
poor
pugillus (L. handful)
pulse
pupil
pureed

$\bar{P}$
mean gas pressure (primary symbol)

P+
poor plus

P-, p-, p
para- (re: chemical formulae)

~P
high-energy phosphate bond

P_1
first parental generation (re: genetics)

P_2, P-2
pulmonic second sound

P_3
luminous flux

P_3, P/3
proximal third

P_{28}, P_{50}, P_{100}, P_0
28th percentile, 50th percentile, 100th percentile, percentile rank of zero (re: statistics)

^{32}P, P 32
radioactive phosphorus

^{33}P
radioactive isotope of phosphorus

P-50
oxygen half-saturation pressure of hemoglobin

P_{700}
pigment in chloroplasts bleached by 700 nm light wavelength (re: botany)

P_{870}
pigment bleached by 870 nm wavelength in bacterial chromatophores (re: bacteriology)

p
atomic orbital with angular momentum quantum number 1
frequency of the more common allele of a pair
momentum
phosphate (re: polynucleotide symbolism)
phosphoric acid molecules (re: genetics)
phosphoric ester (re: polynucleotide symbolism)
pico-(prefix; Sp., a small amount—one trillionth of a unit or 10^{-12})
proton
sample proportion (re: statistics)
short arm of a chromosome

p.
papilla (optic)
probable

$\bar{p}$
after, or post

PA
paper advance
paralysis agitans
paranoia
passive aggressive (re: psychiatry)
paternal aunt
periarteritis
peridural artery
periodontal abscess
permeability-area product
phakic-aphakic (re: Ophth)
phenylalanine
phosphatidic acid
photoallergenic (response)
Picture Arrangement (re: Psychol)
pineapple (test for butyric acid in stomach—if present, odor of pineapple will be given off)
pituitary-adrenal
plasma aldosterone
plasminogen activator
platelet adhesiveness
platelet aggregation
platelet associated
polyarteritis
postaural
posteroanterior
prealbumin
predictive accuracy
pregnancy associated
primary amenorrhea

primary anemia
proactivator
procainamide (an antiarrhythmic)
prolonged action
prophylactic antibiotic
propionic acid
proprietary association
prostate antigen
proteolytic activity
prothrombin activity
Pseudomonas aeruginosa
psychoanalysis
psychoanalyst
psychogenic aspermia
pulmonary artery
pulmonary atresia
pulpo-axial (re: Dent)

PA, P.A.
pernicious anemia

PA, P-A
posterior-anterior

PA, pa
pathology

PA, p.a.
per annum (L. by the year; yearly)

P/A
percussion and auscultation
position and alignment

P$_A$
alveolar pressure

P$_A$
partial pressure in arterial blood

P & A, P&A
percussion and auscultation
position and alignment
present and active (re: reflexes)

Pa
pascal (SI unit of stress; pressure)
protactinium (element)
pulmonary arterial (pressure)

P$_2$>A$_2$
pulmonic second heart sound greater
than aortic second heart sound

P$_2$<A$_2$
pulmonic second heart sound less than
aortic second heart sound

P$_2$=A$_2$
pulmonic and aortic second heart
sounds physiologically split

^{233}Pa
radioactive isotope of protactinium

pA$_2$
affinity constant (re: binding drug to
drug receptor)

p.a.
post applicationem (L. after [the]
application)
pro anno (L. for the year)

PAA
partial agonist activity
phenylacetic acid
physical abilities analysis
plasma angiotensinase activity
polyacrylamide
premarket approval application
Prueba de Aptitude Acadèmia (Spanish
version of Scholastic Aptitude Test)
3-pyridineacetic acid (homonicotinic
acid—vasodilator)

3-PAA1
3-pyridineacetic acid (homonicotinic
acid—vasodilator)

Paa, p.a.a
parti affectae applicandus (L. apply to
the affected parts)

p.a.a.
parti affectase applicetur (L. let it be
applied to the affected region)

P(A-aDO$_2$)
alveolar-arterial oxygen tension
difference

PAB
para-aminobenzoic acid (vitamin B$_x$)
Positive Attention Behavior
premature atrial beat(s)
purple agar base (medium)

PABA
p-aminobenzoic acid (vitamin B$_x$—
antirickettsial; sunscreen agent)

PAC
Parent-Adult-Child (re: Transactional
Analysis)
phenacetin (acetophenetidin), aspirin,
caffeine
Platinol (cisplatin), Adriamycin
(doxorubicin), and cyclophosphamide
(re: chemotherapy)
premature atrial contraction
premature atrial contracture
premature auricular contraction
Progress Assessment Chart of Social
and Personal Development

PACC
protein A immobilized in collodion
charcoal

PACE
Personal Assessment for Continuing
Education
personalized aerobics for
cardiovascular enhancement
Professional and Administrative Career

403

Examination (re: psychological testing)

promoting aphasics' communicative effectiveness

pulmonary angiotensin I converting enzyme

Pa_CO
mean alveolar volume of gas

Pa_CO2, Pa_CO2, PaCO2, Pa_CO2, pACO2
arterial carbon dioxide pressure, or tension

partial pressure of oxygen in arterial blood

PACP
pulmonary artery counterpulsation

PACT
precordial acceleration tracing

PAD
percutaneous abscess drainage

phenacetin, aspirin, desoxyephedrine (methylamphetamine)

phonological acquisition device

pre-aid to the disabled

primary affective disorder (re: psychiatry)

psychoaffective disorder (re: psychiatry)

pulsatile assist device

PAd
pulmonary artery diastolic

PADDS
photon-activated drug delivery system

PADP
pulmonary artery diastolic pressure

PAD pressure
pulmonary artery diastolic pressure

PAE
progressive assistive exercise

p. ae.
partes aequales (L. equal parts)

paed.
paediatrics

PAEDP
pulmonary artery end-diastolic pressure

PAF
paroxysmal auricular fibrillation

platelet-activating factor

platelet-aggregating factor

platelet aggregation factor

pollen adherence factor

Premenstrual Assessment Form

pseudoamniotic fluid

pulmonary arteriovenous fistula

PA&F
percussion, auscultation, and fremitus

PA + F
percussion, auscultation, and fremitus

PAF-A
platelet-activating factor of anaphylaxis

PAFD
pulmonary artery filling defect

PAFI
platelet-aggregation factor inhibitor

PAFIB
paroxysmal atrial fibrillation

PAG
periaqueductal gray (matter—re: Neuro)

polyacrylamide gel (electrophoresis)

pregnancy-associated alpha-glycoprotein

pregnancy-associated globulin

pAg
protein A gold (technique)

PAGE
polyacrylamide gel electrophoresis

PAgF
platelet-aggregating factor

PAGIF
polyacrylamide gel isoelectric focusing

PAGMK
primary African green monkey kidney

PAH
para-aminohippurate (a salt of para-aminohippuric acid)

para-aminohippuric acid (re: kidney function tests)

polycyclic aromatic hydrocarbon

pulmonary artery hypertension

pulmonary artery hypotension

PAHA
para-aminohippuric acid (re: kidney function tests)

PAHT
phosphotungstic acid hematoxylin

PAHVC
pulmonary alveolar hypoxic vasoconstriction

PAI
Pair Attraction Inventory (re: Psychol)

PAIgG
platelet-associated immunoglobulin G

P-A interval
P wave to A wave in His bundle

electrogram (the intra- arterial
conduction time—re: cardiology)

PAIR
Personal Assessment of Intimacy in
Relationships

PAIS
Psychosocial Adjustment to Illness
Scale

PAJ
paralysis agitans juvenilis

PAK
phytohemagglutinin-activated killers
Pseudomonas aeruginosa (strain) K

PAL
Pathology Laboratory (test)
posterior axillary line
product of activated lymphocyte
Profile of Adaptation to Life
pyogenic abscess of the liver

PA & Lat
posteroanterior and lateral

palp.
palpable
palpate
palpation
palpitation

palpi.
palpitations

palpit.
palpitations

PALS
periarteriolar lymphocyte sheaths

PA-LS-ID
pernicious anemia-like syndrome and
immunoglobulin deficiency

PALST
Picture Articulation and Language
Screening Test (re: Psychol)

PAM
crystalline penicillin G in 2% aluminum
monostearate
pancreatic acinar mass
L-phenylalanine mustard (L-PAM,
melphalan, Alkeran— an
antineoplastic)
p-methoxyamphetamine
pralidoxime chloride (2-PAM chloride—
a cholinesterase reactivator)
pregnancy-associated alpha-
macroglobulin
primary amoebic (amebic)
meningoencephalitis
pulmonary alveolar macrophage(s)
pulmonary alveolar microlithiasis

pulse amplitude modulation (re:
computers)
pyridine aldoxime methiodide (2-PAM
iodide—a cholinesterase reactivator)

2-PAM
pralidoxime chloride (cholinesterase
reactivator; antidote for nerve gases;
cholinesterase-inhibitor- type
insecticides)

pam.
pamphlet

2-PAM chloride
2-pyridine aldoxime methyl chloride
(pralidoxime chloride—antidote for
nerve gases; cholinesterase-inhibitor
insecticides)

PAME
primary amoebic (amebic)
meningoencephalitis

2-PAM iodide
2-pyridine aldoxime methyl iodide
(pralidoxime iodide— antidote for
nerve gases; cholinesterase-inhibitor
insecticides)

PAMP
pulmonary arterial mean pressure
pulmonary artery mean pressure

PAN
panarteritis nodosa
periarteritis nodosa
periodic alternating nystagmus
peroxyacetyl nitrate (a specific
compound)
peroxyacylnitrates (re: class of
compounds)
polyarteritis nodosa
positional alcohol nystagmus

pancreat.
pancreatic

panendo.
panendoscopy

PANESS
Physical and Neurological Examination
for Soft Signs

PANS
puromycin aminonucleoside

P antigens
P blood group antigens

PAO
peak acid output

PAo
pulmonary artery occlusion pressure
(wedge pressure)

Pao
ascending aortic pressure

P$_{ao}$
airway opening pressure

PAo$_2$, P$_{AO_2}$, PaO$_2$
alveolar pO$_2$ (oxygen pressure tension)
arterial pO$_2$ (partial pressure of oxygen
  in arterial blood; arterial oxygen
  concentration or tension)

PAOD
peripheral arterial occlusive disease
peripheral arteriosclerotic occlusive
  disease

PAOI
peak acid output insulin-induced

PAP
passive-aggressive personality
Patient Assessment Program
peak airway pressure
peroxidase-antiperoxidase
placental acid phosphatase
placental alkaline phosphatase
positive airway pressure
primary atypical pneumonia
prostatic acid phosphatase
pulmonary alveolar proteinosis
pulmonary arterial pressure
pulmonary artery pressure
purified alternate pathway

PAP, Pap
Papanicolaou smear (stain, test)

Pap
papillary

pap.
papilla(e)

PAP complex
peroxidase-antiperoxidase complex

PAPF
platelet adhesiveness plasma factor

Pap in. canthus
papilloma, inner canthus

PAPP
para-aminopropiophenone (antidote for
  cyanide)
pregnancy-associated plasma protein

PAPPC
pregnancy-associated plasma protein C

PAPS
3′-phosphoadenosine-5′-
  phosphosulfate (also called
  phosphoadenosine diphosphosulfate;
  adenosine-3′-phosphate-5′-
  sulfonatophosphate;
  phosphoadenosylphosphosulfate)

Pap sm.
Papanicolaou smear

PAP technique
peroxidase-antiperoxidase technique

PAPUFA
physiologically active polyunsaturated
  fatty acids

Pa-Pv
pulmonary arterial pressure-pulmonary
  venous pressure

PAPVC
partial anomalous pulmonary venous
  connection

PAPVR
partial anomalous pulmonary venous
  return

PAPW
posterior aspect of the pharyngeal wall

PAQ
Personal Attributes Questionnaire
Position Analysis Questionnaire (job
  analysis—re: Psychol)

PAR
perennial allergic rhinitis
photosynthetically active radiation
physiological aging rate
positive attention received
postanesthesia recovery (room)
postanesthesia (recovery) room
postanesthetic recovery (room)
probable allergic rhinitis
proximal alveolar region
pulmonary arteriolar resistance

par.
paraffin
parallel

Para, para
paraplegic
parous (having borne one or more
  children)

para.
paraparesis
paraplegia

Para I, II, III, etc.
unipara (having borne one child),
  bipara, tripara, etc. (having borne two,
  three children, etc.)

I-para
primipara (first pregnancy)

II-para
secundipara (second pregnancy)

III-para
tertipara (third pregnancy)

para C, para c
paracervical

paracent.
paracentesis

paradox.
paradoxical

Par aff., par. aff.
pars affecta (L. to the part affected)

para L
paralumbar

Parapsych, parapsych.
parapsychology

Parasit
parasitology

parasym. div.
parasympathetic division (of autonomic
   nervous system)

para T
parathoracic

paravert.
paravertebral

PARD
platelet aggregation as a risk of
   diabetes

parent.
parenteral
parenterally

parox.
paroxysmal

PARR
Postanesthesia Recovery Room

PARS
Personal and Role Skills

PaRS
pararectal space

PARS Scale
Personal Adjustment and Role Skills
   Scale

part.
partim (L. partly)
partis (L. of a part)
parturition

part. aeq.
partes aequales (L. equal parts)

part. dolent.
partes dolentes (L. painful parts)

part. vic.
partitis vicibus (L. in divided doses)

PARU
postanesthetic recovery unit

parv.
parvus (L. small)

PAS
para-aminosalicylic acid (for TB)
Parent Attitude Scale
periodic acid-Schiff (method, stain,
   technique, test, reaction)
peripheral anterior synechia
personality assessment system
phosphatase acid serum
photoacoustic spectroscopy
Physician's Activity Study
pregnancy advisory service
professional activity study
progressive accumulated stress
pseudoachievement syndrome
pulmonary artery stenosis

PASA
para-aminosalicylic acid (for TB)

PAS-C
para-aminosalicylic acid crystallized
   (with ascorbic acid)

P'ase
alkaline phosphatase

PASH
periodic acid-Schiff hematoxylin

PASM
periodic acid-silver methenamine

PAS/MAP
Professional Activities Study Medical
   Audit Program (re: medical records)

pass.
passim (L. here and there)
passive

Past.
Pasteurella (genus)

past.
paste

PASVR
pulmonary anomalous superior venous
   return

PAT
Pain Apperception Test
paroxysmal atrial tachycardia
paroxysmal auricular tachycardia
1-phenyl-5-aminotetrazole (fenamole—
   anti-inflammatory)
Photo Articulation Test (re: Psychol)
physical abilities test
picric acid turbidity
platelet aggregation test
polyamine acetyltransferase

preadmission (screening and)
    assessment team
preadmission testing
Predictive Ability Test (re: Psychol)
pregnancy at term
prism adaptation test
psychoacoustic testing
pulmonary artery trunk

PAT, pat.
patient

pat
paternal origin (re: cytogenetics)

pat.
patella
patent
patented

PATCO
prednisone, ara-C (cytarabine),
    thioguanine, cyclophosphamide, and
    Oncovin (vincristine) (re:
    chemotherapy)

PATE
pulmonary artery
    thromboendarterectomy

pat. gf.
paternal grandfather

pat. gm.
paternal grandmother

PATH
pituitary adrenotropic hormone

Path
Pathology (Department of)

path.
pathogen
pathogenesis
pathogenic
pathological
pathologist
pathology

path. fx
pathological fracture

PATLC
Progressive Achievement Tests of
    Listening Comprehension (re:
    Psychol)

pat. med.
patent medicine

PATS
priority activity tracking system

pat. T
patellar tenderness

PAV
partial atrioventricular
Pavulon (pancuronium bromide—re:
    Anesth)
poikiloderma atrophicans vasculare
posterior arch vein

Pa Va Ex
passive vascular (or veno-arterial)
    exercise (a negative pressure—re:
    orthopaedics and physiatry)

PAVe
procarbazine, Alkeran, Velban (re:
    chemotherapy)

PA-VF
pulmonary arteriovenous fistula

PAVN
paraventricular nucleus

PAW
peripheral airways
pulmonary artery wedge

PAWP
pulmonary artery wedge pressure

PB
pancreaticobiliary
paraffin bath(s) (re: physical therapy)
Paul-Bunnell (antibodies, test)
perineal body
periodic breathing
peripheral blood
peroneus brevis
phenobarbital
phenobarbitone
pinealoblastoma
polymyxin B
posterior baffle
powder bed
premature beat
pressure balanced
pressure breathing
protein binding
protein bound
punch biopsy

PB, P.B.
Pharmacopoeia Britannica

P$_B$, P$_B$
barometric pressure

PB, Pb, pb.
phenobarbital

PB, p.b.
phonetically balanced (word lists—re:
    Audio)

PB%
phonetic balanced percent (re: Audio)

P & B
pain and burning
phenobarbital and belladonna

Pb
plumbum (L. lead—element)
presbyopia

Pb.
probenecid (uricosuric)

PBA
phenylboronate agarose
polyclonal B-cell activities
pressure breathing assister
prolactin-binding assay (buffer)
pulpobuccoaxial (re: Dent)

P$_{BA}$
brachial arterial pressure

PBB
polybrominated biphenyls (flame
retardant)

Pb-B
lead (plumbum) level in blood

PBBs
polybrominated biphenyls (flame
retardant)

PBC
peripheral blood cells
point of basal convergence
prebed care
pregnancy and birth complications
primary biliary cirrhosis
progestin-binding complement

PBE
Perlsucht Bacillenemulsion

PBF
peripheral blood flow
phosphate-buffered formalin
placental blood flow
pulmonary blood flow

PB-Fe
protein-bound iron

PBG
porphobilinogen

PBI
Parental Bonding Instrument
phenformin (oral hypoglycemic agent—
withdrawn from market in 1978)
protein-bound iodine

PBI, PbI
lead (plumbum) intoxication

PB^{131}I
protein-bound iodine (now rarely used;
superseded by T_3, T_4)

PBK
phosphorylase *b* kinase
pseudophakic bullous keratopathy (re:
Ophth)

PBL
peripheral blood leukocyte
peripheral blood lymphocytes

PB list
phonetically balanced (words) list (re:
Audio)

PBM
peripheral basement membrane
peripheral blood mononuclear (cells)

PBMC
peripheral blood mononuclear cell(s)

PBMV
pulmonary blood mixing volume

PBN
paralytic brachial neuritis
peripheral benign neoplasm

PBNA
partial body neutron activation

PBO
penicillin in beeswax and oil

PBO, pbo.
placebo

PbO
lead (plumbum) monoxide

PBP
penicillin-binding protein
porphyrin biosynthetic pathway
prostate-binding protein
pseudobulbar palsy

PBQ
Preschool Behavior Questionnaire

PBRT
Phonetically Balanced Rhyme Test

PBS
phenobarbital sodium
phosphate-buffered saline
phosphate-buffered sodium
pulmonary branch stenosis

PbS
lead (plumbum) sulfide

PBSP
prognostically bad signs during
pregnancy

PBT
Paul Bunnell test
phenacetin breath test
profile-based therapy

PBT₄
protein-bound thyroxin(e)

PBV
Platinol, bleomycin, vinblastine (re: chemotherapy)
predicted blood volume
pulmonary blood volume

PBW
posterior bite wing (re: Dent)

PBZ
phenylbutazone (anti-inflammatory)

PBZ, Pbz
Pyribenzamine (tripelennamine—an antihistaminic)

PC
packed cells
panting center
paper chromatography
parent cell(s)
parent to child
particulate component
partition coefficient
pelvic cramps
pentose cycle
peritoneal cell
phone call
phosphate cycle
phosphatidylcholine (lecithin)
phosphocreatine
phosphorylcholine
photoconductive
Phrase Construction (test)
Picture Completion (test)
pill counter
piriform cortex
plasma concentration
plasma cortisol
plasmacytoma
platelet concentrate
platelet concentration
platelet count
pneumotaxic center
polycentric
poor condition
popliteal cyst
portacaval (shunt)
portal cirrhosis
postcoital
posterior cervical
posterior chamber
posterior commissure
posterior cortex
precaution category
precordium
prepiriform cortex
present complaint
presenting complaint
primary cleavage
primary closure
printed circuit (re: computers)

privilege card
procollagen
producing cell
productive cough
Professional Corporation (physician)
proliferative capacity
prostatic carcinoma
provisional cortex
proximal colon
pseudoconditioning control
pseudocyst
pubococcygeus (muscle)
pulmonary capillary
pulmonary circulation
pulmonic closure
pure clairvoyance (re: Parapsychol)
Purkinje cell
pyloric canal
pyruvate carboxylase

PC, P.C., p.c.
pondus civile (L. avoirdupois weight)

PC, Pc
penicillin

P-C
phlogistic corticoid

P & C
prism and (alternative) cover-test (cross-over test; screen and cover test—re: Ophth)

pc
per cent
piece

pc, pc.
picocurie (pCi preferred)

p.c.
post cibos (L. after meals)
post cibum (L. after a meal)

PCA
parietal cell antibody
passive cutaneous anaphylaxis
patient care area
patient care audit
patient-controlled analgesia
perchloric acid
percutaneous carotid arteriogram
photocontact allergic
portacaval anastomosis
posterior cerebral artery
posterior communicating aneurysms
posterior communicating artery
posterior cricoarytenoid
precoronary care area
principal components analysis
procoagulant activity
prostatic carcinoma
2-pyrrolidone-5-carboxylic acid (glutimic acid—re: racemic amines resolution)

PCAS
Psychotherapy Competence
  Assessment Schedule

PCB
page control block (re: computers/data
  processing)
paracervical block
polychlorinated biphenyl(s)
portacaval bypass
procarbazine
process control block (re: computers/
  data processing)

PCB, PcB
near point of convergence to the
  intercentral baseline (re: Ophth)

Pcb
puncta convergentis basalis (L. point of
  convergence to the baseline—re:
  Ophth)

PC-BMP
phosphorylcholine-binding myeloma
  protein

PCBs
polychlorinated biphenyls (toxic
  industrial chemical)

PCC
Pasteur Culture Collection
phenol, (meta)cresol, chloroform
pheochromocytoma
phosphate carrier compound
plasma catecholamine concentration
Poison Control Center
precoronary care
prematurely condensed chromosome
primary care curriculum
prothrombin-complex concentration

PCC, p.c.c.
premature chromosome condensation

PCc, P.Cc.
periscopic concave

PCCS
parent-child communication schedule

PCD
paroxysmal cerebral dysrhythmia
phosphate, citrate, dextrose
plasma cell dyscrasia
polycystic disease
posterior corneal deposits (re: Ophth)
prolonged contractile duration
pulmonary clearance delay

PCDC
plasma clot diffusion chamber (culture)

PCDUS
plasma cell dyscrasia of unknown
  significance

PCE
pseudocholinesterase
pulmocutaneous exchange

P cells
special cells with probable pacemaker
  function (re: cardiology)

PCF
peripheral circulatory failure
pharyngoconjunctival fever
posterior cranial fossa
prothrombin conversion factor

PCFT
platelet complement fixation test

PCG
paracervical ganglion
phonocardiogram
Planning Career Goals (re:
  psychological testing)
primate chorionic gonadotrop(h)in
pubococcygeus (muscle)

PCH
paroxysmal cold hemoglobinuria
polycyclic hydrocarbons

PCHE
pseudocholinesterase

PCI
intermediate posterior curve (cornea)
pneumatosis cystoides intestinalis
Premarital Communication Inventory
prophylactic cranial irradiation

pCi
picocurie

PCILO
perturbative configuration interaction
  (using) localized orbitals

PCIS
postcardiac injury syndrome

PCK
polycystic kidney (disease)

PCKD
polycystic kidney disease

PCL
persistent corpus luteum (re: OB-GYN)
plasma cell leukemia
posterior cruciate ligament

P closure
plastic closure

PCM
process control monitor (re: computers)
protein-calorie malnutrition
protein-carboxyl methylase
pulse code modulation (re: computers/
  data processing)

punched card machine (re: computers/ data processing)

_p_CM3
p-chloromercuribenzoate

PCMB, _p_-CMB
parachloromercuribenzoate (*p*- chloromercuribenzoic acid—now replaced by ClHgBzOH)

PCMC
Primary Children's Medical Center

PCMF
perceptual cognitive motor function

PCN
penicillin
pregnenolone-16α-carbonitrile
primary care network

PCNA
proliferating cell nuclear antigen

PCNB
pentachloronitrobenzene (fungicide)

PCO
patient complains of
polycystic ovary
predicted cardiac output

P_CO_
carbon monoxide pressure or tension

PCO_2_, pCO_2_
partial pressure or tension of carbon dioxide

PCoA
posterior communicating artery

PCO_2_A
partial pressure, alveolar carbon dioxide

PCO_2_ art
partial pressure, arterial carbon dioxide

PCOD
polycystic ovarian disease

PCO(D,S)
polycystic ovarian (disease, syndrome)

PCO_2_E, pCO_2_E
partial pressure, expiratory carbon dioxide (torr)

PCOS
polycystic ovarian syndrome

PCP
pentachlorophenate (sodium salt of pentachlorophenol—a topical antibacterial)
pentachlorophenol (toxic herbi-, fungi-, bacteri-, and algicide—a wood preservative)

peripheral coronary pressure
1-(1-phencyclohexyl)piperidine (phencyclidine—angel dust, HOG— an anesthetic; veterinary analgesic; also bromide, hydrochloride forms)
pneumocystic pneumonia
Pneumocystis carinii pneumonia
primary care physician
pulmonary capillary pressure

PCPA
DL-3-(*p*-chlorophenyl)alanine (fenclonine—a serotonin inhibitor)

pcpn.
precipitation

pcpt.
perception
precipitate
precipitation

PCR
patient contact record
phosphocreatine
plasma clearance rate
protein catabolic rate

PCS
palliative care service
portacaval shunt
postcardiac surgery
postcardiotomy syndrome
postcholecystectomy syndrome
precordial stethoscope
primary cancer site
print contrast signal (re: computers/data processing)
Priority Counseling Survey
proportional counter spectrometer
proximal coronary sinus
pseudomotor cerebri syndrome

Pcs, pcs.
preconscious (re: Psychol)

PCSM
percutaneous stone manipulation

P-C syndrome
posterior cervical syndrome

P-C syndrome c̄ ch. tens.
posterior cervical syndrome with much tension

PCT
patient clotting time
Physiognomic Cue Test (re: Psychol)
plasma clotting time
plasmacrit test (syphilis)
plasmacytoma
platelet hematocrit
polychlorinated triphenyl
porcine calcitonin
porphyria cutanea tarda
portacaval transportation

position computed tomography
postcoital test
progestogen challenge test
prothrombin consumption time
proximal convoluted tubule (of nephron)
pulmonary care team

p ct, pct.
per cent

PCU
patient care unit
primary care unit
Progressive Care Unit
protective care unit
protein-calorie undernutrition
pulmonary care unit

p. cut.
percutaneous

PCV
packed cell volume
parietal cell vagotomy
polycythemia vera
postcapillary venule

PCV-M
myeloid metaplasia with polycythemia
vera

PCW
Paul C. Williams (re: braces/exercises)
pulmonary capillary wedge

PCWP
pulmonary capillary wedge pressure

PCW pressure
pulmonary capillary wedge pressure

PCx, P Cx, P. Cx.
periscopic convex

PCZ
pancreozymin
procarbazine

PD
Paget's disease
pancreatic duct
paralytic dose
paralyzing dose
parkinsonism dementia
Parkinson's disease
paroxysmal discharge
pars distalis (pituitary)
patent ductus
patient demonstration
pediatrics
percentage difference
peritoneal dialysis
personality disorder
pharmacodynamics
phenyldichlorarsine (a war gas)
phosphate dehydrogenase
phosphate dextrose (media)

Pick's disease
plasma defect
poorly differentiated
Porak-Durante (syndrome)
porphobilinogen deaminase
posterior division
postnasal drainage
postural drainage
potential difference
potential differential
pregnanediol
present disease
pressor dose
primary dendrite
problem drinker
Process Diagnostic (re: Psychol)
progression of disease
protein degradation
protein deprived
protein diet
psychopathic deviate
psychotic depression
pulmonary disease
pulpodistal (re: Dent)
pulse duration
pyloric dilator

PD, P.D.
patient day

PD, pd, p.d., p-d
prism diopter

PD, p.d.
papilla diameter
(inter)pupillary distance

P(D+)
probability of having disease

P(D−)
probability of not having disease

PD$_{\infty}$
paralytic dose
paralyzing dose

PD$_{50}$
median paralysis

Pd
palladium (element)

^{103}Pd
radioactive isotope of palladium

^{109}Pd
radioactive isotope of palladium

p.d.
per diem (L. by the day)
pro die (L. for the day)

pd.
period

p/d
packs per day

PDA
patent ductus arteriosus
patient distress alarm
pediatric allergy
predialyzed human serum
pulmonary disease anemia

PDAB
paradimethylaminobenzaldehyde

PDB
Paget's disease of bone
p-dichlorobenzene (paracide)
phosphorus-dissolving bacteria

PDC
pediatrics cardiology
3-pentadecylcatechol (diagnostic aid—
    re: allergens)
physical dependence capacity
plasma digoxin concentration
plasma disappearance curve
postdecapitation convulsion
preliminary diagnostic clinic
private diagnostic clinic
pyridinol carbamate (an anti-
    arteriosclerotic)

3-PDC
3-pentadecylcatechol (diagnostic aid—
    re: allergens)

PDCD
primary degenerative cerebral disease

PDD
pervasive developmental disorder
phorbol didecanoate
primary degenerative dementia
pyridoxine-deficient diet

PDDB
phenododecinium bromide (topical anti-
    infective)

PDE
paroxysmal dyspnea on exertion
phosphodiesterase
pulsed Doppler echocardiography

PDF
peritoneal dialysis fluid

PDG
phosphogluconate dehydrogenase

PDGA
pteroyldiglutamic acid (diopterin—
    antineoplastic)

PDGF
platelet-derived growth factor

PDH
past dental history

phosphate dehydrogenase
postdental history
pyruvate dehydrogenase

PDHC
pyruvate dehydrogenase complex

P-DHP
16,17-[(1-phenylethylidene)bis(oxy)]
    pregn-4-ene-3,20-dione (algestone—
    a progestin; contraceptive)

PDI
Periodontal Disease Index
Psychomotor Development Index

Pdi
transdiaphragmatic pressure

P-diol
pregnanediol

PDL
poorly differentiated lymphocytic
    (lymphoma)
population doubling level
primary dysfunctional labor

Pdl, pdl
pudendal

pdl
poundal (name for force which can
    accelerate a one-pound mass by one
    foot per second per second)

PDLC
poorly differentiated lung cancer

PDLL
poorly differentiated lymphocytic
    lymphoma

PDL-N
poorly differentiated (lymphocytic)
    lymphoma-nodular

PDLP
predigested liquid protein

PDM
pulse-duration modulation (re:
    computers)

P-DMEA
phosphoryldimethylethanolamine
    (demanyl phosphate—psychotonic)

PDMS
pharmacokinetic drug monitoring
    service

PDP
pattern disruption point
platelet-depleted plasma
primer-dependent DNA polymerase
product development protocol

PD & P
postural drainage and percussion

PDPD
prolonged dwell peritoneal dialysis

PDPI
primer-dependent DNA polymerase
    index

PDQ
immediately; at once (pretty damn
    quick)
Prescreening Developmental
    Questionnaire
Protocol Data Query

PDR
pandevelopmental retardation
pediatrics radiology
peripheral diabetic retinopathy
Physicians' Desk Reference
pleiotropic drug resistance
post-delivery room
post-drug repetition
primary drug resistance
progress direct report
proliferative diabetic retinopathy (re:
    Ophth)

pdr.
powder
powdered

PDRB
Permanent Disability Rating Board

PDS
pain dysfunction syndrome
paroxysmal depolarizing shift
patient data system
pediatric surgery
peritoneal dialysis system
predialyzed human serum
primary dependence study

PdS
psychiatric deviate, subtle

PDT
photodynamic therapy
population doubling time

PDUF
pulsed Doppler ultrasonic flowmeter

PDV
peak diastolic velocity

PDW
platelet distribution width

PE
pancreatic extract
paper electrophoresis
parallel elastic (component—re:
    muscle)

partial epilepsy
Pel-Ebstein (disease)
pelvic examination
penile erection
percentage of estimated normal value
pericardial effusion
peritoneal exudate
pharyngoesophageal
phenylephrine (hydrochloride—an
    adrenergic)
phosphatidylethanolamine (cephalins,
    kephalins—re: local hemostatic;
    reagent in liver function tests)
photographic effect
physical education
physical evaluation
physical exercise
pigment(ed) epithelium (retinal)
pilocarpine hydrochloride with
    epinephrine
plasma exchange
plating efficiency
pleural effusion
polyethylene
polynuclear eosinophil
potential energy
powdered extract
preeclampsia
present examination
pressure equalization
prior to exposure
probable error
probe excision
protein excretion
pulmonary edema
pulmonary embolism
pulmonary embolus
pyramidal eminence

PE, P.E.
physical examination

PE, P/E
point of entry

P$_E$, Pe
expiratory pressure

PE2
secondary plating efficiency

Pe
Peclet number (re: transfer of thermal
    energy in fluids)
perylene (dibenz[*de,kl*]anthracene;
    peri-dinaphthalene—occurs in coal
    tar)

p.e.
per exemplum (L. for example)

PEA
pelvic examination under anesthesia
phenethyl alcohol (blood agar)
phenethylamine
polysaccharide egg antigen

PE ↓ A
pelvic examination under anesthesia

PEACH
Preschool Evaluation and Assessment
for Children with Handicaps

PEAQ
Personal Experience and Attitude
Questionnaire

PEARLA
pupils equal and react to light and
accommodation

PEBC
propyl ethyl-*n*-butylthiolcarbamate
(pebulate—herbicide)

PEBG
1-phenethylbiguanide (phenformin—
toxic antidiabetic, no longer used in
U.S.)

PEC
parallel elastic component
peduncle of cerebrum
peritoneal exudate cells
photoelectric cell
pyogenic exotoxin C

Pecho
prostatic echogram

PeCO₂
mixed expired carbon dioxide

PECT
positron emission computed
tomography

PED
pediatrician
peduncle (cerebral)
pharyngoesophageal diverticulum
pollution and environmental
degradation
post-entry day
postexertional dyspnea

PED, Ped, ped.
pediatrics

PEd, P Ed
physical education

ped.
pedangle
pedestrian

ped. ed.
pedal edema

PEDG
phenylethyldiguanide (phenformin—
toxic antidiabetic no longer used in
U.S.—withdrawn from market in
1978)

Peds
Pediatrics (Department of)

Peds, peds
pediatrics

PEE
parallel elastic element

PEEP
positive end-expiratory pressure (re:
Resp)

PEER
Pediatric Examination of Educational
Readiness

PEF
peak expiratory flow (re: Resp)
pharyngoepiglottic fold
Psychiatric Evaluation Form
pulmonary edema fluid

PEFR
peak expiratory flow rate (re: Resp)

PEFR$_n$
peak expiratory flow rate through the
nose

PEFSR
partial expiratory flow—static recoil
curve (re: Resp)

PEFT
Preschool Embedded Figures Test

PEFV
partial expiratory flow volume (re: Resp)

PEG
pneumoencephalogram
pneumoencephalograph
pneumoencephalography
polyethylene glycol (ointment and
suppository base)

PEI
phosphate excretion index
phosphorus excretion index
physical efficiency index

PEL
peritoneal exudate lymphocytes

Pel
pelvic (amputation level, upper limb—
re: Ortho)

PELISA
paper enzyme-linked immunosorbent
assay

PELS
propionylerythromycin lauryl sulfate
(erythromycin estolate—antibacterial)

PEM
peritoneal exudate macrophage
polyethylene matrix
precordial electrocardiographic
  mapping
prescription-event monitoring
primary enrichment medium
probable error of measurement (re:
  statistics)
production engineering measures
protein energy malnutrition
pulmonary endothelial membrane

PEMA
phenylethylmalonamide

PEMF
pulsating electromagnetic field

Pen, pen.
penicillin

pen.
penis

pend.
pendulous

penic.
penicillin

penic. cam.
penicillum camelinum (L. camel's tail
  [camel's hair brush])

PEN-O
Penner serotype-O

pens.
pension

Pent, pent.
penthiobarbital sodium (thiopentone
  sodium—IV anesthesia)

PEO
progressive external ophthalmoplegia

PEP
performance evaluation procedure (re:
  Psychol)
phosphoenolpyruvate (high energy
  ester of pyruvic acid)
physiologic evaluation of primates
polyestradiol phosphate (re: prostatic
  cancer)
positive expiratory pressure
postencephalitic parkinsonism
pre-ejection period (re: Cardio)
Procytox (cyclophosphamide),
  epipodophyllotoxin derivative (VM-
  26), and prednisolone (re:
  chemotherapy)
Psychiatric Evaluation Profile
Psycho-Epistemological Profile

Pep
peptidase

PEPA, Pep A
peptidase A

PEPB, Pep B
peptidase B

PEPC, Pep C
peptidase C

PEP$_c$
pre-ejection period corrected

PEPD, Pep D
peptidase D

PEPI
pre-ejection period index

PEPP
positive expiratory pressure plateau

PEPR
precision encoder and pattern
  recognizer

PEPS, Pep S
peptidase S

PER
pediatrics emergency room
Period Evaluation Record
protein efficiency ratio
pudendal evoked response

Per
permission

per.
perineal
period
periodic
person

PERC
potential erythropoietin-responsive cell

Perc
Percodan

percus.
percussion

Percuss. & ausc.
percussion and auscultation

PERD
photoelectric registration device

perf.
perfect
perfected
perforated
perforating
perforation
performed

PERI
Psychiatric Epidemiology Research
  Interview

peri.
perineal
perineum

periap.
periapical

perim.
perimeter

periorb.
periorbital

periph.
peripheral
periphery

periumb.
periumbilical

PERL
pupils equal and reactive to light

PERLA
pupils equal, react to light and
  accommodation

perm.
permanent
permutation

per. op. emet.
peracta operatione emetici (L. when the
  action of the emetic is over)

perp.
perpendicular

perpad, per. pad
perineal pad

PERRLA
pupils equal, round, react to light and
  accommodation
pupils equal, round, regular to light and
  accommodation

PERS
patient evaluation rating scale

pers.
person
personal
personality

persp.
perspiration

PERT
program evaluation and review
  technique (re: computers)
Program Evaluation Review Technique

pert.
pertaining to

pertinent
pertussis (whooping cough)

per. unc.
period of unconsciousness

PES
photoelectron spectroscopy
polyethylene sulfonate (anticoagulant)
postextrasystolic
pre-epiglottic space
pre-excitation syndrome
programmed electrical stimulation
programmed extrastimulus
Psychiatric Emergency Service
  (Department of)

PESP
postextrasystolic potentiation

PESS, pess.
pessus (Gr. oval stone [re: OB-GYN;
  pessary—an oval device to support
  the uterus])

PEST
point estimation by sequential testing

PET
Parent Effectiveness Training (re:
  Psychol)
peak ejection time
pear-shaped extension tube
polyethylene terephthalates (re: arterial
  grafts)
polyethylene tube
poor exercise tolerance
positron-emission tomography
pre-eclamptic toxemia
progressive exercise test
Psychiatry Emergency Team

pet.
petrolatum

petech.
petechiae

PETELS
peritoneal exudate T-enriched
  lymphocyte system

PETH
pink-eyed, tan-hooded (re: rat strain)

PETN
pentaerythritol tetranicontinate
  (niceritrol—an anti- lipemic)
pentaerythritol tetranitrate
  (pentaerythrityl—a vasodilator)

petr.
petroleum

PETT
positron-emission transaxial
  tomography

positron-emission transverse
tomography

PE tube
polyethylene tube

PEU
plasma equivalent unit

PEV
peak expiratory velocity (re: Resp)

PeV
peripheral vein

pev
peak electron volts

PEVN
periventricular nucleus

PEWV
pulmonary extravascular water volume

PEx
physical examination

p. ex.
per exemplum (L. for example)

PF
page footing (re: computers)
pair fed
parallel fiber
parotid fluid
partially follicular
past findings
peak flow
perfusion fluid
pericardial fluid
peripheral fields
peritoneal fluid
personality factor
pertinent findings
picture frustration (study—re: Psychol)
plantar flexion
plasma fibronectin
Plasmodium falciparum
platelet factor
pleural fluid
prostatic fluid
protection factor
pterygoid fossa
pulmonary factor
pulmonary (blood) flow
pulmonary function
Purkinje fiber
purpura fulminans
push fluids

PF, pf
permeability factor
power factor

P$_F$
final pressure (re: intraocular glaucoma)

P/F
pass-fail system

PF3, PF 3, PF$_3$
platelet factor 3

PF4, PF 4, PF$_4$
platelet factor 4

16 PF
Sixteen Personality Factor
Questionnaire

Pf.
Pfeifferella (genus)

pF
picofarad (one trillionth [10^{-12}] plus
farad— a practical unit of electrical
capacity)

pf
point of fusion

PFA
1-phosphofructaldolase

P-FAD
prosthetic (group) flavine-adenine
dinucleotide

PFAGH
penalty, frustration, anxiety, guilt,
hostility

PFC
pelvic flexion contracture
perfluorocarbons
pericardial fluid culture
persistence of fetal circulation
plaque-forming cells

PFD
polyostotic fibrous dysplasia
primary flash distillate

PFFD
proximal femoral focal deficiency

PFG
peak flow gauge

PFGS
phosphoribosyl formylglycinamide
synthetase

PFH
perifornical hypothalamus

PFIB
perfluoroisobutylene

PFK
phosphofructokinase

PFK1
phosphofructokinase-1

PFL
profibrinolysin

PFM
peak flow meter
pulse frequency modulation (re:
  computers)

PFN
partially functional neutrophil

PFO
patent foramen ovale (cordis—re:
  Cardio)

PFP
platelet-free plasma
preceding foreperiod

PFQ
Personality Factor Questionnaire

PFR
peak filling rate
peak flow rate (reading)

PFRC
predicted functional residual capacity

PFS
pulmonary function score

PFST
positional feedback stimulation trainer

PFT
pancreatic function test
phenylalanine mustard (melphalan),
  fluorouracil, tamoxifen (re:
  chemotherapy)
posterior fossa tumor
pulmonary function test

PFT$_4$
proportion free thyroxin(e)

PFU
plaque-forming unit

PFUO
prolonged fever of unknown origin

PFV
physiological full value

PFW
peak flow whistle

PG
paralysie générale (Fr. general
  paralysis)
paregoric
parotid gland
pentagastrin
pepsinogen
phosphatidylglycerol (in amniotic fluid—
  re: fetal lung maturity; hyaline
  membrane disease)

phosphogluconate
pigment granule
pituitary gonadotrop(h)in
plasma gastrin
plasma triglyceride
postgraduate
postgraft
pregnanediol glucuronide
pressure of gas
progesterone
propyl gallate (anti-oxidant)
prostaglandin
proteoglycans
pyoderma gangrenosum

PG, P$_G$
plasma glucose

PG, Pg, pg
pregnant

2-PG
2-phospho-D-glycerate (re: glucose
  metabolism)

3-PG
3-phosphoglycerate (re: glucose
  pathways)

6-PG
6-phosphogluconate (re: glucose
  metabolism)

Pg
gastric pressure

pg, pg.
picogram (one trillionth [10^{-12}] of a
  gram)

pg.
pregnancy

PGA
prostaglandin A (15-hydroxy-9-
  oxoprostanoic acid)
pteroylglutamic acid (folic acid)

PGA$_1$
prostaglandin A$_1$

PGA$_2$
prostaglandin A$_2$

PGA$_3$
prostaglandin A$_3$

PGB
prostaglandin B (15-hydroxy-prostanoic
  acid)

PGC
percentage of goblet cells
primordial germ cell
prostaglandin C

PGD
phosphogluconate dehydrogenase

phosphoglyceraldehyde
dehydrogenase
prostaglandin D

PGD$_2$
prostaglandin D$_2$

6-PGD, 6-P-GD
6-phosphogluconate dehydrogenase

PGDH
phosphogluconate dehydrogenase

PGDR
plasma glucose disappearance rate

PGE
platelet granule extract
posterior gastroenterostomy
primary generalized epilepsy
prostaglandin E

PGE$_1$
prostaglandin E$_1$ (alprostadil—
vasodilator)

PGE$_2$
prostaglandin E$_2$ (dinoprostone—
oxytocic)

PGEM
prostaglandin E metabolite

PGF
paternal grandfather
prostaglandin F

PGF$_{1\alpha}$
prostaglandin F$_{1\alpha}$ (less potent than
PGF$_{2\alpha}$)

PGF$_{2\alpha}$
prostaglandin F$_{2\alpha}$ (dinoprost—oxytocic)

PGG
polyclonal gamma globulin
prostaglandin G

PGG$_2$
prostaglandin G$_2$ (15-hydroperoxy-9α-
11α-peroxido-prosta-5,13-dienoic
acid; prostaglandin endoperoxide)

PGH
pituitary gonadotropic hormone
(pituitary growth hormone)
pituitary growth hormone (pituitary
gonadotropic hormone)
plasma growth hormone
porcine growth hormone
prostaglandin H

PGH$_2$
prostaglandin H$_2$ (15-hydroxy-9,11-
peroxidoprosta-5,13-dienoic acid)

PGI
potassium, glucose, insulin

PGI, PG I
(serum) pepsinogen I
(radioimmunoassay)

PGI$_2$
prostaglandin I$_2$ (prostacyclin)

PGK
phosphoglycerate kinase

PGM
paternal grandmother
phosphoglucomutase
phosphoglyceromutase (important step
in Emden-Meyerhof pathway)

PGM1
phosphoglucomutase-1

PGM2
phosphoglucomutase-2

PGM3
phosphoglucomutase-3

PGN
proliferative glomerulonephritis

PGO
pontogeniculo-occipital (rapid eye
movements—re: Neuro)

PGP
3-phosphoglyceroyl phosphate
phosphoglycollate phosphatase
postgamma proteinuria
prepaid group practice (plan)
progressive general paralysis

PGR
psychogalvanic response

PGR, PgR
progesterone receptor

PGS
pineal gonadal syndrome
plant growth substance
prostaglandin synthetase
proteoglycans subunits

PGSI
prostaglandin synthetase inhibitor

PGSR
psychogalvanic skin resistance

PGT
play group therapy

PGTR
plasma glucose tolerance rate

PGU
peripheral glucose uptake
postgonococcal urethritis

PGV
proximal gastric vagotomy

PGX
prostaglandin X

PGY
postgraduate year

PGYE
peptone, glucose, yeast extract
  (medium)

PH
page heading (re: computers)
parathyroid hormone
partially hepatectomized
passive hemagglutination
patient history
peliosis hepatitis
persistent hepatitis
personal history
physical history
polycythemia hypertonica
porphyria hepatica
porta hepatis
posterior hypothalamus
previous history
prolactin hormone
prostatic hypertrophy
pseudohermaphroditism
pubic hair
public health
pulmonary hypertension
punctate hemorrhage

PH, P.H.
past history

PH, Ph, ph.
pharmacopoeia
phenyl

PH₃
phosphine (H_3P—a poisonous gas)

Ph
phalangeal (amputation level, upper
  limb—re: Ortho)
pharmacy
phenanthrene (toxic substance found in
  coal tar)

Ph, ph.
phosphate

Ph¹
Philadelphia chromosome

pH
acid-base scale
hydrogen ion concentration (measure of
  alkalinity and acidity)
logarithm of hydrogen ion concentration
  reciprocal

pH₁
isoelectric point

ph
phote (unit of illumination of a surface)

ph.
phase
phial

PHA
passive hemagglutination
peripheral hyperalimentation (solution)
phenylalanine
phytohemagglutin
phytohemagglutinin
pulse height analyzer

pHa
arterial pH

PHAL
phytohemagglutinin-stimulated
  lymphocyte

phal.
phalanges
phalanx

PHAlb
polymerized human albumin

PHA-M, PHA-m
phytohemagglutinin-
  mucopolysaccharide (fraction)

PHA-P
phytohemagglutinin-protein (fraction)

PHAR, Phar, phar.
pharmacy

Phar, phar.
pharmacist

phar.
pharmaceutical
pharmacopoeia
pharyngeal
pharyngitis
pharynx

PHARM, pharm.
pharmacist
pharmacy

pharm.
pharmaceutical
pharmacopoeia

pharmacol.
pharmacological

pH art.
arterial pH (alkalinity-acidity measure)

pharyn.
pharyngeal
pharyngitis

Ph B
British Pharmacopoeia

Ph BC
phenylbutylcarbinol (fenipentol—
   choleretic)

PHC
posthospital care
premolar aplasia, hyperhidrosis, and
   (premature) canities
premolar aplasia, hyperhidrosis, and
   canities prematura (Böök
   syndrome—re: genetics)
primary health care
primary hepatic carcinoma
primary hepatocellular carcinoma

Ph′c
Philadelphia chromosome

PHCC
primary hepatocellular carcinoma

PHC syndrome
premolar aplasia, hyperhidrosis,
   (premature) canities (Böök
   syndrome—re: genetics)

PHD
packaged hospital disaster
photoelectron diffraction
pinhole disk (re: Ophth)
potentially harmful drug
pulmonary heart disease

PHDPE
porous high density polyethylene

PHE
periodic health examination
post-heparin esterase

Phe, phe.
phenylalanine (nutrient)

PhEEM
photoemission electron microscope

Phen
phenformin (withdrawn from market in
   1978)

phen.
phenobarbital

pheno.
phenotype

phenobarb.
phenobarbital

Pheo
pheochromocytoma

PHF
paired helical filaments

PHFG
primary human fetal glia

PHGA
pteroylhexaglutamylglutamic acid

PhGABA
β-phenyl-γ-aminobutyric acid
   (tranquilizer; mood elevator)

Phgly
phenylglycine

Φ, φ
phi (the 21st letter of the Greek
   alphabet)

Φ
magnetic flux

φ
an angular coordinate variable (re:
   mathematics)

PHI
passive hemagglutination inhibitor
past history of illness
phosphohexoisomerase
physiological hyaluronidase inhibitor

phial.
phiala (Gr. bottle)

PHIM
posthypoxic intention myoclonus

PHK
platelet phosphohexokinase
postmortem human kidney

PHK cells
postmortem human kidney cells

PHLA
post-heparin lipolytic activity

PHM
posterior hyaloid membrane (limiting
   membrane)
psyllium hydrophilic mucilloid
pulmonary hyaline membrane

PhM
pharyngeal musculature

PHN
Public Health Nurse

PhNCS
phenyl isothiocyanate ($C_6H_5N{=}C{=}S$;
   phenylisothiocyanate—a reagent—
   this abbreviation preferred over PITC)

phos.
phosphatase
phosphate
phosphorus

phot.
photophobia

photocoag.
photocoagulation

PHP
passive hyperpolarizing potential
post-heparin phospholipase
prehospital program
prepaid health plan
primary hyperparathyroidism
pseudohypoparathyroidism

pHPPA
p-hydroxyphenylpyruvic acid

PHPT
pseudohypoparathyroidism

PHPV
persistent hyperplasia of the primary
   vitreous (re: Ophth)
persistent hyperplastic primary vitreous
   (re: Ophth)

PHR
peak heart rate
photoreactivity

PHS
patient-heated serum
pooled human serum
posthypnotic suggestion
Public Health Service

PHSC
pluripotent hemopoietic stem cell

PHSQ
Psychosocial History Screening
   Questionnaire

PHT
phenytoin (diphenylhydantoin—
   anticonvulsant; anti- epileptic)
portal hypertension
primary hyperthyroidism
pulmonary hypertension

PHV
peak height velocity

pHv
mixed venous pH

PHX
pulmonary histiocytosis X

P Hx
past history

PHY
pharyngitis
physical

PHY, phy.
phytohemagglutinin

PHYS
physiological

PHYS, phys.
physiology

PhyS
physiological saline

Phys, phys.
physician

phys.
physical
physics

Phys Dis, phys. dis.
physical disability

PhysEd, Phys Ed
physical education

physio.
physiological
physiotherapist
physiotherapy

Physiol, physiol.
physiological
physiology

PhysMed, Phys Med
physical medicine

phys. sol.
physiological (saline) solution

PhysTher, phys. ther.
physical therapy

PI
international protocol
pacing impulse
pancreatic insufficiency
pars intermedia (re: Neuro/Endo)
patient's interests
performance index
performance intensity
perinatal injury
Periodontal Index (classification of
   periodontal diseases—re: Dent/
   Periodont)
peripheral iridectomy (re: Ophth)
permanent incidence
permeability index
personal injury
phagocytic index
phosphatidylinositol
Phospholine Iodide (echothiophate
   iodide—re: Ophth)
physically impaired
pineal (body—re: Endo)
pneumatosis intestinalis
poison ivy
ponderal index
post infectionem (L. after infection)
post inoculation

pregnancy induced
pre-induction (examination)
premature infant
prematurity index
preparatory interval
pressure on inspiration
primary infarction
proactive inhibition (re: Psychol)
proactive interference
programmed instruction
proinsulin
prolactin inhibitor
proximal intestine
pulmonary incompetence
pulmonary infarction

PI, P.I.
present illness
protamine insulin

PI, P/I
post injury

PI, Pi
protease inhibitor (a gene)

P$_I$
inspiratory pressure

Π, π
pi (16th letter of Greek alphabet)

Pi
pressure of inspiration

Pi, P$_i$
inorganic phosphate

pI
pH of a given substance at its iso-
    electric point
pH of a solution containing a solute at
    its isoelectric point

PIA
peripheral interface adaptor
photoelectronic intravenous
    angiography
plasma insulin activity
porcine intestinal adenomatosis
preinfarct angina

PIAPACS
psychological information, acquisition,
    processing and control system

PIAT
Peabody Individual Achievement Test

PIB
psi-interactive biomolecules

π bond
one of the bonding molecular orbitals

PIC
Personality Inventory for Children

postinflammatory corticoid
postintercourse

PICA
Porch Index of Communicative Ability
    (re: aphasic adults)
posterior inferior cerebellar artery

PICAC
Porch Index of Communicative Ability in
    Children

PICD
primary irritant contact dermatitis

π complex
pi complex (re: molecular bonds)

picornavirus
pico + ribonucleic acid + virus

PICSI
Picture Identification for Children-
    Standardized Index

PICU
pediatric intensive care unit
pulmonary intensive care unit

PID
pain intensity difference
pelvic inflammatory disease
2-phenyl-1H-indene-1,3(2H)-dione
    (phenindione—anticoagulant)
photoionization detector
plasma-iron disappearance
post-inertia dyskinesia
prolapsed intervertebral disc
prolapsed intervertebral disease
proportional-integral-derivative
protruded intervertebral disc

PIDRA
portable insulin dosage-regulating
    apparatus

PIDT
plasma-iron disappearance time

PIE
postinfectious encephalomyelitis
preimplantation embryo
pulmonary infiltrate with eosinophilia
pulmonary infiltration (associated with)
    eosinophilia
pulmonary interstitial edema
pulmonary interstitial emphysema

PIEF
isoelectric focusing in polyacrylamide

PIEP
peripheral infarct epicardium

PIES
Picture Interest Exploration Survey (re:
    Psychol)

PIF
peak inspiratory flow (re: Resp)
pigment-inducing factor
point of identical flow
premorbid inferiority feeling (re:
    Psychol)
pro-insulin free
prolactin-inhibiting factor
prolactin release-inhibiting factor
proliferation inhibiting factor
proliferation inhibitory factor
prostatic interstitial fluid

PIFG
poor intrauterine fetal growth

PIFR
peak inspiratory flow rate (re: Resp)

PIFT
platelet immunofluorescence test

Pig
pigmentation

pig.
pigmented

pigm.
pigmentum (L. paint)

PIGPA
pyruvate, inosine, glucose, phosphate,
    adenine

PIH
β-phenylisopropylhydrazine
    (pheniprazine—antihypertensive)
pregnancy induced hypertension
prolactin (release-) inhibiting hormone

PIHH
postinfluenza-like hyposmia and
    hypogeusia (re: ENT)

PII
plasma inorganic iodine
primary irritation indices

PIIP
portable insulin infusion pump

PIIS
posterior inferior iliac spine

PIL
patient information leaflet
Purpose in Life Test (re: Psychol)

pil.
pilula(e) (L. pill[s])

PIM
penicillamine-induced myasthenia

ping.
pinguis (L. fat)

PINN
proposed international nonproprietary
    name

PINS
person in need of supervision

PiO$_2$
partial pressure of inspiratory oxygen

PIP
paralytic infantile paralysis
peak inspiratory pressure
piperacillin
posterior interphalangeal (joint—re:
    podiatry)
probable intrauterine pregnancy
proximal interphalangeal (joint)
Psychotic Inpatient Profile

PIPA
platelet ^{125}I-labeled (staphylococcal)
    protein A

PIPJ
proximal interphalangeal joint

PIQ
performance intelligence quotient

PIR
piriform (muscle)
postinhibitory rebound

P-IRI
plasma immunoreactive insulin

PIRS
plasma immunoreactive secretion
    (level)

PIT
pacing-induced tachycardia
patellar inhibition test
perceived illness threat
Picture Identification Test (re: Psychol)
plasma iron turnover

pit.
Pitocin (an oxytocic—re: OB)
pituitary
Pituitrin

Pit Aug
Pitocin augmentation (re: OB)

PITC
phenylisothiocyanate (Edman's reagent)

Pit Ind
Pitocin induction (re: OB)

PITR
plasma iron turnover rate

PIU
path information unit (re: computers/
  data processing)
polymerase-inducing unit

PIV
parainfluenza virus

PIVD
protruded intervertebral disc

PIVH
peripheral intravenous
  hyperalimentation

PIVKA
protein in vitamin K absence
protein induced by vitamin K absence
protein induced by vitamin K antagonist

PIXE
proton-induced x-ray emission

pixel
picture element (re: CT display image)

PJ
pancreatic juice
Peutz-Jeghers (syndrome)

PJB
premature junctional beat

PJC
premature junctional contraction

P-J interval
time elapsed from beginning of P wave
  to end of QRS complex (J = junction
  between QRS and S-T segments—
  re: electrocardiogram)

PJP
pancreatic juice protein

PJS
peritoneojugular shunt

PJT
paroxysmal junctional tachycardia

PK
Parrot-Kaufmann (syndrome)
Paterson-Kelly (syndrome)
penetrating keratoplasty (re: Ophth)
pericardial knock
pharmacokinetic
Piringer-Kuchinka (syndrome)
protein kinase
psychokinesis
psychokinetic
pyruvate kinase (assay)

PK, P-K
Prausnitz-Küstner (reaction)

pK
negative logarithm of ionization
  (dissociation) constant

pK'
negative logarithm of the dissociation
  constant of an acid (-log $K_{a'}$)

PKA
prekallikrein activator

pKa, pK_a
measure of strength of an acid defined
  as the negative logarithm of the acid
  ionization constant (K_a)

PKAR
protein kinase activation ratio

PKase
protein kinase

PKD
polycystic kidney disease

PKF
phagocytosis and killing function

PKK
prekallikrein

PKM2
pyruvate kinase (M2)

PKN
parkinsonism

PKP
penetrating keratoplasty

PKR
phased knee rehabilitation
Prausnitz-Küstner reaction

PKSAP
Psychiatric Knowledge and Skills Self-
  Assessment Program

PK test
Prausnitz-Küstner test

PKU
phenylketonuria

PKV
killed poliomyelitis vaccine
peak kilovolts

pkV
peak kilovoltage

PL
palmaris longus
palm leaf (reaction)
pancreatic lipase
peroneus longus
phospholipid
photoluminescence
placebo

placental lactogen
plantar
plasmalemma
plastic surgeon
plastic surgery
preleukemia
problem list
prolymphocytic leukemia
psychosocial-labile
pulpolingual (re: Dent)
Purkinje layer

PL, P.L.
perception (of) light (light perception)

P$_L$
pulmonary venous pressure
transpulmonary pressure

pl
picoliter

pl.
place
plasma
plate
platelets
pleural
plexus
plural

PLA
phospholipase A
plasminogen activator
platelet antigen
polymer of lactic acid
posterior lip of acetabulum (re: Ortho)
posterior wall, left atrium (re: Cardio)
procaine and lactic acid
pulpolinguoaxial (re: Dent)

PLA, PLa
pulpolabial (re: Dent)

Pla
left atrial pressure

plac. praev.
placenta praevia

plant-flex
plantar flexion

PLAP
placental alkaline phosphatase

plat.
platelets

PLB
phospholipase B
porous layer bead (re: chromatography)

PLBO
placebo

PLC
Personal Locus of Control (re: Psychol)

phospholipase C
primary liver (cell) cancer
proinsulin-like component
proinsulin-like compound
protein-lipid complex
pseudolymphocytic choriomeningitis

PLCC
primary liver cell cancer

PLD
peripheral light detection
phospholipase D
platelet defect
posterior latissimus dorsi
postlaser day
potentially lethal damage

PLDH
plasma lactic dehydrogenase

PLDR
potentially lethal damage repair

PLE
panlobular emphysema
pleura
polymorphic light eruption
protein-losing enteropathy
pseudolupus erythematosus
    (syndrome)

PLED
periodic lateralized epileptiform
    discharge (re: EEG)

PLEDS
periodic lateral epileptiform discharges
    (re: EEG)

PLES
parallel-line equal-space (re:
    scintillating cameras)

pleth.
plethoric

Pleur Fl
pleural fluid

PLEVA
pityriasis lichenoides et varioliformis
    acuta (re: Derma)

PLF
posterior lung fiber

PLG
plasminogen
pregnandiol-like glycuronides

P-LGV
psittacosis-lymphogranuloma venereum

PLH
placental lactogenic hormone

PL/I
programming language one (re: computers)

PLL
peripheral light loss
pressure length loop

PLM
percent labeled mitoses (re: cell cycle)
plasma level monitoring
polarized light microscopy

PLMV
posterior-leaf mitral valve

PLN
peripheral lymph node
popliteal lymph node
posterior lip nerve

PLND
pelvic lymph node dissection

PLP
plasma leukapheresis
polystyrene latex particles
pyridoxal 5-phosphate

PLPD
pseudoperiodic lateralized paroxysmal discharge

PLR
pupillary light reflex

PLS
Preschool Language Scale (re: Psychol)
prostaglandin-like substance

pls.
please

PLT
platelet
primed lymphocyte test
primed lymphocyte typing
psittacosis-lymphogranuloma venereum-trachoma (Chlamydia-related group of diseases)

PLTS
platelets

plumb.
plumbum (L. lead)

PLV
live poliomyelitis vaccine
panleukopenia virus
phenylalanine, lysine, vasopressin
posterior left ventricle (re: Cardio)

plx.
plexus

PM
mean pressure (of a gas)
pacemaker
papillary muscle
papular mucinosis
partial meniscectomy
partial musculature
Pelizaeus-Merzbacher (syndrome)
peritoneal macrophages
petit mal
phenylalanine and methotrexate
photomultiplier (tube)
Physical Medicine (Department of)
plasma membrane
platelet membrane
platelet microsome
pneumomediastinum
poliomyelitis
polymorphonuclear
polymorphs
polymyositis
posterior mitral
post menstrua
post mortem (L. after death)
postmortem (L. adj. occurring or performed after death)
premamillary nucleus
premarketing approval
premolar
presystolic murmur
pretibial myxedema
preventative medicine (preventive)
Progressive Matrices
prostatic massage
protein methylesterase
pterygoid muscle
pulmonary macrophage
pulpomesial (re: Dent)
purple membrane (protein)

PM, P.M., p.m.
post meridiem (L. after noon—used as evening, night)

Pm
promethium (element—formerly illinium)

147Pm
radioactive isotope of promethium

149Pm
radioactive isotope of promethium

151Pm
radioactive isotope of promethium

pM
picomolar

pm
picometer

p.m.
punctum maximum (L. largest point)

PMA
papillae, marginal or attached gingivae
(re: Dent)
P = papillary portion of gingiva;
M = marginal portion; A = attached
portion (re: Dent)
phenylmercuric acetate (an herbicide,
fungicide)
phosphomolybdic acid (a reagent)
p-methoxyamphetamine
positive mental attitude
Primary Mental Abilities (test)
progressive muscular atrophy

PMAC
phenylmercuric acetate (herbicide;
fungicide)

PMB
papillomacular bundle
polychrome methylene blue
polymyxin B
postmenopausal bleeding

PMB, P.M.B.
polymorphonuclear basophil
(leukocytes)

PMC
phenylmercuric chloride (antimicrobial
agent)
physical medicine clinic
pleural mesothelial cell
premature mitral closure
pseudomembranous colitis

PM clinic
physical medicine clinic

PMD
posterior mandibular depth
primary myocardial disease
private medical doctor
programmed multiple development (re:
chromatography)
progressive muscular dystrophy

PMD, P.M.D., PMd
private medical doctor (physician)

PME
progressive myoclonus epilepsy

PME, P.M.E.
polymorphonuclear eosinophil
(leukocytes)

PMF
progressive massive fibrosis
proton motive force
pterygomaxillary fossa

PMH
past medical history
pemoline magnesium hydroxide
(mixture—central stimulant)
posteromedial hypothalamus

previous medical history
programmed medical history

PMHR
predicted maximal heart rate

PMHY
past medical history

PMI
past medical illness
patient medical instructions
patient medication instruction
perioperative myocardial infarction
petition of mental illness
point of maximal intensity
point of maximum impact
point of maximum impulse
point of maximum intensity
posterior myocardial infarction
post-myocardial infarction (syndrome)
present medical illness
previous medical illness

PMI, P.M.I.
point of maximal impulse

PMK
primary (rhesus) monkey kidney

PML
polymorphonuclear leukocytes
posterior mitral leaflet
progressive multifocal leukodystrophy
progressive multifocal leukoencephalopathy
pulmonary microlithiasis

PMLE
polymorphous light eruption

PM lividity
postmortem lividity

PMM
pentamethylmelamine
protoplast maintenance medium

PMMA
polymethylmethacrylate (re: optics)

PMN
polymorphonuclear
polymorphonuclear neutrophil(ic)
(leukocytes)
polymorphonucleotides

PMNC
percentage of multinucleated cells

PMNG
polymorphonuclear granulocyte

PMNL
polymorphonuclear leukocyte

PMNN
polymorphonuclear neutrophil

PMNR
periadenitis mucosa necrotica
  recurrens

PMNs
polymorphonucleocytes

PMO
postmenopausal osteoporosis
Principal Medical Officer

PMP
past menstrual period
patient management problem
patient medication profile
persistent mentoposterior (position of
  fetus)
previous menstrual period

PMPO
postmenopausal palpable ovary
  (syndrome)

PMR
perinatal morbidity rate
perinatal mortality rate
periodic medical review
physical medicine and rehabilitation
polymyalgia rheumatica
prior medical record
proportionate morbidity ratio
proportionate mortality rate
proportionate mortality ratio
proton magnetic resonance

PM&R
Physical Medicine and Rehabilitation
  (service)

PM + R
Physical Medicine and Rehabilitation
  (service)

PMRS
Physical Medicine and Rehabilitation
  Service

PM & RS
Physical Medicine and Rehabilitation
  Service

PMS
phenazine methosulfate (re:
  biochemistry)
poor miserable soul
post-marketing surveillance
postmenopausal syndrome
postmitochondrial supernatant
pregnant mare serum (chorionic
  gonadotrop[h]in)
premenstrual syndrome

PMSC
pluripotent myeloid stem cell

PMSG
pregnant mare serum gonadotrop(h)in

PM splint
posterior molded splint

PMT
photoelectric multiplier tube
photomultiplier tube
Porteus Maze Test (re: Psychol)
premenstrual tension

PMTS
premenstrual tension syndrome

PMTT
pulmonary mean transit time

PMV
paralyzed, mechanically ventilated
prolapse of the mitral leaflet

pMVL
posterior mitral valve leaflet

PMW
pacemaker wires

PN
papillary necrosis
parenteral nutrition
perceived noise
periarteritis nodosa
peripheral nerve
peripheral neuropathy
peripheral nodes
phrenic nerve
plaque neutralization
Polenské number
polyneuritis
pontine nucleus (re: Neuro)
positional nystagmus (re: Neuro/Ophth)
posterior nares
postnatal
predicted normal
progress note
Psychiatry-Neurology
psychoneurologist
psychoneurology
psychoneurotic (individual)
pyelonephritis
pyrrolnitrin (antifungal)

PN, P.N.
percussion note

PN, P/N
post nausea

PN, Pn, pn.
pneumonia

P.N.
polynuclear neutrophil(e)s

P/N
positive to negative (ratio)

P & N, P&N
psychiatry and neurology

P_{N2}
partial pressure of nitrogen

Pn
pneumatic

P_{*n*}
Poisson probability of obtaining a count
   of n

pn.
pain
pneumothorax

PNA
Nomina Anatomica (Paris) (re:
   anatomical nomenclature)
pentosenucleic acid

P_{NA}
plasma sodium

PNAvQ
positive-negative ambivalent quotient
   (re: Psychol)

PNB
perineal needle biopsy
p-nitrobiphenyl
polymyxin, neomycin, bacitracin

PNBT
para-nitroblue tetrazolium

PNC
penicillin
peripheral nucleated cell
pneumotaxic center
postnecrotic cirrhosis
premature nodal contraction
pseudonurse cells
purine nucleotide cycle

PND
paroxysmal nocturnal dyspnea
partial neck dissection
postnasal drainage
postnasal drip
postneonatal death
purulent nasal drainage

pnd.
pound

PNdB
perceived noise decibel

PNDMA
(para or) *p*-nitroso-*N,N*-dimethylaniline
   (manufacturing chemical)

PNE
plasma norepinephrine
pneumoencephalogram
pseudomembranous necrotizing
   enterocolitis

PNET
peripheral neuroepithelioma
primitive neuroectodermal tumor

pneu.
pneumatic
pneumonia

pneumo.
pneumonia

PNF, P N F
proprioceptive neuromuscular
   facilitation (re: Neuro)

pnfl.
painful

PNG
penicillin G
pneumogram

PNH
paroxysmal nocturnal hemoglobinuria
polynuclear hydrocarbons

PNI
peripheral nerve injury
postnatal infection
pseudoneointimal (re: Cardio)
psychoneuroimmunology

PNK
polynucleotide kinase

PNL
peripheral nerve lesion
polymorphonuclear neutrophilic
   leukocyte

PNM
perinatal mortality
postneonatal mortality

PNMT
phenylethanolamine-*N*-methyl
   transferase

PNP
peripheral neuropathy
pneumoperitoneum
polyneuropathy
psychogenic nocturnal polydipsia
   (syndrome)
purine nucleotide phosphorylase

PNP, P-NP
p-nitrophenol (re: alkaline phosphatase
   assay)

PNPB
positive-negative pressure breathing

PNPG
p-nitrophenyl-β-galactoside
p-nitrophenylglycerine

PNPP
p-nitrophenylphosphate (re: alkaline
phosphatase assay)

PNPR
positive-negative pressure respiration
positive-negative pressure respirator

PNS
parasympathetic nervous system
peripheral nerve stimulator
peripheral nervous system

PNT
partial nodular transformation
patient

pnt.
point

pnth.
pneumothorax

pnthx.
pneumothorax

pnts.
points

PNU
protein nitrogen unit

PNX
pneumonectomy

PNX, Pnx, pnx.
pneumothorax

PNZ
posterior necrotic zone

PO
parapineal organ
parietal operculum
parieto-occipital
percentage of observed value
perceptual organization
period of onset
perioperative
physician only
posterior
predominating organism

PO, P.O., p.o.
per os (L. through the mouth [by mouth;
orally])

PO, P-O, P/O
postoperative

PO, P/O
phone order

P/O
oxidative phosphorylation ratio
protein to osmolar ratio

P$_O$
opening pressure

PO I, II, III, etc.
postoperative day 1, 2, 3, etc.

PO$_2$, P$_{O_2}$, pO$_2$, pO$_2$
arterial oxygen pressure
oxygen partial pressure

PO$_4$
phosphate radical

Po
polonium (element)

P$_o$
intraocular pressure

^{208}Po
radioactive isotope of polonium

p.o.
predominant organism

POA
pancreatic oncofetal antigen
phalangeal osteoarthritis
point of application
preoptic area
primary optic atrophy

POA-AH
preoptic anterior hypothalamic area

POB
penicillin in oil and beeswax
phenoxybenzamine
place of birth

POBE
Profile of Out-of-Body Experiences

POC
particulate organic carbon
position of comfort
postoperative care
procarbazine, Oncovin, CCNU (re:
chemotherapy)
products of conception
purgeable organic carbon

POCA
prednisone, Oncovin (vincristine),
cytarabine, and Adriamycin
(doxorubicin) (re: chemotherapy)

POCC
procarbazine, Oncovin (vincristine),
cyclophosphamide, and CCNU
(lomustine) (re: chemotherapy)

pocill.
pocillum (L. a small cup)

pocul.
poculum (L. cup)

POCY
postoperative chronologic year

POD
peroxidase
place of death
polycystic ovarian disease

POD, P-O-D
postoperative day

PODQ
Perceptual Organization Deviation
   Quotient (re: Psychol)

PODx
preoperative diagnosis

POE
pediatric orthopaedic examination
point of entry
polyoxyethylene
portal of entry
postoperative endophthalmitis

P of E
point of entry

P of E, PofE
portal of entry

POEMS
polyneuropathy, organomegaly
   (hepatosplenomegaly),
   endocrinopathy, M protein, and skin
   changes (syndrome)

POF
position of function
pyruvate oxidation factor

POG
polymyositis ossificans generalisata

pOH
approximate concentration of hydroxide
   ions in a solution (hydroxyl
   concentration)

POHI
physically or otherwise health-impaired

POHS
per os hora somni (L. through the
   mouth at the hour of sleep [by mouth
   at bedtime])
presumed ocular histoplasmosis
   syndrome

POI
Personal Orientation Inventory

poik.
poikilocyte
poikilocytosis

pois.
poison
poisonous

pol.
polish (re: Dent)

polio.
poliomyelitis

POLL
pollex (L. thumb)

POLY, poly
polymorphonuclear (leukocyte)

polyA, poly-A
polyadenylate

poly A:U
polyadenylate:polyuridylate

polyIC
polyinosinic-polycytidylic (acid)

poly I:C
polyriboinosinic:polyribocytidylic

polys
polymorphonuclear (leukocytes)

polyU, poly(U)
polyuridylic acid

POM
pain on motion
prescription only medicine

POMC
pro-opiomelanocortin

POMP
prednisone, Oncovin (vincristine),
   methotrexate, and Purinethol (6-
   mercaptopurine) (re: chemotherapy)
principal outer material protein

POMR
problem-oriented medical record

POMS
Profile of Mood States (re: Psychol)

POMS-V
Profile of Mood States, Vigor (re:
   Psychol)

PON
particulate organic nitrogen
(brachium) pontis

pond.
pondere (L. by weight)
ponderosus (L. heavy)

PONS
Profile of Nonverbal Sensitivity (re:
   Psychol)

POP
2,5-diphenyloxazole (a primary
   scintillator)
persistent occipitoposterior (position of
   fetus)
pituitary opioid peptide
plasma oncotic pressure
plasma osmotic pressure
polycystic ovarian syndrome
polymyositis ossificans progressiva

POP, p.o.p.
plaster of paris

P.O.P.
paroxypropione (hormone inhibitor,
   pituitary)

POp, P Op, P-op
postoperative

Pop, pop.
popliteal
population

pop.
popular

poplit.
popliteal

POPOP
1,4-bis(5-phenyloxazol-2-yl)benzene (a
   secondary scintillator)

POR
post-occlusive oscillatory response
problem-oriented record

P/O ratio
measure of oxidative phosphorylation
   (re: cell metabolism)

PORH
postocclusive reactive hyperemia

PORP
partial ossicular replacement prosthesis
   (re: Oto)

port.
portable

POS
parosteal osteosarcoma

POS, Pos, pos.
positive

Pos, pos.
position

POSC
Problem Oriented System of Charting

POSM
patient-operated selector mechanism
patient-operated sensing mechanism

pos. pr.
positive pressure

pos. press.
positive pressure

POSS
percutaneous on-surface stimulation
proximal over-shoulder strap

poss.
possibility
possible

POST, post.
post mortem

post
post mortem (autopsy)

post.
posterior

post aur.
post aurem (L. behind the ear)

post cib.
post cibos (L. after meals)
post cibum (L. after a meal)

postgangl., post gangl.
postganglionic

Postinoc
postinoculation

postop., post-op
postoperative

post part.
post partum (L. occurring after
   childbirth)

postred., post-red
postreduction

post. sag. D
posterior sagittal diameter

post sing. sed. liq.
post singulas sedes liquidas (L. after
   every loose stool)

post. tib.
posterior tibial

post traum.
post trauma

POT
periostitis ossificans toxica

POT, pot.
potus (L. a drink, draught)

pot.
potassa
potassium
potential

435

POTAGT
potential abnormality of glucose
  tolerance

potass.
potassium

poten.
potential

POU
placenta, ovaries, uterus

POV
privately owned vehicle

PoV
portal vein

POVT
puerperal ovarian vein thrombophlebitis

POW
Powassan encephalitis
prisoner of war

powd.
powder
powdered

POX
point of exit

P. OX-2
Proteus vulgaris antigen strain (re: Weil-
  Felix test)

P. OX-19
Proteus vulgaris antigen strain (re: Weil-
  Felix test)

P. OX-K
Proteus vulgaris antigen strain (re: Weil-
  Felix test)

PP
pacesetter potential
pancreatic polypeptide
paradoxical pulse
parietal pleura
partial pressure
pathology point
pentose pathway
perfusion pressure
peripheral pulses
permanent partial
per pro (L. instead of)
Peyer's patch (re: aggregation of
  lymphatic follicles)
pink puffers (re: emphysema)
pinpoint
pinprick
placement problem
placenta praevia (previa)
placental protein
plane polarization
plasma pepsinogen

plasmapheresis
plasma protein
plaster of paris
polypropylene
porcine pancreatic (disease)
posterior papillary (disease)
posterior pituitary (disease)
post partum (L. after childbirth or
  delivery)
postpartum (L. adj. occurring after
  childbirth or delivery—re: the mother)
presenting problem
primipara
private patient
private practice
proactivator plasminogen
prothrombin-proconvertin
protoporphyria
protoporphyrin
proximal phalanx
pterygoid process
pulmonary pressure
pulse pressure
pulsus paradoxus
purulent pericarditis
(inorganic) pyrophosphatase
pyrophosphate

PP, P.P.
per primam (intentionem—L. by first
  [intention]—re: healing by first
  intention; fibrous adherence of wound
  without suppuration or granulation
  tissue formation)

PP, P-P
pellagra-preventing factor
pellagra preventive

PP, pp
postprandial (L. after an early meal)

P.P., Pp, p.p.
punctum proximum (L. nearest point [of
  accommodation]—re: Ophth)

P&P
prothrombin and proconvertin (test)

PP5
placental protein 5

P-5-P, P-5'-P
pyridoxal-5'-phosphate (enzyme co-
  factor vitamin)

pp
pedal pulses
pluripara
polyphosphate

PPA
palpation, percussion, auscultation
phenylpyruvic acid
Pittsburgh pneumonia agent

postpartum amenorrhea
postpill amenorrhea

PPA, Ppa, p.p.a.
phiala prius agitata (L. the bottle having
first been shaken)

PP&A, pp&a
palpation, percussion, and auscultation

pp + a
palpation, percussion, and auscultation

PPACK
D-phenyl-alanyl-prolyl-arginine
chloromethyl ketone (diagnostic tool;
re: blood thrombin level)

PPA pos.
phenylpyruvic acid positive

PPAS
peripheral pulmonary artery stenosis

PPAT
phosphoribosylpyrophosphate
amidotransferase

PPB
platelet poor blood
positive pressure breathing (re: Resp)

PPB, ppb
parts per billion

PPBE
proteose-peptone beef extract

PPBS
postprandial blood sugar

PPC
pentose phosphate cycle
peripheral posterior curve (cornea)
plasma prothrombin conversion
platinum-palladium colloid
progressive patient care
proximal palmar crease

PPCA
plasma prothrombin conversion
accelerator
proserum prothrombin conversion
accelerator

PPC(A,F)
plasma prothrombin conversion
(acceleration, factor)

PPCF
peripartum cardiac failure
plasma prothrombin conversion factor

PPCM
postpartum cardiomyopathy

PPD
paraphenylenediamine (p-

phenylenediamine [hydrochloride] —
blood reagent)
percussion and postural drainage
permanent partial disability
postpartum day
primary physical dependence

PPD, P.P.D.
progressive perceptive deafness
purified protein derivative (of tuberculin)

PPD, Ppd, p.p.d.
packs per day (tobacco)

P&PD
percussion and postural drainage

PPD-B
purified protein derivative-Battey

PPDR
preproliferative diabetic retinopathy

PPDS, PPD-S
purified protein derivative-standard

PPE
permeability pulmonary edema
polyphosphoric ester
porcine pancreatic disease
programmed physical examination

PPF
pellagra preventive factor (niacinamide;
nicotinic acid)
plasma protein fraction

P.P. factor, P-P factor
pellagra preventive factor (nicotinic
acid)

PPG
photoplethysmography
polymorphonuclear cells per
glomerulus
polyurethane-polyvinyl graphite
pretragal parotid gland

ppg., ppg
picopicogram

PPGA
postpill galactorrhea/amenorrhea

PPGF
polypeptide growth factor

PPGIR
psychophysiological gastrointestinal
reaction

PPGP
prepaid group practice

ppGpp
guanosine-5'-diphosphate-3'-
diphosphate

PPH
past pertinent history
persistent pulmonary hypertension
postpartum hemorrhage
primary pulmonary hypertension
protocollagen proline hydroxylase

PPHN
persistent pulmonary hypertension of
the newborn

PPHP
pseudo-pseudohypoparathyroidism

PPI
partial permanent impairment
patient package insert
Plan-Position-Indication
preceding preparatory interval
Present Pain Intensity
purified porcine insulin

PP$_i$
inorganic pyrophosphate

PPIM
postperinatal infant mortality

P-P interval
distance between consecutive P waves
in EKG (re: Cardio)

PPK
palmoplantar keratosis

PPL
penicilloyl polylysine (diagnostic aid
[allergen])
phospholipid

Ppl
(intra)pleural pressure

PPLF
postperfusion low flow

PPLO
pleuropneumonia-like organism(s)

PPL test
penicilloyl polylysine test (re:
intradermal diagnosis of penicillin
sensitivity)

PPM
permanent pacemaker
phosphopentomutase
posterior papillary muscle

PPM, ppm, ppm.
parts per million

p.p.m.
pulses per minute

PPMM
postpolycythemia myeloid metaplasia

PPMS
Purdue Perceptual-Motor Survey (re:
Psychol)

PPN
partial parenteral nutrition
pedunculopontine nucleus (re: Neuro)
peripeduncular nucleus (re: Neuro)

PPNA
peak phrenic nerve activity

PPNG
penicillinase-producing *Neisseria
gonorrhoeae*

PPO
2,5-diphenyloxazole (POP—a
scintillator)
peak pepsin output
platelet peroxidase
pleuropneumonia organisms
Preferred Provider Organization
prepatient periods to oocyst

PPP
palmoplantar pustulosis
paraoxypropiophenone (POP;
paroxypropione—pituitary
gonadotrop[h]ic hormone inhibitor)
pentose phosphate pathway
Pickford Projectives Pictures (re:
Psychol)
plasma protamine precipitating
platelet-poor plasma
polyphoretic phosphate
porcine pancreatic polypeptide
portal perfusion pressure
purified placental protein
pustulosis palmaris et plantaris (re:
Derma)

PPPH
purified placental protein, human

PPPI
primary private practice income

PPR
patient-physician relationship
photopalpebral reflex (blink response to
light)
poor partial response
posterior primary rami
Price's precipitation reaction

PPr
paraprosthetic

PPRF
paramedian pontine reticular formation
(horizontal gaze center)
postpartum renal failure

PPRibP
phosphoribosylpyrophosphate (5-
phospho-α-D-ribosyl pyrophosphate)

PPRP
5-phospho-α-D-ribosyl pyrophosphate

PPRPE
preserved para-arteriolar retinal pigment epithelium

PPRWP
poor precordial R-wave progression (re: EKG)

PPS
pepsin (hydrolase class enzyme)
Personal Preference Scale
polyvalent pneumococcal polysaccharide
postpartum sterilization
postperfusion syndrome
postpericardiotomy syndrome
postsump syndrome

PPS, p.p.s.
pulses per second

PPSB
prothrombin, proconvertin, Stuart factor, antihemophilic B factor

PPSH
pseudovaginal peritoneoscrotal hypospadias

PPT
parietal pleural tissue
partial prothrombin time
peak-to-peak threshold
plant protease test

PPT, Ppt, ppt.
precipitate

Ppt
pneumoperitoneum

Ppt, ppt
praeparatus (L. prepared)

ppt.
praecipitatus (L. precipitated)

ppta.
precipitation

pptd.
precipitated

P&P test
prothrombin-proconvertin test

PPTL
postpartum tubal ligation

ppt. LBP
precipitates low back pain

pptn.
precipitation

PPTT
postpartum painless thyroiditis with transient thyrotoxicosis

PPT vib. pos.
pinprick, touch, vibration, and position

PPV
positive pressure ventilation (re: Resp)
progressive pneumonia virus

pp60v-src
phosphoprotein (molecular weight of) 60 (kd), (encoded by) viral (gene) src (the protein encoded by the Rous sarcoma virus oncogene—re: genetics)

PPVT
Peabody Picture Vocabulary Test (re: Psychol)

PPVT-R
Peabody Picture Vocabulary Test-Revised (re: Psychol)

PQ
paraquat (highly poisonous nonselective herbicide)
permeability quotient
personal quality
physician's questionnaire
plastoquinone
pronator quadratus (muscle)
pyrimethamine-quinine (antimalarial)

PQ$_3$
γ-tocotrienol

PQ-9
plastoquinone-9 (one of a group of E and K vitamins and coenzyme Q)

PQ-3-al
γ-tocotrienol

PQD
Protocol Data Query

PR
Panama red (variety of marijuana)
parallax and refraction
pars recta
partial reinforcement
partial remission
partial response
patient relations
peer review
pelvic rock (re: PM&R)
percentile rank (re: statistics)
perfusion rate
peripheral resistance
phenol red (an indicator)
photoreacting
photoreaction
physical rehabilitation
pityriasis rosea

pleiotropic resistance
polymyalgia rheumatica
postural reflex
potency ratio
potential relation
preference record
pregnancy rate
pressoreceptor
pressure
prevention
Preyer's reflex
production rate
professional relations
progesterone receptor
progressive relaxation
progressive resistance
progress report
prolonged release
prolonged remission
propranolol
prosthion (re: Dent)
psychotherapy responder
public relations
Puerto Rican
pulmonary regurgitation
pulse rate
pulse repetition
pulse/respirations
pyramidal response

PR, P.R., P.r., pr.
punctum remotum (L. farthest point [of
accommodation]— re: Ophth)

PR, Pr
presbyopia
proctologist
prolactin
propyl (normal)
protein

PR, Pr, Pr.
prism

PR, pr., p.r.
per rectum (L. through the rectum)

P/R
productivity-to-respiration ratio

P&R
pelvic and rectal
pulse and respiration(s)

Pr
Prandtl number (re: fluid mechanics)
praseodymium (element)
premature
presentation
proctology

[142]Pr
radioactive isotope of praseodymium

[143]Pr
radioactive isotope of praseodymium

pr.
pair

PRA
phonation, respiration, articulation-
resonance
5-phosphoribosyl-1-amine
plasma renin activity
progesterone receptor assay
progressive resistance to arms

prac.
practice

PRACT
practitioner

pract.
practical

prand.
prandium (L. late breakfast or lunch; an
early meal)

PRAS
phosphoribosylaminoimidazole
synthetase
prereduced anaerobically sterilized
(media)

p. rat. aetat.
pro ratione aetatis (L. in proportion to
age)

PRBC
packed red blood cells

PRBS
pseudorandom binary signal

PRBV
placental residual blood volume

PRC
packed red cells
panretinal cryotherapy (re: Ophth)
peer review committee
phase response curve
physician's review committee
plasma renin concentration
prime responder cell
professional review committee

PRCA
pure red cell agenesis
pure red cell aplasia

PRD
partial reaction of degeneration
phosphate restricted diet
polycystic renal disease
postradiation dysplasia

PrDptr
prism diopter (re: Ophth)

PRE
photoreacting enzyme

pigmented retinal epithelial (cells)
progressive resistive exercises (re:
  PM&R)

Pre, pre.
preliminary

PREB
Pupil Record of Education Behavior (re:
  Psychol)

prec.
preceding

p. rec.
per rectum (L. through the rectum)

precip.
precipitate
precipitation

precord.
precordial

Prec steth.
precordial stethoscope

PRED, pred.
prednisone

PreD$_3$
previtamin D$_3$

pred.
predicted
prednisolone

prednis.
prednisolone
prednisone

PREE
partial reinforcement extinction effect

pref.
prefer
preference

prefd.
preferred

preg.
pregnancy
pregnant

pregang.
preganglionic (re: Neuro)

pregn.
pregnancy
pregnant

Preinoc
preinoculation

prelim.
preliminary

prelim. diag.
preliminary diagnosis

prem.
premature
premature infant

premie
premature infant

prenat.
prenatal

Pre-O$_2$
preoxygenated

Preop, preop., pre-op
preoperative

prep.
preparation
prepare

prepd.
prepared

prepn.
preparation

PRERLA
pupils round, equal, react to light and
  accommodation

PREs
progressive resistive exercises

pres.
pressure

preserv.
preservation
preserve

PRESS
PreReading Expectancy Screening
  Scales (re: psychological testing)

press.
pressure

prev.
prevent
preventative
prevention
preventive
previous

PREVAGT
previous abnormality of glucose
  tolerance

prev. hx
previous history

PrevMed
preventative medicine (preventive)

prevoc., pre-voc
pre-vocational

PR ex., pr. ex.
progressive resistive exercises (re: PM&R)

PRF
partial reinforcement
patient report form
Personality Research Form
pontine reticular formation (re: Neuro)
progressive renal failure
prolactin-releasing factor
pyrogen-releasing factor

pRF
polyclonal rheumatoid factor

PRFA
plasma recognition factor activity

PRFM
prolonged rupture of fetal membranes

PRFR
pressure-retaining flow-relieving

PRG
phleborheography
purge

PRGI
percutaneous retrogasserian glycerol injection

PRGS
phosphoribosylglycineamide synthetase

PRH
past relevant history
preretinal hemorrhage (re: Ophth)
prolactin-releasing hormone

PRHBF
peak reactive hyperemia blood flow

PRI
phosphate reabsorption index
phosphoribose isomerase
plexus rectales inferiores
Prescriptive Reading Inventory (re: psychological testing)

PRIH
prolactin release-inhibiting hormone

prim.
primary

prim. diag.
primary diagnosis

PRIME
procarbazine, isophosphamide, and methotrexate (re: chemotherapy)

primip.
primipara (woman bearing first child)

prim. luc.
prima luce (L. at first light [early in the morning])

prim. m.
primo mane (L. first [thing] in the morning)

prin.
principal

princ.
principal
principle

PRIND
prolonged reversible ischemic neurologic deficit

PRIST
paper radioimmunosorbent technique
paper radioimmunosorbent test

priv.
private
privilege

PRK
primary rabbit kidney

PRL
progressive resistance to leg (re: physical therapy)
prolactin

PRLA
pupils react to light and accommodation

PRM
phosphoribomutase
photoreceptor membrane
prematurely ruptured membrane
preventive medicine

PRN
polyradiculoneuropathy
principalization

p.r.n.
pro re nata (L. according as circumstances may require; as required; whenever necessary; as occasion arises; as needed)

PRNT
plaque reduction neutralization test

PRO
projection
pronation

PRO, Pro
proline (an amino acid)

PRO, Pro, pro.
prothrombin

PRO, pro.
protein

Pro
prophylactic

prob.
probability
probable
probably
problem

proc.
procedure
proceeding
process

Procs
proceedings

Proct
proctologist

Proct, proct.
proctology

PROCTO
proctology
proctoscopic

procto.
proctoclysis
proctoscopy

prod.
produce
produced
product

pro dos.
pro dose (L. for a dose)

Prof, prof.
professor

prof.
profession
professional

prog.
prognosis
program
progress
progressive

progn.
prognosis

progr.
progress

proj.
project
projection (re: Radio)

prol.
proline (an amino acid)

prolong
prolonged

prolong.
prolongatus (L. prolonged)

PROM
passive range of motion
premature rupture of membranes
preventative rupture of membranes
    (preventive)
programmable read only memory (re:
    computers)
prolonged rupture of membranes

ProMACE
prednisone, methotrexate, Adriamycin,
    cyclophosphamide, etoposide (VP-16-
    213) (re: chemotherapy)

PROMACE-MOPP
procarbazine, methotrexate,
    Adriamycin, Cytoxan, etoposide (VP-
    16-213), Mustargen, Oncovin,
    procarbazine, prednisone (re:
    chemotherapy)

PROMIN
programmable multiple ion monitor

PROMIS
Problem-Oriented Medical Information
    System

pron.
pronate
pronated
pronation

pron/sup
pronation/supination

prop.
propranolol

proph.
prophylactic

PROPLA
prophospholipase A

pro rat. aet.
pro ratione aetatis (L. according to
    [patient's] age; in proportion to age)

pro rect.
pro recto (L. by rectum)

pros.
prostate
prosthesis
prosthetic

prost.
prostate

prostat.
prostatic

prosth.
prosthesis
prosthetic

PROT, Prot
Protestant

PROT, prot.
protein

prothr. cont.
prothrombin content

prothrom.
prothrombin

proth. time
prothrombin time

pro-time, pro. time
prothrombin time

PROTO
protoporphyrin

pro us. ext.
pro usu externo (L. for external use)

PROVIMI
proteins, vitamins, and minerals

Pro-X
prothrombin time

Prox, prox.
proximal

PRO-XAN
protein-xanthophyll

prox. luc.
proxima luce (L. the next morning)

PRP
panretinal photocoagulation (re: Ophth)
pityriasis rubra pilaris
platelet-rich plasma
polymer or ribose phosphate
postreplication repair
pressure rate product
Problem Reporting Program
progressive rubella panencephalitis
Psychotic Reaction Profile

PRPP
5-phosphoribosyl-1-pyrophosphate

PRPS
phosphoribosylpyrophosphate
  synthetase

PRR
proton relaxation rate
pulse repetition rate

PRRE
pupils round, regular, and equal

PR-RSV
Prague strain Rous sarcoma virus

PRS
Parent's Rating Scale
Personality Rating Scale
plasma renin substrate
positive rolandic sharp (wave—re: EEG)
Pupil Rating Scale: Screening for
  Learning Disabilities

PRSA
plasma renin substrate activity

P-R segment
portion of electrocardiogram between
  end of P and beginning of QRS

PRT
OISE Picture Reasoning Test
pharmaceutical research and testing
phosphoribosyltransferase
photoradiation therapy
postoperative respiratory treatment

PRTase
phosphoribosyltransferase

PRTH-C
prothrombin time control

PRU
peripheral resistance unit

PRV
polycythemia rubra vera
pseudorabies virus

PRVA
peripheral vein renin activity

PRVEP
pattern reversed visual evoked potential

PrVS
prevesical space

PRW
polymerized ragweed

PS
chloropicrin (a war gas)
Paget-Schroetter (syndrome)
paired stimulation
paradoxical sleep
paralaryngeal space
paraspinal
paraspinous
parasternal
parasympathetic
partial shoulder
pathologic state
pathological state
patient's serum
pediatric surgery
Pellegrini-Stieda (syndrome)
perceptual speed (test)

performing scale (re: IQ)
periodic syndrome
peripheral smear
peritoneal spread
permeability surface
phosphate saline (buffer)
phosphatidylserine
photosystems
phrenic (nerve) stimulation
physical status
pigeon serum
plastic surgeon
plastic surgery
point of symmetry
polysaccharides
polystyrene
population sample
postmaturity syndrome
postscriptum
pregnancy serum (taken from pregnant
    woman)
present symptoms
prestimulus
principal sulcus
prostatic secretion
protective service
protein synthesis
psychiatric
pulmonary stenosis
pulmonic stenosis
pyloric stenosis

PS, P-S
Porter-Silber (chromogen)

PS, Ps
prescription (re: drugs requiring a
    prescription)
Pseudomonas (genus)

PS, ps, p.s.
per second

P-S
pancreozymin-secretin
pyramid surface

P/S
polyunsaturated/saturated (fatty acid
    ratio)
polyunsaturated-to-saturated (fatty
    acids ratio)

P&S
paracentesis and suction
Physicians and Surgeons

P & S, p & s
permanent and stationary (re:
    disabilities)

Ps
pseudocyst
psoriasis

ps
picosecond
pseudo- (prefix)

PSA
polyethylene sulfonic acid (polyethylene
    sodium sulfonate; PES—an
    anticoagulant)
pone (ad) situm affectum (L. apply to
    the affected parts)
progressive spinal ataxia
prolonged sleep apnea
prostate-specific antigen

PSAGN
poststreptococcal acute
    glomerulonephritis

PSAn, PsAn
psychoanalytic
psychoanalytical

PSAn, PsAn, Ps An
psychoanalysis
psychoanalyst

PSAT/NMSQT
Preliminary Scholastic Aptitude Test/
    National Merit Scholarship Qualifying
    Test

PSB
phosphorus-solubilizing bacteria
protected specimen brush

PSC
partial subligamentous calcification
physiologic squamocolumnar
pluripotential stem cell
Porter-Silber chromogen
posterior semicircular canal
posterior subcapsular cataract
primary sclerosing cholangitis
pulse synchronized contractions

PSCC
posterior subcapsular cataract

PSCI
Primary Self-Concept Inventory

PS closure
plastic surgery closure

PSCM
pokeweed activated spleen-conditioned
    medium

PSD
particle size distribution
peptone-starch-dextrose
periodic synchronous discharge
phosphate supplemented diet
photon-stimulated desorption
poststenotic dilation
postsynaptic density (re: Neuro)

PSDES
primary symptomatic diffuse
  esophageal spasm

PSE
paradoxical systolic expansion
partial splenic embolization
penicillin-sensitive enzyme
point of subjective equality (re: Psychol)
portal systemic encephalopathy
postshunt encephalopathy
Present State Examination (re: Psychol)
purified spleen extract

PSEC
picosecond (one-trillionth of a second)
poststress ethanol consumption

PSF
peak scatter factor (re: electron
  microscopic image)
point spread function
prostacyclin production stimulating
  factor
pseudosarcomatous fasciitis

p.s.f.
pounds per square foot

PSG
peak systolic gradient
phosphate-saline-glucose (buffer)
polysomnogram (re: sleep and
  neurological disorders)
presystolic gallop

PSGN
poststreptococcal glomerulonephritis

PSH
plastic surgical history
postspinal (anesthesia) headache

P & SHy
personal and social history

Ψ, ψ
psi (23rd letter of the Greek alphabet)

ψ
pseudo- (prefix)
wavelength

PSI
per secundam intentionem (L. by
  second intention [re: healing by
  second intention—two granulating
  surfaces uniting with suppuration and
  delayed closure])
posterior sagittal index
Problem Solving Information
  (apparatus)
prostaglandin synthetic inhibitor
Psychological Screening Inventory
psychosomatic inventory

psi, p.s.i.
pounds per square inch

psia
pounds per square inch absolute

PSI apparatus
Problem Solving Information apparatus

PSIFT
platelet suspension
  immunofluorescence test

psig
pounds per square inch (on the) gauge

PSIL
preferred-frequency speech
  interference level

PSIS
posterior sacroiliac spine
posterosuperior iliac spine

P site
prokaryote attachment site (re: protein
  synthesis)

PSK, PS-K
polysaccharide-K (antineoplastic)

PSL
parasternal line
percent stroke length
potassium, sodium chloride, sodium
  lactate (solution)

PSL sol.
potassium, sodium chloride, sodium
  lactate solution

PSLT
Picture Story Language Test

PSM
presystolic murmur

PSMA
progressive spinal muscular atrophy

PSMed
Psychosomatic Medicine

PSMF
protein-sparing modified fast

PSMRD
post-surgical minimum residual disease

PSNS
parasympathetic nervous system

PSO
physostigmine salicylate ophthalmic
proximal subungual onychomycosis (re:
  Derma)

P sol., p. sol.
partly soluble

PSOR
psoralen

P/sore
pressure sore

PSP
pace-setting potential
paralytic shellfish poisoning
parathyroid secretory protein
periodic short pulse
Personnel Security Preview (re:
   Psychol)
phenolsulfonphthalein (diagnostic aid—
   re: renal function)
positive spike pattern (re: EEG)
posterior spinous process
prednisolone sodium phosphate
professional simulated patient
progressive supranuclear palsy
pseudopregnancy

PSP, ps.p, p.s.p.
postsynaptic potential (re: Neuro)

PSPF
prostacyclin synthesis stimulating
   plasma factor

PSPLV
posterior superior process of left
   ventricle

PSQ
Patient Satisfaction Questionnaire

PSR
pain sensitivity range
(extrahepatic) portal systemic
   resistance
proliferative sickle (cell) retinopathy
pulmonary stretch receptors

PSRI
Professional Sexual Role Inventory (re:
   Psychol)

PSRO
Professional Standards Review
   Organization

PSS
painful shoulder syndrome
physiologic saline solution
physiological saline solution
progressive systemic sclerosis
psoriasis severity scale
Psychiatric Services Section
Psychiatric Status Schedule

PSSO
peer specialist second opinion

PST
pancreatic suppression test
paroxysmal supraventricular
   tachycardia

penicillin, streptomycin, and tetracycline
perceptual span test
peristimulus time
phonemic segmentation test
poststenotic
poststimulus time
prefrontal sonic treatment
protein-sparing therapy
proximal straight tubule (re: kidneys)

PST, p.s.t.
platelet survival time

PSt
punctum sternale (L. sternal puncture)

P + st
poor plus start

PSTA
Predictive Screening Test of Articulation
   (re: Psychol)

PSTH
poststimulus time histogram
poststimulus time histograph

PSTI
pancreatic secretory trypsin inhibitor

PSTO
Purdue Student-Teacher Opinionaire
   (re: Psychol)

PSTV
potato spindle tuber viroid

PSU
photosynthetic unit
primary sampling unit

P subst.
protein substance

PSurg, P. Surg., P surg.
plastic surgery

PSV
psychological, social, and vocational
   (adjustment factors)

PSVER
pattern-shift visual-evoked response

PSVT
paroxysmal superventricular
   tachycardia
paroxysmal supraventricular
   tachycardia

PSW
past sleepwalker
primary surgical ward
program status word (re: computers)

Psy, psy.
psychiatry
psychology

PSYCH, Psych, psych.
psychiatry

Psych, psych.
psychology

PSYCHEM
psychiatric chemistry

psychiat.
psychiatric
psychiatry

psychoan.
psychoanalysis

PSYCHOL, psychol.
psychology

psychopath.
psychopathic
psychopathological

psychopathol.
psychopathological
psychopathology

psychophys.
psychophysics

psychophysiol.
psychophysiology

PsychosMed
Psychosomatic Medicine

psychosom.
psychosomatic

psychother.
psychotherapy

psy-path
psychopath
psychopathic

psy-som
psychosomatic

PT
parathormone
parathyroid
paroxysmal tachycardia
pericardial tamponade
permanent and total
pharmacy and therapeutics
phenytoin
phonation time
photophobia
phototoxicity
physical therapist
physical training
physiotherapy
planum temporale (re: cranium)
plasma thromboplastin
pneumothorax
polyvalent tolerance
posterior tibial

post transfusionem (L. after transfusion)
premature termination
preterm
pronator teres (muscle)
propylthiouracil
prothrombin time
pulmonary thrombosis
pulmonary trunk
pulmonary tuberculosis
pure tone (audiometry)
pyramidal tract (re: Neuro)

PT, P.T.
physical therapy

PT, pt.
patient
pint

P & T
permanent and total (disability)

Pt
platinum (element)

193Pt
radioactive isotope of platinum

197Pt
radioactive isotope of platinum

pt.
part
perstetur (L. let it be continued)
point

PTA
parathyroid adenoma
percutaneous transluminal angioplasty
peroxidase labeled antibodies (test)
persistent trigeminal artery
persistent truncus arteriosus
phosphotungstic acid
plasma thromboplastin antecedent
  (Factor XI)
posttraumatic amnesia
prior to admission
prior to arrival
prothrombin activity
pure tone acuity
pure tone average

P-TAG
target-attaching globulin precursor

PTAH
phosphotungstic acid hematoxylin

PTAP
purified (diphtheria) toxoid (precipitated
  by) aluminum phosphate

p'tase
phosphatase

PTB
patellar tendon bearing (re: prosthesis)

prior to birth
prothrombin
pulmonary tuberculosis

PTBA
percutaneous transluminal balloon
   angioplasty

PTB cast
patellar tendon-bearing cast

PTBD
percutaneous transhepatic biliary
   drainage

PTB prosth.
patellar tendon-bearing prosthesis

PTBS
posttraumatic brain syndrome

PTB-SC
patellar tendon bearing-supracondylar
   (re: lower limb prostheses)

PTB-SC-SP
patellar tendon bearing-supracondylar-
   suprapatellar (re: lower limb
   prostheses)

PTC
patient to call
patient to clinic
percutaneous transhepatic
   cholangiogram
percutaneous transhepatic
   cholangiography
phase-transfer catalyst
phenylthiocarbamide (phenylthiourea—
   re: genetics)
phenylthiocarbamoyl (re: protein
   degradation)
pheochromocytoma, thyroid carcinoma
   (syndrome)
plasma thromboplastin component
   (Factor IX—Christmas factor)
posterior trabeculae carneae (heart
   ventricle muscle bundle)
premature tricuspid closure
prior to conception
propionyl thiocholine
prothrombin complex
pseudotumor cerebri

PTCA
percutaneous transluminal coronary
   angioplasty

PtcCO$_2$
transcutaneous carbon dioxide tension

PtcO$_2$
transcutaneous oxygen tension

PTCP
pseudothrombocytopenia

PTC peptide
phenylthiocarbamoyl peptide

PTCR
percutaneous transluminal coronary
   recanalization

PTD
permanent (and) total disability
personality trait disorder
prior to delivery

Ptd
phosphatidyl

PtdCho
phosphatidylcholine

PtdEth
phosphatidylethanolamine

PtdIns
phosphatidylinositol

PtdSer
phosphatidylserine

PTE
parathyroid extract
pretibial edema
pulmonary thromboembolism

PTED
pulmonary thromboembolic disease

PteGlu
pterolyglutamic acid (folic acid)

PTF
plasma thromboplastin factor (Factor X)
program temporary fix (re: computers)

PTFA
prothrombin time fixing agent

PTFE
polytetrafluoroethylene (resin—re:
   prosthetics)

PTG
parathyroid gland

PTGA
pteroyltriglutamic acid (former
   antineoplastic)

PTH
parathormone (parathyroid hormone)
parathyroid hormone
phenylthiohydantoin (re: protein
   degradation)
post-transfusion hepatitis
prior to hospitalization

PTh
primary thrombocythemia

Pth
pathology
pneumothorax

PTHS
parathyroid hormone secretion (rate)

PTI
pancreatic trypsin inhibitor
persistent tolerant infection
Personnel Tests for Industry (re:
   Psychol)
Pictorial Test of Intelligence
pressure time index

PTL
perinatal telencephalic
   leukoencephalopathy
pharyngotracheal lumen (re: ENT)
plasma thyroxin(e) level
posterior tricuspid leaflet (re: Cardio)

PTLC
precipitation thin-layer chromatography
preparative thin-layer chromatography

PTLD
prescribed tumor lethal dose

PTM
phenyltrimethylammonium
post-transfusion mononucleosis
post-traumatic meningitis
pressure time per minute
preterm milk
pulse time modulation (re: computers)

PTMA
phenyltrimethylammonium (selective
   stimulant—re: motor end plates of
   skeletal muscle nerves)

PTMD
pupils, tension, media, disks (re: Ophth)

PTMDF
pupils, tension, media, disks, fundi (re:
   Ophth)

PTMFD
pupils, tension, media, fundi, disks (re:
   Ophth)

PTN
pain transmission neuron

PTO
percutaneous transhepatic obliteration
please turn over
Purdue Teacher Opinionaire (re:
   Psychol)
2-pyridinethiol-1-oxide (pyrithione—
   fungicide; bactericide)

PTO, P.T.O., Pto
Perlsucht Tuberculin Original (Ger.—re:
   Spengler's tuberculin)

PTP
percutaneous transhepatic portography
posterior tibial pulse
post-tetanic potentiation
post-transfusion purpura
prior to program

Ptp
transpulmonary pressure

PTPI
post-traumatic pulmonary insufficiency

PTQ
Parent-Teacher Questionnaire

PTR
patella tendon reflex
patient termination record
patient to return
peripheral total resistance
plasma transfusion reaction
post-tetanic repetition
psychotic trigger reaction

PTR, P.T.R., Ptr
Perlsucht Tuberculin Rest

PTr
porcine trypsin

P$_{Tr}$
inspiratory triggering pressure

PTRA
percutaneous transluminal renal
   angioplasty

P trx
pelvic traction

PTS
painful tonic seizure
para-toluenesulfonic acid
patella tendon socket
permanent threshold shift
phosphotransferase system

PTS, pts
patients

PTSA
patient's surface area

PTSD
post-traumatic stress disorder

PTT
particle transport time
patellar tendon transfer
posterior tibial transfer
pulmonary transit time
pulse transmission time

PTT, ptt
partial thromboplastin time

PTTH
prothoracicotropic hormone (re: insects)

PTU
propylthiouracil (antithyroid drug)

PTWTKG
patient's weight in kilograms

PTX
palytoxin (re: evaluation of anti-anginal
    chemotherapeutic agents)
phototoxic (reaction)
pneumothorax

PTX, PTx
parathyroidectomy

P Tx, ptx, p. tx
pelvic traction

PTXA
parathyroidectomy and
    autotransplantation

PTY
proprietary

PTZ
pentylenetetrazol (central nervous
    system stimulant)

PU
pass urine
passed urine
paternal uncle
pepsin unit
peptic ulcer
per urethra
precursor uptake
pregnancy urine
prostatic urethra

Pu
plutonium (element)
purple (an indicator color)

^{237}Pu
radioactive isotope of plutonium

^{239}Pu
radioactive isotope of plutonium

^{240}Pu
radioactive isotope of plutonium

pub.
pubic
public
published
publisher

PUC
pediatric urine collector

PUD
peptic ulcer disease

possible ulcer, duodenal
pudendal (block)

PUD, PuD, Pu D
pulmonary disease

PUE
pyrexia (fever) of unknown etiology

puerp.
puerperium (re: OB)

PUF
pure ultrafiltration

PUFA
polyunsaturated fatty acid

PUH
pregnancy urine hormone

PUL
pubourethral ligament

PUL, Pul, pul.
pulmonary

pul.
pulvinar (L. pulvinus—cushion—re:
    nucleus lateralis thalamus)

pul. gros.
pulvis grossus (L. a coarse powder)

PULM, pulm.
pulmentum (L. gruel)
pulmonary

pulm.
pulmonic

Pulse VAC
vincristine, actinomycin D
    (dactinomycin), and
    cyclophosphamide (re:
    chemotherapy)

pul. tenu.
pulvis tenuis (L. a fine powder)

PULV, pulv.
pulveres (L. powders)
pulvis (L. powder)

pulv.
pulverize

pulv. gros.
pulvis grossus (L. a coarse powder)

pulv. subtil.
pulvis subtilis (L. a smooth powder)

pulv. tenu.
pulvis tenuis (L. a fine powder)

PUMS
permanently unfit for military service

PUN
plasma urea nitrogen

punct.
puncture

PUO, P.U.O.
pyrexia (fever) of unknown origin

PUPP
pruritic urticarial papules and plaques
  (of pregnancy)

PUR
polyurethane

pur.
purulent

purg.
purgativus (L. cathartic, purgative)

PUT
putamen

PUV
pelvic urethral valve

PUVA
psoralen plus ultraviolet light of the A
  wavelength (re: psoriasis)

PUVD
pulsed ultrasonic (blood) velocity
  detector

PU walker
pick-up walker

PV
pancreatic vein
papillomavirus
paraventricular (nucleus—re: Neuro)
paravertebral
paromomycin-vancomycin blood agar
pemphigus vulgaris
peripheral vascular
peripheral vascular (plasma volume)
peripheral vein
peripheral venous
peripheral vessels
phonation volume
photovoltaic
pinocytotic vesicle
plasma viscosity
plasma volume
Plummer-Vinson (syndrome)
pneumococcus vaccine
polycythemia vera
polyoma virus
polyvinyl
portal vein
post vaccinationem (L. after
  vaccination)
postvasectomy
postvoiding
pressure/volume

Proteus vulgaris
pulmonary vein
pulmonic valve
pure vegetarian

PV, p.v.
per vaginam (L. through the vagina)

P/V
pressure-to-volume ratio

P&V
pyloroplasty and vagotomy

PVA
partial villous atrophy
Personal Values Abstract
polyvinyl acetate
polyvinyl alcohol (fixative)
Prinzmetal's variant angina

P value
significance probability (re: statistics)

PVB
paravertebral block
Platinol (cisplatin), vinblastine, and
  bleomycin (re: chemotherapy)
premature ventricular beat(s)

PVBS
possible vertebral-basilar system

PVC
polyvinyl chloride
postvoiding cystogram
predicted vital capacity
premature ventricular complex
premature ventricular contraction
primary visual cortex
pulmonary venous capillary
pulmonary venous congestion

Pv_{CO_2}
venous carbon dioxide pressure

P$\bar{v}_{CO_2}$
partial pressure of carbon dioxide in
  mixed venous blood

PVD
patient very disturbed
peripheral vascular disease
portal vein dilation
posterior vitreous detachment (re:
  Ophth)
postvagotomy diarrhea
pulmonary vascular disease

PVD c̄ ASO
peripheral vascular disease with
  arteriosclerosis obliterans

PVE
premature ventricular extrasystole
prevocational evaluation
prosthetic valve endocarditis

PVF
peripheral visual field
portal venous flow
primary ventricular fibrillation

PVG
pulmonary valve gradient

PVH
periventricular hemorrhage

PVI
peripheral vascular insufficiency
periventricular inhibitor
personal values inventory

P-VL
Panton-Valentine leukocidin

PVM
pneumonia virus of mice
proteins, vitamins, minerals

PVMed
Preventative Medicine (preventive)

PVMT
Primary Visual Motor Test (re: Psychol)

PVN
paraventricular nucleus (re: Neuro)
predictive value of a negative test

p.v.n.
per vias naturales (L. by natural ways)

PVNPS
Post-Viet Nam Psychiatric Syndrome

PvO₂
partial pressure of venous oxygen

P$\bar{v}$O₂
mixed venous pressure of oxygen

PVOD
peripheral vascular occlusive disease

PVP
penicillin V potassium
peripheral vein plasma
peripheral venous pressure
portal venous pressure
predictive value of a positive test
pulmonary venous pressure

PVP, P.V.P.
polyvinylpyrrolidone (povidone—
    pharmaceutic aid)

PVP-I
povidone-iodine (polyvinylpyrrolidone
    iodine complex— re: topical anti-
    infective)

PVR
paraventricular nuclear stratum (re:
    Neuro)

peripheral vascular resistance
pulmonary vascular resistance
pulse volume recording

PVRI
pulmonary vascular resistance index

PVS
paravesical space
percussion, vibration, suction
persistent vegetative state
pigmented villonodular synovitis
plexus visibility score
polio virus sensitivity
polyvinyl sponge
premature ventricular systole
programmed ventricular stimulation
pulmonary valvular stenosis
pulmonary vein stenosis

PVT
paroxysmal ventricular tachycardia
physical volume test
portal vein thrombosis
pressure, volume, temperature
private (patient)

pvt.
private

PVW
posterior vaginal wall

pvz.
pulverization (re: cytogenetics)

PW
Parkes Weber (syndrome—Frederick
    Parkes Weber)
peristaltic wave
pinwheel
plantar wart (re: podiatry)
posterior wall
psychological warfare
pulmonary wedge (pressure)
pulsed wave

PW, P-W
Prader-Willi (syndrome)

Pw
progesterone withdrawal

pw
pinworms

PWB
partial weight-bearing
Paul Williams brace

PWBC
peripheral white blood cells

PWBRT
prophylactic whole brain radiation
    therapy

PWC
peak work capacity
Pfeifer-Weber-Christian (syndrome)
physical work(ing) capacity

PWD
precipitated withdrawal diarrhea

pwd.
powder

PWE
posterior wall excursion

PWI
posterior wall infarct

PWLV
posterior wall of left ventricle

PWM
pokeweed mitogen

PWMP
pulmonary wedge mean pressure

PWP
pulmonary wedge pressure

PWR
pressurized water reactor

PWS
port wine stain
pulse-wave speed

PWV
peak weight velocity
posterior wall velocity
pulse wave velocity

PX
pancreatectomized
peroxidase

PX, Px
past history
physical examination

PX, Px, px.
pneumothorax

P/X, px
point of exit

Px, px
prognosis

px
prescription

PXE
pseudoxanthoma elasticum (Grönblad-
    Strandberg syndrome)

PXM
projection x-ray microscope

PY
person year

Py
polyoma (virus)
pyrene (occurs in coal tar)
pyridoxal
(any) pyrimidine (such as thymine,
    cytosine, or uracil)

PYC
proteose-yeast, castione (medium)

PyC
pyogenic culture

PYE
peptone yeast extract (medium)

PYG
peptone yeast (extract) glucose (agar/
    broth)

PYGM
peptone-yeast glucose maltose (agar/
    broth)

PYP
pyrophosphate

PYR
person-year rad
pyramid

Pyr
pyruvate

Pyr, pyr.
pyridine

Pyro
pyrophosphate

PyrP
pyridoxal 5-phosphate (enzyme co-
    factor vitamin)

PZ
pancreozymin
prazosin
pregnancy zone (protein)
proliferative zone

pz
pieze (basic unit of pressure in meter-
    ton-second system)

PZA
pyrazinamide (pyrazinoic acid amide;
    D-50—antibacterial, tuberculostatic)

PZ-B, PzB
parenzyme, buccal

PZ-CCK
pancreozymin-cholecystokinin

PZE
piezoelectric

PZI
protamine zinc insulin

PZP
pregnancy zone protein

Q

Q
cardiac output
clerical perception (re: General Aptitude Test Battery)
coenzyme Q (ubiquinone)
coulomb (unit of charge—re: electricity—abbreviation C is preferred)
glutamine (Gln is IUPAC abbreviation)
perfusion
quantitative
quantity
quantity of heat
quart
quartile
query (fever—Queensland fever)
question
quinacrine (fluorescent method)
quinidine
quinone (oxidizing agent)
quotient
volume of blood flow

Q, q
quarter

Q, q.
quantity of electric charge
quaque (L. each, every)

Q̇
perfusion
rate of blood flow
time derivative

Q°, q°
every hour

Q', q'
every hour

Q1°
every hour around the clock

Q$_1$, Q$_2$, Q$_3$
first or lowest quartile, second quartile, third, etc. (re: statistics)

Q2°
every two hours around the clock

Q2°, q2°
every two hours

Q2', q2'
every two hours

Q-6, Q$_6$
ubiquinone-6; ubiquinone-Q$_6$ (one of the naturally occurring Q coenzymes—re: cardiovascular agent)

Q$_9$
ubichromanol-9 (chroman form of ubiquinol-10)
ubichromenol-9 (chromene form of ubiquinone-10)

Q-10, Q$_{10}$
ubiquinone-50 (a naturally occurring Q coenzyme)

Q$_{10}$
increase in rate of a process when temperature is raised 10°C (temperature coefficient)

q
frequency of the rarer allele of a pair
long arm of a chromosome

QA
quality assurance

Qa
a series of loci close to H-2 (a major histocompatibility complex in the mouse—re: genetics)

QAC
quaternary ammonium compound

QAM
Quality Assurance Monitor (re: medical records)

Qa.m., q.a.m.
quaque ante meridiem (L. every morning)

Q angle
Quatrefage's angle (parietal angle)

QAP
Quality Assurance Program
quinine, Atabrine (quinacrine hydrochloride), pamaquine, naphthoate (antimalarial)

QAR
quality assurance reagent
quantitative autoradiographic

QAS
quality assurance standards

QAT
quality assurance technical (material)

QB
Quantitative (Electrophysiological)
  Battery
whole blood

Q_B
total body clearance

Q banding
quinacrine banding (re: chromosomal
  banding)

Q bands
A bands (anisotropic discs—re: muscle
  fiber)

QBC
quality buffy coat

QBV
whole blood volume

QC
quality control
quinine and colchicine

Qc
pulmonary capillary blood flow

QCB
queue control block (re: computers)

QCD
quantum chromodynamics

Q_{CO_2}
microliters of carbon dioxide given off/
  mg (of tissue)/hr

Q_{CSF}
rate of bulk flow of cerebrospinal fluid
  from CSF space by arachnoid villi
  uptake

Qd, q.d.
quaque die (L. every day)

Q2d, q2d, q. 2 d.
quaque secunda die (L. every second
  day)

QDPR
quinoid dehydropteridine reductase
  (dihydro-)

q.d.s.
quater die sumendum (L. to be taken
  four times a day)

QED
quantum electrodynamics
quod erat demonstrandum (L. that
  which is to be demonstrated)

QEE
quadriceps extension exercise (re:
  PM&R)

Q-enzyme
1,4-α-glucan branching enzyme

QF
quality factor (re: relative biological
  effectiveness)

Q factor
quality (or selectivity of a circuit) factor

Q fever
Australian Q fever (Q for query—also
  hibernovernal bronchopneumonia;
  nine-mile fever; Queensland fever)

Q fract.
quick fraction (re: membrane potentials)

Q-H_2
ubihydroquinone (ubiquinol—a
  reduction product of ubiquinone)

Qh, q.h.
quaque hora (L. every hour)

Q2h, q2h, q. 2 h.
quaque secunda hora (L. every second
  hour)

Q3h, q3h, q. 3 h.
quaque tertia hora (L. every three
  hours)

Q4h, q4h, q. 4 h.
quaque quater hora (L. every four
  hours)

QHS, q.h.s.
quaque hora somni (L. every hour of
  sleep; each bedtime)

q.i.d.
quater in die (L. four times a day)

QISAM
queued indexed sequential access
  method (re: computers/ data
  processing)

q.l.
quantum libet (L. as much as you
  please; as much as wanted)

qlty.
quality

Qm, q.m.
quaque mane (L. every morning)

Q-M sign
Quénu-Muret sign (re: aneurysm)

QMT
quantitative muscle testing

Qn, q.n.
quaque nocte (L. every night)

QNB
3-quinuclidinyl benzilate (*dl*-form
   benzilate ester—chemical warfare;
   hypotensive; cholinergic)

QNS, q.n.s.
quantum non sufficiat (L. quantity would
   not suffice)

Qo
oxygen consumption

QO₂, Q_{O_2}
oxygen consumption
oxygen quotient

QOC
Quality of Contact

Qod, q.o.d.
quaque (other) die (L. q.a.d.—quaque
   altera die—every other day)

Qoh, q.o.h.
quaque (other) hora (L. q.a.h.—quaque
   altera hora— every other hour)

Qon, q.o.n.
quaque (other) nocte (L. q.a.n.—
   quaque altera nocte— every other
   night)

QP
quadrant pain

QP, Q.P.
quanti-Pirquet (reaction)

Qp
pulmonary blood flow

q.p.
quantum placeat (L. as much as
   desired)

QPC
quality of patient care

Qpc
pulmonary capillary blood flow

QPEEG
quantitative pharmaco-electro-
   encephalography

Qpm., q.p.m.
quaque post meridiem (L. each
   evening)

Qp/Qs
left-to-right shunt ratio

QPVT
Quick Picture Vocabulary Test

q.q.
quaque (L. each or every)
quoque (L. also)

Qqh, q.q.h.
quaque quarta hora (L. every fourth
   hour)

Qq hor., qq. hor.
quaque hora (L. every hour)

QR
quantum rectum (L. quantity is correct)
quieting reflex
quinaldine red

QR, qr
quadriradial (re: cytogenetics)

qr.
quarter
quarterly

Q-RB interval
EKG time-wave interval

QRN
quasiresonant nucleus

QRS
segment of electrocardiogram

QRS-ST junction
re: segment of electrocardiogram

QRS-T angle
re: segment of electrocardiogram

QRZ
Quaddel Reaktion Zeit (Ger. wheal
   reaction time)

QS
quiet sleep

QS2
total electromechanical systole

Q-S₂
EKG time-wave interval

Qs
systemic blood flow

q.s.
quantum satis (L. a sufficient quantity)
quantum sufficiat (L. as much as may
   suffice)
quantum sufficit (L. as much as
   suffices)

q.s. ad
quantum satis ad (L. to a sufficient
   quantity)

QSAM
queued sequential access method (re:
   computers/data processing)

QSAR
quantitative structure-activity
  relationship

QSC
quasistatic compliance

QS₂I
shortened electrochemical systole

QSPV
quasistatic pressure volume

Qs/Qt
intrapulmonary shunt fraction
right-to-left shunt ratio

QSS
quantitative sacroiliac scintigraphy

Q's sign
Quant's sign (re: rickets)

Q-S test
Queckenstedt-Stookey test (re: spinal
  fluid pressure)

q. suff.
quantum sufficit (L. as much as
  suffices)

QT
blood volume (quantity) per unit of time
cardiac output
Queckenstedt's test
Quick Test (re: Psychol)
Quick's test (for pregnancy or
  prothrombin)

qt.
quantitative
quantity
quart
quiet

QTAM
queued telecommunications access
  method (re: computers/ data
  processing)

qt. dx
quantities duplex

Q-T interval
re: segment of electrocardiogram

qtr.
quarter
quarterly

quad.
quadrant
quadriceps
quadrilateral
quadriplegia

quad, quad.
quadriplegic

quad. atrophy
quadriceps atrophy

quad. ex.
quadriceps exercises

quadrupl.
quadruplicato (L. four times as much)

quads.
quadriceps

qual.
qualitative
quality

qual. anal.
qualitative analysis

quant.
quantitative
quantity

quant. anal.
quantitative analysis

quant. suff.
quantity sufficient

quar.
quarantine

quart.
quarterly
quartus (L. fourth)

quat.
quater (L. four times)
quattuor (L. four)

quer.
querulous (re: chart note)

quest.
question
questionable

QuF
(Australian) Q (Queensland) fever

QUICHA
quantitative inhalation challenge
  apparatus

quinq.
quinque (L. five)

quint.
quintus (L. fifth)

quor.
quorum (L. of which)

quot.
quotient
quoties (L. as often [as necessary; as
  needed])

QUOTID, quotid.
quotidie (L. daily)

quot. op. sit
quoties opus sit (L. as often as
  necessary)

quot. o. s.
quoties opus sit (L. as often as
  necessary)

q.v.
quantum vis (L. as much as you please;
  as much as you wish)
quantum volueris (L. as much as you
  wish)

q.v., *qv*
quod vide (L. which see)

Q-value
disintegration energy (re: nuclear
  reaction)

QW
quality of working life

Q wave
re: electrocardiogram segment

R

R
arginine
chemical radical (used to show position
    of unspecified radical—re: organic
    compounds)
drug-resistant plasmid
gas constant (8.315 joules)
indicates number in reference file
metabolic respiratory quotient
ohm
organic radical (usually alkyl or aryl
    groups)
race
radioactive (mineral)
radiologist
radiology
radius
ramus
rate
rationale
raw
reading
recessive
recipe (L. take)
rectal
rectally
rectified (average)
rectum
red (an indicator color)
regimen
regression coefficient
regulator (gene)
Reiz (Ger. stimulus)
rejection factor
relapse
relations (products—re: Psychol;
    Aptitudes Research Project testing
    within structure of intellect model)
remainder (of chemical formula)
remission
remote point of convergence
repressor
resazurin
residue
residuum
resistance (electrical)
resistance unit (re: cardiovascular
    system)
resistant (re: disease)
respirations
respiratory
respiratory exchange ratio (primary
    symbol)
respond

response
rest (re: cell cycle)
resting
restricted
reticulocyte
reverse Giemsa method
review
Rhabdomonas (genus)
Rhipicephalus (genus of cattle ticks)
Rhizobium (genus)
Rhizopus (genus)
Rhodomicrobium (genus)
Rhodopseudomonas (genus)
Rhodospirillum (genus)
Rhodotorula (genus)
Rhus (genus)
rhythm
rib
right (eye)
roentgenologist
roentgenology
rough (re: bacterial colonies)
routine
rub
side chain (re: amino acid formulae)

R, R.
Behnken's unit (of roentgen-ray
    exposure)
Rankine (temperature scale)
Réaumur (temperature scale)
Rickettsia (genus)
Rinne test (hearing test)

R, r
racemic (re: naming compounds,
    sometimes replacing *dl*)
rare
ratio
remotum (L. far)
roentgen (unit of radiation exposure;
    small r is former symbol—cap R now
    used)
rounded

R, r.
ribose

R+, +R
Rinne's test positive (re: Oto/Audio)

R−, −R
Rinne's test negative (re: Oto/Audio)

R-
stereodescriptor (re: asymmetric carbon
    atoms)

(R)
rectal
right

(R)-
rectus (L. right—re: spatial arrangement
  about an asymmetric carbon)

®
registered trademark
right

°R
degree Rankine

R#1
good risk (re: anesthesia)

R$_1$
good risk (re: anesthesia)

R#2
fairly good risk (re: anesthesia)

R$_2$
fairly good risk (re: anesthesia)

R#3
poor risk (re: anesthesia)

R$_3$
poor risk (re: anesthesia)

R#4
very poor risk (re: anesthesia)

R$_4$
very poor risk (re: anesthesia)

r
angle of refraction
correlation coefficient
observed count rate ($=n/t$)
radius (of a circle)
reproductive potential
ring chromosome
round

ρ
correlation coefficient
electric charge density
mass density
rho (Greek lower case)

RA
radioactive
radioactivity
radionuclide angiography
radium (re: x-ray examination)
ragweed antigen
Raynaud's (phenomenon)
reading age
refractory anemia
refractory ascites
renal artery
renin activity
renin angiotensin
repeat action (drugs)

residual air
rheumatic arthritis
rheumatoid agglutinins
rheumatoid arthritis
right angle (re: Ortho)
right angulation (re: Ortho)
right arm
right atrial
right atrium
right auricle

RA, R/A
room air

R$_A$
airway resistance

Ra
radial
radium (element)
Rayleigh number

Ra, ra.
radius

^{226}Ra, Ra 226
radium-226 (an isotope)

RAA
renin angiotensin aldosterone
right atrial appendage

RAAGG
rheumatoid arthritis agglutinin

RAAS
renin-angiotensin-aldosterone system

RABA
rabbit antibladder antibody

RABCa
rabbit antibladder cancer

RAbody
right atrium body

RAC
radial artery catheter
right atrial contraction

rac.
racemic (an optically inactive mixture—
  re: chemistry)

RA cell
ragocyte cell

RAD
radical
reactive airway disease
right atrial diameter
right axis deviation
roentgen administered dose

RAD, rad
radiation absorbed dose

Rad
radiologically
radiologist
radiology
radiotherapy

rad
radian (a unit of angular measure)

rad.
radial
radiate
radiating
radical
radicular
radiculitis
radius
radix (L. root)

RADA
radioactive
right acromiodorsoanterior (position of
  fetus)

rad. imp.
radium implant

RADIO
radiotherapy

Radiol.
radiologist
radiology

RadLV
radiation leukemia virus

RADP
right acromiodorsoposterior (position of
  fetus)

RADS
reactive airway disease syndrome
retrospective assessment of drug safety

rad/s
radians per second

Rad Ther
radiotherapy

RADTS
rabbit antidog-thymus serum

RADWASTE
radioactive waste

RAE
right atrial enlargement

RaE
rabbit erythrocyte

RAEM
refractory anemia with excess
  myeloblasts

RAF
rheumatoid arthritis factor

Ra-F
radium-F

RA factor
rheumatoid arthritis factor

RAG
ragweed (pollen antigen)

Ragg
rheumatoid agglutinator

RAH
radioactive Hippuran (test)
regressing atypical histiocytosis
right anterior hemiblock
right atrial hypertrophy

RAHO
rabbit antibody to human ovary

RAHTG
rabbit antihuman thymocyte globulin

RAI
radioactive iodine
resting ankle index

RAID
radioimmunodetection

RAIS
reflection-absorption infrared
  spectroscopy

RAIU
radioactive iodine uptake

RAL
resorcylic acid lactone (zearalenone—
  re: veterinary anabolic)

RALs
resorcylic acid lactones (zearalenone—
  re: veterinary anabolic)

RALT
Riley Articulation and Language Test
routine admission laboratory tests

RAM
rabbit antimouse
random access memory (re: computers)
rapid alternating movements
right anterior measurement

ramb.
rambling

RAMP
radioactive antigen microprecipitin
right atrial mean pressure

RAMT
rabbit antimouse thymocyte

RAN
resident admit note
resident's admission notes
resident's admitting note

ran.
random

RANA
rheumatoid arthritis-associated nuclear
antigen

RAO
right anterior oblique

RAP
recurrent abdominal pain
regression-associated protein
Relative Aspects of Potential (re:
Psychol)
renal artery pressure
rheumatoid arthritis precipitin
right arterial pressure
right atrial pressure

RAPE
right atrial pressure elevation

RAPM
refractory anemia with partial
myeloblastosis

RAPO
rabbit antibody to pig ovary

RAR
right arm resting

RAR, rar, r.a.r.
right arm reclining
right arm recumbent

RARLS
rabbit antirat-lymphocyte serum

RARTS
rabbit antirat-thymocyte serum

RAS
rapid atrial stimulation
recurrent aphthous stomatitis
reflex-activating stimulus
renal artery stenosis
renin-angiotensin system
reticular activating system
rheumatoid arthritis serum (factor)

RAS, RA-S
right arm, sitting

ras.
rasurae (L. scrapings or filings)

RA slide
rheumatoid arthritis slide (test)

RASP
rapidly alternating speech

RAST
radioallergosorbent technique
radioallergosorbent test

RASV
recovered avian sarcoma virus

RAT
rat aortic tissue
Remote Associates Test (re: Psychol)
repeat-action tablet
right anterior thigh

RATA
radioimmunologic assay (anti)thyroid
antibody

RATG, R-ATG
rabbit antithymocyte globulin

RATHAS
rat thymus antiserum

RATS
rabbit antithymocyte serum

RATx
radiation therapy

RAU
radioactive uptake

RAUC
raw area under the curve

RAV
Rous associated virus

RAW, R_{AW}, Raw
airway resistance (re: Resp)

RAZ
razoxane (antineoplastic)

RB
rating board
rebreathing
Red Blanket
Renaut's bodies
respiratory bronchiole
respiratory burst
reticulate body
retinoblastoma
rice body
right bundle
right buttock
Roth-Bernhardt (disease)
round body

Rb
rubidium (element)

⁸¹Rb
radioactive isotope of rubidium

⁸²Rb
radioactive isotope of rubidium

^{83}Rb
radioactive isotope of rubidium

^{84}Rb
radioactive isotope of rubidium

^{86}Rb
radioactive isotope of rubidium

RBA
relative binding activity
relative binding affinity
rescue breathing apparatus
right basilar artery
rose bengal antigen

RBAF
rheumatoid biologically active factor

R banding, R-banding
reverse banding (re: chromosome
   banding)

RBAP
repetitive burst of action potentials

RBB
right bundle branch (re: Cardio)

RBBB
right bundle-branch block (re: Cardio)

RBBSB, RBBsB, RBB$_s$B
right bundle-branch system block (re:
   Cardio)

RBBX
right breast biopsy examination

RBC, R.B.C.
red blood cell (count)
red blood corpuscle (cell)
red blood count

r.b.c.
red blood cell(s)

RBC-ADA
red blood cell adenosine deaminase

RBC/hpf
red blood cells per high-power field

RBCM
red blood cell mass

RBC/P
red blood cell to plasma (ratio)

RBCV
red blood cell volume

RBD
relative biological dose
right border of dullness (of heart to
   percussion)

RBE
relative biological effectiveness

RBF
regional blood flow
renal blood flow
rice bran factor

Rb Imp, RbImp
rubber base impression (re: Dent)

r_{bis}
biserial correlation coefficient (re:
   statistics)

RBL
rat basophilic leukemia
Reid's base line

RBM
regional bone mass

RBME
regenerating bone marrow extract

RBN
retrobulbar neuritis

RBP
retinol-binding protein

RBR
radiation bowel reaction

RBS
random blood smear
random blood sugar
rutherford backscattering (method—re:
   radioactivity)

RbSA
rabbit serum albumin

RB-V
right bundle, ventricular

RBW
relative body weight

RC
radiocarpal
Raymond-Céstan (syndrome)
reaction center
receptor chemoeffector
recrystallized
red cell
red (cell) casts
red corpuscle
Red Cross
referred care
reflection coefficient
regenerated cellulose
resistance and capacitance
respiration ceases
Respiratory Care (unit)
respiratory center
rest cure
retention catheter
retrograde cystogram
rib cage

Roman Catholic
root canal
Roussy-Cornil (syndrome)
routine cholecystectomy

RC, Rc
response, conditioned

Rc
receptor

RCA
red cell adherence
red cell agglutination
relative chemotactic activity
renal cell carcinoma
retrograde conduction to the atria
right carotid artery
right coronary artery

rCBF
regional cerebral blood flow

RCBV, rCBV
regional cerebral blood volume

RCC
radiographic coronary calcification
receptor chemoeffector complex
red cell cast
red cell concentrate
red cell count
renal cell carcinoma
right common carotid
right coronary cusp

Rcc
radiochemical

RC circuit
resistor and capacitor in series (re:
    electronic circuits)

RCCT
randomized controlled clinical trial
results of clinical controlled trial

RCD
relative (area of) cardiac dullness

RCDR
relative corrected death rate

RCE
reasonable compensation equivalent

RCF
red cell filterability
red cell folate
relative centrifugal force

RCG
radioelectrocardiograph

RCH
rectocolic hemorrhage

RCHF
right-sided congestive heart failure

RCI
rate change induced
respiratory control index

RCIA
red cell immune adherence

RCIT
red cell iron turnover

RCITR
red cell iron turnover rate

RCL
range of comfortable loudness
renal clearance

RCLAAR
red cell-linked antigen-antiglobulin
    reaction

RCM
radiocontrast material
radiocontrast media
radiographic contrast media
red cell mass
reinforced clostridial medium
replacement culture medium
rheumatoid cervical myelopathy
right costal margin
Roux conditioned medium

rCMRO$_2$
regional cerebral metabolic rate for
    oxygen

RCN
right caudate nucleus

RCO—
aliphatic acyl radical

R colony
rough colony (re: bacteria)

RCP
recognition and control processor (re:
    computers/data processing)
riboflavin(e) carrier protein

RCPH
red cell peroxide hemolysis

RCQG
right caudal quarter ganglion

RCR
relative consumption rate
respiratory control ratio

RCRS
Rehabilitation Client Rating Scale

RCS
rabbit aorta-contracting substance

red cell suspension
reticulum cell sarcoma
right coronary sinus
Royal College of Surgeons (strain of rat)

RCSi
radioactivity per cell in S (a DNA
  synthetic period— re: cell cycle)

RCT
randomized clinical trial
red colloidal test
retrograde conduction time
Rorschach Content Test (re: Psychol)

RCTL
resistor-capacitor-transistor logic (re:
  computers)

RC TNTC
red cells too numerous to count

RCU
respiratory care unit

RCV
red cell volume

RD
radial deviation
Raynaud's disease
reaction of denervation
renal disease
Rénon-Delille (syndrome)
resistance determinant
respiratory disease
respiratory distress
retinal detachment
Reye's disease
right deltoid
right dorso-anterior
Riley-Day (syndrome)
rubber dam
ruptured disc

RD, R.D.
reaction of degeneration

R&D
research and development

Rd, rd
reading
rutherford (unit of radioactivity)

RDA
recommended daily allowance
recommended dietary allowance
right dorso-anterior (position of fetus)

RdA, Rd A
reading age

RDB
randomized double blind (trial)
research and development board

RDC
Research Diagnostic Criteria

RDDA
recommended daily dietary allowance

RDDP
RNA-dependent DNA polymerase
RNA-directed DNA polymerase

RDE
receptor-destroying enzyme

RDEB
recessive dystrophic epidermolysis
  bullosa

R determinant
resistant determinant (re: plasmid)

RDFS
ratio of decayed and filled surfaces (re:
  Dent)

RDFT
ratio of decayed and filled teeth (re:
  Dent)

RDHBF
regional distribution of hepatic blood
  flow

RDI
recommended daily intake
recommended dietary intake
rupture delivery interval

RDIH
right direct inguinal hernia

RDLS
Reynell Development Language Scales
  (re: psychological testing)

RDM
rod disk membrane

RDM, Rdm
readmission

rDNA
recombinant deoxyribonucleic acid
ribosomal deoxyribonucleic acid

RDP
right dorsoposterior (position of fetus)

RDPase
RNA-dependent DNA polymerase

RDQ
respiratory disease questionnaire

RDQ, RdQ
reading quotient

RDRV
rhesus diploid rabies vaccine

RDS
respiratory distress syndrome
reticuloendothelial depressant
    substance

RDSI
Revised Developmental Screening
    Inventory

RDT
regular dialysis treatment
retinal damage threshold
right dorsotransverse (position of fetus)

RDVR
RD114 virus receptor

RDW
red (cell) distribution width

RE
racemic epinephrine
readmission
re-education
reflux esophagitis
regional enteritis
renal excretion
resistive exercises
resting energy
reticuloendothelial
reticuloendothelium
retinol equivalent
right ear
ring enhancement
rostral end

RE, R.E.
radium emanation
right eye

RE, R/E
rear end (re: motor vehicle accident)
rectal examination

R_E
respiratory exchange (ratio)

R/E
round and equal (re: Ophth)

R & E
research and education
round and equal (re: Ophth)

R ↑ E
right upper extremity

R ↓ E
right lower extremity

Re
rhenium (element)

^{182}Re
radioactive isotope of rhenium

^{186}Re
radioactive isotope of rhenium

^{188}Re
radioactive isotope of rhenium

Re
Reynolds' number (re: nondimensional
    parameters of fluid motion)

R_e
Reynolds' number (used to predict
    turbulent flow of gas or fluid
    molecules through a tube)

re.
regarding

r.e.
radiographic effect

REA
radio-enzymatic assay (radioenzymatic)
renal anastomosis
right ear advantage

react.
reaction
reactive

READ
Reading Evaluation—Adult Diagnosis

readm.
readmission
readmit

REAS
reasonably expected as safe

REB
roentgen equivalent biological
roentgen equivalent, biological
roentgen-equivalent-biological

R-EBA-GH
recessive epidermolysis bullosa
    atrophicans generalisata gravis
    Herlitz

R-EBA-L
recessive epidermolysis bullosa
    atrophicans localisata

R-EBA-mitis
recessive epidermolysis bullosa
    atrophicans generalisata mitis

R-EBD-HS
recessive epidermolysis bullosa
    dystrophica-Hallopeau Siemens

R-EBD-I
recessive epidermolysis bullosa
    dystrophica inversa

R-EBP
recessive epidermolysis bullosa
    progressiva

REC
radioelectrocomplexing
rear end collision
receptor
right external carotid

rec
recombinant (re: cytogenetics)

rec.
recens (L. fresh; recent)
recessive
recipe
recommend
recommendation(s)
record
recovery
recreation
recur
recurrence
recurrent

RECA
right external carotid artery

recd.
received

RECG
radioelectrocardiography (telemetry)

re. ch.
recheck

Recip, recip.
recipient
reciprocal

recog.
recognition
recognize

Recomm, recomm.
recommendation

recomm.
recommend

recond.
recondition
reconditioning

reconstr.
reconstruction

reconstru.
reconstruction

recryst.
recrystallize

recrystn.
recrystallization

rect.
rectal
rectificatus (L. rectified)
rectify

rectum
rectus (muscle)

recumb.
recumbent

recur.
recurrence
recurrent

RED
radiation experience data
rapid erythrocyte degeneration
Research and Experimental
    Department

red.
reduce
reducing
reduction

redig. in pulv.
redigatur in pulverem (L. let it be
    reduced to powder)

red. in pulv.
redactus in pulverem (L. reduced to [a]
    powder)
redige in pulverem (L. reduce to a
    powder [imperative])

redox.
reduction-oxidation

REE
rapid extinction effect
rare earth element
resting energy expenditure

re-ed
re-educate
re-education

REEG
radioelectroencephalograph

R-EEG
resting electroencephalogram

REEL
Receptive-Expressive Emergent
    Language (Scale)

REEP
right end-expiratory pressure

re-eval
re-evaluate
re-evaluation

re-ex
re-examination

REF
ejection fraction at rest
renal erythropoietic factor

REF, ref.
reference

ref.
refer
referred

ref→
refer to

ref. doc.
referring doctor

Ref Dr
referring doctor

REFI
regional ejection fraction image

ref. ind.
refractive index

refl.
reflect
reflection
reflex

reflx.
reflex

ref. phys.
referring physician

REFRAD
released from active duty

REG
Radiation Exposure Guide
radioencephalogram
radioencephalograph
rheoencephalography

Reg
registered

reg.
regarding
region
regular

regen.
regenerate
regeneration

reg. rhy.
regular rhythm

reg. R & R
regular rate and rhythm

REG UMB, reg. umb.
regio umbilici (L. umbilical region)

REH
renin essential hypertension

Rehab, rehab.
rehabilitation

rehabil.
rehabilitation

REL
rate of energy loss
resting expiratory level

rel.
related
relation
relative
relatively

RELE
resistive exercises, lower extremities

reliq.
reliquus (L. remainder)

REM
rapid eye movement(s) (re: Neuro)
recent event memory
reticular erythematous mucinosis
return electrode monitor

REM, rem
radiation equivalent, man (mammal)
roentgen equivalent, man
roentgen-equivalent-man

Re_m
magnetic Reynolds' number (re:
  magnetohydrodynamics)

rem.
remarks
removal
remove

REMA
repetitive excess mixed anhydride
  (method)

REMAB
radiation equivalent manikin absorption

REMCAL
radiation equivalent manikin calibration

remg.
remaining

remit.
remittent

REMP
roentgen-equivalent-man period

REMS
rapid eye movement, sleep

REN
renal

ren.
renoveatur (L. renew)

ren. sem.
renoveatum semis (L. renewed only
  once)
renoveatur semel (L. renew once; shall
  be renewed [only] once)

REO
Receptive-Expressive Observation (re:
  Psychol)

REO virus, reovirus
respiratory and enteric orphan virus

REP
rest-exercise program

REP, ReP
retrograde pyelogram

REP, rep.
repetatur (L. let it be repeated)
report

REP, rep
roentgen equivalent physical (formerly
  tissue roentgen)
roentgen-equivalent, physical
roentgen-equivalent-physical

rep.
repetendum (L. to be repeated)

REPC
reticuloendothelial phagocytic capacity

repetat.
repetatus (L. repeated)

REPS
reactive extensor postural synergy

reps.
repetitions

rept.
repeat
repetatur (L. let it be repeated)
report

reptd.
reported

Rep Test
(Role Construct) Repertory Test (re:
  Kelly personality theory)

req.
request

RER
renal excretion rate
respiratory exchange ratio

RER, rER
rough (surfaced) endoplasmic reticulum

RES
remote entry services (re: computers/
  data processing)

respiratory emergency syndrome
reticuloendothelial system

Res, res.
research
reserve
residence
resident
resistance

res.
resect
resection
residue

resched.
reschedule(d)

resid.
residual

Resid vol.
residual volume

resis.
resistance

resist.
resistance
resistive

RESP, Resp, resp.
respiration(s)

resp.
respective
respectively
respirator
respiratory
respond
response
responsible

resp. → ext. stimuli
responds to external stimuli

resp. → nox. stim.
responds to noxious stimuli

resp. → pn. stim.
responds to painful stimuli

resp. → verb. stim.
responds to verbal stimuli

REST
regressive electroshock treatment
reticulospinal tract

resus.
resuscitation

RET
rational emotive therapy (re: psychiatry)
reticular (formation)
right esotropia

Ret, ret.
retarded (delayed)

ret
rad (radiation absorbed dose)
   equivalent therapeutic

ret.
retained
retention
reticulocyte
retina
retire
retired
return

retard.
retarded (delayed)

RETC
rat embryo tissue culture

ret. cath.
retention catheter

retic.
reticulocyte

retic. count
reticulocyte count

retic. ct.
reticulocyte count

retics
reticulocytes

retr.
retract
retracted
retraction

retro.
retrograde

REUE
resistive exercises to upper extremities

REV
reticuloendotheliosis virus
reversal

rev.
reverse
review
revise
revision
revolution

rev/min
revolutions per minute

Rev of Sym
review of symptoms

Rev of Sys
review of systems

re-x
re-examination

RF
radial fiber
receptive field (of visual cortex)
receptor floor
recognition factor
reflecting (platelet)
regurgitant fraction
relative flow (rate)
relative fluorescence
release (-ing) factor (re: protein
   synthesis)
renal failure
replicative form
resistance factor
respiratory failure
respiratory frequency
reticular formation
retroflexed
rheumatic fever
rheumatoid factor(s)
riboflavin(e)
Riga-Fede (syndrome)
root canal, filling of
rosette forming
Rundles-Falls (syndrome)

RF, R_F
rate of flow (re: chromatography)

RF, R_f
retardation factor

R_F, R_F
ratio of movement of the band to the
   front of the solvent (re: paper
   chromatography)

RF, rf
radiofrequency

Rf
rutherfordium (radioactive element
   #104)

RFA
right femoral artery
right fronto-anterior (position of fetus)

R factor
resistance factor (resistance plasmids—
   re: bacteriology)

RFB
retained foreign body
rheumatoid factor binding

RFC
retrograde femoral catheter
right frontal craniotomy
rosette-forming cells

rfd.
referred

RFE
relative fluorescence efficiency

RFFIT
rapid fluorescent focus inhibition test

RFFSH
releasing factor of follicle-stimulating
hormone

RFI
radiofrequency interference (re:
computers)
recurrence-free interval

RFL
Reiter-Fiessinger-Leroy (syndrome)
releasing factor of luteinizing (hormone)
restriction fragment length
(polymorphisms)
right frontolateral (position of fetus)

RFLA
rheumatoid factor-like activity

RFLC
resistant Friend leukemia cell

RFLP
restriction fragment length
polymorphisms

RFLS
rheumatoid factor-like substance

RFM
rifampin

Rfm
rifampicin

RFP
request for payment
request for proposal
right frontoposterior (position of fetus)

RFR
rapid filling rate
refraction

RFS
rapid frozen section
relapse-free survival
relaxing factor system
renal function study(ies)

RFT
right fibrous trigone
right frontotransverse (position of fetus)
rod-and-frame test

RFTWS
right foot switch

RFV
right femoral vein

RFVC
reason for visit classification (re:
medical records)

RFVII
Reading-Free Vocational Interest
Inventory (re: educable mentally
retarded)

RFW
rapid filling wave

RG
right gluteal
right gluteus

R/G
red/green

$_r$G
regular gene

RGBMT
renal glomerular basement membrane
thickness

RGC
radio-gas chromatography
remnant gastric cancer
retinal ganglial cells
retinal ganglion cell(s)
right giant cell

RGD
range-gated Doppler

RGE
relative gas expansion
respiratory gas equation

RGEPS
Rucker-Gable Educational
Programming Scale (re: Psychol)

RGH
rat growth hormone

RGM
Rietti-Greppi-Micheli (syndrome)

RGMT
reciprocal geometric mean titer

RGP
retrograde pyelogram
rural general practitioner

RGR
relative growth rate

RGT
reversed gastric tube

RH
radial hemolysis
radiant heat
radiological health
reactive hyperemia

recurrent herpes
regional heparinization
relative humidity
releasing hormone
report heading (re: computers)
retinal hemorrhage
Richner-Hanhart (syndrome)
right hand
right handed
right hemisphere
right hyperphoria

Rh
rhesus blood factor
rhesus blood group
Rhipicephalus (genus of cattle ticks)
rhodium (element)

Rh +
rhesus positive (blood)

Rh −
rhesus negative (blood)

^{102}Rh
radioactive isotope of rhodium

^{105}Rh
radioactive isotope of rhodium

^{106}Rh
radioactive isotope of rhodium

rh.
rheumatic
rhonchus, rhonchi (pl) (Gr. rhonchos—a
    snoring—[used by some to denote
    rales])

r/h
roentgens per hour

RHA
right hepatic artery

RhA
rheumatoid arthritis

Rh agglut.
rheumatoid agglutinins

RHB
right heart bypass

RHBF
reactive hyperemia blood flow

RHBV
right heart blood volume

RHC
resin hemoperfusion column
respirations have ceased
right heart catheterization
right hypochondrium

RHD
radial head dislocation

relative hepatic dullness
renal hypertensive disease
rheumatic heart disease
round heart disease

RhD
rhesus (hemolytic) disease

RHE
respiratory heat exchange

RHEED
reflection high-energy electron
    diffraction

rheo.
rheostat

rheu. fev.
rheumatic fever

rheu. ht. dis.
rheumatic heart disease

rheum.
rheumatic
rheumatism
rheumatoid

rheum fev.
rheumatic fever

rheum. ht. dis.
rheumatic heart disease

RHF
right heart failure

Rh factor
rhesus factor

RHG
radial hemolysis in gel
right hand grip

r_{hh}
correlation of half-test (re: Spearman-
    Brown formula)

Rhi
rhinology

RhIg
rhesus immune globulin

Rhin
rhinologist
rhinology

rhin.
rhinitis

rhino.
rhinoplasty

Rhiz
Rhizobium (genus)

RHL
right hepatic lobe

Rhl-A
rhesus leukocyte antigen

RHLN
right hilar lymph node

RHM, rhm
roentgen per hour at one meter (re: quantitative comparison of radioactive sources)

RhMK
rhesus monkey kidney (cells)

RHMV
right heart mixing volume

Rh neg
rhesus (factor) negative

Rh_null
rare blood type in which all Rh factors are lacking

RHP
Rhodospirillum heme protein

RHPA
reverse hemolytic plaque assay

Rh pos
rhesus (factor) positive

RHR
renal hypertensive rat

r/hr
roentgens per hour

RHS
right hand side
rough hard sphere

RHT
renal homotransplantation
right hypertropia

Rhu
rheumatology

RI
radiation intensity
radioimmunology
radioisotope
refractive index
regenerative index
regional ileitis
relative intensity
release inhibiting
remission induced
remission induction
replicative intermediate
respiratory illness
respiratory index
retroactive inhibition (re: Psychol)

retroactive interference
ribosome
right injured
right involved
rooming in
rosette inhibition

RIA
radioimmunoassay
remittent ischemic attacks
reversible ischemic attack

RIA-DA
radioimmunoassay double antibody (test)

RIB
riboflavin

Rib
D-ribose

RIBS
rutherford ion backscattering

RIC
renomedullar interstitial cell
right internal carotid

RICA
reverse immune cytoadhesion

RICE
rest, ice, compression, elevation

RICM
right intercostal margin

RICS
right intercostal space

RICU
Respiratory Intensive Care Unit

RID
radial immunodeficiency
radial immunodiffusion
radioimmunodetection
remission-inducing drug
reversible intravascular device
right (ventricular) internal diameter
ruptured intervertebral disc

RIEP
rocket immunoelectrophoresis

RIF
release-inhibiting factor
resistance-inducing factor
rifampicin (rifampin)
right index finger
rosette inhibitory factor

RIF, R.I.F.
right iliac fossa

RIFA
radioiodinated fatty acid

RIFC
rat intrinsic factor concentrate

RIg
rabies immune globulin

RIgH
rabies immune globulin, human

RIH
right inguinal hernia

RIHSA
radioactive iodinated human serum albumin

RI lines
recombinant inbred lines

RILT
rabbit ileal loop test

RIM
recurrent induced malaria
relative intensity measure

RIMA
right internal mammary artery

RIMS
resonance ionization mass spectrometry

RIND
reversible ischemic neurologic deficit

RINN
recommended international non-proprietary name

RIO
right inferior oblique

RIOJ
recurrent intrahepatic obstructive jaundice

RIP
radioimmunoprecipitation
radioimmunoprecipitin (test)
reflex-inhibiting pattern
reflex-inhibiting posture
respiratory inductance plethysmography

RIPIS
Rhode Island Pupil Identification Scale (re: Psychol)

RIPP
resistive intermittent positive pressure

RIR
right iliac region
right inferior rectus

RIRB
radioiodinated rose bengal

RIS
resonance ionization spectroscopy

RISA
radioactive iodinated serum albumin (iodinated I 125 serum albumin [human]; radioactive iodine serum albumin; radioiodinated serum albumin)
radioimmunosorbent assay

RISB
Rotter Incomplete Sentences Blank (re: Psychol)

RIST
radioimmunosorbent test

RIT
radioiodinated triolein
rosette inhibition titer

RITC
rhodamine isothiocyanate

RIU
radioactive iodine uptake

RIV
ramus interventricular

RIVC
right inferior vena cava

RIVD
ruptured intervertebral disc

RI virus
respiratory illness virus

RIVS
ruptured interventricular septum

RJE
remote job entry (re: computers/data processing)

RJI
radionuclide joint imaging

RK
rabbit kidney
radial keratotomy
right kidney

RKG
radio(electro)kardiogram (radio[electro]cardiogram)

RKS
renal kidney stone
retrograde kidney study

RKV
rabbit kidney vacuolating (virus)

RKW
renal kalium (potassium) wasting

RKY
roentgenkymography

RL
coarse rales (re: auscultation of chest)
reduction level (of respiratory quotient—
    re: Resp)
(stimulus) Reiz limen
resistive load
resting length
reticular lamina
right lateral
right leg
right lower
right lung
Ringer's lactate
Roussy-Lévy (syndrome)

R$_L$
pulmonary resistance

R/L
right/left

R & L
right and left

R-L, R→L
right to left

R>L
right greater than left
right more than left

R<L
right less than left

RL$_1$
few coarse rales

RL$_2$
moderate coarse rales

RL$_3$
many coarse rales

Rl
medium rales

Rl$_1$
few medium rales

Rl$_2$
moderate number of medium rales

Rl$_3$
many medium rales

rl
fine rales

rl$_1$
few fine rales

rl$_2$
moderate fine rales

rl$_3$
many fine rales

RLA
radiographic lung area
react to light and accommodation (re:
    Ophth)

RLB
right lateral bending

RLBCD
right lower border of cardiac dullness

RLC
rectus and longus capitus (muscles)
residual lung capacity

RLD
related living donor
resistive load detection
ruptured lumbar disc

RLE
Recent Life Events (re: Psychol)
right lower extremity

RLF
retrolental fibroplasia (retinopathy of
    prematurity [less than 1500 g] placed
    in high oxygen environment—re:
    Ophth)
right lateral femoral (site of injection)
right lateral flexion

RLL
right liver lobe
right lower lateral
right lower limb

RLL, R.L.L.
right lower lobe (lung)

R LL brace
right long leg brace

RLLE
right lower lid, eye

RLLLNR
right lower lobe lung, no rales

R & LLQ
right and left lower quadrants

RLM
right lower medial

RLMD
rat liver mitochondria (and
    submitochondrial particles derived
    by) digitonin (treatment)

RLN
recurrent laryngeal nerve
regional lymph node

RLNC
regional lymph node cell

RLND
regional lymph node dissection
retroperitoneal lymph node dissection

RLO
residual lymphocyte output

RLP
radiation-leukemia protection
ribosome-like particle

RLQ
right lower quadrant (of abdomen)

RLR
right lateral rectus

RLR muscle
right lateral rectus muscle (of eye)

RLS
person who stammers having difficulty
   in enunciating R, L, and S
rat lung strip
restless legs syndrome
Ringer's lactate solution

RLSB
right lower scapular border

rl-sh
right-left shunt

RLT
right lateral thigh

RLV
Rauscher leukemia virus

RLWD
routine laboratory work done

RLX
right lower extremity

RM
radical mastectomy
random migration
range of motion (re: Ortho)
range of movement (re: Ortho)
red marrow
regional myocardial
repetition maximum (re: PM&R)
resistive movement (re: PM&R)
respiratory metabolism
respiratory movement
right median
Rosenthal-Melkersson (syndrome)
Rothmann-Makai (syndrome)
ruptured membranes

R&M
routine and microscopic (re: urine test)

Rm
relative mobility
remission

rm.
room

RMA
relative medullary area (of kidney)
right mentoanterior (position of fetus)

RMB
right main-stem bronchus

RMBF
regional myocardial blood flow

RMC
right middle cerebral (artery)

RMCA
right middle cerebral artery

RMCAT
right middle cerebral artery thrombosis

RMCL
right midclavicular line

RMCP I
rat mast cell protease I

RMCP II
rat mast cell protease II

RMCT
rat mast cell technique

RMD
ratio of midsagittal diameters
retromanubrial dullness
right manubrial dullness

RME
resting metabolic expenditure
right mediolateral episiotomy

R-meter
radiation meter
roentgen-meter

RMF
right middle finger

RMI
Reading Miscue Inventory (re: Psychol)

RMK
rhesus monkey kidney

RML
radiation myeloid leukemia
right mentolateral

RML, R.M.L.
right middle lobe (of lung)

RML, rml
right mediolateral

RMLB
right middle lobe bronchus

RML scar W/O H
right midline scar without hernia

RMLV
Rauscher murine leukemia virus

RMM
rapid micromedia method
read mostly memory (re: computers)

RMP
rapidly miscible pool
Regional Medical Programs
resting membrane potential
rifampin
right mentoposterior (position of fetus)

RMR
resting metabolic rate
right medial rectus (muscle—re: Ophth)

RMR muscle
right medial rectus muscle (of eye)

RMS
respiratory muscle strength
rheumatic mitral stenosis
rhodomyosarcoma
root-mean-square (square root of mean
  square)

RMSD
root-mean-square deviation

RMSF
Rocky Mountain spotted fever

RMT
relative medullary thickness (of kidney)
retromolar trigone
right mentotransverse (position of fetus)

RMTC
rhesus monkey tissue culture

RMUI
relief medication unit index

RMV
respiratory minute volume

RN
radionuclide
reactive nitrogen
red nucleus (re: Neuro)
residual nitrogen
reticular nucleus

RN, R.N.
Registered Nurse

Rn
radon (element)

RNA
radionuclide angiography
ribonucleic acid

rough, noncapsulated, avirulent (re:
  bacteria)

RNAA
radiochemical neutron activation
  analysis

RNase
ribonuclease

RND
radical neck dissection
reactive neurotic depression

RNm
red nucleus, magnocellular (division)

r$_{nn}$
estimated coefficient (re: statistics;
  Spearman-Brown formula)

RNP
ribonucleoprotein

RNS
reference normal serum

RN5S
5S ribonucleic acid

RNT
radioassayable neurotensin

Rnt
roentgenologist
roentgenology

RNTC
rat nephroma tissue culture

rNTP
ribonucleoside 5'-triphosphates

RNV
radionuclide venography

RNVG
radionuclide ventriculogram

RO
ratio of
reality orientation (re: Psychol)
relative odds
reverse osmosis
Ritter-Oleson (technique)
routine order

RO, R/O
rule out

R$_o$
resting radium

ROA
rat ovarian augmentation
right occipito-anterior (position of fetus)

ROAD
reversible obstructive airway disease

ROAP
Rubidazone, Oncovin (vincristine),
    ara-C (cytarabine), and prednisone
    (re: chemotherapy)

ROATS
rabbit ovarian antitumor serum

rob
robertsonian translocation (re:
    cytogenetics)

ROC
receiver operating characteristic (re:
    diagnostic tests)
relative operating characteristic
resident on call
residual organic carbon

roc
reciprocal ohm centimeter (re: electrical
    conductivity)

ROE
roentgen

Roent
roentgenologist

Roent, roent.
roentgenology
roentgen (ray)

ROH
rat ovarian hyperemia (test)

ROI
region of interest (re: scintiphotography)

ROIH
right oblique inguinal hernia

ROL
right occipitolateral (position of fetus)

ROM
range of motion
range of movement
read-only memory (re: computers)
right otitis media
rupture of membranes

↓ **ROM**
decreased range of motion

Rom
Romberg (sign—re: Neuro)

rom
reciprocal ohm meter (re: electrical
    conductivity)

Romb
Romberg (sign—re: Neuro)

ROM C P
range of motion complete and pain-free

ROMI
rule out myocardial infarction

ROMSA
right otitis media, suppurative, acute

ROMSCh
right otitis media, suppurative, chronic

ROM WNL
range of motion within normal limits

ROP
retinopathy of prematurity (retrolental
    fibroplasia)
right occipitoposterior (position of fetus)

ROPP
receive only page printer (re:
    computers)

Ror
Rorschach (test—re: psychiatry)

ROS
read-only storage (re: computers/data
    processing)
review of symptoms
review of systems
rod outer segments

RoS
rostral sulcus (rostrum—shaped like a
    beak)

ROSS
review of subjective symptoms
review other subjective symptoms

ROT
remedial occupational therapy
right occiput transverse (position of
    fetus)
rotating
rule of thumb

Rot
Roth's (Rot's) disease

Rot, rot.
rotate

rot.
rotated
rotating
rotation
rotator

rot. ny.
rotatory nystagmus

rot. nystag.
rotatory nystagmus

rotoscol.
rotoscoliosis

rout.
routine

ROV
respiratory orphan virus

ROW
rat ovarian weight
Rendu-Osler-Weber (disease)

ROWTHT
ratio of weight to height

RP
radial pulse
radiographic planimetry
rapid processing (film)
reaction product
reactive protein
rectal prolapse
red pulp
re-entrant pathway
refractory period (re: Neuro)
regulatory protein
relapsing polychondritis
relative potency
respirations
respiratory rate: pulse rate (index)
resting potential
resting pressure
rest pain
retinitis pigmentosa (re: Ophth)
retinitis proliferans (re: Ophth)
retractor penis
retrograde pyelogram
retrograde pyelography
retroperitoneal
reversed phase
rheumatoid polyarthritis
ribose phosphate
ristocetin polymyxin (antibacterial)

R-P
radiologist, pediatric

R-1-P
ribose-1-phosphate

R-5-P
ribose-5-phosphate

Rp, R$_p$
pulmonary resistance

RPA
resultant physiological acceleration
reverse passive anaphylaxis
right pulmonary artery

RPAW
right pulmonary artery withdrawal

RPC
relapsing polychondritis
relative proliferative capacity
reticularis pontis caudalis (re: Neuro)

RPCF
Reiter protein complement fixation
(test—for syphilis)

RPCFT
Reiter protein complement fixation test
(for syphilis)

RPDSI
Riley Preschool Developmental
Screening Inventory

RPE
rating of perceived exertion
recurrent pulmonary emboli
retinal pigment epithelium (re: Ophth)

RPF
Reiter protein (complement) fixation
(test—for syphilis)
relaxed pelvic floor
renal plasma flow
retroperitoneal fibrosis

RPF^a
renal plasma flow, arterial

RPFS
Rosenzweig Picture-Frustration Study

RPF^v
renal plasma flow, venous

RPG
report program generator (re:
computers/data processing)
retrograde pyelogram
rheoplethysmography

RPG, rpg
radiation protection guide

RPGG
retroplacental gamma globulin

RPGN
rapidly progressive glomerulonephritis
right pedal giant neuron

RPHA
reverse(d) passive hemagglutination

RPHAMCFA
reversed passive hemagglutination (by)
miniature centrifugal fast analysis
(test)

RP-HPLC
reversed phase high-performance liquid
chromatography

RPI
Racial Perceptions Inventory (re:
Psychol)
Relative Percentage Index
reticulocyte production index

RP index
respiratory (rate)/pulse (rate) index

RPIPP
reversed phase ion-pair partition

RPLAD
retroperitoneal lymphadenopathy

RPLC
reversed phase liquid chromatography

RPLD
repair of potentially lethal damage

RPLND
retroperitoneal lymph node dissection

RPM
radical pair mechanism
right posterior measurement

RPM, rpm
revolutions per minute

RPO
right posterior oblique (view—re:
    radiology)

RPP
rate-pressure product
retropubic prostatectomy

RPPC
regional pediatric pulmonary center

RPPI
Role Perception Picture Inventory

RPPR
red (cell) precursor production rate

RPR
rapid plasma reagent (test)
rapid plasma reagin (re: syphilis test)

R.Pr.
retinitis proliferans (re: Ophth)

RPRCF
rapid plasma reagin complement
    fixation

RPRCT
rapid plasma reagin card test

RPS
renal pressor substance

RPS, rps
revolutions per second

RPT
rapid pull-through
refractory period of transmission

Rpt
report

Rpt, rpt.
repeat

RPTA
renal percutaneous transluminal
    angioplasty

RPTC
regional poisoning treatment center

RPTD
ruptured

rptd.
repeated
reported

RPV
right portal vein
right pulmonary vein(s)

RQ
reading quotient

RQ, R.Q.
recovery quotient
respiratory quotient

RR
radial rate
radiation reaction (cells)
radiation response
rapid radiometric
reacting record
reading retarded
Recovery Room
regular rate
relative response
relative risk
renin release
respiratory reserve
response rate
rest room
retinal reflex
rheumatoid rosette
right rotation
risk ratio
Riva-Rocci (sphygmomanometer)
ruthenium red

RR, R/R
respiratory rate

R&R
rate and rhythm (of pulse)
rest and recuperation

R + R
recess-resect (re: Ophth)

(no) R or R
no rales or rhonchi (re: Resp)

RRA
radioreceptor activity
radioreceptor assay

RRBC
rabbit red blood cell

RRC
Risk Reduction Component
routine respiratory care

RR cells
radiation reaction cells

RRCFCPD
recirculating, regenerating, continuous-
flow, chronic peritoneal dialysis

RRCT,no(m)
regular rate, clear tones, no murmurs
(re: Cardio)

RRE
radiation-related eosinophilia
regressive resistive exercise (re: PM&R)
round, regular, equal (re: Ophth)

RR&E
round, regular and equal (re: Ophth)

RRF
residual renal function

RRf
right ring finger

RR-HPO
rapid recompression-high pressure
oxygen

RRI
reflex relaxation index
relative response index

R-R interval
time elapsing between two QRS
complexes in EKG

rRNA
ribosomal RNA (ribonucleic acid)

RRP
relative refractory period
(neuromuscular)

RRpm
respiratory rate per minute

RRQG
right rostral quarter ganglion

RRR
regular rate and rhythm (re: Cardio)
renin-release rate
risk rescue rating (re: Psychol)

RR & R
regular rate and rhythm (re: Cardio)

RRS
retrorectal space
Riva-Rocci sphygmomanometer

RRT
randomized response technique
relative retention time (re: gas
chromatography)
resazurin reduction time

RRU
respiratory resistance unit

RR = VR
radial rate equals ventricular rate (re:
Cardio)

RS
random sample
rapid smoking
rating schedule
Rauwolfia serpentina
Raynaud's syndrome
reading of standard
recipient's serum
record separator (character—re:
computers/data processing)
rectal sinus
rectal suppository
rectosigmoid
reducing sugar
Reed-Sternberg (cell—re: Hodgkin's
disease)
reinforcement of stimulus
reinforcing stimulus
Reiter's syndrome
relative survival
remnant stomach
renal specialist
Repression-Sensitization (Scale)
reproductive success
resolved sarcoidosis
resorcinol-sulfur
respiratory syncytial (virus)
respiratory system
response to stimulus (ratio)
resting subject
review of symptoms
review of systems
Reye's syndrome
rhinal sulcus
rhythm strip
right sacrum
right septal (surface)
right septum
right side
right stellate (ganglion)
right subclavian
Riley-Shwachman (syndrome)
Ringer's solution
Ritchie sedimentation

R-S
reticulated siderocytes

Rs
(total) systemic resistance

r of s
review of systems

RSA
rabbit serum albumin
rat serum albumin
regular spiking activity (re: EEG)
relative specific activity
relative specific (radio)activity
relative standard accuracy
respiratory sinus arrhythmia
reticulum (cell) sarcoma
right sacro-anterior (position of fetus)
right subclavian artery

RSA→SA
right sacro-anterior to sacro-anterior

Rsa
(total) systemic arterial resistance

RSB
reticulocyte standard buffer
right sternal border

RSBT
rhythmic sensory bombardment therapy

RSC
rat spleen cell
rested-state contraction
reversible sickle cell
right side colon (cancer)

RScA, R ScA
right scapulo-anterior (position of fetus)

rsch.
research

RScP
right scapuloposterior (position of fetus)

RSD
ratoon stunting disease (a basal shoot
    sprouting from a plant; i.e., banana,
    sugar cane, pineapple)
reflex sympathetic dystrophy
relative sagittal depth
relative standard deviation (coefficient
    of variation— re: statistics)

RSE
rat synaptic ending
reverse sutured eye

RSEP
right somatosensory evoked potential

RSES
Rosenberg Self-esteem Scale

RSF
raw soybean flour

R-SICU
Respiratory-Surgical Intensive Care
    Unit

RSIVP
rapid-sequence intravenous pyelogram

RSL
right sacrolateral (position of fetus)

R SL brace
right short leg brace

RSLD
repair of sublethal damage

RSM
risk-screening model

RSMR
relative standardized mortality ratio

RSN
right substantia nigra (re: Neuro)

RSO
right salpingo-oophorectomy (re: GYN)
right superior oblique (muscle)

RSP
recirculating single pass
removable silicone plug
right sacroposterior (position of fetus)

RSPK
recurrent spontaneous psychokinesis

RSR
regular sinus rhythm (re: Cardio)
relative survival rate
right superior rectus (muscle)

RSR ratio
response-stimulus ratio

RSR s̄(m)
regular sinus rhythm without murmur
    (re: Cardio)

RSS
rat stomach strip
rectosigmoidoscope
Russian spring-summer (encephalitis)

RSSE
Russian spring-summer encephalitis

RSSR
relatively slow sinus rate (re: Cardio)

RST
radiosensitivity test(ing)
rubrospinal tract

RST, R.S.T.
right sacrotransverse (position of fetus)

RSTL
relaxed skin tension lines

RSV
respiratory syncytial virus
right subclavian vein
Rous sarcoma virus

RSVC
right superior vena cava

RSVCEF
Rous sarcoma virus-transformed chick
embryo fibroblast

rsvd.
reserved

RS virus
respiratory syncytial virus

RSVM
ram seminal vesicle microsome

RT
rabbit trachea
radiation therapy
radiotelemetry
radiotherapy
radium therapy
random transfusion
raphe transection
rational therapy (re: psychiatry)
reaction time
reading task
reading time
receptor transforming
reciprocal tachycardia
recreational therapy
rectal temperature
red tetrazolium (reagent)
reduction time
renal transplant
reptilase time
resistance transfer
respiratory technology
respiratory therapy
resting tension
rest tremor
retransformed (re: cell lines)
return to
right thigh
room temperature
Rubinstein-Taybi (syndrome)

RT, R.T.
reading test

RT, Rt, rt.
right

RT$_3$
increased resin T$_3$ uptake

RT$_3$, rT$_3$
reverse triiodothyronine

Rt
total resistance

rt.
routine

RTA
renal tubular acidosis

renal tubular antigen
renal tubule acidosis
road traffic accident

RTAVI
Risk-Taking, Attitude, Values Inventory

RTC
randomized trial, controlled
rape treatment center
renal tubular cell
return to clinic

RTCA
1-β-D-ribofuranosyl-1H-1,2,4-triazole-3-
carboxamide (ribavirin—antiviral)

RTCS
Roske-De Toni-Caffey-Smyth (disease)

RTD
routine test dilution

Rtd, rtd.
retarded (delayed)

RTE
rabbit thymus extract

R test
reductase test

rt. ↑ ext.
right upper extremity

rt. ↓ ext.
right lower extremity

RTF
replication and transfer
resistance transfer factor
respiratory tract fluid

rtg.
roentgen

rtgn.
roentgen

RTHCP
Ross Test of Higher Cognitive
Processes

rtl.
rectal

rt. lat.
right lateral

RTM
registered trademark

RTN
renal tubular necrosis

rtn.
return

RTO
return to office

rt. ↑ OQ
right upper outer quadrant

RTP
renal transplant patient
reverse transcriptase-producing (agent)

RTPS
radiation therapy planning system

RTR
red (blood cell) turnover rate
retention time ratio
return to room

RTRR
return to Recovery Room

RTS
real time scan (re: ultrasound)
relative tumor size

rTSAb
rodent thyroid-stimulating antibody

rt. scap. bord.
right scapular border

r$_{tt}$
obtained coefficient (re: statistics;
  Spearman-Brown formula)
reliability coefficient

RTU
relative time unit

rTU
rRNA (ribosomal ribonucleic acid)
  transcription unit

RTV
room temperature vulcanizing

RTW
return to work

RU
reading of unknown
reading unknown
recurrent ulcer
residual urine
resin uptake
resistance unit
retrograde urogram
retroverted uterus
right uninjured
right uninvolved
right upper
rodent ulcer
roentgen unit
routine urinalysis

RU, R.U.
rat unit

Ru
ruthenium (element)

^{97}Ru
radioactive isotope of ruthenium

^{103}Ru
radioactive isotope of ruthenium

^{106}Ru
radioactive isotope of ruthenium

ru
radiation unit (re: measurement of
  cosmic-ray absorption)

rub.
ruber (L. red)

RUBIDIC
Rubidazone/DTIC (re: chemotherapy)

RUE
right upper extremities
right upper extremity

RUL
right upper lateral
right upper (eye)lid
right upper limb
right upper lung

RUL, R.U.L.
right upper lobe (lung)

RUM
right upper medial

R unit
roentgen unit

RUO
right ureteral orifice

RUOQ
right upper outer quadrant

RUP
right upper pole

Ru5-P
ribulose-5-phosphate (re: pentose
  phosphate pathway)

rupt.
rupture(d)

rupt'd
ruptured

rupt. memb.
ruptured membrane

RUQ
right upper quadrant (of abdomen)

RUR
resin uptake ratio

RURTI
recurrent upper respiratory tract infection

RUS
radioulnar synostosis
recurrent ulcerative stomatitis

RUSB
right upper scapular border
right upper sternal border

RUSS
recurrent ulcerative scarifying stomatitis

RUV
residual urine volume

RUX
right upper extremity

RV
random variable
rat virus
Rauscher virus
rectovaginal
reinforcement value
renal venous
reovirus
residual volume
respiratory volume
retinal vasculitis
retroversion
retroverted
return visit
rheumatoid vasculitis
rhinovirus
right ventricle
right ventricular (cavity)
rubella vaccine
rubella virus

R_v
radius of view (re: collimator)

RVA
recorded voice announcement (re: computers/data processing)
re-entrant ventricular arrhythmia
right ventricular activation
right ventricular apical
right vertebral artery

RVAW
right ventricular anterior wall

RVB
red venous blood

RVbody
right ventricle body

RVC
radioactivity of vegetative cells
responds to verbal commands

$R = VCO_2/VO_2$
respiratory exchange ratio

RVD
rat vas deferens
relative vertebral density
relative volume decrease
right ventricular dimension

RVDO
right ventricular diastolic overload

RVDV
right ventricular diastolic volume

RVE
right ventricular enlargement

RVECP
right ventricular endocardial potential

RVEDP
right ventricular end-diastolic pressure

RVEDV
right ventricular end-diastolic volume

RVEDVI
right ventricular end-diastolic volume index

RVEF
right ventricular ejection fraction
right ventricular end-flow

RVESV
right ventricular end-systolic volume

RVESVI
right ventricular end-systolic volume index

RVET
right ventricular ejection time

RVE-VOL
reserve volume

RVF
renal vascular failure
Rift Valley fever
right ventricular failure
right visual field

RV fist.
rectovaginal fistula

RVFV
Rift Valley fever virus

RVG
relative value guide
right ventral gluteus (muscle)
right visceral ganglion

RVH
renal vascular hypertension

RVH, R.V.H.
right ventricular hypertrophy

RVHD
rheumatic valvular heart disease

RVI
relative value index

RVID
right ventricular internal dimension

RVIDd
right ventricular internal dimension
    diastole

RVIT
right ventricular inflow tract

RVLG
right ventrolateral gluteal (muscle—site
    of injection)

RVM
right ventricular mean

RVmid
right ventricle (mid)

RVO
relaxed vaginal outlet
right ventricular outflow

RVOFT recons.
right ventricular outflow tract
    reconstruction

RVOT
right ventricular outflow tract

RVP
rat ventral prostate
red veterinary petrolatum
renovascular pressure
resting venous pressure
right ventricular pressure

RVPEP
right ventricular pre-ejection period

RVPRA
renal vein plasma renin activity

RVR
reduced vascular response
reduced vestibular response
renal vascular resistance
renal vein renin
repetitive ventricular responses
resistance to venous return

RVRA
renal venous renin assay

RVRA, RV/RA
renal vein renin activity (ratio)

RVRC
renal vein renin concentration

RVS
relative value scale
Relative Value Schedule
Relative Value Study
reported visual sensation
retrovaginal space
Rokeach Value Survey (re:
    psychological testing)

RVSO
right ventricular stroke output

RVSW
right ventricular stroke work

RVT
renal vein thrombosis
Russell viper time (Stypven time—a
    prothrombin test)

RVTE
recurring venous thromboembolism

RV-TLC, RV/TLC
residual volume to total lung capacity

RVU
relative value unit

RVV
rubella vaccine-like virus
Russell's viper venom

RVWD
right ventricular wall device

RW
radiological warfare
ragweed
read-write (head—re: computers)
respiratory work
Romano-Ward (syndrome)
round window

RW, R/W
return to work

R-W
Rideal-Walker (phenol coefficient test)

RWAGE
ragweed antigen E

R wave
upward deflection of QRS in
    electrocardiogram

RWD
rewind (re: computers)

RWM
regional wall motion

RWP
ragweed pollen

RWS
ragweed sensitivity

RWT
R-wave threshold (re: EKG)

RX, Rx
drugs
medication

RX, Rx, ℞
prescription
recipe (L. take)
therapy
treatment

Rxd
treated

Rx'd US, diath., trx.
treated with ultrasound, diathermy,
　　traction

RXLI
recessive X-linked icthyosis

RXN, rxn.
reaction

rxns.
reactions

Rx Phys
treating physician

RXT
right exotropia

R-Y
Roux-en-Y (anastomosis)

S

S
area
denotes attachment to sulfur (re: chemistry)
designation of a rare human antigen (genetically related to the MNS blood group)
DNA synthesis phase of cell cycle
entropy (re: thermodynamics)
exposure time (re: radiology)
mean dose per unit cumulated activity
percentage of saturation (of hemoglobin with oxygen or carbon dioxide)
relative storage capacity
response to white space
Saccharomyces (genus)
sacral (in vertebral formulae)
sacrum
saline
Salmonella (genus)
same
Saprospira (genus)
Sarcocystis (genus of itch mite—re: scabies)
Sarcophaga (genus of flies)
Sarcoptes (genus)
saturated
saturation
Schistosoma (genus)
schizophrenia
screen-containing cassette
senile
sensitive
septum
sequential (analysis)
serine (an amino acid)
Serratia (genus)
serum
serving
Shigella (genus)
sick
siderocyte
siemens (SI unit of electrical conductance)
signa (L. mark; write on [label])
signature
signetur (L. let it be written, labeled; it shall be written [as instruction to the patient])
silicate
Silurian (re: geologic time)
single (marital status)
Siphunculina (genus—eye fly of India—re: trachoma)

smooth (re: bacterial colonies)
soft (re: diet)
soft (re: abdomen, muscle bodies, etc.)
soil
solid
soluble
solute
space
spasm
spatial aptitude (re: General Aptitude Test Battery)
special preparations necessary for test
specific activity
spherical
spherical lens
Spirillum (genus)
Spirometra (genus of tapeworm)
spleen
sporadic
Sporothrix (genus)
Sporotrichum (genus)
standard normal deviate (re: statistics)
Staphylococcus (genus of imperfect fungi)
stemline (number—re: tumor cell population)
stimulus
Stomoxys (genus of flies)
storage
Streptobacillus (genus)
Streptococcus (genus)
streptomycin
Strongyloides (genus)
subject (of an experiment)
subjective (findings)
substrate (general)
substrate (specific—in Michaelis-Menton hypothesis)
sulcus
sulfur (element)
sum of an arithmetic series
supervision
supravergence
surface
surgeon
surgery
surgical
suture
symbolic contents
sympathetic
synthesis (of DNA in cell cycle)
systems (products—re: Psychol; Aptitudes Research Project testing within structure of intellect model)

systole
S wave (re: EKG)

S, S.
svedberg (sedimentation coefficient—
  re: analytical centrifuges)

S, s
scruple (apothecaries')
second (fundamental unit of time in all
  systems of units)
section
see
semis (L. half)
sensation
series
sign
signed
singular
sinister (L. left)
sinus
sister
son
symmetrical

S, s, $\bar{\text{s}}$
sine (L. without)

(S)-
sinister (L. left—opposite of R)

/S/, /s/
signature
signed

S1
lethal antigen-1 (Ala-1) (re: genetics)

S1, S_1
first heart sound

S1, S2, etc.; S_1, S_2, etc.
first sacral vertebra, second sacral
  vertebra (or nerve), etc.

S_1, S_2, S_3, S_4
suicide risk

S_1
stage in cycle of cell growth

S2
lethal antigen-2 (Ala-2) (re: genetics)

S2, S_2
second heart sound

S3
lethal antigen-3 (Ala-3) (re: genetics)

S_3
third heart sound (an abnormal heart
  sound)
ventricular gallop sound

S4
species antigen-4 (SA 1) (re: genetics)

S_4
fourth heart sound (an abnormal heart
  sound)

S5
surface antigen-5 (SA-6) (re: genetics)

S6
species antigen-6 (SA 7–1)
  (re:genetics)

S7
surface antigen-7 (SA 7-2) (re: genetics)

S8
surface antigen-8 (SA 12-1) (re:
  genetics)

S9
surface antigen-9 (SA 17-1) (re:
  genetics)

S10
surface antigen-10 (SAX-1) (re:
  genetics)

S11
surface antigen-11 (SAX-2) (re:
  genetics)

S12
surface antigen-12 (SAX-3) (re:
  genetics)

^{35}S
sulfur-35

Σ
foaminess (Σ is initial of Gr. word
  meaning lather)
sigma (capital 18th letter of the Greek
  alphabet)
sum
summation of all quantities following the
  symbol
syphilis (a euphemism for)

σ
population standard deviation (re:
  statistics)
sigma (18th letter of Greek alphabet)
standard deviation (re: statistics)
Stefan-Boltzmann constant
stigma (proposed [1944] unit of length
  equaling 10^{-12}m—re: atomic
  measurements)
surface tension
type of molecular orbital or bond
wavenumber

s
atomic orbital with angular momentum
  quantum number zero
distance
sample standard deviation (re:
  statistics)
sample variance (re: statistics)

satellite (chromosomal)
selection coefficient (re: genetics)
steady state (when written as a
   subscript)

s-
symmetric isomer

s̈, s, š
sine (L. without)

s^2
sample deviation (re: statistics)

SA
salicylic acid
saline
salt added
sarcoma
scalenus anticus
second antibody
secondary amenorrhea
secondary anemia
secondary arrest
self-agglutinating
self-analysis
semen analysis
senile atrophy
sensitizing antibody
serum albumin
serum aldolase
sialic acid
siblings (raised) apart
sinus arrest
sinus arrhythmia
skeletal age
slightly active
social acquiescence (re: Psychol)
social age (re: Psychol)
soluble in alkaline (solution)
Spanish American
spatial average
specific activity
spectrum analyzer
sperm abnormality
spermagglutinin
spiking activity
standard accuracy
Staphylococcus aureus
Stokes-Adams (disease or syndrome;
   Adams-Stokes; Morgagni's;
   Morgagni-Adams-Stokes; Spens)
suicide attempt
surface antigen
surface area
sustained action (re: drugs)
sympathetic activity
systemic arterial (pressure)
systemic aspergillosis

SA, S.A., s.a.
secundum artem (L. according to the
   art; by skill)

SA, S-A
sinoatrial (node)

SA, S/A
short arm

S-A
sinoauricular (sino-auricular)

S/A
same as above
sugar and acetone

S&A
sugar and acetone

S_2A
second heart sound, aortic component

Sa
samarium (element)
saturation

^{153}Sa
radioactive isotope of samarium

SAA
serum amyloid-A (protein)
Stokes-Adams attacks

SAARD
slow-acting antirheumatic drug

SAAST
self-administered alcohol screening test

SAB
Sabouraud (dextrose agar)
serum albumin
significant asymptomatic bacteriuria
sinoatrial block
spontaneous abortion
subarachnoid block

SABHI
Sabouraud (dextrose) agar and brain
   heart infusion

SABP
spontaneous acute bacterial peritonitis

SAC
saccharin
screening and acute care
short arm cast (re: Ortho)
splenic adherent cell

sac.
sacral
sacrum

SACC
short arm cylinder cast

sacc.
saccades (Fr. to jerk—cogwheel
   respiration)

sacch.
saccharin

SACD
subacute combined degeneration

SACE
serum angiotensin converting enzyme
(activity)

SACH
solid ankle, cushion heel (re: Ortho)

SACH foot
solid ankle cushion heel (foot
component— re: Ortho)

sac-il
sacro-iliac

SACS
secondary anticoagulation system

SACSF
subarachnoid cerebrospinal fluid

SACT
sinoatrial conduction time

SAD
Self-Assessment Depression (Scale)
separation anxiety disorder (re:
Psychol)
small airway dysfunction
social avoidance and distress (re:
Psychol)
source-to-axis distance
sugar, acetone, diacetic acid (test)
suppressor-activating determinant

SADD
Standardized Assessment of
Depressive Disorders

SADL
simulated activities of daily living

SADQ
Self-Administered Dependency
Questionnaire

SADR
suspected adverse drug reaction

SADS
Schedule for Affective Disorders and
Schizophrenia
Shipman Anxiety Depression Scale

SADS-C
Schedule for Affective Disorders and
Schizophrenia— Change

SADS-L
Schedule for Affective Disorders and
Schizophrenia— Lifetime (Version)

SAE
short above elbow (cast)
specific action exercise
supported arm exercise

SAEB
sinoatrial entrance block

SAF
serum accelerator factor
simultaneous auditory feedback

SAFA
soluble antigen fluorescent antibody
(test)

SAFE
simulated aircraft fire and emergency

SAG
Swiss (-type) agammaglobulinemia

SAGM
sodium chloride, adenine, glucose,
mannitol

SAH
S-adenosyl-L-homocysteine
subarachnoid hemorrhage

SAHS
sleep apnea hypersomnolence
syndrome

SAI
Social Adequacy Index
systemic active immunotherapy

SAICAR
5-amino-4-imidazole-N-
succinocarboxamide ribonucleotide
(or ribotide; succino-AICAR [an
important purine precursor])

SAID
sexually acquired immunodeficiency
(syndrome)

SAIDS
simian acquired immunodeficiency
syndrome

SAL
sensorineural acuity level
specified antilymphocytic

SAL, Sal.
Salmonella (genus)

SAL, sal.
saline

S.A.L., s.a.l.
secundum artis legis (L. according to
the rules of the art)

sal.
salicylate
saliva

sal. acid
salicylic acid

salicyl.
salicylate

Salm
Salmonella (genus)

SAM
S-adenosylmethionine ("active"
    methionine—re: mouse tumor
    antagonist)
scanning acoustic microscope
sex arousal mechanism
sulfated acid mucopolysaccharide
surface active material
synthetic, adhesive, moisture (vapor
    permeable)
systolic anterior motion
systolic anterior movement

SAMF
single antibody Millipore filtration

SAMI
socially acceptable monitoring
    instrument

SAMS
Study Attitudes and Methods Survey
    (re: Psychol)

SAN
sinoatrial node (re: Cardio)
sinoauricular node (re: Cardio)
slept all night
solitary autonomous nodule

SANC
short arm navicular cast

sanit.
sanitarium
sanitary
sanitation

S-A node
sinoatrial node (re: Cardio)

SANS
Scale for the Assessment of Negative
    Symptoms

S antigen
soluble antigen

SAO
small airway obstruction

Sa$_{O_2}$
oxygen percent saturation (arterial)

SAP
seminal acid phosphatase
sensory action potential
serum acid phosphatase
serum alkaline phosphatase
serum amyloid-P
Staphylococcus aureus protease

sulfosalicylic acid protein
systemic arterial pressure

sap.
saponification
saponify

SAPD
self-administration of psychoactive
    drugs

saph.
saphenous (vein)

sapon.
saponification
saponify

SAQ
School Atmosphere Questionnaire (re:
    Psychol)
short arc quadriceps

SAQC
statistical analysis and quality control

SAR
sexual attitude reassessment
sexual attitude restructuring
structure activity relationship (re: Dent)
sympathomimetic ratio

Sar
sulfarsphenamine (antisyphilitic)

SART
sinoatrial recovery time (re: Cardio)

SAS
School Attitude Survey (Feelings I Have
    About School)
self-rating anxiety scale
short arm splint
Situational Attitude Scale
Sklar Aphasia Scale (for adults)
sleep apnea syndrome
small animal surgery
Social Adaptation Status (re: Psychol)
statistical analysis system
sterile aqueous suspension
subaortic stenosis
subarachnoid space
supravalvular aortic stenosis
surface-active substance

SASDRA
sample acquisition system for
    dissolution rate analysis

SAS-RS
Social Adjustment Self-Report Scale

SAST
serum aspartate aminotransferase
    (serum glutamic-oxaloacetic
    transaminase—re: myocardial infarct;
    liver cell disease)

SAT
satellite
Scholastic Aptitude Test
School Ability Test (re: Psychol)
School Attitude Test
Senior Apperception Technique
Shapes Analysis Test (re: Psychol)
single agent (chemo)therapy
Slide Agglutination Test
sodium ammonium thiosulfate
specified antithymocytic
speech awareness threshold
spermatogenic activity test
spontaneous activity test
Stanford Achievement Test
structural atypia
subacute thyroiditis
systematized assertive therapy (re:
    Psychol)
systemic assertive therapy (re: Psychol)

SAT, sat.
saturate
saturated
saturation

sat.
satisfactory
saturatus (L. saturated)

s.a.t.
sine acido thymonucleinico (L. without
    thymonucleic acid)

SATA
spatial average/temporal average

SATB
Special Aptitude Test Battery

SAT chromosome
a chromosome with a satellite

sat. cond.
satisfactory condition

sat'd
saturated

sat. DNA
satellite DNA (deoxyribonucleic acid)

satis.
satisfactory

SATL
surgical Achilles tendon lengthening

satn.
saturation

SATP
spatial average temporal peak

sat. sol.
saturated solution

sat. sol. KI
saturated solution of potassium iodide

SAU
statistical analysis unit

SB
sandbag
Schwartz-Bartter (syndrome)
serum bilirubin
shortness of breath
sick bay (Navy)
sideroblast
Silvestroni-Bianco (syndrome)
single blind
single breath
sinus bradycardia
small bowel
sodium balance
southbound (re: motor vehicle accident)
soybean
spina bifida
spontaneous blastogenesis
spontaneously breathing
stereotyped behavior
sternal border
stillbirth
surface-binding (protein)

SB, S-B
Stanford-Binet (intelligence test)

SB, S/B
stillborn

S of B
short of breath

S/β
sickle cell beta ($\beta°$ type of sickle cell)

Sb
stibium (element—antimony)

Sb, Sb.
strabismus

^{122}Sb
radioactive isotope of stibium
    (antimony)

^{124}Sb
radioactive isotope of stibium
    (antimony)

^{125}Sb
radioactive isotope of stibium
    (antimony)

sb
stilb (centimeter-gram-second unit of
    luminous intensity—formerly called
    brightness)

SBA
serum bile acid

shared batch area (re: computers/data
   processing)
soybean agglutinin
spina bifida aperta
stand-by assistance
summary basis for approval

SBB
simultaneous binaural, bithermal
stimulation-bound behavior

SBC
serum bactericidal concentration
special back care
strict bed confinement
sunburn cell

SBCl$_3$
antimony trichloride (butter of
   antimony—escharotic, dehorning
   agent for calves, goats—re:
   veterinary)

SBD
senile brain disease
suggested brain dysfunction
Supervisory Behavior Description

SBDP
standard dose beclomethasone
   dipropionate

SBE
self-examination, breast
short below elbow (cast)
shortness of breath on exertion
subacute bacterial endocarditis

SBF
serologic-blocking factor
serum-blocking factor
specific blocking factor
splanchnic blood flow

SBFT
small bowel follow-through

SBG
selenite brilliant green

SBH
sea blue histiocytosis

SBI
soybean (trypsin) inhibitor

SBIS
Stanford-Binet Intelligence Scale

SBL
soybean lectin

SBMV
southern bean mosaic virus

SBN
single-breath nitrogen (test)

SBN$_2$
single-breath nitrogen (test)

SBNT
single-breath nitrogen test

SBNW
single-breath nitrogen washout

SBO
small bowel obstruction
spina bifida occulta

Sb$_2$O$_3$
antimony trioxide (industrial chemical)

Sb$_2$O$_5$
antimony pentoxide (fire retardant—
   clothing)

Sb$_4$O$_6$
antimony trioxide (in vapor phase)

SBOM
soybean oil meal

SBP
serotonin-binding protein
spontaneous bacterial peritonitis
steroid-binding plasma (protein)
systemic blood pressure
systolic blood pressure

S-BP line
sella (to) Bolton point line (re:
   cephalometrics)

SBQ
Smoking Behavior Questionnaire

SBR
spleen-to-body-weight ratio
stillbirth rate
stimulus-bound repetitive
strict bedrest
styrene-butadiene rubber

SBS
short bowel syndrome
side-by-side (structure)
side to back to side
social-breakdown syndrome (re:
   Psychol)

SBT
serum bactericidal test
serum bactericidal titer
serum bacteriological titers
single-breath test

SBTI
soybean trypsin inhibitor

SBV
singular binocular vision

SC
sacrococcygeal

schedule change
Schüller-Christian (disease)
Schwann cell
Scianna (blood group)
sciatic (nerve)
scrupulus (L. scruple [a weight])
secondary cleavage
secretory component
self-care
semicircular
semiclosed
serum complement
serum creatinine
service connected
sex chromatin
shallow compartment
short circuit
sick call
sickle cell (anemia)
sickle cell (test)
silicone coated
single chemical
skin conductance
slow component (re: Neuro)
Smeloff-Cutter (prosthesis, valve—re:
   Cardio)
Snellen chart (re: Ophth)
special care
specific characteristic
spinal cord
spleen cell
squamous cancer
statistical control
stellate cell
sternoclavicular
stimulus, conditioned
stratum corneum
Streptococcus
stroke count
subcellular
subclavian
subcorneal
subcortical
succinylcholine
sugar coated
sulfur colloid
sulfur containing
superior colliculus (nucleus of)
superior constrictor (muscles of
   pharynx)
superior cornu
supportive care
suppressor cell
surface colony
surgical cone
systemic candidiasis
systolic click

SC, S.C.
closure of the semilunar valves (re:
   Cardio)

SC, S-C
sickle cell-(hemoglobin) C (disease)

SC, sc.
science
scientific
scilicet (L. it is permitted to know
   [namely])
subcutaneous

SC, s.c.
sine correctione (L. without correction)

S&C
sclerae and conjunctivae (re: Ophth)
singly and consensually (re: Ophth)

Sc
scandium (element)
scapular

Sc, sc.
scapula

^{43}Sc
radioactive isotope of scandium

^{44}Sc
radioactive isotope of scandium

^{46}Sc
radioactive isotope of scandium

^{47}Sc
radioactive isotope of scandium

Sc
Schmidt number (dimensionless
   transport number)

sc.
scant
sclera

s.c.
subcutaneously

$\dot{\bar{s}}$ c
sine (without) correction

SCA
School and College Ability (tests)
self-care agency
severe congenital anomaly
sickle cell anemia
sperm-coating antigen
spleen colony assay
subclavian artery
superior cerebellar artery
suppressor cell activity

SCAb
autoantibody to stratum corneum

SCABG
single coronary artery bypass graft

SCAG
Sandoz Clinical Assessment for
   Geriatrics
single coronary artery graft

SCAL
Self-Concept as a Learner (Scale)

SCAMIN
Self-Concept and Motivation Inventory

SCAN
scantiscan
suspected child abuse/neglect
systolic coronary artery narrowing

Scand
Scandinavian

Scanz
Scanzoni (maneuver)

scap.
scapula
scapular

SCAS
semicontinuous activated sludge

SCAT
School and College Ability Test
sheep cell agglutination test
sickle cell anemia test

SCAT-III
School and College Ability
Test-Series III

scat.
scatula (L. box)

scat. orig.
scatula originalis (L. original package
[manufacturer's package and label])

SCB
sedative cabinet bath
stratum corneum basic
strictly confined to bed

SCBA
self-contained breathing apparatus

SCBH
systemic cutaneous basophil
hypersensitivity

SCBP
stratum corneum basic protein

SCBU
special care baby unit

ScBU
screening bacteriuria

SCC
sequential combination chemotherapy
short circuit current
short-course chemotherapy
small cell cancer
small cleaved cell

squamous carcinoma of the cervix
squamous cell carcinoma

SCCB
small cell carcinoma of the bronchus

SCCHN
squamous cell carcinoma of the head
and neck

SCCL
small cell (oat cell) carcinoma of the
lung

SCCM
Sertoli's cell culture medium

SCD
service-connected disability
sickle cell disease
spinocerebellar degeneration
subacute combined degeneration (of
the spinal cord)
subacute coronary disease
sudden cardiac death
sudden coronary death
surgeon's certificate of disability

ScDA, Sc DA
scapulodextra anterior (position of
fetus)

S-C disease
sickle cell-(hemoglobin) C disease

ScDP, Sc DP
scapulodextra posterior (position of
fetus)

SCE
saturated calomel electrode
secretory carcinoma of the
endometrium
sister chromatid exchange
somatic cell (re: genetics)
subcutaneous emphysema

SCEP
sandwich counterelectrophoresis

SCER
sister chromatid exchange rate

SCF
supercritical fluid

SCFA
short-chain fatty acid

SCFE
slipped capital femoral epiphysis

SCFI
specific clotting factors and inhibitors

scf/min
standard cubic feet per minute

SCG
serum chemistry graph
serum chemogram
sodium cromoglycate
superior cervical ganglion (re: Neuro)

SCH
Schirmer (test—re: Ophth)
succinylcholine
suprachiasmatic (re: Neuro)

SChE
serum cholinesterase

sched.
schedule
scheduled

schiz.
schizophrenia

SCHL
subcapsular hematoma of the liver

SCI
short crus of incus (re: Oto)
spinal cord injury
structured clinical interview

Sci, sci.
science
scientific

SCIBTA
stem cell indicated by transplantation
    assay

SCID
severe combined immunodeficiency
    disease

SCII
Strong-Campbell Interest Inventory (re:
    Psychol)

scint.
scintigram

SCIPP
sacrococcygeal to inferior pubic point

SCIS
Spinal Cord Injury Service

SCIU
Spinal Cord Injury Unit

SCJ
squamocolumnar junction
sternoclavicular joint

SCK
serum creatine kinase

SCL
scleroderma
serum copper level
soft contact lens

spinocervicolemniscal
symptom checklist

Scl, scl.
sclerosis
sclerotic

ScLA, Sc.L.A.
scapulolaeva anterior (position of fetus)

SCLC
small cell lung cancer

SCLC-v
small cell lung cancer variants

SCLC-V cells
large cell variants of small cell
    carcinoma

Scler
sclerosis

sclero.
scleroderma

ScLP, Sc.L.P.
scapulolaeva posterior (position of
    fetus)

SCM
Schwann cell membrane
sensation, circulation, and motion
soluble cytotoxic medium
spleen cell-conditioned medium
spondylotic caudal myelopathy
steatocystoma multiplex
sternocleidomastoid
streptococcal cell membrane
structure of the cytoplasmic matrix
surface-connecting membrane

SC & M
sensation, circulation, and motion

ScM
scalene muscle

SCMC
spontaneous cell-mediated cytotoxicity

SCN
Special Care Nursery
suprachiasmatic nucleus

SC node
supraclavicular node

SCNS
subcutaneous nerve stimulation

SCO
subcommissural organ

SCOP, scop.
scopolamine

SCP
single-cell(ed) protein

sodium cellulose phosphate
soluble cytoplasmic protein
Standardized Care Plan
submucous cleft palate
superior cerebral peduncle

scp.
scruple

scp, s.c.p.
spherical candle power

SCPK, S-CPK
serum creatine phosphokinase

SCR
Schick Conversion Rate
silicon-controlled rectifier
skin conductance response
spondylotic caudal radiculopathy

SCR, scr.
scruple

SCr
serum creatinine

SCRAM
speech controlled respirometer for
ambulation measurement

SCRAP
Simple-Complex Reaction-Time
Apparatus

Scripts, scripts
prescriptions

SCRS
Short Clinical Rating Scale

scrup.
scruple

SCS
Shared Computer Systems (re: medical
records)
silicon-controlled switch (a
semiconductor device used as a
switch)
Social Climate Scales (re: Psychol)
surface-connecting system
systolic click syndrome

SCSIT
Southern California Sensory Integration
Tests

SCSP
supracondylar, suprapatellar

sc. sp.
scapular spine

SCT
salmon calcitonin
Sentence Completion Test
sex chromatin test

Sexual Compatibility Test
sickle cell trait
special characters table (re: computers/
data processing)
sperm cytotoxic
spinal computed tomography
spinocervicothalamic
staphylococcal clumping test
sugar-coated tablet

SCT, S.C.T.
Sentence Completion Test (re: Psychol)

SCTAT
sex cord tumor with anular tubules

SCTx
static cervical traction

SCU
Self-Care Unit
Special Care Unit

SCUD
septicemic cutaneous ulcerative
disease

SCUM
secondary carcinoma of the upper
mediastinum

SCV
sensory conduction velocity
smooth, capsulated, virulent (re:
bacteria)
squamous cell carcinoma of the vulva
subclavian vein

SCV-CPR
simultaneous compression ventilation-
cardiopulmonary resuscitation

SD
Sandhoff's disease
Scotch douche (alternating hot and cold
water)
secretion droplet
segregation distortion
senile dementia
septal defect
serologically defined (antigen)
serologically detected
serologically determined
serum defect
severe disability
short (time) dialysis
shoulder disarticulation
shoulder dislocation
Shy-Drager (syndrome)
skin destruction
social desirability
socialized delinquency
somadendritic
specially denatured (alcohol)
sphincter dilatation
spontaneous delivery

Sprague-Dawley (rat)
spreading depression
Stensen's duct
stone disintegration
streptodornase
sudden death
superoxide dismutase
systolic discharge

SD, S.D.
skin dose
standard deviation (re: statistics)

SD, Sd
stimulus drive (re: Psychol)

S.D.
sagittal depth (cornea—re: optics or
    contact lens)

S-D
sickle cell-(hemoglobin) D (disease)
strength-duration

S/D
sharp/dull
systolic to diastolic (ratio)

S^d
stimulus, discriminative

SDA
Sabouraud's dextrose agar
sacrodextra anterior (position of fetus)
salt-dependent agglutinin
sialodacryoadenitis (virus)
source-data automation (re: computers)
specific dynamic action
succinic dehydrogenase activity
superficial distal axillary (node)

SDAT
senile dementia, Alzheimer type

SDB
sleep disordered breathing

SDBP
seated diastolic blood pressure
standing diastolic blood pressure
supine diastolic blood pressure

SDC
sensitivity depth compensation (ramp)
serum digoxin concentration
sodium deoxycholate
succinyldicholine

SDCL
symptom distress check list

S-D curve
strength-duration curve

SDD
sporadic depressive disease
sterile dry dressing

SDE, S.D.E.
specific dynamic effect

SDEEG
stereotactic depth
    electroencephalogram

SDES
symptomatic diffuse esophageal spasm

SDF
slow death factor
stream dilution factor
stress distribution factor

SDG
short distance group
sucrose density gradient

SDGC
sucrose density gradient centrifugation

SDGU
sucrose density gradient
    ultracentrifugation

SDH
serine dehydrase
sorbitol dehydrogenase
spinal dorsal horn
subdural hematoma
subjacent dorsal horn
succinate dehydrogenase

SDH1
succinate dehydrogenase-1

SDHD
sudden death heart disease

SDI
selective dissemination of information
    (re: computers)
standard deviation interval (re:
    statistics)
Surtees' Difficulties Index

SDIHD
sudden-death ischemic heart disease

SDL
self-directed learning
serum digoxin level
speech discrimination loss

sdly
sidelying

SDM
sensory detection method
single, divorced, married

SDM, sdm
standard deviation of the mean (re:
    statistics)

SDMT
Symbol Digit Modalities Test

SDN
sexually dimorphic nucleus

SDNA
single-stranded deoxyribonucleic acid

SDO
sudden-dosage onset

SDP
sacrodextra posterior (position of fetus)
stomach, duodenum, pancreas

SDPC
S-D (suicide-depression) Proneness
Checklist

SDR
spontaneously diabetic rat
surgical dressing room

SDRT
Stanford Diagnostic Reading Test

SDS
Self-Directed Search (re: Psychol)
Self-Rating Depression Scale
sensory deprivation syndrome
sexual differentiation scale
Shy-Drager syndrome
simple descriptive scale
single dose suppression
sodium dodecyl sulfate (a detergent)
Student Disability Survey (re: Psychol)
sudden-death syndrome
sustained depolarizing shift

Sds, sds.
sounds

SD sequence
Shine-Dalgarno sequence (re: genetics)

SD-SK
streptodornase-streptokinase

SDS-PAGE technique
sodium dodecyl sulfate-polyacrylamide
gel electrophoresis technique

SDT
sacrodextra transversa (position of
fetus)
sensory decision theory
single donor transfusion
speech detection threshold

SD$_t$
standard deviation of total scores (re:
statistics)

SDU
short double upright (brace)
standard deviation unit

SDUB
short double upright brace

SDV
specific desensitizing vaccine

SDW
separated, divorced, or widowed

SE
saline enema
sanitary engineering
self-explanatory
series elastic (component [muscle])
sheep erythrocyte
side effect
smoke exposure
smoke extract
soft exudate
solid extract
sphenoethmoidal (suture—re: cranium)
spherical equivalent
spongiform encephalopathy
Spurway-Eddowes (syndrome)
squamous epithelium
stage of exhaustion (re: GAS—general
adaptation syndrome)
status epilepticus
subendothelial
supernormal excitability
sustained engraftment

SE, S.E.
standard error (re: statistics)

SE, S-E
Starr-Edwards (prosthesis—re: Cardio)

S & E
safety and efficacy (data)
skeletal and extremities

Se
secretor (gene)
selenium (element)

^{75}Se, Se 75
selenium-75 (reactor-produced
radionuclide)

SEA
sheep erythrocyte agglutination (test)
shock-elicited aggression
soluble egg antigen
spontaneous electrical activity
staphylococcal enterotoxin A

SEAT
sheep erythrocyte agglutination test

SEA test
sheep erythrocyte agglutination test

SEB
Scale for Emotional Blunting
staphylococcal enterotoxin B

SEBA
staphylococcal enterotoxin B antiserum

Seb Derm
seborrheic dermatitis

SEBL
self-emptying blind loop

SEC
secretin
secundum (L. according to)
series elastic component (re: muscles)
size exclusion chromatography
soft elastic capsules
strong exchange capacity (re: resin)

Sec
Seconal

sec.
secant
second (unit of time)
secondary
secretary
section
sectioned
sections

sec. a.
secundum artem (L. according to the art
[by skill])

SECG
stress electrocardiography

sech
hyperbolic secant

SECSY
spin-echo correlated spectroscopy

sect.
section
sectioned
sections

secy
secretary

SED
spondyloepiphyseal dysplasia
standard error of difference (re:
statistics)
staphylococcal enterotoxin D
strain energy density
suberythemal dose

SED, S.E.D.
skin erythema dose

SED, Sed, sed.
sedimentation (rate)

sed.
sedate
sedated
sedative
sedes (L. stool)

SEDD
Szondi's Experimental Diagnostics of
Drives

Sed rate, sed. rate
sedimentation rate

sed. rt.
sedimentation rate

sed. time
sedimentation time

SEE
scopolamine-Eukodal-Ephetonin
series elastic element
standard error of the estimate (re:
statistics)

SEER
Surveillance, Epidemiology, and End-
Result (re: National Cancer Institute
program)

SEF
somatically evoked field
staphylococcal enterotoxin F

SEG
soft elastic gelatin (capsule)
sonoencephalogram

Seg, seg.
segment

seg.
segmented (neutrophil)

segm.
segmented

SEGS, Segs, segs
segmented neutrophils
(polymorphonuclear leukocytes)

SEH
subependymal hemorrhage

SEI
Self-Esteem Inventory

SEM
(verbal) sample evaluation method
scanning electron microscope
scanning electron microscopy
secondary enrichment medium
smoke exposure machine
systolic ejection murmur

SEM, sem
standard error (of the) mean (re:
statistics)

sem.
semen (L. seed)
semi; semis (L. one-half)
seminal

semel in d.
semel in die (L. once a day)

SEMI
subendocardial myocardial infarction
subendocardial myocardial injury

semid.
semidrachma (half a drachm—
apothecaries' weight)

semidr.
semidrachma (half a drachm—
apothecaries' weight)

semih.
semihora (L. half an hour)

SEMLSB
systolic ejection murmur, left sternal
border

sem. ves.
seminal vesicles

sen.
sensation
sensitive

↓ **sen.**
decreased sensation
diminished sensation

SENS
sensitivities (test)

SENS, sens.
sensorium

sens.
sensation
senses
sensitive
sensitivity
sensitivity (pattern—re: antibiotics)
sensory

sens. decr.
sensation decreased

sens. defic.
sensory deficit

sens. lat.
sensu lato (L. in the broad sense)

sens. str.
sensu stricto (L. in the strict sense)

SEP
sensory evoked potential
sepultus (L. buried)
somatosensory evoked potential
sperm entry point
spinal evoked potential
surface epithelium
systolic ejection period

sep.
separate
separated
separately
separation

separ.
separatum (L. separately)

SEPS
selenium-containing protein saccharide

sept.
septem (L. seven)
septum

septo.
septoplasty

SEQ
Side-Effects Questionnaire
simultaneous equation

Seq
sequential

seq.
sequela (L. that which follows)
sequence
sequestrum

seq. luce
sequenti luce (L. the following morning)

seqq.
sequentiae (L. the following)

SER
sebum excretion rate
service
somatosensory evoked response(s)
systolic ejection rate

SER, sER
smooth endoplasmic reticulum

Ser
seryl (radical of serine)

Ser, ser
serine (an amino acid)

Ser, ser.
serology

ser.
serial
serially
series
serological
serous
serum

ser. Cl.
serum chloride

SERI
Spondee Error Index

ser. ind.
serum index

serol.
serology

serosang.
serosanguineous

ser. sect.
serial sections

SERT
sustained ethanol release tube

serv.
serva (L. keep, preserve)
service(s)

SES
socioeconomic status
spatial emotional stimuli
subendothelial space

sesquih.
sesquihora (L. an hour and a half)

sesquiunc.
sesquiuncia (L. an ounce and a half)

Sess
sessile

SET
systolic ejection time

sev.
sever
several
severe
severed

SE valve
Starr-Edwards (heart) valve

SEWHO
shoulder-elbow-wrist-hand orthosis

sex.
sexual

SEXAF
surface extended x-ray absorption fine
(structure— re: spectroscopy)

SeXO
serum xanthine oxidase

s. expr.
sine expressione (L. without expressing
or pressing)

SF
Sabin-Feldman (dye test)
safety factor
salt free
scarlet fever
Schilder-Foix (disease)
seizure frequency

seminal fluid
serosal fluid
serum factor
serum fibrinogen
sham feeding
shell fragment
shipping fever
shrapnel fragment
shunt flow
skin fibroblast
skin fluorescence
slow (initial) function
snack food
sodium azide, fecal (medium)
soft feces
spinal fluid
spontaneous fibrillation
spontaneous fluctuation
spontaneous fracture
stable factor
sterile female
Streptococcus faecalis
stress formula
sulfation factor (of blood serum)
superior facet
suppressor factor
suprasternal fossa
survival fraction
surviving factor
synovial fluid

SF, Sf
svedberg flotation (units)

S.F.
spontaneous fission (re: radioactive
isotopes)

SF%
shortening fraction percent

S_f, S_f
negative sedimentation svedberg unit

SFA
saturated fatty acid
seminal fluid assay
serum folic acid
stimulated fibrinolytic activity
superficial femoral artery

SFB
surgical foreign body

SFBL
self-filling blind loop

SFC
soluble fibrin-fibrinogen complex
spinal fluid count

SFD
sheep factor delta
short foot drape
small for dates (gestational age—re:
OB)

soy-free diet
spectral frequency distribution

SFD, sfd
skin-film distance (re: radiology)

SF def.
silver fork deformity (re: Ortho)

SFEMG
single-fiber electromyography

SFF
speaking fundamental frequency

SFFF
sedimentation field flow fractionization

SFFV
spleen focus-forming virus
spleen focus Friend virus

SFFV-F
spleen focus-forming virus in Friend
   virus complex

SFG
spotted fever group

SFGS
stratum fibrosum et griseum superficiale
   (re: Neuro)

SFH
schizophrenia family history
stroma-free hemoglobin (solution)

SFI
Sexual Functioning Index
Social Function Index

SFLE
Stress From Life Experience

SFM
serum-free medium
soluble fibrin monomer

SFMC
soluble fibrin monomer complex

SFP
screen filtration pressure
simultaneous foveal perception
spinal fluid pressure
stop flow pressure

SFR
screen filtration resistance
stroke(s) with full recovery

s. fr.
spiritus frumenti (L. spirit of grain
   [whiskey])

SFS
serial focal seizures (re: Neuro)
serum fungistatic

skin and fascia stapler
split function study

SFT
Sabin-Feldman (dye) test (re:
   toxoplasmosis)
sensory feedback therapy
serum-free thyroxin(e)
skinfold thickness

SFTAA
Short Form Test of Academic Aptitude

SFTR
sagittal, frontal, transverse, rotation

SFU
surgical follow-up

SFV
Semliki forest virus
shipping fever virus
squirrel fibroma virus

SFW
shell fragment wound
shrapnel fragment wound
slow filling wave

SG
secretory granule
serous granule
serum globulin
serum glucose
sialidase and galactosidase (re: gene
   locus)
signs
skin graft
soluble gelatin (re: capsules)
Strandberg-Groenblad (syndrome)
substantia gelatinosa (of Rolando—re:
   Neuro)
Surgeon General

SG, S-G, S.-G.
Sachs-Georgi (test—re: syphilis)

SG, Sg, s.g., sg
specific gravity

S-G
Swan-Ganz (catheter—re: Cardio)

s-g
subgenus

SGA
small for gestational age (re: OB)

SGa
specific conductance (airway)

SGAW, SGaw, SG$_{aw}$
specific airway conductance (re: Resp)

SGB
sparsely granulated basophil

SGC
spermicide-germicide compound

SG-C
serum gentamicin concentration

SG cath.
Swan-Ganz catheter (re: Cardio)

SGE
secondary generalized epilepsy

SGF
sarcoma growth factor
silica gel filtered
skeletal growth factor

SGFR
single-nephron glomerular filtration rate

s-gg
subgenera

SGH
subgaleal hematoma

SGO
Surgery, Gynecology, and Obstetrics

SGO, S.G.O.
Surgeon General's Office

SGOT
serum glutamic-oxaloacetic
   transaminase

SGP
serine glycerophosphatide
sialoglycoprotein
soluble glycoprotein

SGPT
serum glutamate-pyruvate
   transaminase (alanine
   aminotransferase—ALT)
serum glutamic-pyruvic transaminase
   (alanine aminotransferase—ALT)

SGR
Sachs-Georgi reaction (re: syphilis)
submandibular gland renin
substantia gelatinosa Rolando (re:
   Neuro)

sgs
signs

S-Gt
Sachs-Georgi test (re: syphilis)

SG test
Sachs-Georgi test (re: syphilis)

SGTT
standard glucose tolerance test

SGV
salivary gland virus

selective gastric vagotomy
small granular vesicle

SH
(percentage) saturation of hemoglobin
Schönlein-Henoch (disease)
self help
serum hepatitis
sex hormone
sexual harassment
sham (operated)
sharp
sick (in) hospital (re: chart note)
sinus histiocytosis
somatotrophic hormone
spontaneously hypertensive
state hospital
sulfhydryl
surgical history
symptomatic hypoglycemia
systemic hyperthermia

SH, S.H.
social history

SH, Sh, sh.
shoulder

S&H
speech and hearing

Sh
sheep (re: veterinary medicine)
Shigella (genus)

Sh, sh.
short

Sh
Sherwood number (re: heat transfer)

SHA
soluble HL (human lymphocyte) antigen
staphylococcal hemagglutinating
   antibody

SHAA
serum hepatitis-associated antigens

SHAA-Ab
serum hepatitis-associated antigen-
   antibody

SHA-Ab
serum hepatitis-associated antibody

SHARES
Standard Hospital Accounting and Rate
   Evaluation System

SHAV
superior hemiazygos vein

SHB
subacute hepatitis with bridging

SHB, S Hb
sulfhemoglobin

SHBD
serum hydroxybutyrate dehydrogenase

SHBG
sex hormone-binding globulin

SHCO
sulfated hydrogenated castor oil

Sh, complete
shoulder (amputation level, upper limb)
    complete (re: Ortho)

SHDI
supraoptical hypophyseal diabetes
    insipidus

SHE
superheavy element
Syrian hamster embryo

SHEENT
skin, head, eyes, ears, nose, throat

SHF
simian hemorrhagic fever

SHF, shf
super high frequency

SHG
synthetic human gastrin

SHHP
semihorizontal heart position

Shig
Shigella (genus)

SHL
sensorineural hearing loss

shl.
shoulder

SHLD, shld.
shoulder

shldr.
shoulder

SHML
sinus histiocytosis with massive
    lymphadenopathy

SHMT
serine hydroxymethyltransferase

SHN
spontaneous hemorrhagic necrosis
subacute hepatic necrosis

SHO
secondary hypertrophic
    osteoarthropathy

sho.
shoulder

S hormone
sugar hormone ([Fuller Albright]
    glycogenic corticoids)

should.
shoulder

SHP
Schönlein-Henoch purpura
secondary hyperparathyroidism
surgical hypoparathyroidism

SHR
spontaneously hypertensive rats

SHRC
shortened, held, resisted, contracted

SHRsp
spontaneously hypertensive rat, stroke
    prone

SHS
Sayre head sling
sheep hemolysate supernatant
super high speed

SHSP
spontaneously hypertensive stroke-
    prone (rat)

SHSS
Stanford Hypnotic Susceptibility Scale

SHT
simple hypocalcemic tetany
Stycar Hearing Tests (re: Psychol)
subcutaneous histamine test

SHV
simian herpes virus

SH virus
(homologous) serum(-transmitted)
    hepatitis virus

SI
sacroiliac
saline infusion
saline injection
saturation index
self-inflicted
seriously ill
serum iron
service index
sex inventory
single injection
small intestine
social introversion
stimulation index
stress incontinence
stroke index
structure of intellect (model—re:
    Psychol)
Systeme International d'Unités
    (International System of Units—[a

redefinition of the meter-kilogram-
second system])
systolic index

SI, S.I.
soluble insulin

Si
silicon (element)

^{31}Si
radioactive isotope of silicon

SIA
serum inhibitory activity
stimulation-induced analgesia
stress-induced anesthesia
subacute infectious arthritis
synalbumin-insulin antagonism
syncytia induction assay

SIADH
syndrome of inappropriate antidiuretic
hormone
syndrome of inappropriate (secretion of)
antidiuretic hormone

SIB
self-injurious behavior

sib.
sibling

sibs
siblings

SIC
serum inhibitory concentration
serum insulin concentration

sic.
siccus (L. dry, dried)

SICD
Sequenced Inventory of
Communication Development
serum isocitric dehydrogenase

SICSVA
sequential impaction cascade sieve
volumetric air (sampler)

SICU
Spinal Intensive Care Unit
Surgery Intensive Care Unit
Surgical Intensive Care Unit

SID
sucrase-isomaltase deficiency
sudden infant death
suggested indication of diagnosis
systemic inflammatory disease

s.i.d.
semel in die (L. once a day)

SIDS
sudden infant death syndrome

SIE
stroke in evolution

SIF
serum inhibitory factor
small intensely fluorescent (ganglia)

Sif
segment inferior (re: OB-GYN)

SIF cells
small intensely fluorescent cells

SIFT
selected ion flow tube

SIG
sigmoidoscope
sigmoidoscopic
special interest group

SIG, Sig
sigmoidoscopy

SIg
serum immune globulin

SIg, sIg
surface immunoglobulin (IgD)

Sig
signature
signed

Sig, sig.
signa (L. write; label)
signetur (L. let it be written, labeled [as
instruction to patient])

sig.
signal
significant

S-IgA
secretory immunoglobulin A

sig. F
significant findings

SIGI
System for Interactive Guidance
Information

sigmo.
sigmoidoscopy

Sigmoid
sigmoidoscopy

sig. n. pro.
signa nomine proprio (L. label with the
proper name)

SIJ
sacroiliac joint

SI jt.
sacroiliac joint

SIL
sister-in-law
speech interference level (noise scale—re: acoustics)

SILA
suppressible insulin-like activity

SILD
Sequenced Inventory of Language Development

SI list
seriously ill list

SILS
Shipley Institute of Living Scale (for Measuring Intellectual Impairment)

SIM
selected ion monitoring
sucrase-isomaltose (deficiency)
sulfide, indole, motility (medium)

Sim
simultaneous

simp.
simplex (L. simple, single)

SIMS
secondary ion mass spectroscopy

SIMV
synchronized intermittent mandatory ventilation

sin.
sine (L. without)
sine (re: trigonometry)
sinus

sine
sinusoid (sine curve—re: statistics)

sine conf.
sine confectione (L. without sweetness)

sing.
single
singular (one)
singuli (L. each)
singulorum (L. of each)

sinh, sin h
hyperbolic sine

si non val.
si non valeat (L. if it is not strong enough)

si n. val.
si non valeat (L. if it is not strong enough)

SIO
sacroiliac orthosis

si op. sit
si opus sit (L. if it is necessary; if necessary)

SIP
segment inertial properties
Sickness Impact Profile (re: Psychol)
slow inhibitory potential
surface inductive plethysmography

sIPTH
serum immunoreactive parathyroid hormone

SIQ
sick in quarters (re: military)

SIR
single isomorphous replacement
specific immune release
standardized incidence ratio (re: statistics)

SIREF
specific immune response-enhancing factor

SIRF
severely impaired renal function

SIRS
soluble immune response suppressor

SIS
sterile injectable suspension

sis.
sister

SISI
short increment sensitivity index (re: Audio)
small increment sensitivity index (re: Audio)

SISS
serum inhibitor of streptolysin S

SiSV
simian sarcoma virus

SIT
serum-inhibiting titers
Slosson Intelligence Test
Sperm Immobilization Test
supraspinatus, infraspinatus, teres minor (muscles)

sitg
sitting

SI units
Systeme International d'Unités

SIV
Survey of Interpersonal Values

511

si vir. perm.
si vires permittant (L. if the strength will permit)

SIW
self-inflicted wound

6/6, 20/20
eye chart seen at 6 meters or 20 feet

SJ, S-J
Stevens-Johnson (syndrome)

SJR
Shinowara-Jones-Reinhart (unit)

SJS
Stevens-Johnson syndrome

SK
senile keratosis
skin (specific)
skin (test)
Sloan-Kettering (Institute)
solar keratosis
spontaneous killer (cell)
streptokinase
striae keratopathy

sk.
skeletal
skimmed

SKA
supracondylar knee-ankle (orthosis)

SKAT
Sex Knowledge and Attitude Test (re: Psychol)

Skel, skel.
skeletal

SKI
skin
Sloan-Kettering Institute

SKL
serum killing level

SKSD, SK-SD
streptokinase-streptodornase

sk. tr.
skeletal traction

sk. trx
skeletal traction

sk. tx
skeletal traction

SKU
stockkeeping unit (re: computers/data processing)

SKW
Sturge-Kalischer-Weber (syndrome)

SL
salt loser
sarcolemma
satellite-like
sensation level (of hearing)
sensory latency
serious list
short leg (cast)
Sibley-Lehninger (unit—re: aldolase activity)
signal level
Sinding Larsen (disease)
Sjögren-Larsson (syndrome)
slit lamp
small leukocyte
small lymphocytes
sodium lactate
solidified-liquid
sound level
Stein-Leventhal (syndrome)
streptolysin
Strümpell-Lorrain (disease)

SL, sl.
sublingual

S/L
sucrase to lactase (ratio)

sl
slyke (a unit of buffer value)

sl.
slice
slight
slightly
slow

s.l.
secundum legem (L. according to the rules)
sensu lato (L. in the broad sense)

SLA
sacrolaeva anterior (position of fetus)
slide latex agglutination
surfactant-like activity

SLAM
scanning laser acoustic microscope

SLAP
serum leucine aminopeptidase

SLB
short leg brace

sl. blad. inf.
slight bladder infection

sl. bt.
slightly better

SLC
short leg cast

Sociopolitical Locus of Control (re:
    Psychol)
sodium lithium countertransport

SLCC
short leg cylinder cast

SLD
serum lactate dehydrogenase
serum lactic dehydrogenase

SLDH
serum lactate dehydrogenase
serum lactic dehydrogenase

SLE
St. Louis encephalitis
slit-lamp examination
systemic lupus erythematosus

SLEA
sheep erythrocyte antibody
sheep erythrocyte antigen

SLEV
St. Louis encephalitis virus

SLHR
sex-linked hypophosphatemic rickets

SLI
secretin-like immunoreactivity
selective lymphoid irradiation
somatostatin-like immunoreactivity
speech and language impaired
splenic localization index

SLIP
Singer-Loomis Inventory of Personality
symmetric list processor (re: computer
    list processing language)

SLKC
superior limbic keratoconjunctivitis

SLM
sound level meter

SLMC
spontaneous lymphocyte-mediated
    cytotoxicity

SLN
sublentiform nucleus
superior laryngeal nerve

SLNWBC
short leg nonweight-bearing cast

SLNWC
short leg non-walking cast

SLO
streptolysin-O (titer)

SLP
sacrolaeva posterior (position of fetus)
subluxation of the patella

SLP, Slp
sex-limited protein (re: genetics)

SLPP
serum lipophosphoprotein

SLP of P cast
short leg plaster of paris cast

SLR
single lens reflex
straight leg raising
Streptococcus lactis R (factor),
    resistant

SLS
segment long-spacing (collagen fibers)
short leg splint
single limb support
Stein-Leventhal syndrome

SLSQ
Speech and Language Screening
    Qustionnaire

SLT
sacrolaeva transversa (position of fetus)
solid logic technology (re: computers)
Stycar Language Test (re: Psychol)

slt.
slight
slightly

SlTr
silent treatment

sl. tr.
slight trace

SLUD
salivation, lacrimation, urination,
    defecation

S-L-V
solid-liquid-vapor

SLW
short leg walking (cast)

SLWC
short leg walking cast

SM
sadomasochism
Scheuthauer-Marie (syndrome)
self-monitoring
semimembranous
Serratia marcescens
sewage microparticulates
Sexual Myths (scale)
Shigella mutant
shine mold
simple mastectomy
skim milk
smoker
smooth muscle
somatomedin (a peptide)

Space Medicine
sphingomyelin
stapedius muscle
staphylococcus medium
streptomycin
Strümpell-Marie (disease)
submandibular
submucosal
submucous
substitute for morphine
substituted metabolites
suckling mice
sucrose medium
suction method
superior mesenteric
supramamillary (nucleus—re: Neuro)
sustained medication
symptoms
synaptic membrane
synovial membrane
systolic mean (pressure)
systolic murmur

S/M
sadism/masochism (re: Psychol)

Sm
samarium (element)

sm.
small

SM-1
Singh's mosquito (tissue culture
    medium)

SMA
sequential multichannel autoanalyzer
Sequential Multiple Analysis
sequential multiple analyzer
serial multiple analysis
simultaneous multichannel
    autoanalyzer
smooth muscle antibodies
smooth muscle autoantibody
spinal muscular atrophy
spontaneous motor activity (re: Neuro)
standard methods agar
superior mesenteric artery
supplementary motor area

SM-A
somatomedin A

SMA-6
Sequential Multiple Analysis—6
    different serum tests

SMA 6/60
Sequential Multiple Analysis—6 tests in
    60 minutes

SMA-12
Sequential Multiple Analysis—12-
    channel biochemical profile

SMA 12/60
Sequential Multiple Analysis—12
    different serum tests in 60 minutes

SMA-20
Sequential Multiple Analysis of 20
    chemical constituents

SMA-60
Sequential Multiple Analysis of 60
    chemical constituents

SMABV
superior mesenteric artery blood
    velocity

SMAC
Sequential Multiple Analyzer Computer

SMAE
superior mesenteric artery embolus

SMAF
smooth muscle activating factor
specific macrophage-arming factor
superior mesenteric artery (blood) flow

SMAL
serum methyl alcohol level

sm. amts.
small amounts

sm. an.
small animal

SMAO
superior mesenteric artery occlusion

SMART
simultaneous multiple-angle
    reconstruction technique

SMAS
submuscular aponeurotic system

SMAST
Short Michigan Alcoholism Screening
    Test

SMAT
School Motivation Analysis Test

SMB
selected mucosal biopsy
suckling mouse brain

Smb
standard mineral base (medium)

SMBFT
small bowel follow-through

SMBP
serum myelin basic protein

SMC
smooth muscle cell
special monthly compensation

special mouth care
succinylmonocholine

SM-C
somatomedin C

SMCA
smooth muscle contracting agent
suckling mouse cataract agent

SMCD
senile macular choroidal degeneration

SMD
senile macular degeneration (re: Ophth)
sternocleidomastoid diameter
submanubrial dullness

SMDC
sodium methyldithiocarbamate (soil
    fumigant)

SMDSep
single, married, divorced, separated

SME
stalk median eminence

SMEDI
stillbirth, mummification, embryonic
    death, infertility

SMEM
supplemented (Eagle's) minimum
    essential medium

SMEPP
subminiature end-plate potential (re:
    neuromuscular)

SMF
streptozotocin, mitomycin C, and 5-
    fluorouracil (re: chemotherapy)

SMG
submandibular gland

SMH
state mental hospital
strongyloidiasis with massive
    hyperinfection

SMI
severely mentally impaired
stress myocardial image
Style of Mind Inventory (re: Psychol)
supplementary medical insurance
sustained maximal inspiration

SMIg
surface membrane immunoglobulin

SML
single major locus

SMM
supplemental minimal medium

SMMD
specimen mass measurement device

SMMI
El Senoussi Multiphasic Marital
    Inventory

SMN
second malignant neoplasm

SMNB
submaximal neuromuscular block

SMO
Senior Medical Officer
slip made out

SMON
subacute myelo-optical neuropathy
subacute myelo-optic neuropathy
subacute myelo-opticoneuritis
subacute myelo-opticoneuropathy

SMP
simultaneous macular perception
slow-moving protease
special monthly pension
standard medical practice
standard medical procedure
submitochondrial particle
sulfamethoxypyrazine (antibacterial)

SMPS
sulfated mucopolysaccharides

SMR
sensorimotor rhythm
skeletal muscle relaxant
somnolent metabolic rate
standardized mortality ratio
standard mortality rate
submucous resection (re: nose)

SMRR
submucous resection and rhinoplasty

SMRV
squirrel monkey retrovirus

SMS
Scheuthauer-Marie-Sainton (syndrome)
senior medical student
serial motor seizures (re: Neuro)
stiff-man syndrome

SMSA
Standard Metropolitan Statistical Area

SMSV
San Miguel sea lion virus

SMT
Sertoli cell/mesenchyme tumor
Snider match test (re: Resp)
spindle microtubule
spontaneous mammary tumor

SMV
slow-moving vehicle
small volume
submentovertical
superior mesenteric vein

SMWDSep
single, married, widowed, divorced,
    separated

SMX
sulfamethoxazole

SMZ
sulfamethoxazole

SN
school of nursing
scrub nurse
sensorineural
sensory neuron
seronegative
serum neutralization
serum neutralizing
single nephron
sinus node
spinal needle
spontaneous nystagmus
standard nomenclature
streptonigrin (antibiotic-antineoplastic
    agent)
subnormal
substantia nigra (re: Neuro)
supernatant
supernormal
suprasternal notch

S/N
signal to noise (ratio)

Sn
stannum (L. tin—element)

^{113}Sn
radioactive isotope of tin (stannum)

^{121}Sn
radioactive isotope of tin (stannum)

S_n
n-fold improper rotation axis (symmetry
    group— re: molecules, crystals)

s.n.
secundum naturam (L. according to
    nature)

sn-
stereospecific numbering

SNA
specimen not available
superior nasal artery

S-N-A
sella-nasion-subspinale (or point A
    [angle]—re: cephalometrics)

SNAFU
situation normal, all fouled up

SNagg
serum normal agglutinator

SNB
scalene node biopsy
Silverman needle biopsy

S-N-B
sella-nasion-supramentale (or point B
    [angle]—re: cephalometrics)

SNBU
switched network backup (re:
    computers/data processing)

SNC
sistema nervosum centrale (L. central
    nervous system)

SND
striatonigral degeneration (re: Neuro)

SNDO
Standard Nomenclature of Diseases
    and Operations

SNE
sinus node electrogram
spatial nonemotional (stimuli)
subacute necrotizing
    encephalomyelopathy

SNF
sinus node formation
skilled nursing facility

SNFH
schizophrenia nonfamily history

SNGBF
single nephron glomerular blood flow

SNGFR
single nephron glomerular filtration rate

SNGPF
single nephron glomerular plasma flow

SNHL
sensorineural hearing loss

S-N line
sella to nasal (junction) line (re:
    cephalometry)

SNM
sulfanilamide

SNOBOL
String-Oriented Symbolic Language (re:
    computers)

SNODO
Standard Nomenclature of Diseases
    and Operations (re: medical records)

SNOMED
systematized nomenclature of medicine (re: medical records)

SNOP
systematized nomenclature of pathology (re: computers)

SNP
seronegative polyneuritis

SNQ
superior nasal quadrant

SNR
signal-to-noise ratio

snRNA
small nuclear ribonucleic acid

snRNPs
small nuclear ribonucleoproteins (pronounced "snurps")

SNRT
sinus node recovery time

SNS
sympathetic nervous system

SNST
sciatic nerve stretch test

SNT
sinuses, nose, and throat

SNV
spleen necrosis virus
superior nasal vein

SO
Schlatter-Osgood (disease)
second opinion
sex offender
sham operated
shoulder orthosis
slow-oxidative (re: muscle fiber)
spheno-occipital (synchondrosis)
sphincter of Oddi (re: hepatopancreatic ampulla)
standing orders
suboccipital
superior oblique (muscle)
supraoptic (nucleus)
supraorbital
sutures out

SO, S-O
salpingo-oophorectomy (re: OB-GYN)

S&O
salpingo-oophorectomy (re: OB-GYN)

SO_2
sulfur dioxide

SO_4
sulfate

$^{35}SO_2$
radioactive-labeled sulfur dioxide

So
socialization

so.
south

SOA
symptoms of asthma

SOAA
signed out against advice

SOAM, SO/a.m.
sutures out in a.m.

SOAMA
signed out against medical advice

SOA-MCA
superficial occipital artery to middle cerebral artery

SOAP
subjective data, objective data, assessment, plan (re: progress notes in problem-oriented records)

SOAPS
suction, oxygen apparatus, pharmaceuticals, saline (anesthetists' mnemonic to confirm presence of necessary equipment)

SOB
see order blank
see order book
short(ness) of breath
suboccipitobregmatic (re: cranial sutures)

SOC
sequential-type oral contraceptive
standard of care
syphilitic osteochondritis

SOC, SoC
state of consciousness

soc.
social
society

SOCD
Separation of Circle-Diamond

Soc Hist
Social History

SocSec, Soc Sec
Social Security

Soc Serv
Social Service

SOD
spike occurrence density

superoxide dismutase (orgotein—anti-
inflammatory)

SOD1
superoxide dismutase, soluble

SOD2
superoxide dismutase, mitochondrial

Sod
sodomy

sod.
soda
sodium

sod. bicar.
sodium bicarbonate

SODH
sorbital dehydrogenase (L-iditol
dehydrogenase)

Sod Pent
sodium pentothal

SOER
special orthopaedic examination and
report

SOF
superior orbital fissure (sphenoidal
fissure)

SOFS
spontaneous osteoporotic fracture of
the sacrum

SOFT
Sorting of Figures Test

SOHN
supraoptic hypothalamic nucleus

SOI
Student Opinion Inventory (re: Psychol)

SOL
soleus

SOL, Sol
space-occupying lesion

SOL, Sol, sol.
solution

Sol
solarium

sol.
solubilis (L. soluble)
soluble
solutio (L. a solution)

SOLER
squarely (face person), open (posture),
lean (toward person), eye (contact),
relaxed

solidif.
solidification

soln.
solution

SOLST
Stephens Oral Language Screening
Test

solu.
solute

Solu B c̄ C
solution of soluble B vitamins with
vitamin C

Solut, solut.
solution

SOLV, solv.
solve (L. dissolve)

solv.
solvent

SOM
secretory otitis media
sensitivity of method
serous otitis media
somatotrophin
somnolent (metabolic rate)
start of message (re: computers)
sulphormethoxine (sulfadoxine;
sulforthomidine—antibacterial)
superior oblique muscle

som.
somatic

somat.
somatic

SOMI
skull occiput mandibular immobilization
(orthosis)
sternal occipital mandibular
immobilization

SOMPA
System of Multicultural Pleuralistic
Assessment (re: Psychol)

SOMT
Spatial Orientation Memory Test

SON
Snijders-Oomen Non-Verbal
(Intelligence Scale for Young
Children)
superior olivary nucleus (re: Neuro)
supraoptic nucleus (re: Neuro)

SONH
supraopticoneurohypophyseal (re:
Neuro)

SONP
soft organs not palpable
solid organs not palpable

SOP
standard operating procedure
standing operative procedure

SOPM, SO/p.m.
sutures out in p.m.

SOPP
splanchnic occluded portal pressure

S. op. s., s. op. s.
si opus sit (L. if it is necessary)

S OP SIT, s. op. sit
si opus sit (L. if it is necessary)

SOQ
Suicide Opinion Questionnaire

SOR, S-O-R
stimulus-organism-response

Sorb
sorbitol

Sorb D
sorbitol dehydrogenase

SORD
sorbitol dehydrogenase

SOREMP
sleep-onset rapid eye movement period

SOS
self-obtained smear
speed of sound
stimulation of senses
Student Orientations Survey (re:
    Psychol)
supplemental oxygen system

SOS, s.o.s.
si opus sit (L. if it is necessary)

SOSAI
Springfield Outpatient Symptom and
    Adjustment Index

SOS repair system
error-prone DNA repair in *E. coli*
    (re: genetics)

SOT
stream of thought (re: Psychol)
systemic oxygen transport

SOTT
synthetic (medium) old tuberculin
    trichloracetic (acid precipitated)

SP
sacral promontory
secretory piece
senile plaques

septal pore
septum pellucidum
seropositive
serum protection
serum protein
shunt pressure
shunt procedure
skin potential
sleep deprived
small protein
soft palate
solid phase
space (character—re: computers/data
    processing)
spatial peak
speech pathology
spike potential (re: EEG)
spirometry
spleen
square planar (complex)
standard of performance
standard practice
standard procedure
staphylococcal protease
staphylococcal protein A
steady potential
stool preservative (Hajna)
subliminal perception
substance P (an undecapeptide)
suprapatellar pouch
suprapubic
suprapubic puncture
symphysis pubis
systolic pressure

SP, S/P
semi-private (room)
status post (L. no change after)

SP, Sp
summation potential

SP, Sp, sp
sacrum to pubis

SP, Sp, sp.
spine (especially spine of scapula)

SP, sp.
species (taxonomy)

S-P
Smith-Petersen (nail)

S_2P
second heart sound, pulmonic
    component

Sp
Spirillum (genus)
spirometer

Sp, sp
sacropubic

sp.
space

spasm
specific
spinal
spiritus (L. spirit)
splint

SPA
salt-poor albumin
schizophrenia with premorbid asociality
sheep pulmonary adenomatosis
sperm penetration assay
spinal progressive amyotrophy
spondylitis ankylopoietica
staphylococcal protein A
stimulation-induced analgesia
suprapatellar amputation
suprapubic aspiration

SpAb
specifically purified antibody

SPAC
sectionally processed, antibody coated

SPAI
steroid protein activity index

SPAM
scanning photo-acoustic microscopy

Span
Spanish

sp. an.
spinal anesthesia

spans.
spansules

SPAR
sensitivity prediction by acoustic reflex

SPBI
serum protein-bound iodine

S-PBIgG
serum-platelet bindable
   immunoglobulin G

SPC
salicylamide, phenacetin
   (acetophenetidin), and caffeine
serum phenylalanine concentration
sickled-shaped (particle) cell
simultaneous prism and cover (test—re:
   Ophth)
single palmar crease
single photoelectron counting
single proton counting
small pyramidal cell
spike-processed contraction
spleen cell
standard platelet count
synthesizing protein complex

SPCA
serum prothrombin conversion

accelerator (Factor VII—
   proconvertin)

sp. cd.
spinal cord

SPCK
serum creatine phosphokinase

SPD
salmon poisoning disease (of dogs of
   the Northwest— re: veterinary)
sociopathic personality disorder
specific paroxysmal discharge
spectral power distribution
standard peak dilution
storage pool deficiency

SPD, Spd
spermidine

SPDT
single pole, double throw

SPE
septic pulmonary edema
serum protein electrophoresis
streptococcal pyrogenic exotoxin
subjective paranormal experience
sucrose polyester (non-absorbable
   lipid—diet food supplement)
sustained physical exercise

SPEC, spec.
specimen

spec.
special
specialist
specific
specification

spec. gr.
specific gravity

specif.
specific
specification
specified

SPECT
single photon emission computed
   tomography

SPEM
smooth pursuit eye movement

SPEP
serum protein electrophoresis

S period
synthesis period (re: cell growth cycle)

SPF
skin protection factor
specific-pathogen free
spectrofluorometry
spectrophotofluorometer

split products of fibrin
standard perfusion fluid
streptococcal proliferative factor
Stuart-Prower factor (Factor X)
sun protective factors
suntan photoprotection factor

sp. fl.
spinal fluid

SPG
sucrose, phosphate, glutamate
symmetrical peripheral gangrene

SP GR, Sp Gr, sp. gr.
specific gravity

SPH
secondary pulmonary hemosiderosis
severely and profoundly handicapped

SPH, Sph
sphingomyelin

Sph
spherocytosis

sph.
spherical
spherical (lens)
sphincter

S phen.
Smith's phenomenon (anaphylaxis)

sp. ht.
specific heat

SPI
Self-Perception Inventory
serum precipitable iodine
serum protein index
Shipley Personal Inventory
single program initiator (re: computers/
data processing)
somatotyping ponderal index
subclinical papillomaviral infection

SPIA
solid-phase immunoabsorbent
solid-phase immunoassay

SPIB
Social and Prevocational Information
Battery

SPID
sum of pain intensity difference

SPIF
solid-phase immunoassay fluorescence

SPIH
superimposed pregnancy-induced
hypertension

sp. indet.
species indeterminata (L. species
indeterminate)

sp. inquir.
species inquirendae (L. species of
doubtful status)

Spir
Spirochaeta (genus)

spir.
spiral
spiritual
spiritus (L. spirit)

spiss.
spissus (L. dried)

SPK
serum pyruvate kinase
spinnbarkeit (Ger. "spinnability"—re:
cervical mucus during ovulation)
superficial punctate keratitis

spkr.
speaker

SPL
skin potential level
sound pressure level
splanchnic
spontaneous lesion

spl.
splint

SPLATT
split anterior tibial tendon (transfer)

SPM
self-phase modulation
shocks per minute
significance probability mapping
suspended particulate matter
syllables per minute
synaptic plasma membrane
synaptosomal plasma membrane

SPMA
spinal progressive muscular atrophy

sp. mening.
spinal meningitis

SPMR
standardized proportionate mortality
ratio

SPMSQ
Short Portable Mental Status
Questionnaire

SPN
solitary pulmonary nodule
supplementary parenteral nutrition
sympathetic preganglionic neuron

sp. n.
species novum (L. new species)

SP nail
Smith-Petersen nail

sp. nov.
species novum (L. new species)

spnt.
spontaneous

Sp Ny
spontaneous nystagmus

sp. o.k.
speech o.k.

spon.
spontaneous

spont.
spontaneous

SPOOL
simultaneous peripheral operation on-line (re: data processing systems)

spork
SPoon and fORK (re: physiatry)

SPP
Sexuality Preference Profile (re: Psychol)
superior patellar pole
suprapubic prostatectomy

SPP, spp.
species (plural)

Sp Path
speech pathology

sp. pr.
spinal process

sp. proc.
spinal process

SPPS
solid phase peptide synthesis
stable plasma protein solution

SPR
scan projection radiography
serial probe recognition
skin potential reflex
solid phase radioimmunoassay

spr.
sprain

SPRIA
solid phase radioimmunoassay

SPROM
spontaneous premature rupture of membranes

SPS
sodium polyanetholesulfonate (reagent, stabilizer, in vitro blood coagulant inhibitor)
sodium polyethylene sulfonate (antibiotic)
sound production sample
special Pap smear
status postsurgery
stimulated protein synthesis
sulfite polymyxin sulfadiazine (agar)
systemic progressive sclerosis

SpS
sphenoid sinus

spSHR
stroke-prone spontaneous hypertensive rat

SPSI
School Problem Screening Inventory (re: Psychol)

SPST
single pole, single throw

SPT
secretin-pancreozymin test
slow pull-through
sound production tasks
spinal tap
Spondee Picture Test
standing pivotal transfer
Supervisory Practices Test (re: Psychol)
Symbolic Play Test (re: Psychol)

spt.
spirits (alcohol)
spiritus (L. spirit)

SPTA
spatial peak temporal average

SP TAP
spinal tap

SPTI
systolic pressure time index

SPTP
spatial peak temporal peak

spts
spirits

SP tube
suprapubic tube

SPTURP
status post transurethral resection of prostate

SPTx
static pelvic traction

Spur
Spurling test (re: Ortho)

SPV
Shope papilloma virus (Shope papilloma caused by a papillomavirus)

sp. xr
special x ray (study)

SPZ
sulfinpyrazone (uricosuric)

SQ
social quotient (re: Psychol)
squalene (spinacene—re: cholesterol biosynthesis)
status quo
survey question
symptom questionnaire

SQ, sq
subcutaneous

sq.
sequentia (L. the following)
squamous (cell)
square

SQC
statistical quality control

Sq cell ca., sq. cell ca.
squamous cell carcinoma

sq. cm
square centimeter

sq. epithl.
squamous epithelium

sq. ft
square foot

sq. in
square inch

sq. m
square meter

sq. mm
square millimeter

sqq, sqq.
sequentia (L. and following)

SQ3R
survey, question, read, review, recite (re: Psychol)

SQUID
superconducting quantum interference device

SR
sacroreticular
sarcoplasmic reticulum
saturation recovery
scanning radiometer
secretion rate

seizure resistant
self-recording
sensitivity response
sensitization response
sentence repetition
service record
sex ratio
shortening range
silicone rubber
simple reaction
sinus rhythm
skin resistance
slow release
soluble, repository (re: penicillin)
specific release
specific resistance
specific response
spontaneous (discharge) rate
spontaneous respiration(s)
stage of resistance (re: general adaptation syndrome)
stimulation ratio
stimulus-response
stomach rumble
Stransky-Regala (syndrome)
stress-relaxation
stretch reflex
sulfonamide resistant
superior rectus (muscle)
supply room
sustained release
systemic reaction
systemic resistance
systems research
systems review

SR, S.R.
sedimentation rate

SR, S/R
schizophrenic reaction
smooth-rough (variation—re: bacterial colonies)

SR, Sr
senior
sigma reaction (re: syphilis)

Sr
strontium (element)
Strouhal number (re: vibrations frequency produced in taut wire by passage of a current of fluid)

^{85}Sr
radioactive strontium

^{89}Sr
strontium-89

^{90}Sr, Sr 90
strontium-90

sr
steradian (a unit of three-dimensional measure)

SRA
saturation of the receiving amplitude
segmental renal artery
serum renin activity
spleen repopulating activity

SR ac. undiff.
schizophrenic reaction, acute,
    undifferentiated

SRA Mechanical Aptitudes
Science Research Associates
    Mechanical Aptitudes (re: Psychol)

SR/AP
schizophrenic reaction, acute, paranoid

SR/AU
schizophrenic reaction, acute,
    undifferentiated

SRAW, SRaw
specific resistance, airway (re: Resp)

SRBC
sheep red blood cells

SRC
sedimented red cells
sensitization response cell
sheep red cells
Student Reactions to College (re:
    Psychol)

SRCA
specific red cell adherence

SRCBC
serum reserve cholesterol binding
    capacity

SR cells
sensitization response cells (re: vaginal
    smears)

SR/CP
schizophrenic reaction, chronic,
    paranoid

SR/CU
schizophrenic reaction, chronic,
    undifferentiated

SRD
service-related disability
sodium-restricted diet
soluble, repository, plus
    dihydrostreptomycin (re: penicillin)
specific reading disability

SRDD
sorbent regenerated dialysate delivery

SRDT
single radial diffusion test

SRE
schedule of recent events
Schedule of Recent Experience

SRF
severe renal failure
skin-reactive factor
skin respiratory factor
somatotropin-releasing factor
split renal function
subretinal fluid

SRF-A
slow-reacting factor of anaphylaxis

SRFC
sheep (red cell) rosette-forming cells

SRFOA
slow-reacting factor of anaphylaxis

SRFS
split renal function study

Srg, srg.
surgery

SRH
signs of recent hemorrhage
single radial hemolysis
somatotropin-releasing hormone
spontaneously responding
    hyperthyroidism
stigmata of recent hemorrhage

SRI
severe renal insufficiency

SRID
single radial immunodiffusion

SRIF
somatotropin release-inhibiting factor

SRM
spontaneously ruptured membranes
spontaneous rupture of membranes
standard reference materials
superior rectus muscle

SRNA, sRNA
soluble ribonucleic acid

SRNM
subretinal neovascular membrane (re:
    Ophth)

SRNS
steroid-responsive nephrotic syndrome

SRNV
subretinal neovascularization (re:
    Ophth)

SRO
single room occupancy
smallest region of overlap

SROM
spontaneous rupture of membranes (re: OB)

SRP
signal recognition protein
simple response paradigm

SRR
slow rotation room
stabilized relative response
Surgical Recovery Room

SRRS
Social Readjustment Rating Scale

SR-RSV
Schmidt-Rupin (strain) Rous sarcoma virus

SRS
schizophrenic residual state
sex reassignment surgery
Silver-Russell syndrome
slow-reacting substance (of anaphylaxis)
Social and Rehabilitation Service
Symptom Rating Scale

SRSA, SRS-A
slow-reacting substance of anaphylaxis

SRT
sedimentation rate test
sick role tendency
simple reaction time
sinus (node) recovery time
social relations test
speech reception test (re: Audio)
speech reception threshold (re: Audio)
spontaneously resolving thyrotoxicosis
sustained-release theophylline
Symptom Rating Test

SRU
structural repeating unit

SRV
superior radicular vein

S-R variation
smooth-rough variation (re: bacterial colonies)

SRVT
sustained re-entrant ventricular tachyarrhythmia

SRW
short ragweed (test)

SS
saline soak
saline solution
saliva sample
Sanarelli-Shwartzman (reaction)
saturated solution

schizophrenia spectrum
seizure sensitive
serum sickness
Sézary syndrome
Shigella and *Salmonella* (agar—Salmonella-Shigella)
Shigella sonnei
short stay
siblings
sickle cell (anemia)
side to side
signs and symptoms
single-stranded (DNA)
Sjögren's syndrome
skull series (re: Radio)
slow (wave) sleep (re: EEG)
soap solution
soapsuds
Social Security
social service(s)
sodium salicylate
somatostatin
sparingly soluble
special senses
special services
stable sarcoidosis
staccato syndrome
standard score (re: statistics)
statistically significant
steady state
sterile solution
steroid sulfurylation
Strachan-Scott (syndrome)
subaortic stenosis
subscapularis
subsegmental
subsequent sibling
substernal
suction socket
sum of squares
supersaturated
surging sine
systemic sclerosis

S&S
signs and symptoms

S by S
symptoms by systems

S or S
signs or symptoms

ss
subjects
symptoms

ss, s̄s̄, ss.
semi- (L. a half [prefix])
semisse (L. a half)
semissem (L. one-half)

s.s.
sacrosciatic
sensu stricto (L. in the strict sense)

s̄s̄, s̄s̄, s̈s̈
semis (L. one-half)

SSA
salicylsalicylic acid (salsalate)
skin-sensitizing antibodies
Smith surface antigen
Social Security Administration
special somatic afferent
sperm-specific antigen
subsegmental airway
sulfosalicylic acid (test)

SS agar
Shigella and *Salmonella* agar

SSAV
simian sarcoma-associated virus

SSB
stereospecific binding

SSBG
sex steroid-binding globulin

SSC
sister-strand crossover (re: genetics)
somatosensory cortex
standard saline citrate
Station Selection Code (re: computers)
Stein Sentence Completion (test)
superior semicircular canal (re: Oto)
syngeneic spleen cells

SSCA
sensitized sheep cell agglutination
spontaneous suppressor cell activity

SSCF
sleep stage change frequency

SSCQT
Selective Service College Qualifying
Test

SSCr
stainless steel crown (re: Dent)

SSD
shock(-induced) suppression of drinking
single saturating dose
source to surface distance
speech-sound discrimination
sudden sniffing death
sum of square deviations (re: statistics)

SSD, S.S.D.
source-skin distance
source to skin distance

S/S (diet)
salt substitute diet

ssDNA
single-stranded deoxyribonucleic acid

SSDW
(significant) sharp spike or delta waves
(re: EEG)

SSE
saline solution enema
skin self-examination
soap solution enema
soapsuds enema
steady state exercise
subacute spongiform encephalopathy

SSEA
sensitized sheep erythrocyte
agglutination
stage-specific embyronic antigen

SS enema
saline solution enema

SSEP
somatosensory evoked potential

s̄ seq.
sine sequela (L. without sequel)

SSER
somatosensory evoked response

SSF
soluble suppressor factor
supplementary sensory feedback

SSFI
social stress and functionability
inventory

SSHA
Survey of Study Habits and Attitudes

SSHL
severe sensorineural hearing loss

SSI
segmental sequential irradiation
stuttering severity instrument
subunit-subunit interface
Supplemental Security Income
symptom-sign inventory
synthetic sentence identification

SSIAM
Structured and Scaled Interview to
Assess Maladjustment

SSIDS
siblings of sudden infant death
syndrome (victims)

SSII
Safran Student's Interest Inventory

SSIT
subscapularis, supraspinatus,
infraspinatus, teres minor (muscles)

SSKI
saturated solution of potassium iodide

SSL
skin surface lipid
synthetic sentence list

SSLI
serum sickness-like illness

SSM
sesquiterpenoid stress metabolites
subsynaptic membrane
superficial spreading (malignant)
 melanoma (formerly called pre-
 malignant melanosis and pagetoid
 melanoma)

SSMS
saturated solution of magnesium sulfate
 ($MgSO_4$)

SSN
severely subnormal

s.s.n.
signetur suo nomine (L. let it be labeled
 with its own name)

ss notch
sacrosciatic notch

SSO
special sense organs

SSOP
Standard System of Psychiatry (re:
 computers)

SSP
Sanarelli-Shwartzman phenomenon
Scientific Subroutine Package
small spherical particle
subacute sclerosing panencephalitis
subspecies (re: taxonomy)
supersensitivity perception

SSPE
subacute sclerosing panencephalitis

SSPG
steady state plasma glucose

SSPI
steady state plasma insulin

SSPL
saturation sound pressure level

SSPP
subsynaptic plate perforation

SSPS
side-to-side portacaval shunt

SSR
steady state rest
steroid-resistant rejection
surgical supply room

SSS
scalded skin syndrome (Ritter's
 disease; bullous impetigo; scarlet
 skin syndrome)
Sensation-Seeking Scale (re: Psychol)
sick sinus syndrome
soluble specific substance (specific
 soluble substance; specific capsular
 substance—re: growth of virulent
 pneumococci)
sterile saline soak
Surgical Staging System
systemic sicca syndrome

sss, s.s.s.
stratum super stratum (L. layer upon
 layer)

SSSS
staphylococcal scalded skin syndrome

SSST
superior sagittal sinus thrombosis

SSSV
superior sagittal sinus (blood) velocity

SST
sodium sulfite titration
somatosensory thalamus
somatostatin

s. str.
sensu stricto (L. in the strict sense)

SSU
Saybolt seconds universal
self-service unit
sterile supply unit

SS & US
surging sine and ultrasound

SSV
Schoolman-Schwartz virus
sheep seminal vesicles
simian sarcoma virus
Stock-Spielmeyer-Vogt (syndrome)

SSV, s.s.v.
sub signo veneni (L. under a poison
 label)

SSW
staggered spondaic word

SSX
sulfisoxazole (sulphafurazole)

ST
Salmonella typhosa
scala tympani
sclerotherapy
sedimentation time
semitendinosus
septal thickness
shock therapy

siblings (raised) together
similarly tested
sinus tachycardia
sinus tympani
skin temperature
skin test
slight trace
slow twitch (re: muscle fiber)
Spanlang-Tappeiner (syndrome)
sphincter tone
(heat)-stable (entero)toxin
standardized test (re: Psychol)
standard treatment
starting time
station
sternothyroid
Stewart-Treves (syndrome)
stress testing
striatum
subtalar (re: Ortho)
subtotal
surface tension
surgical therapy
survival time
systolic time

ST, st
stimulus
stomach

S.T.
Speech Therapy (Department)

S-T
sickle cell thalassemia

↓ ST
depressed ST segment (re: EKG)

St
Stanton number (re: forced convection
    studies)
stated
stokes (centimeter-gram-second unit of
    kinematic viscosity)
subtype

St, st.
stent (L. let them stand)
stet (L. let it stand)

st.
stage (of disease)
standing
status
sterile
stimulation
stimuli
stone
straight
strength
stretch

STA
second trimester abortion
serum thrombotic accelerator

serum tobramycin assay
superficial temporal artery

S-Ta
atrial S-T segment change

sta.
station

stab
"stabkernige" (staff or band neutrophils)

STABS
Suinn Test Anxiety Behavior Scale

stabs
"stabkernige" (staff or band neutrophils)

STACL
Screening Test For Auditory
    Comprehension of Language (re:
    Psychol)

St AE
standard above elbow (cast)

STAG, S-TAG
slow (binding) target-attaching globulin

STAI
State-Trait Anxiety Inventory

STAIC
State-Trait Anxiety Inventory for
    Children

STAIRS
Storage and Information Retrieval
    System (re: computers/ data
    processing)

STA-MCA
superficial temporal artery to middle
    cerebral artery

stand.
standard
standardized

standard.
standardization
standardized

StanPsych
Standard Psychiatric (nomenclature)

Stapes mob.
stapes mobilization

STAPH, Staph
Staphylococcus (genus)

staph.
staphylococcal
staphylococcus (species not named)

Staph. aur.
Staphylococcus aureus

Stap mob.
stapes mobilization

STARS
Short Term Auditory Retrieval and
   Storage (re: Psychol)

START
Screening Test for the Assignment of
   Remedial Treatments (re: Psychol)

STAS
State-Trait Anger Scale

STAT
Suprathreshold Adaptation Test

stat.
statim (L. immediately)
statistics

statist.
statistical
statistics

stats.
statistics

Stb, stb.
stillborn

STC
serum theophylline concentration
sexually transmitted condition
soft tissue calcification
somatotropin, L-thyroxine (levothyroxine
   sodium), corticosterone
Stroke Treatment Center

STD
sexually transmitted disease
skin test dose
skin to tumor distance
sodium tetradecyl sulfate
standard test dose

std.
saturated
stand
standard
standardization
standardized

stdg.
standing

STDH
skin test for delayed-type
   hypersensitivity

STDT
standard tone decay test

STD TF
standard tube feeding

STEAM
streptonigrin, thioguanine,

cyclophosphamide, actinomycin,
   mitomycin C (re: chemotherapy)

STEM
scanning and transmission electron
   microscope (combination in a single
   instrument)

STEP-III
Sequential Tests of Educational
   Progress, Series III

STEPS
sequential treatment employing
   pharmacologic supports

ster.
sterile

Stereo, stereo.
stereogram

stern. punct.
sternal puncture

STESS
subject's treatment emergent symptom
   scale

STET
submaximal treadmill exercise test

STF
serum thymus factor
slow twitch fiber
small third-trimester fetus
special tube feeding
sudden transient freezing

STG
short-term goals (re: Psychol)
split-thickness graft

STGC
syncytiotrophoblastic giant cell

STH
somatotrop(h)ic (growth) hormone
somatotrop(h)ic hormone
subtotal hysterectomy
supplemental thyroid hormone

S-Thal
sickle (cell) thalassemia

STHRF
somatotrop(h)ic hormone-releasing
   factor

STI
serum trypsin inhibitor
soybean trypsin inhibitor
systolic time interval

STIC
serum trypsin inhibitory capacity

stillat.
stillatim (L. by drops [in small
   quantities])

Still B, stillb.
stillborn

stim.
stimulate
stimulation
stimulus

stimn.
stimulation

STK
streptokinase

STL
serum theophylline level
swelling, tenderness, limitation (of
   movement)

STLOM
swelling, tenderness, and limitation of
   motion

STM
scanning tunneling microscope
short-term memory (re: Neuro/Psychol)
streptomycin

StMPM
syncytiotrophoblast microvilli plasma
   membrane

STN
subthalamic nucleus
supratrochlear nucleus

STNR
symmetrical tonic neck reflex

STNS
sham transcutaneous nerve stimulation

STNV
satellite tobacco necrosis virus

stom.
stomach

stom. lav.
stomach lavage

stom. lav. → cl.
stomach lavage to clear

STP
scientifically treated petroleum
serenity, tranquility, peace (2,5-
   dimethoxy-4-methylamphetamine
   [users' term for hallucinogen])
Sibling Training Program
sodium thiopental (thiopental sodium)
standard (normal) temperature and
   pulse

STP, s.t.p.
standard temperature and pressure

STPD
standard temperature and pressure, dry
   (0°C 760 mmHg)

STPI
State-Trait Personality Inventory

ST platform
sustentaculum tali platform (re: Ortho)

STPP
sodium tripolyphosphate (industrial
   chemical)

St pr.
status praesens (L. present status)

STPS
specific thalamic projection system
standard temperature and pressure,
   saturated

STQ
superior temporal quadrant

STR
soft tissue relaxation
synchronous transmitter receiver (re:
   computers)

STR, str.
Streptococcus (genus)

Str
striatum

str.
straight
strain
strained
strength
stretch
strong (re: heart sounds)

Strab, strab.
strabismus

STREP, Strep
Streptococcus (genus)

strep.
streptococcus (species not named)
streptomycin

strept.
streptococcus (species not named)

streptoc.
streptococcus (species not named)

STRT
skin temperature recovery time

struc.
structural
structure

struct.
structural
structure

STS
sexual tubal sterilization
short-term storage
steroid sulfatase

STS, S.T.S.
serologic(al) test for syphilis
standard (serologic) test for syphilis

STSG
split-thickness skin graft

STT
sensitization test
serial thrombin time
skin temperature test
standard triple therapy (for
   hypertension)

sttg.
sitting

STU, S.T.U.
skin test unit

STV
superior temporal vein

STVA
subtotal villose (villous) atrophy

STVB
Strong Vocational Interest Blank

STVS
short-term visual storage

STX
saxitoxin (re: neurochemical research)

STYCAR
Screening Tests for Young Children and
   Retardates

S. typhi
Salmonella typhi

STZ
streptozocin (antineoplastic)

SU
salicyluric acid
secretory units
Senear-Usher (syndrome)
sensation unit
sigma units
solar urticaria
sorbent unit
spectrophotometric unit
status uncertain
strontium unit
subunit
supine

su.
subject
sumat (L. let the patient take)
surgeon
surgery
surgical

SUA
serum uric acid
single umbilical artery
single unit activity

SUB
subroutine (re: computers)
substitute (character—re: computers/
   data processing)

SUB, sub.
substitute

subac.
subacute

subclav.
subclavian
subclavicular

subclin.
subclinical

subcr.
subcrepitant

subcrep.
subcrepitant

subcu.
subcutaneous
subcutaneously

subcut.
subcutaneous
subcutaneously

sub fin. coct.
sub finem coctionis (L. toward the end
   of cooking)

subgen.
subgenus

subind.
subinde (L. immediately after)

subj.
subject
subjective

subj. sx
subjective symptoms

subl.
sublimate
sublimation
sublime
sublimes (re: chemistry)
sublingual

subling.
sublingual

sublux.
subluxation

submand.
submandibular

SubN
subthalamic nucleus

suboccip.
suboccipital

suborb. stim.
suborbital stimulation

Sub-Q, subq., sub-q
subcutaneous (injection site)

subsc.
subscapular

subscap.
subscapular

subsp.
subspecies

subst.
substance
substitute

substd.
substandard

suc.
succus (L. juice)

Succ
succinate

succ.
succinylcholine

SUD
skin unit dose
sudden unexpected death
sudden unexplained death

SUDH
succinodehydrogenase

SUDI
sudden unexpected death of infant
sudden unexplained death of infant

sue mutations
suppressor-enhancing mutations (re: genetics)

suf.
sufficient

suff.
sufficient

sug.
sugar
suggest

SUHT
subject's height (in inches)

SUI
stress urinary incontinence

SUID
sudden unexpected infant death
sudden unexplained infant death

sulf.
sulfate

sulfa
sulfonamide(s)

sum.
sumantur (L. let them be taken)
sumat (L. let [the patient] take)
sume (L. take)
sumendum (L. to be taken)
summation

SUMIT
streptokinase-urokinase myocardial infarction trial

sum. tal.
sumat talem (L. let [the patient] take one like this)

SUN
serum urea nitrogen
Standard Units and Nomenclature

SUO
syncope of unknown origin

SUP, sup.
superficial
superior
supinator (muscle)

sup.
supination
supine
supra (L. above; over)

superf.
superficial

superfic.
superficial

superimp.
superimpose(d)

sup. mes.
superior mesenteric (arteriogram)

Supp, supp.
suppository

supp.
suppositorium (L. that which is placed
   under [suppository])
suppurative

sup. pat. (pole)
suprapatellar pole

suppl.
supplement
supplemental
supplementary

suppos.
suppositorium (L. that which is placed
   under [suppository])
suppository

supra cit.
supra citato (L. cited above)

supra pat.
suprapatellar

supt.
superintendent

supv.
supervision
supervisor

SURG, Surg, surg.
surgery

Surg
surgeon

Surg, surg.
surgical

SUS
stained urinary sediment
suppressor sensitive

susc.
susceptibility
susceptible

susp.
suspension

sut.
suture

SUTI
symptomatic urinary tract infection

SUUD
sudden unexpected unexplained death

SUV
small unilamellar vesicles (type of
   liposome)

SUX
succinylcholine

SV
saphenous vein

sarcoma virus
satellite virus
scalp vein
selective vagotomy
semilunar valve
seminal vesicle
Sendai virus
severe
simian virus
single ventricle
single vessel
sinus venosus
snake venom
Spielmeyer-Vogt (disease)
splenic vein
spontaneous ventilation
stimulus valve
stroke volume
Study of Values (re: Psychol)
subclavian vein
subventricular
supraventricular
supravital

S/V
surface to volume (ratio)

SV 40, SV40
simian vacuolating virus 40

Sv
sievert (SI unit of radioactive dose
   equivalent— 100 rems)

sv, s.v.
single vibrations

s.v.
spiritus vini (L. alcoholic spirit)

SVA
selective vagotomy with antrectomy
selective visceral angiography
spatial voltage (at maximum) anterior
   (force)
special visceral afferent (nerve)
subtotal villous atrophy

SVAS
subvalvular aortic stenosis
supravalvular aortic stenosis

SVC
segmental venous capacitance
selective venous catheterization
slow vital capacity
subclavian vein catheterization
superior vena cava
suprahepatic vena cava

SVCG
spatial vectorcardiogram

SVCO
superior vena cava obstruction

SVC-PA
superior vena cava to pulmonary artery

SVCR
segmental venous capacitance ratio

SVC-RPA shunt
superior vena cava-right pulmonary
 artery shunt

SVCS
superior vena cava syndrome

SVD
single vessel disease
small vessel disease
spontaneous vaginal delivery
spontaneous vertex delivery
swine vesicular disease

SVE
soluble viral extract
special visceral efferent (nerve)
Streptococcus viridans endocarditis
supraventricular ectopic (beat)

SVG
saphenous vein graft

s.v.g.
spiritus vini gallici (L. brandy)

SVI
stroke volume index

SVIB
Strong Vocational Interest Blank

SVM
seminal vesicle microsome
spatial voltage (at) maximum (posterior
 force)
syncytiovascular membrane

S$_{VO_2}$
venous oxygen saturation

SVOM
sequential volitional oral movement

SVP
selective vagotomy with pyloroplasty
small volume parenteral (re: solution)
spatial voltage (at maximum) posterior
 (force)
standing venous pressure
static volume pressure
superficial vascular plexus

SVPB
supraventricular premature beats

SVR
sequential vascular response
systemic vascular resistance

S$_1$VR, S$_2$VR
sacral ventral root

s.v.r.
spiritus vini rectificatus (L. rectified spirit
 of wine [distilled])

SVRI
systemic vascular resistance index

SVSe
supravaginal septum

SVT
sinoventricular tachyarrhythmia
sinoventricular tachycardia
STYCAR (Screening Tests for Young
 Children and Retardates) Vision Tests
 (re: Psychol)
supraventricular tachyarrhythmia
supraventricular tachycardia

s.v.t.
spiritus vini tenuis (L. thin spirit of wine
 [diluted])

SW
Schwartz-Watson test (re: acute
 porphyria)
seawater
seriously wounded
short wave
sine wave (wavelength)
slow wave (re: EEG)
social worker
spherule wall (re: *Coccidioides*)
spike wave (re: EEG)
spiral wound
stab wound
sterile water
stroke work
Sturge-Weber (syndrome)

SW, Sw
swine (re: veterinary medicine)

sw.
sweet
swelling
switch

s$_{20,w}$
sedimentation coefficient in water at
 20°C

SWA
seriously wounded in action

Sw^a antigen
low frequency blood group antigen

SWAMP
swine-associated mucoprotein

SWC
submaximal working capacity

SWD
short wave diathermy (re: physical
 therapy)
sine wave diathermy

SW dia.
short wave diathermy (re: physical
   therapy)
sine wave diathermy

SW diath.
short wave diathermy (re: physical
   therapy)
sine wave diathermy

SWE
slow wave encephalography

S&W enema
soap and water enema

SWFI
sterile water for injection

SWG
silkworm gut
standard wire gauge

SWI
sterile water for injection
stroke work index
surgical wound infection

SWIM
sperm-washing insemination method

SWJ
square wave jerk

SWM
segmental wall motion

SWO
superficial white onychomycosis

SWR
serum Wassermann reaction

SWS
slow wave sleep (re: EEG)
spike wave stupor (re: EEG)
steroid wasting syndrome
Sturge-Weber syndrome (trigeminal
   encephaloangiomatosis)

SWT
sine wave threshold

Sx, sx
signs
symptoms

sx ↑
symptoms increased

sx ↓
symptoms decreased

Sx Hx
social history

Sxr
sex-reversed (re: genetics)

sx & sx
signs and symptoms

SXT
sulfamethoxazole

SY
syphilis

SYA
subacute yellow atrophy (of the liver)

Sym, sym.
symmetrical

sym.
symmetry
symptoms

symb.
symbol
symbolic

symp.
sympathetic
symptom(s)

sympat.
sympathetic (nervous system)

sympath.
sympathetic

symp. sys.
sympathetic system

sympt.
symptom(s)

SYN
synchronous (idea character—re:
   computers/data processing)
synthetic

Syn
synchondrosis

syn.
synergist
synergy
synonym
synovial (fluid)
synovitis

syn-
stereochemical opposite of *anti*

sync.
synchronous

synch.
synchronous

synd.
syndrome

Syn Fl
synovial fluid

synov.
synovectomy
synovial
synovitis

synth.
synthetic

syph.
syphilis
syphilitic
syphilologist
syphilology

syr.
syrup

SYS
stretching and yawning syndrome

sys.
system
systemic

SYSLOG
system log (re: computers/data
  processing)

Syst, syst.
systolic

syst.
systemic

syst. m.
systolic murmur

SZ
Skevas-Zerfus (disease)
streptozocin (antineoplastic)

SZ, Sz
schizophrenia

Sz
skin impedance

Sz, sz.
seizure

SZD
streptozocin diabetes

T

T
congenital limb absence—terminal
intraocular tension (Tn = normal;
    T + 1, T + 2, etc., increased tension;
    T − 1, T − 2, etc., decreased
    tension)
obtained under test conditions
resolving time of a nuclear particle
    detector
Tabanus (genus of gadfly)
tablespoonful
Taenia (genus of carnivore-infecting
    tapeworm)
tamoxifen (anti-estrogen)
tanycytes (ependymal cells—re: Neuro)
tau (capital 19th letter of the Greek
    alphabet)
T-bandage
T-bar
temperature
temporary
tender
tenderness
tension (especially intraocular)
tera- (one trillion, a metric prefix—10^{12})
term
tertiar- (third—prefix)
testosterone
tetracycline
Tetrahymena (genus of protozoa)
T-fiber
theophylline
therapist
thoracic (in vertebral formulae)
thorax
threonine (an amino acid)
thrombus
thymidine
thymine
thymus
thymus-derived (lymphocyte)
thyroid
tidal gas (secondary symbol—re: Resp)
tidal volume (when written as a
    subscript)
time period
timing
tincture
tocopherol
tone
topical (re: administration of drugs)
torque
total
toxicity

Toxoplasma (genus)
trace
transformation (products—re: Psychol;
    Aptitudes Research Project testing
    within structure of intellect model)
transition point
transmittance (re: spectrophotometry)
transverse
tray
Treponema (genus)
triangulation
Triatoma (genus of Chagas disease)
Trichinella (genus of nematode
    parasites)
Trichomonas (genus)
Trichophyton (genus)
Trichosporon (genus)
Trichostrongylus (genus of nematode
    worms)
Trichuris (genus of intestinal nematode
    parasites)
triggered
Trombicula (genus of acarine mites)
Trypanosoma (genus of protozoan
    parasites)
tuberculin
tuberculosis
tuberculous
tuberculum
tuberosity
tumor
Tunga (genus of fleas)
T wave (re: EKG)
type

T, T.
tesla (meter-kilogram-second system
    unit of magnetic flux density—equal
    to one weber per square meter)

T, *T*
temperature, absolute (Kelvin, Rankine)

T, t
tertiary
time (life)

T, t, t.
temporal

T, *t*
tritium—hydrogen 3

T +
increased tension

T –
decreased tension

T/
than
then
transfers

T ↑
tension increased (intraocular)
tourniquet inflated

T ↓
tension decreased (intraocular)
tourniquet released

T ↓ ↓
testicles both descended

T½, t½
symbol for half-life of radioactive isotope
terminal half-life (re: isotopes)

T1, T2, T₁, T₂...
first thoracic vertebra, second thoracic
    vertebra, etc.
thoracic nerves

T + 1, T + 2 ...
stages of increased intraocular tension

T – 1, T – 2 ...
stages of decreased intraocular tension

T₁
tricuspid first heart sound

T₂
diiodothyronine
tricuspid second heart sound

T₃
triiodothyronine (3,5,3′-triiodothyronine;
    TITh)

T₄
thyroxin(e) (levothyroxine,
    tetraiodothyronine)

T-28
trapezoid 28 (total hip prosthesis)

T-1824
Evans blue

2,4,5-T
(2,4,5-trichlorophenoxy)acetic acid (a
    herbicide)

t
student's test variable (re: statistics)
teaspoonful
temperature, customary (Celsius,
    Fahrenheit)
terminal
test of significance (re: statistics)
translocation (re: cytogenetics)

t, t.
ter (L. three times)

t½
reaction half-time
time taken for ½ of the initial
    concentration of DNA to renature

τ
Greek lower-case letter tau
relaxation time
time (life—re: radioactive isotopes)

τ½
symbol for half life (time—re:
    radioactive isotopes)

TA
tactile afferent
teichoic acids
temporal arteritis
temporal average
tendo achillis (official alternative for
    tendo calcaneus; Achilles tendon)
tendon of Achilles
tension (by) applanation (re: Ophth)
tension, arterial
terminal antrum
test age
therapeutic abortion
thermophilic *Actinomyces*
thymocytotoxic autoantibody
thyroglobulin autoprecipitation
thyroid antibody
thyroid autoantibody
tibialis anterior
titratable acid
total alkaloids
traffic accident
Transactional Analysis (re: Psychol)
transaldolase
transantral
transplantation antigen
trapped air
treatment assignment
tricuspid annuloplasty (re: Cardio)
tricuspid atresia (re: Cardio)
trophoblast antigen
true anomaly
truncus arteriosus
tryptophan acid (reaction)
tryptose agar
tube agglutination
tuberculin, alkaline
tumor associated

TA, T.A.
toxin-antitoxin

TA, T(A)
temperature, axillary

T/A
time and amount

T&A
tonsillectomy and adenoidectomy
tonsillitis and adenoiditis
tonsils and adenoids

T of A
transposition of aorta

TA$_4$
tetraiodothyroacetic acid

Ta
T-amplifier
tantalum (element)
tarsal (amputation level, lower limb)

^{182}Ta
radioactive isotope of tantulum

TAA
thioacetamide (analytical reagent)
transverse aortic arch
tumor-associated antibodies
tumor-associated antigens

TAAF
thromboplastic activity of amniotic fluid

TAB
therapeutic abortion
typhoid, paratyphoid A, and paratyphoid
  B (vaccine)

TAB, tab.
tabella (L. a [medicated] tablet)
tabellae (L. [medicated] tablets)
tablet

TABC
total aerobic bacteria count
typhoid-paratyphoid A, B, and C
  (vaccine)

tabs
tablets

TABT
combined typhoid-paratyphoid A and B
  (vaccine), tetanus (toxoid)

TABTD
combined typhoid-paratyphoid A and B
  (vaccine), tetanus (toxoid) and
  diphtheria (toxoid)

TAC
terminal antrum contraction
tetracaine, epinephrine, cocaine
thyroid-adrenocortical (syndrome)
total aganglionosis coli
triamcinolone acetonide cream (topical
  anti-inflammatory; glucocorticoid)

TACE
teichoic acids crude extract

TACE, Tace
tri-*p*-anisylchloroethylene (therapy for
  prostate cancer)

tach.
tachycardia

tachy.
tachycardia

TACL
Test For Auditory Comprehension of
  Language (re: Psychol)

TAD
Test of Auditory Discrimination (re:
  Psychol)
6-thioguanine, ara-C (cytarabine), and
  daunorubicin (re: chemotherapy)
thoracic asphyxiant dystrophy

TADAC
therapeutic abortion, dilation, aspiration,
  curettage

TADs
Technical Assistance Documents (re:
  medical records)

TAF
tissue angiogenesis factor
trypsin, aldehyde, fuchsin
tuberculin, albumose-free
tumor angiogenesis factor
tumor angiogenic factor

TAF, T.A.F.
toxoid-antitoxin floccules
Tuberculin Albumose frei (Ger.
  albumose-free tuberculin)

TAG
target-attaching globulin
thymine, adenine, guanine

TAGH
triiodothyronine, amino acids, glucagon,
  heparin

TAH
total abdominal hysterectomy
total artificial heart
transabdominal hysterectomy

TAHBSO; TAH, BSO; TAH-BSO
total abdominal hysterectomy, bilateral
  salpingo-oophorectomy

TAI
Teacher Attitude Inventory (re: Psychol)
Test Anxiety Inventory
tissue antagonist of interferon

TAL
tendo-achillis lengthening
tendon Achilles lengthening
thymic alymphoplasia

tal.
tales (L. such ones)
talia (L. such)
talis (L. such a one)

talc.
talcum (powder)

T-ALL
T-cell acute lymphoblastic leukemia

TALPS
Transactional Analysis Life Position
Survey (re: Psychol)

TAM
tamoxifen (anti-estrogen)
teenage mother
thermoacidurans agar modified

TAM, T.A.M.
toxoid-antitoxoid mixture

TAMe
toxoid-antitoxoid mixture esterase

TAMIS
Telemetric Automated Microbial
Identification System

TAMVEC
Texas A & M variable energy cyclotron

TAN
tonically autoactive neuron
total adenine nucleotides
total ammonia nitrogen

tan
tangent

tanh., tan h.
hyperbolic tangent

TANI
total axial lymph node irradiation

T antigens
tumor antigens

TAO
thromboangiitis obliterans
triacetyloleandomycin (antibacterial—
obsolete term for troleandomycin or
oleandomycin triacetate ester)
turning against object

TAP
tension (by) applanation (re: Ophth)

TAPS
training and placement service
trial assessment procedure scale

TAPVC
total anomalous pulmonary venous
connection

TAPVD
total anomalous pulmonary venous
drainage

TAPVR
total anomalous pulmonary venous
return

TAQW
transient abnormal Q waves (re: Cardio)

TAR
thrombocytopenia-absent radius
(syndrome)
thrombocytopenia (with) absence (of
the) radius
tissue-to-air ratio
total abortion rate

TARA
total articular replacement arthroplasty
tumor-associated rejection antigen

TAS
test for ascendance-submission
tetanus antitoxic serum
turning against self (re: Psychol)

TASA
tumor-associated surface antigen

T'ASE
tryptophan synthetase

TAT
Tell a Tale (re: psychiatry)
tetanus antitoxin
Thematic Aptitude Test (re:
psychological testing)
thromboplastin activation test
total antitryptic (activity)
transaxial tomogram
transverse axial tomography
tray agglutination test
tumor activity test
turn-around time
tyrosine aminotransferase

TAT, T.A.T.
Thematic Apperception Test (re:
Psychol)
toxin-antitoxin

TATA
tumor-associated transplantation
antigen

TATBA
triamcinolone acetonide *tert*-butyl
acetate (glucocorticoid)

TATD
thiamine 8-(methyl 6-
acetyldihydrothioctate) disulfide (oral
thiamine)

TATR
tyrosine aminotransferase regulator

TATST
tetanus antitoxin skin test

TAV
trapped air volume

TB
Taussig-Bing (syndrome)
terminal bronchiole
thromboxane B (thromboxane
    B_2,TXB_2—compound derivation of
    prostaglandin endoperoxides)
thymol blue (an indicator)
toluidine blue
total base
total bilirubin
total body
tracheal bronchiolar (region)
tracheobronchitis
trapezoid body
trigonal bipyramid (re: complexes)
tuberculin
tumor bearing

TB, Tb, T.b., tb
tubercle bacillus

TB, T.b., tb
tuberculosis

Tb
terbium (element)

^{160}Tb
radioactive isotope of terbium

^{161}Tb
radioactive isotope of terbium

T_b
body temperature

T_b
biologic half-life

TBA
tertiary butyl acetate (*tert*-butyl
    acetate—empirical formula gasoline
    additive)
testosterone-binding affinity
thiobarbituric acid
thyroxin(e)-binding albumin
to be added
to be admitted
to be adopted
total bile acid
trypsin-binding activity
tubercle bacillus
tumor-bearing animal

TBAB
tryptose/blood/agar base

TBACA, TB-ACA
3,4,5-trimethoxybenzoyl-ε-aminocaproic
    acid (capobenic acid—anti-
    arrhythmic)

T banding
telomere or terminal banding (re:
    chromosomes)

TBB
transbronchial biopsy

TBBC
total B_{12} binding capacity

TBBM
total body bone mineral

TBC
thyroxin(e)-binding coagulin
total body calcium
total body clearance
total body counting
tubercidin

TBC, Tbc, tbc.
tuberculosis

Tbc
tubercle bacillus

tbcn.
tuberculin

TBD
total body density

TBE
tick-borne encephalitis

TBE, T.B.E.
Tuberculin-Bacillen-Emulsion
    (tuberculin bacillary emulsion)

TBF
total body fat

TBFB
tracheobronchial foreign body

TBG
testosterone-binding globulin
thyroglobulin
thyroid-binding globulin
thyroxin(e)-binding globulin
tracheobronchogram
tris-buffered Gey's (solution)

TBG cap.
thyroxin(e)-binding capacity

TBGE
thyroxin(e)-binding globulin estimated

TBGI
thyroxin(e)-binding globulin index

TBGP
total blood granulocyte pool

TBH
total body hematocrit

TBI
thyrobinding index
thyroid-binding index
thyroxin(e)-binding index
tooth brushing instruction (re: Dent)
total body irradiation

TBII
thyroid-stimulating hormone-binding
inhibitory immunoglobulin

T bili
total bilirubin (assay)

TBK
total body kalium (potassium)

Tbl
tablet

TBLB
transbronchial lung biopsy

TBLC
term birth, living child

TBLI
term birth, living infant

TBM
thyroxin(e)-binding meningitis
total body mass
tuberculous meningitis
tubular basement membrane

TBN
total body nitrogen

TBNA
total body neutron activation
treated but not admitted

TBNAA
total-body neutron activation analysis

TBP
testosterone-binding protein
2,2'-thiobis[4,6-dichlorophenol]
(bithionol—topical anti-infective;
veterinary—anthelmintic; antiseptic)
thyroxin(e)-binding protein
total bypass
tributyl phosphate
tuberculous peritonitis

TBPA
thyroxin(e)-binding prealbumin

TBPT
total body protein turnover

TBR
tumor-bearing rabbit

TB-RD
tuberculosis-respiratory disease

TBRS
Timed Behavioral Rating Sheet

TBS
4-*tert*-butylphenyl salicylate (industrial
chemical)
total body solids
total body solute
total body surface
tracheal bronchial submucosa(l)
tracheobronchoscopy
tribromosalicylanilide (tribromsalan—
bacteriostat)
tribromsalan (bacteriostat)
triethanolamine-buffered saline

tbs.
tablespoon

TBSA
total body surface area

tbsp.
tablespoonful

TBSV
tomato bushy stunt virus

TBT
tolbutamide test
tracheobronchial toilet
tracheobronchial tree

TBTT
tuberculin tine test

TBUT
tear break-up time

TBV
total blood volume

TBVp
total blood volume predicted (from body
surface)

TBW
total body washout
total body water
total body weight

TBWA
total body water

TBX
total-(whole) body irradiation

TBZ
tetrabenazine (tranquilizer)
thiabendazole (anthelmintic)

TC
target cell
taurocholate
temperature compensation

teratocarcinoma
tertiary cleavage
therapeutic community
thermal conductivity
thiocarbanilidin (antibacterial;
    tuberculostatic)
thoracic cage
throat culture
thyrocalcitonin
tissue culture
to contain
total calcium
total capacity (lung)
total cholesterol
total colonoscopy
total correction
transcobalamin
transcutaneous
transplant center
transverse colon
tubocurarine (neuromuscular blocking
    agent)
tumor cell
tumor cerebri
type and crossmatch

TC, T.C.
tuberculin contagious

TC, T/C, Tc, t.c.
telephone call

TC, Tc
tetracycline

T/C
to consider

T & C, T&C
test and crossmatch
turn and cough
type and crossmatch

TC$_{50}$
median toxic concentration

2,4,5-TC
2-(2,4,5-trichlorophenoxy)propionic acid
    (plant hormone)

T$_4$(C)
serum thyroxin(e) measured by column
    chromatography

Tc
core temperature
T (cell) cytolytic
technetium (element)
temporal complex

Tc, T$_c$
cytotoxic T cell

^{99}Tc
technetium-99

TCA
terminal cancer
thyrocalcitonin (calcitonin—calcium
    regulator)
time, color, amount
total cholic acid
total circulating albumin
total circulatory arrest
tricalcium aluminate
tricarboxylic acid (cycle)
(monuron) trichloroacetate (herbicide)
trichloroacetic acid (caustic)
tricyclic antidepressant
tricyclic antipsychotics

TCABG
triple coronary artery bypass graft

TCAD
tricyclic antidepressant

TCAG
triple coronary artery graft

TCAM
telecommunications access method (re:
    computers/data processing)

T-CAP III
triazinate, cyclophosphamide,
    Adriamycin (doxorubicin), and Platinol
    (cisplatin) (re: chemotherapy)

TCB
total cardiopulmonary bypass
transcatheter biopsy
tumor cell burden

TCBS
thiosulfate citrate bile (salt) sucrose
    (agar)

TCC
thromboplastic cell component
toroidal coil chromatography
transitional cell carcinoma
trichlorocarbanilide (triclocarban—
    disinfectant)
triclocarban (trichlorocarbanilide—
    disinfectant)

TCCA
transitional cell cancer associated
    (virus)

TCCAV
transitional cell cancer associated
    (virus)

TCCL
T cell chronic lymphocytic (leukemia)

TCC$_O$
total cardiac cost above zero

TCD
thermal conductivity detector

tissue culture dose
transverse cardiac diameter

TCD∞
tissue culture dose

TCD$_{50}$
median tissue culture dose

TCDB
turn, cough, deep breathe

TC & DB; T, C & DB
turn, cough, and deep breathe

TCDBD
2,3,6,7-tetrachlorodibenzodioxin (highly
toxic and teratogenic; contaminant of
2,4,5-trichlorophenol; contaminant
created in the manufacture of Agent
Orange)

TCDC
taurochenodeoxycholate

TCDD
tetrachlorodibenzodioxin (2,3,7,8-
tetrachlorodibenzo-p-dioxin—[a
chlorophenoxy herbicide, highly
toxic])
2,3,6,7-tetrachlorodibenzodioxin (highly
toxic and teratogenic; contaminant of
2,4,5-trichlorophenol; contaminant
created in the manufacture of Agent
Orange)

2,3,7,8-TCDD
2,3,7,8-tetrachlorodibenzo[b,e][1,4]
dioxin

TC detector
thermal conductivity detector (re: gas
chromatography)

TCE
T-cell enriched
tetrachlorodiphenylethane (insecticide
[now called 1,1-dichloro-2,2-bis(p-
chlorophenyl)ethane])
tetrachloroethylene (solvent)
trichloroethanol (hypnotic; anesthetic)
trichloroethylene (inhalation anesthetic;
industrial solvent)

T cell
thymus (-derived) cell

TCES
transcutaneous cranial electrical
stimulation

TCESOM
trichloroethylene-extracted soybean-oil
meal

TCET
transcerebral electrotherapy

TCF
tissue-coding factor
total coronary flow

TCFU
trichlorofluoromethane (aerosol
propellant)
tumor colony-forming units

TCG
time compensation gain

TCGF
thymus cell growth factor (interleukin 2)

TCGP
taenia coli muscle of the guinea pig

TCH
tanned cell hemagglutination
total circulating hemoglobin
turn, cough, hyperventilate

TChE
total cholinesterase

Tchg
teaching

Tchr
teacher

TCI
to come in (to hospital)
total cerebral ischemia
transient cerebral ischemia
Trotman's Change Index

TCID
tissue culture infective dose
tissue culture inoculated dose

TCID$_{50}$
median tissue culture infective dose

TCIE
transient cerebral ischemic episode

TCIPA
tumor cell induced platelet aggregation

T$_{cis}$
cytotoxicity and suppression T cells

T-CLL
T-cell chronic lymphatic leukemia

TψC loop
re: transfer RNA—genetics

TCM
tissue culture medium
transcutaneous monitor

Tc 99m
technetium-99m (re: nuclear medicine)

TcMAA
99mTc macroaggregated albumin (re:
nuclear medicine)

Tc-99m-DMSA
technetium Tc-99m dimercaptosuccinic
acid (re: nuclear medicine)

Tc-99m-DTPA
technetium Tc-99m pentetic acid (re:
nuclear medicine)

Tc-99m-HSA
technetium Tc-99m human serum
albumin (re: nuclear medicine)

Tc-99m-MAA
technetium Tc-99m macroaggregated
albumin (99mTc-MAA—re: nuclear
medicine)

TCMP
Thematic Content Modification Program
(re: Psychol)

Tc-99m-Sn-DTPA
technetium Tc-99m pentetic acid
(pertechnetate reduced by stannous
chloride and chelated by pentetate
[diethylenetriaminepentaacetic
acid]—re: nuclear medicine)

TCN
tetracycline

TCNE
tetracyanoethylene (re: spiro compound
synthesis; in modified Diels-Alder
reactions)

TC̄NM
tumor with node metastasis

TC + NP
throat culture + nasopharyngeal
culture

TCNS
transcutaneous nerve stimulator

T$_{CO_2}$
carbon dioxide, total

TCP
teacher-child-parent (re: Psychol)
technical consulting panels (re: medical
records)
Test of Creative Potential (re: Psychol)
therapeutic class profile
therapeutic continuous penicillin
total circulating protein
tricalcium phosphate
trichlorophenol
tricresyl phosphate (flame retardant,
solvent, sterilizer of certain surgical
instruments)

TC p.
to contain pipet(te) (re: Lab)

TCPO$_2$, TCpO$_2$
transcutaneous (partial) pressure of
oxygen

TCPP
tris(1,3-dichloroisopropyl)phosphate
(flame retardant)

TCR
T-cell reactivity
thalamocortical relay
total cytoplasmic ribosome

T & CrM
type and cross-match (crossmatch)

tcRNA
translation control ribonucleic acid

TCRP
total cellular receptor pool

TCS
T-cell supernatant
total cellular score
total coronary score

Tcs
T-cell (mediating) contact sensitivity

TCSA
tetrachlorosalicylanilide

TCSW
Thinking Creatively With Sounds and
Words (re: psychological testing)

TCT
thrombin clotting time
thyrocalcitonin (calcitonin—calcium
regulator)
transmission computed tomography

Tct
tinctura (L. tincture)

TCU
Test of Concept Utilization (re: Psychol)

TCu
copper T (an intrauterine device)

TCV
thoracic cage volume

TD
tardive dyskinesia
T-cell dependent
temporary disability
teratoma differentiated
terminal device
therapy discontinued
thoracic duct
three times a day
threshold dose

threshold of detectability
threshold of discomfort
thymus dependent (cells)
timed disintegration
tocopherol deficient
to deliver (re: pipet[te]s)
tone decay (re: Audio)
torsion dystonia
total disability
total discrimination
total dose (of radiation)
touch-down (gait)
toxic dose
tracheal diameter
tracking dye
transdermal
transverse diameter
treating distance
tubero-infundibular dopaminergic
tumor dose
typhoid dysentery

TD, T/D
treatment discontinued

TD, Td
tetanus-diphtheria (toxoid—adult)

TD50, TD$_{50}$
median toxic dose

T$_4$(D)
thyroxin(e) measured by displacement
　(analysis)

t.d.
ter die (L. three times daily)

TDA
thyrotropin displacing activity
TSH-(thyroid stimulating hormone)
　displacing antibody

TDC
taurodeoxycholate
total dietary calories

TDD
thoracic duct drainage
total digitalizing dose

TDDA
tetradecadiene acetate (prodlure—
　insect sex attractant)
thoracic duct drainage

TDE
tetrachlorodiphenylethane (larvicide—
　now called 1,1-dichloro-2,2-bis (*p*-
　chlorophenyl)ethane)
time-delayed exponential
total digestible energy
triethylene glycol diglycidyl ether
　(etoglucid— antineoplastic)

TDF
testis-determining factor

Thinking Disturbance Factor (re:
　Psychol)
thoracic duct fistula
thoracic duct flow
time-dose fractionation (factor)
tissue-damaging factor
tris-disrupted fraction
tumor dose fractionation (re:
　radiotherapy)

TDH
total decreased histamine
toxic dose, high

TDI
temperature difference integrator
toluene 2,4-diisocyanate (re:
　manufacture of elastomers; industrial
　chemical)
total-dose infusion
total-dose insulin
triacetyldiphenolisatin (cathartic)

t distribution
(re: statistical sampling distribution)

TDL
thoracic duct lymph
thoracic duct lymphocytes
thymus-dependent lymphocytes
toxic dose, low

TDM
therapeutic drug monitoring
trehalose dimycolate

TDN
total digestible nutrients

t-DNA
transfer deoxyribonucleic acid

TDP
ribothymidine 5′-diphosphate
thermal death point
thoracic duct pressure
thymidine diphosphate

TD p.
to deliver pipet(te) (re: Lab)

TdR
thymidine (thymine-2-desoxyriboside)

TDS
temperature, depth, salinity
temperature-determined sex
thiamine disulfide

t.d.s.
ter die sumendum (L. to be taken three
　times a day)

TDT
tentative discharge tomorrow
thermal death time
tumor-doubling time

TDT, TdT
terminal deoxynucleotidyl transferase
tone decay test (re: Audio)

TDZ
thymus-dependent zone (of lymph
node)

TE
tennis elbow
test ear
tetracycline
threshold energy
thromboembolism
thymus epithelial (cell)
thyrotoxic exophthalmos
time estimation
tissue-equivalent
tonsillectomy
tonsils excised
tooth extracted
total estrogen (excretion)
trace element
tracheoesophageal
transepithelial elimination (terminated)
treadmill exercise
trial (and) error

TE, Te
tetanus

T$_E$
expiratory phase time

T&E
testing and evaluation
training and experience
trial and error

Te
tellurium (element)
tetanic (contraction—re:
electrodiagnosis)

T$_e$
effective half-life

T-e
erythrocyte triiodothyronine

^{132}Te
radioactive isotope of tellurium

TEA
tetraethylammonium (bromide or
chloride—ganglion-blocking agents)
thermal energy analyzer
thromboendarterectomy
transient emboligenic aortoarteritis
transversely excited atmospheric
(pressure)
triethanolamine (alkalizing agent;
intermediate agent in manufacture of
herbicides)

TEAB
tetraethylammonium bromide (ganglion-
blocking agent)

TEAC
tetraethylammonium chloride (ganglion-
blocking agent)

TEAE
triethylaminoethyl

TEAE-cellulose
triethylaminoethyl-substituted cellulose
(re: ion-chromatography)

teasp.
teaspoonful

TEBG, TeBG
testosterone-estradiol-binding globulin

TeBG
testosterone-binding globulin

TEC
total electron count
total (blood) eosinophil count
total exchange capacity (re: resin)
transient erythroblastopenia of
childhood

T&EC
Trauma and Emergency Center

tech.
technical
technician
technique

techn.
technician

TECV
traumatic epiphyseal coxa vara

TED
thromboembolytic disease
tracheoesophageal dysraphism

TED, T.E.D.
Tasks of Emotional Development (test)
threshold erythema dose
thromboembolic disease

TEDs
thromboembolic disease support (hose)

TEE
thermic effect of exercise
tyrosine ethyl ester

TEEM
tanned erythrocyte electrophoretic
mobility

TEEP
tetraethyl pyrophosphate (insecticide;
cholinesterase inhibitor)

TEF
thermic effect of food
tracheo-esophageal fistula

T_{eff}
effective half-life (re: radioisotopes)

TE fist.
tracheo-esophageal fistula

T-E fistula
tracheo-esophageal fistula

TEFS
transmural electrical field stimulation

TEG
thromboelastogram
thromboelastograph
triethyleneglycol (used in air
    disinfection)

TEL
tetraethyl lead (tetraethyllead;
    tetraethylplumbane— toxic if inhaled
    or absorbed through skin)

TELE, Tele, tele.
telemetry

Tele
telephone

TEM
transmission electron microscope
transmission electron microscopy
transverse electromagnetic
triethanolamine
triethylenemelamine (antineoplastic)

Temp, temp.
temperature

temp.
temple
temporal
temporary

temp. dext.
tempori dextro (L. to the right temple)
tempus dextrum (L. the right temple)

temp. sinist.
tempori sinistro (L. to the left temple)
tempus sinistrum (L. the left temple)

TEN
total excretory (or excreted) nitrogen
transepidermal neurostimulation

TEN, T.E.N.
toxic epidermal necrolysis
toxic epidermal necrosis

ten.
tense
tension

tenac.
tenaculum

tend.
tender
tenderness

TENS
transcutaneous electrical nerve stimu-
    lation
transcutaneous electrical nerve stimu-
    lator

tens.
tension

tent.
tentative

tent. diag.
tentative diagnosis

TENVAD
Test of Nonverbal Auditory
    Discrimination

TEP
tetraethylpyrophosphate (insecticide;
    cholinesterase inhibitor)
thromboendophlebectomy
tracheal-esophageal puncture

TEPA
triethylenephosphoramide
    (antineoplastic)

TEPP
tetraethylpyrophosphate (insecticide;
    cholinesterase inhibitor)

TER
total endoplasmic reticulum
transcapillary escape rate
transcapillary escape route

ter
terminal end of a chromosome
    (telomere—re: cytogenetics)

ter.
tere (L. rub)
tertiary

Terleu
tertiary leucine

term.
terminal
terminate
termination

ter. sim.
tere simul (L. rub at the same time
    [together])

tert.
tertiary

TES
(Supervisor-Executive) Tri-Dimensional
    Evaluational Scales
Team Effectiveness Survey (re:
    Psychol)
toxic epidemic syndrome
transcutaneous electrical stimulation
transmural electrical stimulation

TESS
treatment emergent symptom scale

TET
total ejection time
total exchangeable thyroxin(e)
treadmill exercise test

Tet
tetralogy of Fallot

Tet, tet.
tetanus

TETA
triethylenetetramine (chelating agent)
triethylenetetramine dihydrochloride

TETD
tetraethylthiuram disulfide (disulfiram—
    for alcoholism)

tet. tox.
tetanus toxoid

TEV
tadpole edema virus
talipes equinovarus

TEWL
transepidermal water loss

TF
free thyroxin(e)
tactile fremitus
tail-flick (reflex)
temperature factor
tetralogy of Fallot
thymidine factor
thymol flocculation
thymus factor
thymus (transfer) factor
tissue-(damaging) factor
total flow
transfer factor
transformation frequency
transfrontal
tube feeding
tubular fluid

TF, T.F.
tuberculin filtrate

TF, Tf, T$_f$
transferrin

TF, t.f.
to follow
tuning fork

T of F
tetralogy of Fallot

TFA
total fatty acids
transverse fascicular area

TFC
transferrin, common form

TFE
tetrafluoroethylene
    (polytetrafluoroethylene—Teflon)
two-fraction fast exchange

TFF
tube-fed food

Tf-Fe
transferrin-bound ferritin (iron)

TFL
tensor fascia lata

TFM
testicular feminization mutation
total fluid movement
3-trifluoromethyl-4-nitrophenol (lamprey
    killer)

TFM, Tfm
testicular feminization (syndrome)

TFN
total fecal nitrogen
totally functional neutrophil
transferrin

TFP
treponemal false positive

TF/P
tubular fluid plasma

TFPZ
trifluoperazine

TFR
total fertility rate
total flow resistance

TFS
testicular feminization syndrome
thyroid function studies
tube-fed saline

TFT
thrombus formation time
thyroid function test
transfer factor test
trifluorothymidine (antiviral eye drops)

TG
tendon graft

testosterone glucuronide
tetraglycine
thioglycolate broth
thioguanine
thyroglobulin
toxic goiter
Toxoplasma gondii
transmissible gastroenteritis (virus of
   swine)
treated group
trigeminal (neuralgia)
triglycerides
tumor growth

TG, Tg
thyroglobulin

6-TG
thioguanine (2-aminopurine-6-thiol—
   [antineoplastic])

Tg
generation time

Tg, tg
type genus

TGA
taurocholate gelatin agar
thyroglobulin antibody
total glycoalkaloids
total gonadotrop(h)in activity
transient global amnesia
transposition of great arteries
tumor glycoprotein assay

TgAb
thyroglobulin antibody

TGAR
total graft area rejected

TGB
thyroid-binding globulin

TGC
time gain compensation
time gain compensator
time-varied gain control (re: ultrasound)

TGD
thermal green dye
transit gastroduodenal

TGE
theoretical growth evaluation
transmissible gastroenteritis (of swine)
tryptone glucose extract (broth or agar)

TGF
transforming growth factor
tubuloglomerular feedback (re: Uro)
tumor growth factor

TGFA
triglyceride fatty acid

TGF-β
transforming growth factors, type beta

TGG
turkey gamma globulin

TGL
triglyceride lipase
triglycerides

TGP
tobacco glycoprotein

TGR
thioguanosine

6-TGR
thioguanine riboside

T-group
(sensitivity)-training group (re: Psychol)

TGT
thromboplastin generation test
thromboplastin generation time
tolbutamide-glucagon test

TGV
thoracic gas volume
transposition of the great vessels

TGY
tryptone (tryptophan peptone), glucose,
   yeast (agar)

TH
Tamm-Horsefall (mucoprotein)
tetrahydrocortisol
theophylline
thrill
thyrohyoid
thyroid hormone (thyroxin[e])
thyrotropic hormone
topical hypothermia
torcular herophili (re: cranial sinuses)
total hysterectomy

TH, Th, th.
thoracic

T&H
type and hold (re: blood typing)

Th
thenar
therapy
thigh (amputation level, lower limb—re:
   Ortho)
thorium (element)
throat
thyroid

Th, th.
thorax

th
thermie (meter-ton-second system
   basic unit of heat)

THA
total hip arthroplasty
total hydroxyapatite (re: tooth enamel
  and bone)

THA, T.H.A.
1,2,3,4-tetrahydro-5-aminoacridine
  (anticholinesterase; respiratory
  stimulant)

ThA
thoracic aorta

Thal
thalassemia

THAM
tris(hydroxymethyl)aminomethane
  (tromethamine—an alkalizer)

THAN
transient hyperammonemia of newborn

THARIES
total hip arthroplasty with internal
  eccentric shells
total hip articular replacement by
  internal eccentric shells

THb
total (amount of) hemoglobin

THC
tetrahydrocannabinol (active principle of
  marijuana)
tetrahydrocortisone
tetrahydrone E
thiocarbanidin (antibacterial;
  tuberculostatic)
transhepatic cholangiogram
transhepatic cholangiography
transplantable hepatocellular carcinoma
Troisier-Hanot-Chauffard (syndrome)

TH & C
terpin hydrate and codeine

THCCRC
tetrahydrocannabinol cross-reacting
  cannabinoids

THD
transverse heart diameter

Thd
ribothymidine

THDOC
tetrahydrodeoxycorticosterone

THE
tetrahydrocortisone
tonic hind-limb extension (re:
  veterinary)
tropical hypereosinophilia

theor.
theoretical

THER, ther.
therapy

ther.
therapeutic
thermometer

THERAP
therapeutic

ther. ex.
therapeutic exercise

therm.
thermal
thermolite
thermometer

th. ex.
therapeutic exercises

THF
tetrahydrofluorenone (1,2,3,4-
  tetrahydro-9-fluorenone—
  phentydrone; amebicidal; fungistatic)
tetrahydrofolate
tetrahydrofolic (acid)
tetrahydrofuran (a solvent)
thymic humoral factor

THFA
tetrahydrofolic acid
tetrahydrofurfuryl alcohol (solvent)

THF glycol
2,5-tetrahydrofurandimethanol (solvent;
  softener; humectant)

Thg
thyroglobulin

THH
telangiectasia hereditaria
  haemorrhagica

THI, Thi
thiamin

**Thio-TEPA, thio-TEPA, Thiotepa,
thiotepa**
thiotriethylene phosphoramide
  (triethylenethiophosphoramide—
  antineoplastic)

THIP
4,5,6,7-tetrahydroisoxazolo
  [5,4-*c*]pyridin-3-ol
  (re: GABA receptors)

THM
total heme mass

THO
tritiated water

Thor
thoracic (surgery)

Thor, thor.
thoracic
thorax

thou
thousandth of an inch (colloquial term)

THP
tetrahydropapaveroline (re: neurological
   biochemistry)
tissue hydrostatic pressure
total hydroxyproline

THPP
2,4,6-trihydroxypropiophenone
   (flopropione—antispasmodic)

THPP, ThPP
thiamine pyrophosphate

THPV
transhepatic portal vein

THQ
tetroquinone (systemic keratolytic)

THR
total hip replacement
transhepatic resistance

THR, Thr, thr.
threonine

thr.
thrill (re: Cardio)

THRF
thyrotrop(h)ic hormone-releasing factor

throm.
thrombosis
thrombus

Thromb, thromb.
thrombosis
thrombus

THS
tetrahydro-compound S (tetrahydro-11-
   deoxycortisol)

THSC
totipotent hematopoietic stem cell

THTH
thyrotrop(h)ic hormone

THU
tetrahydrouridine

THUG
thyroid uptake gradient

THVO
terminal hepatic vein obliteration

Thy
thymine

thym. turb.
thymol turbidity (obsolete test—re:
   hepatic function)

THz
terahertz (unit of frequency—1 trillion
   Hz—10^{12})

TI
congenital limb absence—tibia,
   complete
temporal integration
terminal ileum
thalassemia intermedia
therapeutic index
thoracic index
threshold of intelligibility
thymus independent (cells)
time interval
tissue invasiveness
translational inhibitor
transverse diameter between ischia
transverse inlet
tricuspid incompetence
tricuspid insufficiency
trunk index

TI, Ti
tumor inducing (plasmid)

T$_I$
inspiratory phase time

Ti
titanium (element)

^{44}Ti
radioactive isotope of titanium

ti
congenital limb absence—tibia,
   incomplete

TIA
transient ischemia attack
transient ischemic attack
tumor-induced angiogenesis
turbidimetric immunoassay

TIAH
totally implanted artificial heart

TIA-IR
transient ischemic attack—incomplete
   recovery

TIAN
Trauma intern admit note

TIB
This I Believe (Test—re: Psychol)

tib.
tibia
tibial

TIBC
total iron-binding capacity

tib.-fib.
tibia-fibula

tib. plat.
tibial plateau

TIC
ticarcillin
trypsin inhibitory capability (assay)
trypsin inhibitory capacity
tumor-inducing complex

TICCC
time interval between cessation of
contraception and conception

TID
time interval difference
titrated initial dose

t.i.d.
ter in die (L. three times a day)

TIDA
tubero-infundibular dopamine

TIE
transient ischemic episode

TIF
tumor-inducing factor
tumor-inhibiting factor

TIFPB
thrombin increasing fibrinopeptide B

TIG, TIg
tetanus immune globulin

TIH
time interval histogram

TIMC
tumor-induced marrow cytotoxicity

TIN
tubulointerstitial nephropathy

t.i.n.
ter in nocte (L. three times nightly; three
times a night)

tinc.
tincture

tinct.
tinctura
tincture

T$_{IND}$, T$_{ind}$
T inducer (cell)

T$_3$ Index
triiodothyroxine index

ting.
tingling

T in m.l.
tongue in midline

TIP
thermal inactivation point
translation-inhibiting protein
tumor-inhibiting principle
tumor insularis pancreatis

Ti plasmid
tumor-inducing plasmid

T.I.P.P.S.
tetraiodophenolphthalein sodium
(diagnostic aid— radiopaque medium
for cholecystograph)

TIR
terminal innervation ratio
total immunoreactive (insulin)

TIS
tetracycline-induced steatosis
transdermal infusion system
trypsin insoluble segment
tumor in situ

TISP
total immunoreactive serum
pepsinogen

TIT
Treponema (*pallidum*) immobilization
test
triiodothyronine

T$_I$/T$_E$
inspiratory-expiratory phase time ratio

TITH, TITh
triiodothyronine

titr.
titrate

TIU
trypsin-inhibiting unit

TIUV
total intrauterine volume (re: OB
ultrasonography)

TIVC
thoracic inferior vena cava

TJ
terajoule (one billion joule—joule: SI
and practical unit of work)
tight junction
triceps jerk
Troell-Junet (syndrome)

Tj antigen
P blood group antigen

TJB
time sharing job (control) block (re:
computers/data processing)

TJR
total joint replacements

TJTA
Taylor-Johnson Temperament Analysis

TK
thymidine kinase
transketolase
Turner-Kieser (syndrome)

TK1
thymidine kinase, soluble

TK2
thymidine kinase, mitochondrial

TKA
total knee arthroplasty
transketolase activity
trochanter, knee, ankle (alignment)

TKD
thymidine kinase deficient
tokodynagraph (re: OB)
tokodynamometer (re: OB)

TKG
tokodynagraph (re: OB)

TKM
thymidine kinase, mitochondrial

TKO
to keep open

TKR
total knee replacement

TKS
thymidine kinase, soluble

TL
team leader
temporal lobe
terminal limen
thermolabile
thermoluminescence
threat to life
thymic (-derived) lymphocyte
thymic lymphoma
thymus leukemia
time lapse
time limited
tolerance level
total lipids
total lung (capacity)

TL. T.L.
tubal ligation

T-L
thymus (-dependent) lymphocyte

Tl
thallium (element)

^{202}Tl
radioactive isotope of thallium

^{204}Tl
radioactive isotope of thallium

TLA
tissue lactase activity
translaryngeal aspiration
translumbar aortogram

TLAA
T lymphocyte-associated antigen

TLAC
Test of Listening Accuracy in Children
    (formerly called Picture Speech
    Discrimination Test)

T lam.
thoracic laminectomy

TL antigen
thymus-leukemia antigen

TLC
tender loving care
thin-layer chromatography
total L-chain concentration
total lung capacity
total lung compliance
total lymphocyte count

TLD
thermoluminescent dose
thermoluminescent dosimeter
thermoluminescent dosimetry
thoracic lymph duct
tumor lethal dose

T/LD$_{100}$
minimum dose which will cause
    malformation or death of 100% of
    fetuses

TLE
temporal lobe epilepsy
thin-layer electrophoresis
total lipid extract

TLI
thymidine-labeling index
tonic labyrinthine inverted
total lymphoid irradiation
Totman's Loss Index
trypsin-like immunoactivity

TLMO
truncated localized molecular orbital
    (method)

TLQ
total living quotient

TLR
tonic labyrinthine reflex

TLSO
thoracolumbosacral orthosis

TLSSO
thoracolumbosacral spinal orthosis

TLT
tryptophan load test

TLU
table look-up (re: computers)

TLV
threshold limit value (re: contaminants
allowed in clean air in factories and
work places)
total lung volume

TLV-STEL
threshold limit value-short-term
exposure limit (re: contaminants
allowed in clean air in factories and
work places)

TLV-TWA
threshold limit value-time-weighted
average (re: contaminants allowed in
clean air in factories and work places)

TLX
trophoblast/lymphocyte cross-reactive
(antigens)

T lymphocyte
thrombocyte-derived lymphocyte (T
cell)

TM
tectorial membrane (re: Neuro)
temperature by mouth
temporalis muscle
temporomandibular
tender midline
teres major (muscle)
term milk
thalassemia major
time-motion (technique)
tobramycin
trademark
transmediastinal
transmetatarsal
transport mechanism
transport messenger
tropical medicine
tubular myelin
tumor
tympanic membrane
tympanometric

TM, T-M
Thayer-Martin (medium)

TM, Tm
transport medium (re: biochemistry/
biology)

TM, Tm, T$_m$
maximal tubular excretory capacity (of
kidney)

T & M
type and crossmatch

Tm
maximum tubular clearance (of kidney)
muscle temperature
thulium (element)
tumor-bearing mice

T_m, t_m
temperature midpoint (Kelvin)

tM
time required to complete M phase of
the cell cycle

t_m
temperature midpoint, Celsius

t.m.
true mean (re: statistics)

TMA
tetramethylammonium
thrombotic microangiopathy
thyroid microsomal antibody
transmetatarsal amputation
trimethoxyamphetamine (hallucinogen)
trimethylamine

TMAb
thyroid microsomal antibody

TMAI
tetramethylammonium iodide
(emergency disinfectant for drinking
water)

TMAS
Taylor Manifest Anxiety Scale

T$_{max}$
time of maximum concentration

TMCA
trimethylcolchicinic acid

TMD
1,1,10-trimethyl-*trans*-2-decalol
(cholinesterase biosynthesis inhibitor)

TME
Technische Mass Einheit (Ger.
Engineering Mass Unit)
total metabolizable energy
transmissible mink encephalopathy
transmural enteritis

TMF
transformed mink fibroblast (cell line)

Tm$_G$, TmG, Tm (g)
maximum tubular glucose (reabsorptive
capacity)

TMI
Test of Motor Impairment
transmural myocardial infarction

TMIF
tumor-cell migratory inhibition factor

TMJ
temporomandibular joint

TMJ-PDS
temporomandibular joint-pain
  dysfunction syndrome

TMJS
temporomandibular joint syndrome

TM jt.
temporomandibular joint

TML
terminal motor latency
tetramethyl lead
tongue in midline

TML, T/ML
tender midline

TMM
tonometer, Mackay-Marg (electronic
  applanation tonometer—re: Ophth)

TMP
ribothymidine 5′-phosphate
terminal monitor program (re:
  computers/data processing)
thymidine monophosphate (thymidine
  5′-monophosphate)
thymine ribonucleoside-5′-phosphate
  (ribothymidylic acid)
thymolphthalein (pH indicator)
transmembrane potential
transmembrane (hydrostatic) pressure
trimethoprim (antibacterial)
4,5′,8-trimethylpsoralen (trioxalen—
  photosensitizer— re: pigment)

TmPAH, Tm$_{PAH}$
maximum tubular excretory capacity for
  para-aminohippurate

TMPD
tetramethyl-p-phenylenediamine
  (Wurster's reagent; Wurster's blue)

TMPDS
thiamine monophosphate disulfide
  (thiamine disulfide— enzyme co-
  factor vitamin)

TMP-SMX
trimethoprim-sulfamethoxazole
  (antibiotic)

TMR
tissue maximum ratio
topical magnetic resonance

trainable mentally retarded (re:
  psychological testing)

TMS
thallium myocardial scintigraphy
ton meter second (metric system)

TMST
treadmill stress test

TMT
tarsometatarsal (re: podiatry)

Tmt, tmt.
treatment

TMTC
too many to count

TMTD
tetramethylthiuram disulfide (thiram—
  topical antifungal)

TMU
tetramethylurea (solvent; reagent)

TMV
tobacco mosaic virus
tracheal mucous velocity

TMZ
transformation zone

TN
talonavicular
tarsonavicular
team nursing
temperature normal
total negatives
transport (medium)
trigeminal nucleus
trochlear nucleus
true negative

TN, Tn
normal intraocular tension

T/N
tar and nicotine

T$_4$N
normal serum thyroxin(e)

Tn
thoron (radon-220—antineoplastic)
transposon (re: bacterial genetics)

TNC
too numerous to count

TND
term normal delivery

TNEE
titrated norepinephrine excretion

Tn element
transposon (re: bacterial genetics)

TNF
2,4,7-trinitrofluorenone (used in
photocopiers—re: study of employee
exposure)
true negative fraction
tumor necrosis factor

TNG
tongue
toxic nodular goiter
trinitroglycerol (nitroglycerin—coronary
vasodilator)

Tng
training

TNH
transient neonatal hyperammonemia

TNI
total nodal irradiation

TNM
tetranitromethane (proposed irritant war
gas)
thyroid node metastasis
tumor, node, metastasis (NOTE: see
appendix for specific areas of
involvement)

TNMR
tritium nuclear magnetic resonance

TNP
total net positive

TNR
tonic neck reflex
true negative rate

TNS
total nuclear score
transcutaneous nerve stimulation
tumor necrosis serum

tns.
tension

tnsn.
tension

TNT
tetranitro blue tetrazolium
2,4,6-trinitrotoluene (an explosive—
toxic when ingested, inhaled, or
absorbed through skin)

TNTC, t.n.t.c.
too numerous to count

t number
photographic lens stop setting (re: light
transmission)

TNV
tobacco necrosis virus

TO
target organ
Theiler's Original (re: mouse
encephalomyelitis virus)
thoracic orthosis
thrown off
thrown out (re: motor vehicle accident)
total obstruction
transfer out
tuberculin ober (supernatant portion)
tubo-ovarian
turned on
turnover (number)

TO, T.O.
original tuberculin (old)

TO, T.O., T/O, t.o.
telephone order

TO, T-O
trachelotomy and oophorectomy

TO, T(O)
temperature, oral

TO, to
tinctura opii (L. tincture of opium)

TO$_2$
oxygen transport rate

TOA
Tuberculin-Original-Alt
tubo-ovarian abscess

TOAP
thioguanine, Oncovin (vincristine),
cytosine arabinoside (cytarabine),
and prednisone (re: chemotherapy)

TOB
tobramycin

TOBE
Tests of Basic Experiences (re:
psychological testing)

TOBE 2
Tests of Basic Experiences, 2nd Edition
(re: psychological testing)

TobRV
tobacco ringspot virus

TOC
test of cure
total organic carbon

TOCP
tri-o-cresyl phosphate (triorthocresyl
phosphate; tri-o-tolyl phosphate—
highly toxic)

TOD
tension of oculus dexter
time of day (re: computers/data
processing)

TOF
tetralogy of Fallot

TOIT
Tien Organic Integrity Test

TOL
trial of labor

TOL, tol.
tolerated

tol.
tolerance
tolerate

tolb.
tolbutamide

TOLD
Test of Language Development

tomo.
tomogram

TONAR
the oral-to-nasal acoustic ratio

tonoc.
tonight (a hybrid term)

tonoct.
tonight (a hybrid term)

TOP
temporal, occipital, parietal
termination of pregnancy
Test Orientation Procedure (re: Psychol)
tissue oncotic pressure
transovarial passage (transovarian)
tri-o-cresyl phosphate (tri-o-tolyl
    phosphate—manufacturing chemical;
    toxic if ingested)

top.
topical
topically

TOPOSS
Tests of Perception of Scientists and
    Self (re: Psychol)

TOPV
trivalent oral poliovirus vaccine

TORCH
toxoplasmosis, other (viruses), rubella,
    cytomegalovirus, herpes (simplex
    viruses)

TORCHS
toxoplasmosis, other (viruses), rubella,
    cytomegalovirus, herpes (viruses),
    syphilis

TORP
total ossicular reconstruction prosthesis
    (re: ENT)

total ossicular replacement prosthesis
    (re: ENT)

TOS
tape operating system (re: computers)
tension of oculus sinister
thoracic outlet syndrome

tosyl-
tolylsulfonyl-

tot.
total

TOTPAR
total pain relief

tot. prot.
total protein

TOV
thrombosed oral varix
trial of voiding

t.o.w.
to other ward

TOWER
Testing, Orientation and Work
    Evaluation for Rehabilitation

Tox, tox.
toxicity

tox.
toxic
toxicology
toxin

TP
posterior tibial
temperature and pressure
temperature probe
temporal peak
terminal phalanx
testosterone propionate
tetanus-pertussis
thickly padded
threshold potential
thrombocytopenic purpura
thrombophlebitis
thymic polypeptide
thymidine phosphorylase
thymus protein
tissue pressure
toilet paper
total positives
total protein
trailing pole
transforming principle (re: bacteriology)
transition point
transpyloric
transverse polarization
transverse process
Treponema pallidum
trigonal prism
triosephosphate

true positive
tryptophan
tuberculin precipitation
tuberculosis pulmonum (L. tuberculosis
  of the lungs)

TP, T-P
temporoparietal

T & P, T + P
temperature and pulse

6-TP
6-thiopurine

Tp
tampon

T_p
physical half-life

+ = PA (cardio vascular)

TPA
tannic acid, polyphosphomolybdic acid,
  amido acid (staining technique)
12-*O*-tetradecanoylphorbol-13-acetate
  (a phorbol diester— co-carcinogen)
tissue plasminogen activator
tissue polypeptide antigen
total parenteral alimentation
total phobic anxiety
Treponema pallidum agglutination (test)
tumor (-derived) polypeptide antigen

TPAL
total pregnancies, abortions, and living
  (children)

TPB
tryptone phosphate broth

TPBF
total pulmonary blood flow

TPC
telopeptide-poor collagen
thromboplastic plasma component
  (Factor XIII)
thromboplastin plasma component
time-to-pulse-height converter
total plasma catecholamines
total plasma cholesterol
treatment planning conference
Treponema pallidum complement
  (fixation test)

TPCC
Treponema pallidum cryolysis
  complement

TPCF, TPC(F)
Treponema pallidum complement
  fixation (test)

TPCV
total packed cell volume

TPD
temporary partial disability

thiamine propyl disulfide (enzyme
  cofactor vitamin)
tumor-producing dose

TPE
therapeutic plasma exchange
total protected environment
typhoid-paratyphoid enteritis

T^{Pe}
expiratory pause time

t. pedis
tinea pedis (athlete's foot)

TPEY
tellurite polymyxin egg yolk (agar)

TPF
thymus permeability factor
time to peak flow
trained participating father
true positive fraction

TPG
therapeutic play group
transmembrane potential gradient
transplacental gradient
tryptophan-peptone-glucose (broth)

TPH
trained participating husband
transplacental hemorrhage

TPHA
Treponema pallidum hemagglutination
  (test)

TPI
time period integrator
treponemal immmobilization (test
  [cardiolipin]
Treponema pallidum-immobilization
  (test)
triose phosphate isomerase
  (triosephosphate isomerase)

TPI1
triosephosphate isomerase-1

TPI2
triosephosphate isomerase-2

T^{Pi}
inspiratory pause time

TPIA
Treponema pallidum immobilization
  (immune) adherence
Treponema pallidum immune
  adherence (test)

TPM
temporary pacemaker
thrombophlebitis migrans
total particulate matter
triphenylmethane
trophopathia pedis myelodysplastica

TPN
thalamic projection neurons
total parenteral nutrition
triphosphopyridine nucleotide

TPNH
triphosphopyridine nucleotide, reduced
   (small hydrogen carrier protein; TPN
   is former name for nicotinamide
   adenine dinucleotide phosphate—
   NADP)

TPP
thiamin(e) pyrophosphate
   (diphosphothiamine)
transpulmonary pressure
triphenyl phosphate (manufacturing
   chemical)

TP & P
time, place, and person

TPR
temperature, pulse, respirations
testosterone production rate
total peripheral resistance
total pulmonary resistance
true positive rat (probability)

TPRI
total peripheral resistance index

TPS
trypsin
tumor polysaccharide substance

TPST
true positive stress test

TPT
tetraphenyl tetrazolium (a histological
   stain)
time-to-peak tension
total protein tuberculin
treadmill performance test
typhoid-paratyphoid (vaccine)

TPTHS
total parathyroid hormone secretion
   (rate)

TPTX
thyroid-parathyroidectomized

TPTX, T-PTX
thyroparathyroidectomy

TPTZ
2,3,5-triphenyl-2H-tetrazolium chloride
   (reagent)
tripyridyltriazine (2,4,6-
   tripyridyltriazine—reagent in
   analytical chemistry)

TPV
tetanus-pertussis vaccine

TPVR
total peripheral vascular resistance
total pulmonary vascular resistance

TPZ
thioproperazine (anti-emetic,
   neuroleptic)

TQ
time questionnaire
tocopherolquinone (tocopherylquinone)
tourniquet

TR
teaching and research
tetrazolium reduction
therapeutic radiology
timed release
total repair
total resistance
total response
trachea
transfusion reaction
tricuspid regurgitation (re: Cardio)
tuberculin R (new tuberculin)
tuberculin residuum
tubular reabsorption (re: Uro)
turbidity reducing (units)
turnover rate

TR, T.R.
tuberculin residue

TR, T(R)
temperature, rectal

TR, Tr, tr.
tinctura (L. tincture)

T$_R$
Triassic (re: geologic time division)

T & R
tenderness and rebound

T or R
tenderness or rebound

Tr
transferrin
trypsin

Tr, tr.
trace
transfer

tr
triradial (re: cytogenetics)

t$_r$
radiologic half-life

tr.
traction
trauma
treatment
tremor

TRA
transaldolase
tumor-resistant antigen

Tr^a antigen
low frequency blood group antigen

TRAb
thyrotrophin receptor antibody

Trach, trach.
tracheotomy

trach.
trachea
tracheostomy
trachoma

trach. asp.
tracheal aspiration

tract.
traction

train.
training

TRAJ
time repetitive ankle jerk

TRAM
Treatment Rating Assessment Matrix
Treatment Response Assessment
 Matrix
Treatment Response Assessment
 Method

trans.
transaction
transfer
transferred
transilluminate
transverse

trans-
stereochemical opposite of *cis-*

trans D, trans. d.
transverse diameter

transm.
transmission

transpl.
transplant
transplantation

trans. sec.
transverse section

trans. sect.
transverse section

transv. proc.
transverse process

TRAP
tartrate-resistant acid phosphatase

trap.
trapezius (muscle)

TRAS
transplant renal artery stenosis

trau.
trauma
traumatic

TRB
terbutaline

TRBF
total renal blood flow

TRC
tanned red cell
therapeutic residential center
total respiratory conductance
total ridge count

TRCA
tanned red cell agglutination

TRCH
tanned red cell hemagglutination
 (inhibition test)

TRCHII
tanned red cell hemagglutination
 inhibition immunoassay

TRCV
total red-cell volume

TRD
tongue-retaining device

TRE
thymic reticuloepithelial
true radiation emission

TREA
thoroughness, reliability, efficiency,
 analytic (ability)

treat.
treatment

TREES
time-resolved europium excitation
 spectroscopy

trem.
trembling

tremb.
trembling

Trend
Trendelenburg (position)

Trep
Treponema (genus)

TRF
T cell replacing factor

thyrotrop(h)in-releasing factor
tubular rejection fraction

TRFC
total rosette-forming cell

trg.
training

TRGI
Teacher's Reading Global Improvement

TRH
tension-reducing hypothesis
thyrotrop(h)in-releasing hormone

TRI
tetrazolium reduction inhibition
total response index (re: Psychol)
trichloroethylene (trichloroethene—an
    analgesic; inhalation anesthetic)

tri.
triceps

T3RIA
triiodothyronine radioimmunoassay

TRIAC, Triac
triiodothyroacetic acid

TRIC
trachoma inclusion conjunctivitis
    (agent)
trachoma inclusion and conjunctivitis

Trich, trich.
Trichomonas (genus)

TRIC ophthalmia neonatorum
(Chlamydia) trachomatis inclusion
    conjunctivitis ophthalmia neonatorum

trid.
triduum (L. three days)

TRIG, Trig, trig.
triglycerides

trig.
trigger
trigonal

trig. pnt.
trigger point

trig. pt.
trigger point

TRIS, tris
tris(hydroxymethyl)aminomethane
    (trometamol; tromethamine—an
    alkalizer)

Tris-BP
tris(2,3-dibromopropyl)phosphate
    (flame retardant)

TRIT
triiodothyronine
trithyronine

TRIT, trit.
tritura (L. triturate)

trityl-
triphenylmethyl-

TRK
transketolase

TRML
terminal

TRN
tegmental reticular nucleus (re: Neuro)

tRNA
transfer ribonucleic acid

TRO
tissue reflectance oximeter
to return to office

TROCA
tangible reinforcement operant
    conditioning audiometry

TROCH, troch.
trochiscus (Gr. trokhiskos—a small
    wheel [a lozenge, troche])

troch.
trochanter

Trol
troland (re: retinal illumination)

Trop Med
tropical medicine

TRP
Tactical Reproduction Pegboard
total refractory period
tubular reabsorption of phosphate

Trp, trp.
tryptophan (and its radicals)

TRPA
tryptophan-rich prealbumin

TrPl
treatment plan

TRPT
theoretical renal phosphorus threshold

TRRP
Thackray Reading Readiness Profile

TRS
total reducing sugars
tuberculosis record system
tubuloreticular structure

TrS
traumatic surgery

TRSV
tobacco ringspot virus

TRT
total reading time

TRT, trt.
treatment

TRU
turbidity reducing unit

T₃RU
triiodothyronine resin uptake (test)

TRV
tobacco rattle virus

TRY, Try
tryptophan (obsolete abbreviation; now Trp or L-Trp)

Tryp
tryptophan (obsolete abbreviation; now Trp or L-Trp)

TRX, trx
traction

trx
treatments

TS
Tay-Sachs (disease)
temperature sensitive
temporal stem
tensile strength
terminal (or greater) sensation
thermostable
thoracic surgery
tissue space
tocopherol supplemented
toe signs
total solids
Tourette syndrome
toxic substance
tracheal sound
tracheal spirals
transitional sleep
transsexual
transverse section
transverse sinus
transverse (tubular) system
treadmill score
trichostasis spinulosa
tricuspid stenosis
triple strength
tropical sprue
tuberous sclerosis
tubular (tracheal) sound
tumor specific
type-specific (antibodies)

TS, T.S.
test solution

TS, T/S
thyroid:serum (radioiodide ratio)

T.S.
thymidylate synthetase

Ts
skin temperature
tosylate

T$_s$
T suppressors (cells)

tS
time required to complete the S phase of the cell cycle

TSA
technical surgical assistance
Test of Syntactic Ability
p-toluenesulfonic acid (test)
Total Severity Assessment
total solute absorption
trypticase soy agar
tumor-specific antigen
tumor-surface antigen
tumor-susceptible antigen
type-specific antibody

T₄SA
thyroxin(e)-specific activity

TSab
thyroid-stimulating antibody

Tsaph
temperature in the saphenous vein

TSAT
tube slide agglutination test

TSB
total serum bilirubin
trypticase soy broth

TSBA
total serum bile acids

TSBB
transtracheal selective bronchial brushing

TSBC
Time-Sample Behavioral Checklist

TSC
technetium sulfur colloid
thiosemicarbazide (reagent; tuberculostatic—re: metal detection)
thiosemicarbazone (compound containing thiosemicarbazide radical; tuberculostatic)
time-sharing control (task—re: computers/data processing)

total static compliance
tryptose-sulfite cyclosterone (agar)

TSCS
Tennessee Self-Concept Scale (re:
    psychological testing)

TSD
target skin distance
Tay-Sachs disease
theory of signal detectability
theory of signal detection

TSE
testicular self-examination
trisodium edetate

T sect., T-sect.
transverse (cross) section

TSEM
transmission scanning electron
    microscopy

TSES
Target Symptom Evaluation Scale

T-set
tracheotomy set

TSF
thrombopoietic-stimulating factor
tissue-coding factor
total systemic flow
triceps skin fold
triceps skin-fold (thickness)
T-suppressor factor

TSG
Touraine-Solente-Golé (syndrome)

TSG(P)
tumor-specific glycoprotein

TSH
thyroid-stimulating hormone (also
    thyrotropin)
thyrotropic-stimulating hormone

TSH-RF
thyroid-stimulating hormone-releasing
    factor

TSH-RH
thyroid-stimulating hormone-releasing
    hormone

TSI
Test of Social Inferences (re: Psychol)
thyroid-stimulating immunoglobulins
triple sugar (lactose, glucose, sucrose)
    iron (agar)

TSIA
total small intestinal allotransplantation
triple sugar iron agar

TSL
terminal sensory latency

TSM
type-specific M (protein)

ts mutation
temperature-sensitive mutation

TSN
tryptophan peptone sulfide neomycin
    (agar)

TSO
time-sharing option (re: computers/data
    processing)

TSP
thrombin-sensitive protein
thyroid-stimulating (hormone of the
    anterior) pituitary
total serum protein
total suspended particulate
tribasic sodium phosphate (industrial
    chemical)

tsp.
teaspoon
teaspoonful

TSPA
thiophosphoramide (Thiotepa)

TSPAP
total serum prostatic acid phosphatase

TSPP
tetrasodium pyrophosphate (industrial
    chemical)

TSR
testosterone-sterilized (female) rat
theophylline-sustained release
thyroid-serum ratio
total systemic resistance
transient situational reaction

TSRBC
trypsinized sheep red blood cell

TSS
toxic shock syndrome
tropical splenomegaly syndrome

TSSA
tumor-specific (cell) surface antigen

TSSE
toxic shock syndrome exotoxin

TSSU
(operating) theater sterile supply unit

TST
thromboplastin screening test
total sleep time
transition state theory

treadmill stress test(ing)
tumor skin test

TSTA
toxoplasmin skin test antigen
tumor-specific transplantation antigen

T state
tension state

T-strain mycoplasma
a strain forming especially tiny colonies

TSU
triple sugar urea (agar)

TSV
total stomach volume

TSY
trypticase soy yeast

TT
tablet triturate
tactile tension (of eye)
talking task
tendon transfer
terminal transferase
test tube
tetanus toxoid
tetrathionate (broth)
tetrazol
thrombin time
thymol turbidity (obsolete test of hepatic
    function)
tibial tubercle
tibial tuberosity
tilt table
tine test
token test
tolerance test
tooth, treatment of
total thyroxin(e)
total time
transferred to
transit time (of blood through heart and
    lungs)
transthoracic
transtracheal
tuberculin tested
tube thoracostomy
tumor thrombus
turnover time

T&T
time and temperature
touch and tone

TT₄
total thyroxin(e)

(no)T or T
(no) thrust or thrill (re: Cardio)

TTA
tetanus toxoid antibody
timed therapeutic absence

transtracheal aspirates
transtracheal aspiration

TTBV
total trabecular bone volume

TTC
triphenyltetrazolium chloride (red
    tetrazolium—reagent and industrial
    chemical)

TTCT
Torrance Tests of Creative Thinking

TTD
temporary total disability
tetraethylthiuram disulfide (disulfiram—
    alcohol deterrent)
tissue tolerance dose
transient tic disorder
transverse thoracic diameter

TTF
time to failure

TTFD
thiamine tetrahydrofurfuryl disulfide
    (enzyme cofactor vitamin)

TTGA
tellurite-taurocholate-gelatin agar

TTH
thyrotrop(h)ic hormone
tritiated thymidine

TTI
tension-time index
time-tension index
transtracheal insufflation

TTL
total thymic lymphocyte
transistor-transistor logic (re: logic
    circuitry)

TTLC
true total lung capacity

TTMS
tetraethylthiuram monosulfide (sulfiram;
    ectoparasiticide—re: veterinary)

TTN
transient tachypnea of newborn

TTNA
transthoracic needle aspiration

TTNB
transthoracic needle (aspiration) biopsy

TTO
to take out

TTP
ribothymidine 5′-triphosphate
thrombotic thrombocytopenia purpura

thrombotic thrombocytopenic purpura
thymidine triphosphate (dTTP;
　　thymidine 5′-triphosphate)
time to peak (flow)
tritolyl phosphate

TTPA
triethylenethiophosphoramide
　　(Thiotepa—antineoplastic)

TTR
transthoracic resistance
triceps tendon reflex
type-to-token ratio

TTS
temporary threshold shift
tilt-table standing
transdermal therapeutic system

TTT
thymol turbidity test (obsolete test of
　　hepatic function)
tolbutamide tolerance test
total twitch time

TTTT
test tube turbidity test

TTV
tracheal transport velocity
transfusion transmitted virus

TTX
tetrodotoxin (toxin from ovaries and liver
　　of many species of *Tetraodontidae,*
　　especially the globe fish)

TTY
teletypewriter (equipment)

TU
thiouracil
thyroidal uptake
Todd units
transurethral
turbidity unit

TU, T.U.
toxic unit
toxin unit
tuberculin unit

TU, T.U., Tu
transmission unit (formerly used—now
　　called decibel)

T₃U
triiodothyronine (resin) uptake (test)

TUB
tubo-uterine (junction)

tuberc.
tuberculosis

TUD
total urethral discharge

TUG
total urinary gonadotropin

TUI
transurethral incision

TUPI
total ulcerous pathology index (of
　　prostate)

T₃ uptake
triiodothyronine uptake

T₄ uptake
thyroxin(e) uptake

TUR
transurethral resection (re: prostate)

tur.
turgor

TURB
transurethral resection, bladder

turb.
turbid
turbidity
turbinate

TURBT
transurethral resection of bladder tumor

turg.
turgor

TURP
transurethral resection, prostate

turp.
turpentine

TUS
take-up strap

tus.
tussis (L. a cough)

tuss.
tussis (L. a cough)

TV
talipes varus (re: Ortho)
television
tetrazolium violet
thoracic vertebrae
tickborne virus
tidal volume
total volume
toxic vertigo
transfer vehicle
transvenous
transvestite
trial visit
Trichomonas vaginalis
trichomoniasis vaginitis
tricuspid valve (apparatus)
trivalent

true vertebra
truncal vagotomy
tuberculin volutin
tubulovesicular
typhus vaccine

TVA
truncal vagotomy plus antrectomy

TVC
third ventricle cyst
timed ventilatory capacity
timed vital capacity (re: Resp)
total viable cells
total volume capacity
transvaginal cone
triple voiding cystogram
true vocal cords

TVD
transmissible virus dementia
triple vessel disease

TVDALV
triple vessel disease with an abnormal
    left ventricle

TVF
tactile vocal fremitus

TVG
time-varied gain (control—re:
    ultrasound)

TVH
total vaginal hysterectomy
turkey virus hepatitis

TVL
tenth value layer (re: radiation)
tunica vasculosa lentis (re: fetal eye)

TVP
tensor veli palatini (re: ENT)
textured vegetable proteins
transvenous pacemaker
tricuspid valve prolapse
truncal vagotomy plus pyloroplasty

TV pacemaker
transvenous pacemaker

TVR
tonic vibration reflex
tricuspid valve replacement

T$_2$VR, TVr$_2$
example of thoracic ventral root nerve
    by number

TVT
transmissible venereal tumor
tunica vaginalis testis

TVU
total volume urine (in 24 hours)

TW
tap water
terminal web
Thibierge-Weissenbach (syndrome)
thymic weight
total (body) water

TWA
time-weighted average

Twb
wet bulb temperature

TWBC
total white blood cells

TWCS
Test of Work Competency and Stability
    (re: Psychol)

TWE
tap water enema
tepid water enema

TWHW ok
toe walking and heel walking ok (all
    right)

TWIS
treatment write-in scale

TWL
transepidermal water loss

TWSb
"antimony dimercaptosuccinate"
    (stibocaptate)

TX
a derivative of contagious tuberculin
thromboxane
thyroidectomy

TX, Tx
transplantation

TX, Tx, tx
treatment

T & X
type and crossmatch

Tx
therapy
transfusion

Tx, tx, tx.
traction

TxA
thromboxane A

TXA$_2$
thromboxane A$_2$ (re: platelets)

TXB$_2$
thromboxane B$_2$ (stable metabolite of
    TXA$_2$)

T & Xmatch
type and crossmatch (cross-match)

Ty
thyroxin(e)
type
typhoid

ty elements
transposon-yeast elements (re:
    genetics)

Tymp
tympanicity (re: auscultation of chest)
tympanitic

Tymp, tymp.
tympany

tymp.
tympanic

tymp. memb.
tympanic membrane

TYMV
turnip yellow mosaic virus

***ty-neg* OCA**
tyrosinase-negative oculocutaneous
    albinism

typ.
typical

***ty-pos* OCA**
tyrosinase-positive oculocutaneous
    albinism

TYR
iodinated tyrosine

Tyr, tyr
tyrosine (and its radicals)

Tyr-Gly-Gly-Phe-Leu
L-tyrosylglycylglycyl-L-phenylalanyl-L-
    leucine) (leu-5-enkephalin—
    pentapeptide)

Tyr-Gly-Gly-Phe-Met
L-tyrosylglycylglycyl-L-phenylalanyl-L-
    methionine) (met-5-enkephalin—
    pentapeptide)

TyRIA
thyroid radioisotope assay

TYS
sclerotylosis

TZ, Tz
tuberculin zymoplastic

TZn
total estrogens after Zn-HCl treatment

U

U
congenital limb absence—ulnar, complete
international unit (of enzyme activity; International Union of Biochemistry unit)
kilurane (1000 radium units—re: radioactivity unit)
ulcus (L. ulcer)
ulnar
umbilicus
unable
uncertain
unerupted (re: Dent)
units (products—re: Psychol; Aptitudes Research Project testing within structure of intellect model)
university
unknown
upper
uracil
uranium (element)
uridine
uridine in polymers
urinary concentration (when followed by subscripts)
urine
urologist
urology
Urtica (genus)
utendus (L. to be used)
uterus
uvula

U, U., u
unit

U, u.
ulna
urea
urethra

U/2
upper one-half (re: long bone)

U/3
upper third (re: long bones)

UII
uranium II (uranium-234)

234U
uranium-234 (uranium II)

235U
uranium-235

238U
uranium-238

u
congenital limb absence—ulnar, incomplete
symbol sometimes used for micron
unified atomic mass unit

UA
Ulex agglutinin
ultra-audible (sound)
ultrasonic arteriogram
umbilical artery
unaggregated
unrelated (children raised) apart
unstable angina
upper airway
upper arm
urethra
uridylic acid
urinary aldosterone
urine aliquot
urocanic acid
uronic acid
user area (re: computers)
uterine aspiration

UA, U/A
uric acid

UA, U/A, Ua
urinalysis

u.a.
usque ad (L. up to; as far as)

UAA
uracil, adenine, adenine (a termination codon in protein synthesis—re: genetics)

UAC
umbilical artery catheter

UA/C
uric acid-creatinine (ratio)

UAE
unilateral absence of excretion

u.a.f.
ut aliquid fiat (L. that something be done)

UAG
uracil, adenine, guanine (a termination

codon in protein synthesis—re: genetics)

UAI
uterine activity interval

UAN
uric acid nitrogen

UAO
upper airway obstruction

UAP
unstable angina pectoris
urinary alkaline phosphate

UAR
upper airway resistance
uric acid riboside

UAS
upper abdominal surgery

UASA
upper airway sleep apnea

UAU
uterine activity unit

UB
ultimobranchial (body—re: embryology)
urinary bladder

UB, Ub
upper back

UBBC
unsaturated (vitamin) B_{12}-binding capacity

UBF
uterine blood flow

UBG
ultimobranchial glands (re: embryology)

UBG, Ubg
urobilinogen

UBI
ultraviolet blood irradiation

UBIP
ubiquitous immunopoietc polypeptide

UBL
undifferentiated B-cell lymphoma

Ubn
urobilin (urohematin)

UBP
ureteral back pressure

UC
ulcerative colitis
ultracentrifugal
umbilical cholesterol
umbilical cord

unchanged
unclassifiable
unconscious
unfixed cryostat
unsatisfactory condition
untreated cell
urea clearance
urethral catheter
urethral catheterization
urinary catheter
uterine contractions

UC, U/C
urine culture

U & C
urethral and cervical
usual and customary

UCB
unconjugated bilirubin

UCBC
umbilical cord blood culture

UCB orthosis
University of California, Berkeley orthosis (re: Ortho)

UCBR
unconjugated bilirubin

UCD
urine collection device
usual childhood diseases

UCD s̄ seq.
usual childhood diseases without sequelae

UCE
urea cycle enzymopathy

UCG
ultrasonic cardiography
urinary chorionic gonadotrop(h)in

UCHD
usual childhood diseases

UCI
urethral catheter in
urinary catheter in
usual childhood illnesses

UCL
ulna collateral ligament
uncomfortable listening level
uncomfortable loudness (sound level)
upper confidence limit (re: statistics)

UCL, U Cl
urea clearance (test)

UCO
urethral catheter out
urinary catheter out

UCP
urinary coproporphyrin
urinary C peptide

UCPP
urethral closure pressure profile

UCPT
urinary coproporphyrin test

UCR
unconditioned reflex
unconditioned response
usual, customary, and reasonable

UCRP
Universal Control Reference Plasma

UCS
unconditioned stimulus
universal character set (re: computers/
data processing)

UCS, Ucs
unconscious

UCT
unchanged conventional treatment

UCU
Urinary Care Unit

UCV
ulcus cruris varicosum
uncontrolled variable

UD
ulcerative dermatosis
ulnar deviation
underdeveloped
undesirable discharge
unit dose
urethral discharge
urethral drainage
uridine diphosphate
urinary drainage
uroporphyrinogen decarboxylase
uterine delivery

u.d.
ut dictum (L. as directed)

UDC
undeveloped countries
usual diseases of childhood

UDCA
ursodeoxycholic acid

UDMH
unsym-dimethylhydrazine (rocket fuel
formulation base; convulsant poison)

UDO
undetermined origin

UDP
uridine 5′-diphosphate (uridine 5′-
pyrophosphate)

UDPAG
uridine-5-diphospho-*N*-
acetylglucosamine

UDPG
uridine diphosphate glucose (uridine 5′-
diphosphoglucose)

UDPGA
uridine diphosphate glucuronic acid

UDPGal, UDP-Gal, UDPgal
uridine diphosphate galactose (uridine
5′-diphosphogalactose)

UDP-galactose
uridine diphosphogalactose

UDP-Glc, UDP-glc
uridine diphosphate glucose (uridine 5′-
diphosphoglucose)

UDP-GlcUA
uridine diphosphoglucuronic acid

UDP-glucose
uridine 5′-diphosphoglucose (uridine
diphosphoglucose)

UDP-glucuronate
uridine diphosphoglucuronate

UDPGT
uridine diphosphoglucuronyl transferase

UdR
uracil deoxyriboside (deoxyuridine)

UDS
unscheduled deoxyribonucleic (acid
[DNA]) synthesis

UE
under elbow
undetermined etiology
uninvolved epidermis
upper esophagus
upper extremities
upper extremity

UEG
ultrasonic encephalogram

UEM
universal electron microscope

UEMC
unidentified endosteal marrow cell

UER
unaided equalization reference

UES
upper esophageal sphincter

U ext., U/ext., u/ext
upper extremity

UF
Ullrich-Feichtiger (syndrome)
ultrafiltrate
ultrafiltration
ultrafine
ultrasonic frequency
unflexed
unknown factor
until finished
urinary formaldehyde

UFA
unesterified fatty acids

UFC
urinary-free cortisol

UFD
ultrasonic flow detector

UFE
uniform food encoding

UFP
ultrafiltration pressure

UFR
ultrafiltration rate
urine filtration rate

UG
urogastrone
urogenital
uteroglobulin (blastokinin)

UGA
uracil, guanine, adenine (a termination
    codon in protein synthesis—re:
    genetics)

UGD
urogenital diaphragm

U-gen
urobilinogen

UGF
unidentified growth factor

UGH syndrome
uveitis, glaucoma, hyphema syndrome
    (re: Ophth)

UGI
upper gastrointestinal (series)

UGIS
upper gastrointestinal series

UGIT
upper gastrointestinal tract

UGP1
uridyl diphosphate glucose
    pyrophosphorylase-1

UGP2
uridyl diphosphate glucose
    pyrophosphorylase-2

UGS
urogenital sinus

UGT
urogenital tuberculosis

UH
umbilical hernia
unfavorable histology
upper half

UHC
ultrahigh carbon

UHF
ultrahigh frequency

UHL
universal hypertrichosis lanuginosa

UHMW
ultrahigh molecular weight

UHMWPE
ultrahigh molecular weight polyethylene
    (re: orthopaedic biomaterials)

UHT
ultrahigh temperature

UHV
ultrahigh vacuum

UHV, uhv
ultrahigh voltage

UI
Ulcer Index
uroporphyrin isomerase
uroporphyrinogen isomerase (reduced
    uroporphyrin)

U/I
unidentified

UIBC
unsaturated iron-binding capacity

UIF
undegraded insulin factor

UIP
usual interstitial pneumonitis

UIQ
upper inner quadrant

UJT
unijunction transistor (a semiconductor
    used in relaxation oscillators)

UK
unknown
urinary kallikrein
urokinase

UL
unauthorized leave
undifferentiated lymphoma
upper limit
upper lobe
utterance length

U & L
upper and lower

ULA
undedicated logic array

ULDH
urinary lactic acid dehydrogenase

ULL
uncomfortable loudness level

ULLE
upper lid, left eye

ULN
upper limits of normal

ULPE
upper lobe pulmonary edema

ULQ
upper left quadrant

ULRE
upper lid, right eye

ULT
ultrahigh temperature (pasteurization)

ult.
ultimate
ultimately
ultime (L. lastly)
ultimus (L. ultimately, last)

ult. praes.
ultimus praescriptus (L. the last ordered
  or prescribed)

ULV
ultralow volume

UM
unmarried
upper motor (neuron)
uracil mustard

UMA
urinary muramidase activity

Umax
maximum urinary osmolality

umb.
umbilical
umbilicus

umb. reg.
umbilical region

UMC
unidimensional chromatography

UMN
upper motor neuron

UMNL, UMN(L)
upper motor neuron lesion

U & M NP
ulnar and median nerve palsy

UMP
uridine monophosphate (uridine-5′-
  phosphate; uridine 5′-
  monophosphate; uridylic acid)

UMPK
uridine monophosphate kinase

UN
ulnar nerve
undernourished
urea nitrogen
urinary nitrogen

un.
unable

UNa
urinary natrium (sodium)

unacc.
unaccompanied

unc.
unconscious

uncert.
uncertain
uncertainties

unchg.
unchanged

uncomp.
uncompensated
uncomplicated

uncompl.
uncomplicated

uncon.
unconscious

uncond.
unconditioned

uncond. ref.
unconditioned reflex

uncond. resp.
unconditioned response

uncoop.
uncooperative

UNCOR, uncor.
uncorrected

uncorr.
uncorrected

UnCS, unCS
unconditioned stimulus

unct.
unctus (L. anointed [smeared])

UNCV
ulnar nerve conduction velocity

undet.
undetermined

undet. etiol.
undetermined etiology

undet. orig.
undetermined origin

UNG, ung.
unguentum (L. ointment)

ungt.
unguentum (L. ointment)

unilat.
unilateral

Univ, univ.
university

univ.
universal
universally

UNK, unk.
unknown

unkn.
unknown

UNL
upper normal limit

unof.
unofficial

unoff.
unofficial

unrem.
unremitting

unremit.
unremitting

UnS, un. s.
unconditioned stimulus

uns.
unsatisfactory
unsymmetrical

uns-
asymmetrical
unsymmetrical

unsat.
unsatisfactory
unsaturated

unst.
unstable
unsteady

unsw.
unsweetened

unsym.
unsymmetrical

UO
undetermined origin
ureteral orifice
urinary output
urine output

UO, U/O
under observation

U/O adeq.
urine output adequate

UOQ
upper outer quadrant

Uosm
urinary osmolality

UOV
units of variance

UP
ulcerative proctitis
ultrahigh purity
under proof
unipolar
Unna-Pappenheim (stain)
upright posture
ureteropelvic
uridine phosphorylase
uroporphyrin

U/P
concentration in urine and plasma (e.g., glucose)
urine/plasma (concentration ratio)

up ad lib.
up ad libitum (L. at pleasure [out of bed or ambulatory as desired])

UPC
usual provider continuity

UPD
urinary production (rate)

UPG
uroporphyrinogen

UPI
uteroplacental insufficiency
uteroplacental ischemia

UPJ
ureteropelvic junction

UPN
unique patient number

up OOB ad lib.
up out of bed ad libitum (L. as desired)

UPOR
usual place of residence

UPP
urethral pressure profile
urethral pressure profilometry

UPPP
uvulopalatopharyngoplasty (re: ENT)

UPPRA
upright peripheral plasma renin activity

UPS
ultraviolet photoelectron spectroscopy
uroporphyrinogen synthetase
uterine progesterone system

UQ
ubiquinone
upper quadrant

UR
unconditional response
unconditioned reflex
unconditioned response
unrelated
unsatisfactory report
upper respiratory
uridine
urinal
urology
Utilization Review

UR, Ur
urologist

UR, Ur, ur.
urine

URA, Ura
uracil

ur. anal.
urine analysis

URC
upper rib cage

URD
upper respiratory disease

URD, Urd
uridine

U.R.D.
unspecific respiratory diseases

URES
University Residence Environment
   Scale (re: psychological testing)

ureth.
urethra
urethral

URF
uterine-relaxing factor

urg.
urgent

URI
upper respiratory infection

URO
urology
uroporphyrin

uro-gen.
urogenital

Urol, urol.
urologist
urology

URQ
upper right quadrant

URT
upper respiratory tract

URTI
upper respiratory tract illness
upper respiratory tract infection

URVD
unilateral renovascular disease

US
ultrasonic
ultrasound
unconditioned stimulus
unconditioned structure
unit separator (character—re:
   computers/data processing)
unknown significance
upper segment

u.s.
ut supra (L. as above)

USAN
United States Adopted Names (Council)

USASCII
USA Standard Code for Information
   Interchange (re: computers)

USBS
United States Bureau of Standards

USBuStand
United States Bureau of Standards

USERID
user identification (re: computers/data
    processing)

USFMS
United States foreign medical (school)
    student

USG
ultrasonography

USI
urinary stress incontinence

US/LS
upper strength/lower strength (ratio of
    growth)

USN
ultrasonic nebulizer

USO
unilateral salpingo-oophorectomy

USP, U.S.P.
United States Pharmacopeia

USPhar
United States Pharmacopeia

USPHS
United States Public Health Service

USR
unheated serum reagin (test)

USS
ultrasound scanning

ust.
ustus (L. burnt)

USVMD
urine specimen volume measuring
    device

USVMS
urine sample volume measurement
    system

USW
ultrashort wave

UT
Ullrich-Turner (syndrome)
universal time (time reference
    coordinate for scientific work—
    replaced Greenwich mean time 1 Jan
    1972)
Unna-Thost (syndrome)
unrelated (children raised) together
untested
untreated
urinary tract
urticaria

UTBG
unbound TBG (thyroxin[e]-binding
    globulin)

UTC
coordinated universal time (time taken
    from atomic clock; also called
    international atomic time)

UTD
up to date

ut dct.
ut dictum (L. as directed)

ut dict.
ut dictum (L. as directed)

utend.
utendus (L. to be used)

utend. mor. sol.
utendus more solito (L. to be used in
    the usual manner)

UTI
urinary tract infection
urinary trypsin inhibitor

UTLD
Utah Test of Language Development

UTOC
upper thoracic outlet compression
    (syndrome)

UTP
unilateral tension pneumothorax
uridine triphosphate (uridine 5′-
    triphosphate)

UTS
ulnar tunnel syndrome
ultimate tensile strength

ut supr.
ut supra (L. as above)

UU
urine urobilinogen

UUN
urinary urea nitrogen
urine urea nitrogen

UUO
unilateral ureteral occlusion

UUP
urine uroporphyrin

UV
ultraviolet
umbilical vein
urinary volume
urine volume

U_V, U v.
Uppsala virus

UVA
ultraviolet light, long wave

UVB
ultraviolet light, midrange sunbeam
  spectrum

UVC
umbilical venous catheter

UVI
ultraviolet irradiation

UVJ
ureterovesical junction

UVL
ultraviolet light

UVP
ultraviolet photometry

UV/P
U = concentration of solute in urine;
  V = quantity of urine excreted in a
  unit of time; P = concentration of

substance in plasma (ratio =
  clearance of the substance)

UVR
ultraviolet radiation

UW
unilateral weakness
Urbach-Wiethe (syndrome)

U/WB
unit of whole blood

UWL
unstirred water layer

UWM
unwed mother

UX$_1$
uranium X$_1$ (thorium-234)

Ux
urinalysis

ux.
uxor (L. wife)

UYP
upper yield point

V

V
coefficient of variation (re: statistics)
roman numeral five (V)
unipolar chest lead (re: cardiography)
vaccinated
vaccine
valine
vanadium (element)
variable
variation
varnish (re: Dent)
vegetarian
vegetation
Veillonella (genus of nonpathogenic
   micro-organisms)
ventilation
verbal (aptitude—re: General Aptitude
   Test Battery)
vertebral
vestibular
view
violet (an indicator color)
viral
virgin
virulence
virulent
virus
visit
visitor
visual
visual capacity
visus (L. seeing; sight)
vitreous
voice
voltage
volume (when written with subscripts,
   denoting location, chemical species,
   conditions)
vomit
vomiting

V, V.
Vibrio (genus)
vision
visual acuity

V, v
valve
vein
velocity (average linear velocity of flow)
venous
ventral
ventricle
ventricular
verbal

vertex
volume (minute—of air or blood)
volume of gas

V, v.
very

V, v, v.
versus (L. turn, towards, in that
   direction)
volt

V, *V*, $V \rightarrow$
vector

V̇
ventilation (frequently with subscript)
volume of gas per unit of time (rate of
   gas flow)

V1, V2 ..., V_1, V_2 ...
chest lead 1, chest lead 2,....

V #1, V #2
vehicle number one, number two, etc.
   (re: motor accident)

V_1
ophthalmic division of fifth cranial nerve

V_2
maxillary division of fifth cranial nerve

V_3
mandibular division of fifth cranial nerve

^{48}V
radioactive isotope of vanadium

^{49}V
radioactive isotope of vanadium

VII$_{Ag}$
Factor VII antigen

VIII$_c$
Factor VIII clotting activity

VIII$_{VWF}$
von Willebrand factor (Factor VIII)

v
mixed venous (pulmonary arterial)
   blood (when written as a subscript)
venous blood (when subscripted)
venule
vitamin
von (Ger. of—used in names)

v.
vel (L. or [take what you will; one or the other])
vena (L. vein)
vide (L. see)

v-
vicinal isomer

v-
vicinal (adjacent)

VA
alveolar volume
anatomical volume
vacuum aspiration
vancomycin
vasodilator agent
(nucleus) ventralis anterior (re: thalamus)
ventricular aneurysm
ventricular arrhythmia
ventro-anterior
vertebral artery
Veterans Administration
viral antigen
visual activity
visual aid
visual axis
volcanic ash
volume averaging

VA, V-A
ventriculoatrial

VA, Va
visual acuity

VA, va
volt ampere

V$_A$, V̇$_A$, Va, V$_a$
alveolar ventilation
volume of alveolar gas

VAB
vinblastine, actinomycin D (dactinomycin), and bleomycin (re: chemotherapy)
voice answer back (re: computers)

VAB-I
vinblastine, actinomycin D, bleomycin (re: chemotherapy)

VAB-II
vinblastine, actinomycin D (dactinomycin), bleomycin, and cisplatin (re: chemotherapy)

VAB-III
vinblastine, actinomycin D (dactinomycin), bleomycin, cisplatin, chlorambucil, and cyclophosphamide (re: chemotherapy)

VAB-V
vinblastine, actinomycin D (dactinomycin), bleomycin, cyclophosphamide, and cisplatin (re: chemotherapy)

VABCD
vinblastine, Adriamycin, bleomycin, CCNU, DTIC (re: chemotherapy)

VABP
venoarterial bypass pumping

VAC
vincristine, actinomycin D (dactinomycin), and cyclophosphamide (re: chemotherapy)
vincristine, Adriamycin (doxorubicin), and cyclophosphamide (re: chemotherapy)

vac.
vaccine
vacuum

VAcc, VA$_{cc}$
visual acuity with correction

vacc.
vaccination
vaccine

V-A conduction
ventriculoatrial conduction (retrograde conduction)

VACTERL
vertebral, anal, cardiac, tracheal, esophageal, renal, and limb (re: pattern of congenital anomalies)

VAD
ventricular assist device
virus-adjusting diluent
vitamin A deficiency

V Ad
vocational adjustment

Vadj
vocational adjustment

V Adm
Veterans Administration

VAFAC
vincristine, amethopterin (methotrexate), 5-fluorouracil, Adriamycin (doxorubicin), and cyclophosphamide (re: chemotherapy)

VAG, Vag, vag.
vagina
vaginal

vag.
vaginitis

VAG HYST, vag. hyst.
vaginal hysterectomy

VAH
vertebral ankylosing hyperostosis
Veterans Administration Hospital
virilizing adrenal hyperplasia

VAHS
virus-associated hemophagocytic
  syndrome

VAIN
vaginal intra-epithelial neoplasia

VAKT
visual, association, kinesthetic, tactile
  (re: reading)

VAL, Val, val.
valine (and its radicals)

val.
valve

VALE
visual acuity, left eye

VAM
ventricular arrhythmia monitor
VP-16-213 (etoposide), Adriamycin
  (doxorubicin), and methotrexate (re:
  chemotherapy)

VAMP
vincristine, amethopterin
  (methotrexate), 6-mercaptopurine,
  and prednisone (re: chemotherapy)

V antigen
viral antigen
virus antigen

VAOD
visual acuity, oculus dexter

VA ↓ OD
visual acuity decreased, oculus dexter

VAOS
visual acuity, oculus sinister

VA ↓ OS
visual acuity decreased, oculus sinister

VAOU
visual acuity, oculi unitas

VA ↓ OU
visual acuity decreased, oculi unitas

VAP
vaginal acid phosphatase
variant angina pectoris
vinblastine, actinomycin D

(dactinomycin), and Platinol
  (cisplatin) (re: chemotherapy)
vincristine, Adriamycin (doxorubicin),
  and prednisone (re: chemotherapy)
vincristine, Adriamycin, procarbazine
  (re: chemotherapy)

VA$_{ph}$
visual acuity with pinhole

Va/Qc
ventilation (alveolar air flow) to
  perfusion (capillary blood flow) ratio

Va/Qc ratio
ventilation-perfusion ratio

VAR
visual-auditory range
visual-aural range

VAR, var.
variety

var
variant or heteromorphic chromosome
  (re: cytogenetics)

var.
variable
variant
variation
varicose
varicosities
variometer
various
varying

VARE
visual acuity, right eye

VAS
vesicle attachment site
viral analog scale
visual analog scale

Vas
vascular

VASC
Verbal Auditory Screen for Children
  (test)
Visual-Auditory Screening (test for)
  Children

VASC, vasc.
vascular

VAsc, VA$_{sc}$
visual acuity without correction

vas. dis.
vascular disease

vasodil.
vasodilatation

VAS RAD
vascular radiology

vas vit.
vas vitreum (L. a glass vessel)

VAT
variable antigen type
ventricular activation time
Vestibular Accommodation Test
visual action therapy
visual action time
visual apperception test
Vocational Apperception Test

VATD, VAT-D
vincristine, ara-C (cytarabine),
  6-thioguanine, and daunorubicin
  (re: chemotherapy)

VATER
vertebral defects, anal atresia,
  tracheoesophageal fistula with
  esophageal atresia, renal defects,
  and radial dysplasia
vertebral defects, imperforate anus,
  tracheoesophageal fistula, and radial
  and renal dysplasia

VATER/VACTERL
vertebral, anal, tracheoesophageal,
  renal and radial limb anomalies,
  including cardiovascular and
  nonradial limb anomalies

VATH
vinblastine, Adriamycin (doxorubicin),
  and thiotepa (re: chemotherapy)
vinblastine, Adriamycin (doxorubicin),
  thiotepa, Halotestin
  (fluoxymesterone) (re: chemotherapy)

VAV
VP-16-213 (etoposide), Adriamycin
  (doxorubicin), and vincristine (re:
  chemotherapy)

V_A/V_P
ratio of additive variance to phenotype
  variance (re: genetics—heritability)

VB
vagina bulbi
valence bond
venous blood
ventrobasal (complex—of thalamus)
veronal buffer
vertebrobasilar (arteries)
viable birth
vinblastine (vincaleukoblastine—
  antineoplastic)
vinblastine, bleomycin (re:
  chemotherapy)
virus buffer
voided bladder

VB_1
first voided bladder specimen

VB_2
second midstream bladder specimen

VB_3
third midstream bladder specimen

VBA
vincristine, BCNU, Adriamycin (re:
  chemotherapy)

VBAIN
vertebrobasilar artery insufficiency
  nystagmus

VBAP
vincristine, BCNU (carmustine),
  Adriamycin (doxorubicin), and
  prednisone (re: chemotherapy)

VBD
vinblastine, bleomycin, and cis-
  diamminedichloroplatinum (cisplatin)
  (re: chemotherapy)

VBG
vagotomy and Billroth
  gastroenterostomy
vein (aortocoronary artery) bypass graft
venous blood gas
veronal-buffered (serum with) gelatin

VBI
vertebrobasilar insufficiency
vertebrobasilar ischemia

VBL
vinblastine (vincaleukoblastine—
  antineoplastic)

VBM
vincristine, bleomycin, methotrexate (re:
  chemotherapy)

VBMCP
vincristine, BCNU (carmustine),
  melphalan, cyclophosphamide,
  prednisone (re: chemotherapy)

VBOS
veronal-buffered oxalated saline
  (barbital)

VBP
venous blood pressure
vinblastine, bleomycin, and Platinol
  (cisplatin) (re: chemotherapy)

VBR
ventricular-brain ratio

VBS
veronal-buffered saline (medium—
  barbital)
vertebral basilar (artery) system

VBS:FBS
veronal-buffered saline:fetal bovine
    serum (barbital)

VC
acuity of color vision (chromatopsia)
vascular change
vasoconstriction
vasoconstrictor
vena cava
venereal case
venous capacitance
venous capillary
ventilatory capacity
ventral column
ventricular contractions
verbal comprehension
vertebral canal
vincristine
vinyl chloride
visual capacity
visual cortex
vital capacity
vomiting center
vowel-consonant

VC, V C
voluntary closing (device—re: upper
    limb prosthesis)

VC, V$_C$, Vc
pulmonary capillary blood volume

VC, v.c.
vocal cord

V/C
ventilation-circulation (ratio)

VCA
vancomycin, colistin, and anisomycin
    (inhibitor)
viral capsid antigen(s) (virion)
virus capsid antigen (virion)

VCAP
vincristine, cyclophosphamide,
    Adriamycin (doxorubicin), and
    prednisone (re: chemotherapy)

V-CAP III
VP-16-213 (etoposide),
    cyclophosphamide, Adriamycin
    (doxorubicin), and Platinol (cisplatin)
    (re: chemotherapy)

VCC
vasoconstrictor center
ventral cell column

VCD
vibrational circular dichroism

VCDQ
Verbal Comprehension Deviation
    Quotient

VCE
vagina, (ecto)cervix, and endocervix
    (re: cytologic smear)

VCF
vincristine, cyclophosphamide, and
    5-fluorouracil (re: chemotherapy)

VCF, V$_{CF}$, Vcf
velocity of circumferential fiber
    (shortening rate)

VCG
vectorcardiogram
vectorcardiography
vector space cardiogram
voiding cystogram
voiding cystourethrogram

VCI
volatile corrosion inhibitor

V-cillin
penicillin V

VCIU
voluntary control of involuntary
    utterances

VCM
vinyl chloride monomer

VCMP
vincristine, cyclophosphamide,
    melphalan, prednisone (re:
    chemotherapy)

VCN
vancomycin hydrochloride,
    colistimethate sodium, nystatin
    (medium)
vibrio cholerae neuraminidase

V$_{CNS}$
volume of central nervous system
    (cerebrospinal fluid plus extracellular
    fluid of brain and spinal cord)

V$_{co}$
carbon monoxide (endogenous
    production)

V$_{CO_2}$
carbon dioxide output
volume, carbon dioxide elimination

VCP
Veterinary Creolin-Pearson (antiseptic;
    parasiticide [except for cats])
vincristine, cyclophosphamide,
    prednisone (re: chemotherapy)

VCR
vasoconstriction rate
vincristine (vincaleukoblastine—
    antineoplastic)

V-C (ratio)
ventilation-circulation (ratio)

VCS
vasoconstrictor substance
vesicocervical space

VCSA
viral cell surface antigen

VCSF
ventricular cerebrospinal fluid

VCT
venous clotting time

VCU
videocystourethrography
voiding cystourethrogram

VCUG
voiding cystourethrogram

VCV
vowel-consonant-vowel

VD
vapor density
vasodilation
vasodilator
venous dilatation
ventricular dilator
ventriculo dextro (L. in the left ventricle)
ventrodorsal
vessel disease
virus diarrhea
volume of dead space
volume of distribution

VD, V.D.
venereal disease

V_D, Vd
physiologic dead space in percent of
    tidal volume

+VD
positive vertical divergence

−VD
negative vertical divergence

Vd, V_d
apparent volume of distribution (V area)

vd
double vibrations (cycles)

vd.
void
voided

VDA
visual discriminatory acuity

VDAC
voltage-dependent anion-(selective)
    channel

Vd alv.
alveolar dead space

Vd anat.
anatomic dead space

VDBR
volume of distribution of bilirubin

VdB test
van den Bergh test

VDC
vasodilator center
Venereal Disease Clinic

VDD
vitamin D dependent (rickets)

VDDR
vitamin D-dependent rickets

V deflection
deflection in His bundle electrogram (re:
    ventricular septum)

VDEL
Venereal Disease Experimental
    Laboratory

VDEM
vasodepressor material

VDF
ventricular diastolic fragmentation

VDG, V.D.G.
venereal disease, gonorrhea

vdg.
voiding

vdg. q.s.
voiding sufficient quantity (L. quantum
    sufficiat)

VDH, V.D.H.
valvular disease of the heart

VDL
vasodepressor lipid
visual detection level

VDM
vasodepressor material

(no) VD or M
(no) venous distention or masses

VDP
ventricular premature depolarization
vincristine, daunorubicin, prednisone
    (re: chemotherapy)

Vd p
physiologic dead space

VDR
venous diameter ratio

VDRL
Venereal Disease Research Laboratory
   (re: test for syphilis)

VDRR
vitamin D-resistant rickets

VDRS
Verdun Depression Rating Scale

VDRT
Venereal Disease Reference Test (of
   Harris)

VDS
vasodilator substance
vindesine (antineoplastic)

VDS, V.D.S.
venereal disease, syphilis

VDT
visual display terminal (re: computers)
visual distortion test

VDU
video display unit

VDV
ventricular end-diastolic volume

VD/VT, Vd/Vt
ratio of dead space ventilation to total
   ventilation

VE
esophageal lead (exploring electrode
   within esophageal lumen)
vaginal efficiency
vaginal examination
Venezuelan encephalitis
venous extension
ventilatory equivalent (index)
ventricular elasticity
ventricular escape
ventricular extrasystole
vesicular exanthema (virus of swine)
viral encephalitis
visual efficiency
vitamin E
volume ejection
volumic ejection
voluntary effort

VE, Ve
ventilation

V$_E$
volume of expired gas (pulmonary
   function test)

V̇$_E$
respiratory minute volume

V & E
Vinethene and ether

VEA
ventricular ectopic activity
ventricular ectopic arrhythmia
viral envelope antigens

VEB
ventricular ectopic beat

VECG
vector electrocardiogram

VECP
visual evoked cortical potential
visually evoked cortical potential

vect.
vector

VED
ventricular ectopic depolarization

VEE
vagina, ectocervix, and endocervix
Venezuelan equine encephalomyelitis
   (virus)

V-EEG
vigilance-controlled
   electroencephalogram

VEF
visually evoked field

Veg
vegetations

vehic.
vehiculum (L. vehicle)

vel.
velocity

Vel antigen
high frequency blood group antigen

veloc.
velocity

VELS
Vane Evaluation of Language Scale
   (also called VANE-L)

VEM
vaso-excitor material

V$_{Emax}$
maximum flow per unit of time

Ven, ven.
venous

Ven antigen
low frequency blood group antigen

VENP
vincristine, Endoxan
   (cyclophosphamide), Natulan,
   prednisone (re: chemotherapy)

VENT, vent.
ventricular

vent.
ventilation
ventilator
ventral
ventricle

vent. fib.
ventricular fibrillation

ventr.
ventral

ventric.
ventricle
ventricular

ventric. fib.
ventricular fibrillation

VEP
visual evoked potential
visually evoked potential

VEPA
vincristine, Endoxan
(cyclophosphamide), prednisolone,
Adriamycin (re: chemotherapy)

VER
visual evoked response
visually evoked (cortical) response

Verb Exp
verbal expression

vert.
vertebra
vertebral
vertical
vertigo

vert. comp.
vertebral compression
vertical compression

vert. compr.
vertebral compression
vertical compression

VES, ves.
vesica (L. bladder)
vesicular (re: chest sounds)

ves.
vesicle
vessel

vesic.
vesicula (L. a little bladder—blister)
vesicular (re: chest sounds)

V-esotropia
convergent strabismus greater in
downward than in upward gaze (re:
Ophth)

vesp.
vesper (L. evening)

vest.
vestibular

ves. ur.
vesica urinaria (L. urinary bladder)

VESV
vesicular exanthema of swine virus

VET
vestigial testis (rat)

Vet
veteran
veterinary

v. et.
vide etiam (L. see also)

Vet Adm
Veterans Administration

VetAdmin
Veterans Administration

VetSci
veterinary science

VEWA
Vocational Evaluation and Work
Adjustment (re: Psychol)

VF
left leg (electrode—aVF)
ventricular fluid (re: Neuro)
ventricular flutter
ventricular fusion
vigil, fatiguing
vitreous fluorophotometry

VF, V.F.
vocal fremitus

VF, Vf
visual field (field of vision)

VF, v.f.
ventricular fibrillation

VF***, VF***
voluntary free breathing capacity at rate
of choice of patient

Vf
video frequency

V$_f$
variant frequency

VFA
volatile fatty acid

V factor
verbal comprehension factor (re:
Psychol)

Vfb
ventricular fibrillation

VFC
ventricular function curve

VFD
visual feedback display

VFDF
very fast death factor

VFI
visual fields intact

Vfib, V fib.
ventricular fibrillation

VFL
ventricular flutter

VFP
ventricular filling pressure
ventricular fluid pressure (re: Neuro)

VFR
voiding flow rate

VFT
venous filling time
ventricular fibrillation threshold

VG
van Gieson (stain)
ventilated group
ventricular gallop
volume of gas

VG, V/G
very good

VGH
very good health

VGL
vinglycinate (analog of vinblastine—
  antineoplastic)

VGM
vein graft myringoplasty
ventriculogram

VGP
viral glycoprotein

V_G/V_P
ratio of total genetic variance to
  phenotypic variance in heritability (re:
  genetics)

VH
vaginal hysterectomy
venous hematocrit
ventricular hypertrophy
Veterans Hospital
viral hepatitis

V_H
variable region (re: heavy chain of IgA
  or IgG)

VHD
valvular heart disease
ventral heart disease
viral hematodepressive disease

VHDL
very high density lipoprotein

VHF
very high frequency (re: radio waves)
viral hemorrhagic fever
visual half-field

VI
vaginal irrigation
variable interval (reinforcement)
vastus intermedius (muscle)
virgo intacta (L. untouched girl)
virulence
viscosity index
Visual Imagery (re: Psychol)
visual impairment
visual inspection
visually impaired
vitality index
volume index

Vi
virginium (former name for element
  francium)
virulent

v.i.
via intermedia (L. intermediate way)

VIA
virus-inactivating agent
virus infection-associated antigen

Vi antigen
"virulence" antigen

VIB
Vocational Interest Blank (re: Psychol)

VIB, vib.
vibration

vib.
vibratory

VIBS, vibs
vocabulary, information, block design,
  similarities (re: Psychol)

VIC
Values Inventory for Children
vasoinhibitory center
visual communication (therapy)
voice intensity controller

vic.
vices (L. times)

VID
visible iris diameter

vid.
vide (L. see)

VIESA
Vocational Interest, Experience, and
  Skill Assessment

VIF
virus-induced interferon

VIG
vaccinia immune globulin

VIH
violence-induced handicap

VIM
video intensification microscopy

VIN
vulvar intra-epithelial neoplasia
vulvar intra-epithelial neoplasm

Vin
vinyl ether

vin.
vinum (L. wine)

VIO
virtual I/O (input/output—re: computers/
  data processing)

VIP
vasoactive intestinal peptide
vasoactive intestinal polypeptide
vasoinhibitory peptide
venous impedance plethysmography
Vital Initial of Pregnancy (in vitro
  fertilization)
voluntary interruption of pregnancy

VIP, V.I.P.
very important person

VIP-oma
vasoactive intestinal polypeptide
  (secreting) tumor

VIQ
verbal intelligence quotient
Vocational Interest Questionnaire

VIR
virology

vir.
viridis (L. green)
virulent

VIS
vaginal irrigation smear
visual information storage
vocational interest schedule

vis.
vision
visiting
visitor(s)
visual

VISA
ventriculum inhibited synchronously
  with the atrium
Vocational Interest and Sophistication
  Assessment

VISAB
Vocational Interest Scale for Adult Blind

VISC
vitreous infusion suction cutter (re:
  Ophth)

visc.
visceral
viscosity
viscous

Vit, vit.
vitamin (when followed by a letter)
vitreous

vit.
vital
vitellus (L. yolk of an egg)

Vit B$_1$
thiamine

Vit B$_2$
riboflavin

Vit B$_3$
nicotinamide

Vit B$_6$
pyridoxine

Vit B$_{12}$
cobalamin, cyanocobalamin

Vit B$_{12b}$
hydroxocobalamin

Vit C
ascorbic acid

VIT CAP, vit. cap.
vital capacity

Vit D$_2$
ergocalciferol

Vit D$_3$
cholecalciferol (natural vitamin D)

Vit E
tocopherol(s)

vitel.
vitellus (L. yolk of an egg)

Vit G
riboflavin

Vit H
obsolete name for biotin

Vit K
coagulation vitamin, antihemorrhagic
factor

vit. ov. sol.
vitello ovi solutus (L. dissolved in yolk of
egg)

Vit PP
B_3 (niacinamide; nicotinic acid amide—
originally called P-P for pellagra
preventing)

vitr.
vitreum (L. glass)

Vit U
cabagin or anti-ulcer vitamin

viz.
videlicet (L. namely)

VJ
ventriculojugular (shunt)
Vogel-Johnson (agar)

VJC
ventriculojugulocardiac (shunt)

VK
Vogt-Koyanagi (syndrome)

VKH
Vogt-Koyanagi-Harada (syndrome)

VL
left arm (electrode—aVL)
vastus lateralis (muscle)
ventralis lateralis (nucleus—re:
thalamus)
ventrolateral
visceral leishmaniasis
vision, left

V_L
variable light (chain)

VLA
virus-like agent

VLB
vincaleukoblastine (vinblastine—
antineoplastic)

VLBR
very low birth rate

VLBW
very low birth weight

VLCFA
very long chain fatty acid

VLD
very low density

VLDL
very low density lipoprotein (prebeta-
lipoproteins)

VLDLC
very low density lipoprotein cholesterol

VLDLP
very low density lipoprotein

VLDTG, VLD-TG
very low density lipoprotein triglyceride

V lead
central terminal chest lead (re: EKG)

VLF
very low frequency

VLG
ventral nucleus of the lateral geniculate
body

VLH
ventrolateral nucleus of the
hypothalamus

VLM
(nucleus) ventralis lateralis pars
medialis (thalamus)
visceral larval migrans

VLP
vincristine, L-asparaginase, and
prednisone (re: chemotherapy)
virus-like particle

VLR
vinleurosine (alkaloid—antineoplastic)

VLSI
very large scale integration (re:
computers)

VM
vasomotor
vastus medialis
ventralis medialis (L. middle belly)
(nucleus) ventralis medialis (re:
thalamus)
ventricular mass
ventricular muscle
ventromedial
Verner-Morrison (syndrome)
vestibular membrane
viral myocarditis
viscous metamorphosis

VM, Vm
viomycin
voltmeter

V/m
volts per minute

589

VMA
vanillylmandelic acid (correctly called 3-methoxy-4-hydroxymandelic acid)

VMAD
vincristine, methotrexate, Adriamycin, actinomycin D (re: chemotherapy)

V_{max}
maximum velocity (re: enzymes; myocardial fiber shortening)

$\dot{V}_{max}$
instantaneous volumetric flow

VMC
vasomotor center
void metal composite

VMCG
vector magnetocardiogram

VMCP
vincristine, melphalan, cyclophosphamide, prednisone (re: chemotherapy)

VMGT
Visual Motor Gestalt Test (re: Psychol)

VMH
ventromedial hypothalamic (neurons; nuclei)

VMI
Visual-Motor Integration (test—re: Psychol)

V-MI
Volpe-Manhold Index (comparing amounts of calculus in individuals)

VMIT
Visual-Motor Integration Test

VMN
ventromedial nucleus (re: hypothalamus)

VMO
vastus medialis oblique (muscle)

VM-26PP
VM-26 (teniposide), procarbazine, prednisone (re: chemotherapy)

VMR
vasomotor rhinitis

VMS
Visual Memory Score (re: Psychol)
visual memory span (re: Psychol)

VMST
Visual-Motor Sequencing Test (re: Psychol)

VMT
vasomotor tone
ventilatory muscle training

VN
vesical neck (re: bladder)
vestibular nucleus (re: Neuro)
virus neutralization
virus neutralizing
visceral nucleus
visual naming
vomeronasal

VNDPT
visual numerical discrimination pre-test

VNE
verbal nonemotional (stimuli)

VNO
vomeronasal organ

VNR
ventral nerve root

V, N, R
verbal, numerical, and reasoning (re: psychological testing)

VO
(ventricular) volume overload

VO, V O
voluntary opening (device—re: upper limb prosthesis)

VO, V/O, v.o.
verbal order

VO$_2$, Vo$_2$
oxygen consumption (uptake)

V_O
standard volume

voc.
vocational

vocab.
vocabulary

VOCAP
VP-16-213 (etoposide), Oncovin (vincristine), cyclophosphamide, Adriamycin (doxorubicin), Platinol (cisplatin) (re: chemotherapy)

VOD
venous occlusive disease (Budd-Chiari syndrome)
visio, oculus dexter (dextra) (L. sight, right eye)

VOGAD
Voice-Operated Gain-Adjusting Device (re: computers/ data processing)

VOI
Vocational Opinion Index (re: Psychol)

VOL, vol.
volume

vol.
volar
volatilis (L. volatile)
volumetric
voluntary
volunteer
volvendus (L. to be rolled)

vol%
volume per cent

Vol Adm
voluntary admission (re: psychiatry)

volt.
volatile
volatize

vol. vent.
volume ventilator

VOM
vinyl chloride monomer
volt-ohm-milliammeter (an electric test
    instrument)

VOP
venous occlusion plethysmography

VOPP
veterinary, optometry, podiatry,
    pharmacy

VOR
vestibulo-ocular reflex (oculocephalic
    reflex)

VOS
visio, oculus sinister (L. vision of left
    eye)
visus, oculus sinister (L. vision, left eye)

v.o.s.
vitello ovi solutus (L. dissolved in yolk of
    egg)

VOT
voice onset time

VOU
visio, oculi utriusque (L. vision of each
    eye)
visus, oculus uterque (L. vision, each
    eye)

voxel
(single) volume element (re: CT image
    display)

VP
physiological volume
variegate porphyria

vascular permeability
vasopressin
velopharyngeal (re: ENT)
venipuncture
venous (volume) plethysmograph
venous pressure
vertex potential
vincristine and prednisone (re:
    chemotherapy)
viral protein
virus protein
Voges-Proskauer (test, reaction)
volume pressure
vulnerable period

VP, V/P
ventriculoperitoneal

VP, vp
vapor pressure

V$_P$
plasma volume

V/P
ventilation and perfusion

V&P
vagotomy and pyloroplasty

↑ VP
increased venous pressure

↓ VP
decreased venous pressure

Vp
ventricular premature (beats)

V$_p$
peak voltage

V-pattern
horizontal misalignment of eye

VPB
ventricular premature beat
vinblastine, Platinol, bleomycin (re:
    chemotherapy)

VPBCPr
vincristine, prednisone, vinblastine,
    chlorambucil, procarbazine (re:
    chemotherapy)

VPC
vapor-phase chromatography
ventricular premature complex
ventricular premature contraction
volume packed cells
volume per cent

VPCMF
vincristine, prednisone,
    cyclophosphamide, methotrexate,
    and 5-fluorouracil (re: chemotherapy)

VP Comp
velopharyngeal competency (re: ENT)

VPCT
ventricular premature contraction
  threshold

VPD
ventricular premature depolarization

VPF
vascular permeability factor

VPG
velopharyngeal gap (re: ENT)

VPI
vapor phase inhibitor
velopharyngeal insufficiency (re: ENT)
ventral posterior inferior
virus structural protein
Vocational Planning Inventory (re:
  Psychol)
Vocational Preference Inventory

VPL
(nucleus) ventralis posterolateral (re:
  thalamus)
ventral posterolateral (nucleus)

VPM
ventilator pressure manometer
(nucleus) ventralis posteromedialis (re:
  thalamus)
ventral posteromedial (nucleus)

vpm
vibrations per minute

VPN
ventral pontine nucleus (re: Neuro)
Vickers pyramid number (unit of
  hardness—solids)

VPO
velopharyngeal opening (re: ENT)

VPP
viral porcine pneumonia

VPR
Voges-Proskauer reaction
volume-to-pressure ratio

V-P ratio
ventilation-perfusion ratio

VPRBC
volume of packed red blood cells

VPRC
volume of packed red cells

VPS
ventriculoperitoneal shunt
visual pleural space

VPS, vps, v.p.s.
vibrations per second

VP shunt, v-p shunt
ventriculoperitoneal shunt

VP test, V-P test
Voges-Proskauer test (re:
  Enterobacteriaceae species
  differentiation)

VPW
ventral prostate weight

VQ
voice quality

V/Q
ventilation-perfusion (quotient) ratio

V/Q scan
ventilation perfusion (quotient) of lung
  scan

VR
right arm (electrode [aVR]—re:
  electrocardiogram)
valve replacement
variable ratio (reinforcement)
vascular resistance
venous rate
venous return
ventilation rate
ventilation ratio
ventricular rate
vision, right
visual reproduction
vital records
vocational rehabilitation

VR, V.R.
vocal resonance

VR, v.r.
ventral root (of a spinal nerve)

Vr
relaxation volume (re: Resp)

VRA
Visual Reinforcement Audiometry

VRBC
red blood cell volume

VRC
venous renin concentration
ventral (nerve) root, cervical
vertical redundancy check (re:
  computers/data processing)

VRC$_1$, VRC$_2$, VRC$_3$, etc.
ventral root, cervical, by number

VRD
ventricular radial dysplasia
vinrosidine (alkaloid—re: antineoplastic)

VR&E
vocational rehabilitation and education

VRI
viral respiratory infection
virus respiratory infection

VRL
ventral (nerve) root, lumbar

VRL$_1$, VRL$_2$, VRL$_3$, etc.
ventral (nerve) root, lumbar, by number

vRMS
van Riper memory span

VRNA
viral ribonucleic acid

VROM
voluntary range of motion

VRP
very reliable product (written on
   prescription)

VRR
ventral root reflex

VRS
Vocational Rehabilitation Services

VRT
variance of residence time
ventral (nerve) root, thoracic
(Benton) Visual Retention Test

VRT$_1$, VRT$_2$, VRT$_3$, etc.
ventral root, thoracic, by number

VRV
ventricular residual volume
viper retrovirus

VS
vaccination scar
vaccine serotype
vagal stimulation
vasospasm
venesection (venisection)
ventral subiculum (re: Neuro)
ventricular septum
verbal scale
vertically selective (re: visual cell)
very sensitive
vesicular sounds (re: auscultation of
   chest)
vesicular stomatitis (virus)
vilonodular synovitis
Vogt-Spielmeyer (syndrome)
volatile solids
voluntary sterilization

VS, V.S., V/S, v.s.
vital sign(s)

VS, V.S.
volumetric solution

Vs
venae sectio (L. venesection
   [venisection])

Vs, vs.
voids

V·s
volt-second

vs, v.s.
vibration seconds

vs, v/s
visited
visitors

vs.
versus (L. a turning toward)

v.s.
single vibration (cycles)
vide supra (L. see above)

VSA
variant-specific surface antigen

VSAM
virtual storage access method (re:
   computers/data processing)

VsB
venae sectio brachii (L. a cutting of a
   vein of the arm [to draw blood from a
   vessel in the arm])

VSBE
very short below elbow (cast)

VSC
voluntary surgical contraception

VSCS
ventricular specialized conduction
   system

VSD
ventricular septal defect
viral safe dose

VSEPR
valence shell-electron pair repulsion

VSFP
venous stop-flow pressure

VSG
variant surface glycoprotein

VSHD
ventricular septal heart defect

VSL
very serious list

VSM
vascular smooth muscle

VSMS
Vineland Social Maturity Scale

vsn.
vision

VSOK
vital signs OK (normal)

VSR
venereal spirochetosis of rabbits

VSS, V/S/S
vital signs stable

VST
ventral spinothalamic tract

V+ substance
kynurenine (an amino acid produced
    from tryptophan in the body)
    substance (re: biochemical
    investigations)

VSULA
vaccination scar, upper left arm

VSV
vesicular stomatitis virus

VSW
ventricular stroke work

VT
gas volume unit time
tetrazolium violet (a histological stain)
vacuum tube
vasotocin
ventricular tachyarrhythmia
ventricular tachycardia
Vero cytotoxin
vertical tabulation (character—re:
    computers/data processing)

VT, V.T.
vacuum tuberculin

VT, V$_T$
total ventilation

V$_T$
physiologic dead space in percent of
    tidal volume

V$_T$, Vt
tidal volume

VT*
voluntary maximum breathing rate
    timed by metronome

V&T
volume and tension (of pulse)

Vt
pulmonary parenchymal tissue volume

VTA
ventral tegmental area (re: Neuro)

VTAM
virtual telecommunications access
    method (re: computers/ data
    processing)

VTE
ventricular tachycardia event
vicarious trial and error (re: Psychol)

V-test
Voluter test (re: radiology)

VTG
volume thoracic gas

VTI
volume thickness index

VTM
variegated translocation mosaicism

VTMoV
(virusoid of) velvet tobacco mottle virus

VTOC
volume table of contents (re:
    computers/data processing)

VTR
videotape recorded

VTS
vesicular transport system

VTSRS
Verdun Target Symptom Rating Scale

VTVM
vacuum tube voltmeter

VTX, vtx
vertex

Vtx
vertex (presentation—re: OB)

VU
varicose ulcer (i.e., stasis ulcer)
very urgent

VU, vu
volume unit (re: telecommunication
    engineering)

VUR
vesicoureteral reflex
vesicoureteric reflex

VUV
vacuum ultraviolet

VV
vagina and vulva
veins
viper venom
vulva and vagina

VV, vv
varicose veins

V/V
volume per volume

V & V
vulva and vagina

vv.
venae (L. veins)

v.v.
vice versa

v/v
percent (%) "volume in volume" (the
  number of milliliters of an active
  constituent in 100 milliliters of
  solution)

VVI
vocal velocity index

V/VI
grade five on a six-grade basis (roman
  numerals—re: cardiac murmur
  [arabic numbers now preferred])

VV lig.
varicose vein ligation

VVQ
Verbalizer-Visualization Questionnaire

VVS
vesicovaginal space

VW
von Willebrand (factor)
von Willebrand's (disease)

VW, V.W., v.w.
vessel wall

v/w
volume per weight

Vw antigen
MNS blood group antigen

V wave
vertex sharp transient wave (re: EEG)

v wave
one of three jugular venous pulse
  waves

VWD, vWD
von Willebrand's disease

VWF
velocity wave form
vibration white finger

VWF, vWF
von Willebrand factor (Factor VIII)

Vx, vx.
vertex

VY
veal yeast

VZ, V-Z
varicella-zoster (antibody)

VZIg
varicella zoster immune globulin

VZV
varicella zoster virus

W

W
tryptophan
tungsten (element—formerly called
   wolfram, wolframium)
ward
weakness
Weber's test (re: Oto)
weight
west
western
wetting
white cell
whole (response)
widowed
Wohlfahrtia (genus of flies—re:
   cutaneous myiasis)
wolframium (wolfram; tungsten)
word fluency (re: Psychol)
work
Wuchereria (genus of roundworms)

W, W.
wehnelt (unit of hardness of roentgen
   rays—penetrating ability)

W, w
water
weak
white
wide
widow
widower
width
wound

W, w.
watt (SI and practical unit of power)
week
wife

W+
weakly positive

181W
radioactive isotope of wolframium
   (tungsten)

185W
radioactive isotope of wolframium
   (tungsten)

187W
radioactive isotope of wolframium
   (tungsten)

w.
with

w/
with

WA
Widal-Abrami (syndrome)
wide awake
Wiskcott-Aldrich (syndrome)

WA, W/A, Wa, w.a.
when awake

W/A
weakness or atrophy
white adult

W or A
weakness or atrophy

w.a.
with average

WAB
Western Aphasia Battery

WAF
weakness, atrophy, fasciculation
white adult female

WAIS
Wechsler Adult Intelligence Scale

WAIS-R
Wechsler Adult Intelligence Scale—
   Revised

WAK
wearable artificial kidney

WAM
white adult male

WAP
wandering atrial pacemaker

WAR
Wassermann antigen reaction

w.a.r.
without additional reagents

WARF
warfarin (WARF compound 42—a
   rodenticide; sodium salt as
   anticoagulant)

WARS
tryptophanyl-tRNA synethetase
(TRPRS—gene-marker symbol)

WAS
Ward Atmosphere Scale (re: Psychol)
weekly activity summary
Wiskott-Aldrich syndrome

WASP
Weber Advanced Spatial Perception
(Test—re: Psychol)

Wass
Wassermann test

WAT
word association test

WB
waist belt (restraint)
washable base
washed bladder
water bottle
Wechsler-Bellevue (Scale—re: Psychol)
weight bearing
west bound (re: motor vehicle accident)
wet-bulb (temperature)
whole blood
whole body
Willowbrook (virus)
Wilson Blair (agar)

WB, Wb
weber (SI and practical unit of magnetic
flux)

Wb
(sense of) well-being (re: California
Psychological Inventory test)

WBA
wax bean agglutinin
whole body activity

WBC
well baby care
Well Baby Clinic

WBC, W.B.C.
white blood cell
white blood corpuscle
white blood (cell) count

WBC diff.
white blood count and differential

WBC/hpf
white blood cells per high-power field

WBCT
whole blood clotting time

WBDS
whole body digital scanner

WBE
whole body extract

WBF
whole blood folate

WBH
whole blood hematocrit
whole-body hyperthermia

WBM
whole boiled milk

WBN
whole blood nitrogen

WBPTT
whole blood partial thromboplastin time

WBR
whole body radiation
whole body retention

WBRS
Ward Behavior Rating Scale

WBRT
whole blood recalcification time

WBS
Wechsler-Bellevue Scale
whole body scan
whole body shower
wound-breaking strength

WBT
wet-bulb temperature

WBTT
weight bearing to tolerance

WC
Weber-Christian (syndrome)
white cell
white count
whooping cough
will call
work capacity
writer's cramp

WC, WC'
whole complement

WC, W/C
white child

WC, W/C, wc, w/c
wheelchair

WC, w.c.
wound check

WCC
Walker's carcinosarcoma cell
white cell count

WCD
Weber-Christian disease

WCL
Wenckebach cycle length

whole cell lysate
word connection list

W/cm²
watts per centimeter squared

WCN
Walthard's cell nests

WCST
Wisconsin Card-Sorting Test

WD
wallerian degeneration (re: Neuro)
well differentiated
wet dressing
Whitney Damon (dextrose agar)
Wilson's disease
with disease
withdrawal dyskinesia
without dyskinesia
Wolman's disease
wrist disarticulation

WD, W/D, w.d., w-d, w/d
well developed

W/D
warm and dry

W4D
Worth four-dot (test—re: Ophth)

Wd, wd.
ward

wd.
wound

WDCC
well-developed collateral circulation

WDHA
watery diarrhea with hypokalemia and
achlorhydria (syndrome—Verner-
Morrison)

WDHHA
watery diarrhea, hypochlorhydria,
hypokalemia, and alkalosis

WDI
warfarin dose index

WDL
well-differentiated lymphocyte

WDLL
well-differentiated lymphatic lymphoma
well-differentiated lymphocytic
lymphoma

WDS
watery diarrhea syndrome
wet-dog shake (behavior)

wds.
wounds

WDWN, WD/WN; WD, WN
well developed, well nourished

WDWNBM
well-developed, well-nourished black
male

WDWNWF
well-developed, well-nourished white
female

WDWNWM
well-developed, well-nourished white
male

WE
wage earner
wax ester
western encephalitis
western encephalomyelitis
whiskey equivalent

WE, W/E
wound of entry

We
weber (number—re: surface tension
waves)

WEE
western equine encephalomyelitis

w.e.f.
with effect from

WEPS
Work Environment Preference
Schedule (re: Psychol)

WER
wheal erythema reaction

WES
Work Environment Scale (re: Psychol)

WEUP
willful exposure to unwanted pregnancy

WF
Waterhouse-Friderichsen (syndrome)
Weil-Felix (reaction)
wet films
Wistar-Furth (rat)
Word Fluency (test—re: Psychol)

WF, W/F, wf
white female

*WF
West gas phase, fractional
concentration

WFE
Williams flexion exercises (re: PM&R)

WFL
within functional limits

WF-O
will follow in office

WFR
Weil-Felix reaction

WFSS
Wolpe Fear Survey Schedule

WG
water gauge
Wegener's granulomatosis
Wright-Giesma (stain)

WGA
wheat germ agglutinin

WGCTA
Watson-Glaser Critical Thinking
Appraisal

WH
walking heel (cast)
well healed
well hydrated
Werdnig-Hoffmann (syndrome)
whole homogenate
wound healing

wh.
whisper
whispered
white

WHA
warmed, humidified air

wh. ch.
wheelchair

WHNS
well healed, nonsymptomatic (re:
wound)

WHO
World Health Organization
wrist-hand orthosis

whp.
whirlpool

whpl.
whirlpool

Whr, W hr, W-hr, whr
watt hour

WHS
Werdnig-Hoffmann syndrome

WHV
woodchuck hepatic virus

WHVP
wedged hepatic vein pressure
wedged hepatic venous pressure

wh/was
which was

WI
walk-in (medicine)
water ingestion
waviness index

WI-38
Wistar Institute 38 (first continuously
cultivated normal human cell)

WIA
waking imagined analgesia
wounded in action

WIC
women, infants, and children

Wid, wid.
widow
widower

wid.
widowed

WII
Work Information Inventory (re:
Psychol)

WILD
What I Like to Do: An Inventory of
Students' Interests

WIPI
Word Intelligibility by Picture
Identification

WIQ
Waring Intimacy Questionnaire

WIS
Ward Initiation Scale

WISC
Wechsler Intelligence Scale for Children

WISC-R
Wechsler Intelligence Scale for
Children—Revised

WIST
Whitaker Index of Schizophrenic
Thinking

WITT
Wittenborn (Psychiatric Rating Scale)

WK
Wernicke-Korsakoff (syndrome)
Wilson-Kimmelstiel (syndrome)

WK, wk.
weak

wk.
week
work

/wk
per week

WKD
Wilson-Kimmelstiel disease

WK dis.
Wilson-Kimmelstiel disease

WKF
well-known fact

wks
weeks

WKY
Wistar-Kyoto rats

WL
waiting list
weight loss
work load

WL, wl
wavelength

WLD
Werner linear dichroism

WLE
wide local excision

WLF
whole lymphocyte fraction

WLI
weight-length index

WLM
work-level month

WLN
Wiswesser Line Notation (Chemical Code)

WLT
whole lung tomography

WL test
waterload test

WM
warm, moist
Weill-Marchesani (syndrome)
Wernicke-Mann (hemiplegia)
whole milk
Wilson-Mikity (syndrome)
woman milk

WM, W/M, w.m.
white male

WM, wm, w.m.
whole mount (re: microscopy)

WMA
wall motion abnormalities

WMC
weight-matched control

WME
Williams' medium E

WMF
white married female

Wm flex. ex.
Williams flexion exercises

WMM
white married male

WMO
ward medical officer

WMR
work metabolic rate

WMS
Wechsler Memory Scale

Wms flex. ex.
Williams flexion exercises (re: PM&R)

WMX
whirlpool, massage, exercise

WN, W/N, w.n., w-n, w/n
well nourished

WNE
west Nile encephalitis

WNF
well-nourished female

WNL
within normal limits

WNM
well-nourished male

WNPW
wide, notched P wave

WNV
west Nile virus

WNWD
well nourished, well developed

WO
washout (re: nitrogen washout curve)

WO, W/O
written order

W/O
water in oil (re: emulsions)
will order

W/O, w/o
without

WOB
work of breathing

WOE
wound of entry

WOP
without pain

WOU
women's outpatient unit

W/O/W
water in oil in water

WOWS
Weak Opiate Withdrawal Scale

WOX
wound of exit

WP
water packed
weakly positive
wedge pressure
wet pack
wettable powder
whirlpool
white pulp
working point

WPAI
Wilson-Patterson Attitude Inventory (re: Psychol)

WPB
whirlpool bath

WPFM
Wright Peak Flow Meter

WPk
Ward's (mechanical issue) pack (re: Dent)
wet pack

WPM
word per minute (re: telegraph systems)

w.p.m.
words per minute

WPN
white (mucosa with) punctation

WP
water packed

WPPSI
Wechsler Preschool and Primary Scale of Intelligence

WPRS
Wittenborn Psychiatric Rating Scale

WPW
Wolff-Parkinson-White (syndrome)

WR
weak response
weakly reactive
whole response
wiping reflex
work rate

WR, W.R., W.r.
Wassermann reaction

WR, wr.
wrist

W/r
with respect to

Wr^a antigen
very rare blood group antigen

WRAT
Wide Range Achievement Test (re: Psychol)

WRC
washed red cells
water-retention coefficient

WRE
whole ragweed extract

W-response
whole response

WREST
Wide Range Employment Sample Test (re: Psychol)

WRIOT
Wide Range Interest-Opinion Test

WRIPT
Wide Range Intelligence and Personality Test

WRVP
wedged renal vein pressure

WS
Wardenburg's syndrome
water soluble
water swallow
Westphal-Strümpell (syndrome)
wet swallow
whole (response plus white) space
Wilder's silver (stain)
Williams syndrome
working storage (re: computers)

W/S, w.s.
well supported (re: abdomen or perineum)

W-s
watt-seconds

WSA
water-soluble antibiotics

WSB
wheat-soy blend

WSDI
Wahler Self-Description Inventory

W-sec
watt seconds

WSS
weight sum of squares

WSSDT
Washington Speech Sound
  Discrimination Test (re: Psychol)

WT
wall thickness
water temperature
wild type (re: cells; strain)
Wilms' tumor
work therapy

WT, wt.
weight

wt.
white

wt. b.
weight bearing

WTD
wet-tail disease

WTE
whole time equivalent

WTO
write-to-operator (re: computers/data
  processing)

WTOR
write-to-operator with reply (re:
  computers/data processing)

WU
Word Understanding (re: Psychol)

W/U, w/u
work-up

WUSCT
Washington University Sentence
  Completion Test (re: Psychol)

WV
walking ventilation
whispered voice

w/v
percent "weight in volume" (the number
  of grams of an active constitutent in

100 milliliters of solution, whether
  water or another liquid is the solvent)

WVI
Work Values Inventory (re: Psychol)

WV-MBC
ratio of walking ventilation to maximum
  breathing capacity

WW
wet weight

w/w
percent "weight in weight" (the number
  of grams of an active constituent in
  100 grams of solution or mixture)

WWI
World of Work Inventory (re: Psychol)

WWII
World War II

W/wo
with or without

W with P
white with pressure (re: skin blanching)

W without P
white without pressure (re: skin
  blanching)

WWTP
wastewater treatment plant

WX, W/X, w/x
wound of exit

WxB
wax bite (re: Dent)

WxP
wax pattern

WXTRN
weak external reference (re: computers/
  data processing)

WY
women years

WZa
wide zone alpha (hemolysis)

X

X
cross or transverse (re: sections)
crossed with
decimal scale of potency of dilution
exophoria (re: Ophth)
exophoria distance (re: Ophth)
exophoric (re: Ophth)
extra
femal sex chromosome
homeopathic symbol for the decimal
  scale of potencies
Kienböck's unit of x-ray exposure
  (dosage)
magnification
multiplication (sign of)
nervus vagus
reactance (re: electric current)
removal of
respirations (re: anesthesia chart)
roman numeral ten (10)
start of anesthesia
times
unknown quantity
Xanthomonas (genus of plant
  pathogenic micro-organisms)
xanthosine (xanthine ribonucleoside;
  9-β-ᴅ-ribosylxanthine—the
  deamination product of guanosine)
Xenopsylla (genus of fleas)
xerophthalmia

X, x
exposure
extremity
unknown factor
x ray

𝑋
electric susceptibility (when written as a
  subscript)

X, χ
capital and lower-case Greek letter chi

X′
exophoria near (re: Ophth)

X̄, x̄
symbol for the sample mean (re:
  statistics)

X¹
exophoric, near viewing

X$_2$
offspring of a first filial generation test
  cross (re: genetics)

X3, X4..., X 3, X 4....
times three, times four

x
axis (of cylindrical lens)
except
thickness of absorber, mg/cm (re:
  radiation)
xanthine

Ξ
Greek capital letter xi

ξ
Greek lower case letter xi

χ^2
chi square

XA
xanthurenic acid

Xa
chiasma

Xam
examination

X-A mixture
xylene-alcohol mixture (for killing insect
  larvae)

XAN
xanthine

XANES
x-ray absorption near-edge structure

Xanth, xanth.
xanthomatosis

Xao
xanthosine (xanthine ribonucleoside—
  the deamination product of
  guanosine, the O replacing —NH$_2$)

"x" axis of Fick
transverse axis of Fick

X-Bein
genu valgum (Ger. bone)

x-bodies
obsolete term for cancer bodies
unknown flecks noted on certain blood
  specimen slides

XC
excretory cystogram

X_C
capacitive reactance

X-chrome
a sex-determinant chromosome

XD
X-line dominant (re: genetics)

x'd
x-rayed

X2d, X3d,..., X 2d, X 3d....
times two days, times three days...

4Xd, 4 X d
four times a day

X-DBM-MC
X-linked dystrophia bullosa hereditaria,
Mendes da Costa

XDH
xanthine dehydrogenase

X disease
morbid symptoms of unknown origin

XDP
xanthine diphosphate
xeroderma pigmentosum

XDR
transducer

Xe
xenon (element)

Xe
electric susceptibility (when written as a
subscript)

^{127}Xe, Xe 127
xenon-127 (accelerator-produced
radionuclide)

^{133}Xe, Xe 133
xenon-133 (accelerator-produced
radionuclide)

XEF
excess ejection fraction

XEQ
execute (re: computers)

XES
x-ray energy spectrometer
x-ray energy spectroscopy

X-esotropia
increasing convergence from primary
position in both upward and
downward gaze (re: Ophth)

X-factor
hemin (oxidized form of heme)

x factor
an unidentified factor

Xfmr
transformer

Xg
Xg blood group

Xg antigen
Xg blood group antigen

XGP
xanthogranulomatous pyelonephritis

XH
extra high

X Hufte
coxa valga (Ger. hip)

XIP
x ray (examination) in plaster

X-ized
crystallized

XKO
not knocked out

XL
excess lactate
xylose lysine (agar)

X_L
inductive reactance

XLD
xylose, lysine, deoxycholate (agar)

XLH
(human) X-linked hypophosphatemia

XLI
X-linked ichthyosis

XLP
X-linked lymphoproliferative (syndrome)

XLR
X-linked recessive

XM
cross-match (cross match, crossmatch)

X-mas
Christmas (factor)

X-match
cross-match (cross match, crossmatch)

X-matching
cross-matching

XMP
xanthosine monophosphate
(xanthosine-5'-phosphate)

XN
night blindness

Xn
Christian

XO
presence of only one sex chromosome
xanthine oxidase

XOAF
X-linked ocular albinism, Forsius-
  Eriksson (re: genetics)

XOAN
X-linked ocular albinism, Nettleship (re:
  genetics)

X-off
transmitter off (re: computers/data
  processing)

XOM
extraocular movements

X-on
transmitter on (re: computers/data
  processing)

XOOP
x rays out of plaster

XOP
x ray (examination) out of plaster

XOR
exclusive OR (re: binary logic)

X-organ
neurosecretory organ in crustacea

XP
xeroderma pigmentosum

XPN
xanthogranulomatous pyelonephritis

X prep.
x-ray preparation

X-protein
antigammaprotein

XPS
x-ray photoemission spectroscopy

XR
X-linked recessive (re: genetics)

XR, xr
x ray (roentgen ray)

x rays
roentgen rays (algebraic x = unknown)

XRD
x-ray (powder) diffraction

XRF
x-ray fluorescence

XRMR
X-linked recessive mental retardation

XRT
x-ray radiation treatment
x-ray therapy

XS
cross section (cross-section)
excess
xiphisternum

XSA
cross-sectional area
xenograph surface area

X-sect, x sect.
cross-section

XSP
xanthoma striatum palmare

XT
constant exotropia
exotropia (divergent strasbismus;
  exodeviation—re: Ophth)
exotropia distance (re: Ophth)
exotropic (re: Ophth)

XT′
exotropia near (re: Ophth)

X(T)
intermittent exotropia (re: Ophth)

Xta
chiasmata

Xtal
crystal

XTE
xeroderma, talipes, enamel (defect)

X test
Xenopus test (for pregnancy)

XTM
xanthoma tuberosum multiplex

XU
excretory urogram
X-unit (equal to approximately 10^{-13}
  meters—re: x-ray wavelength)

Xu
x-unit (re: x-ray wavelength)

X unit
siegbahn unit (re: describing
  wavelength in x-ray spectroscopy)

X walk
cross-walk

XX
any expiratory gas
double strength
normal female chromosome type (re:
    genetics)

XY
normal male chromosome type (re:
    genetics)

XYL, Xyl
Xylocaine

Xyl
xylose

Xyl & cort.
Xylocaine and cortisone

Y

Y
male sex chromosome
tyrosine
yellow
Yersinia (genus—some species
  pathogenic to man)
yttrium (element)

Y, y
symbol for one of the coordinate axes in
  a plane (re: statistics)
years
young

^{87}Y
radioactive isotope of yttrium

^{88}Y
radioactive isotope of yttrium

^{90}Y
radioactive isotope of yttrium

^{91}Y
radioactive isotope of yttrium

ϒ
Greek capital letter upsilon

y
yield

υ
Greek lower case letter upsilon

Y/A
years ago
years of age

YACP
young adult chronic patient

YADH
yeast alcohol dehydrogenase

YAG
yttrium aluminum garnet

"y" axis of Fick
longitudinal axis of Fick (re: Ophth)

Y/B
yellow/blue

Yb
ytterbium (element)

^{169}Yb, Yb 169
ytterbium-169 (a cyclotron produced
  radionuclide)

^{175}Yb
radioactive isotope of ytterbium

Y band
iliofemoral band

Y body
fluorescent spot seen on long arm of
  chromosome (re: genetics)

YBR
Yellow Brick Road (re: Psychol)

YBT
Yerkes-Bridges test (re: Psychol)

YCB
yeast carbon base

Y chrom.
male sex chromosome

YCT
Yvon coefficient test

yd.
yard

yd^2
square yard

YE
yeast extract
yellow enzyme

YEH$_2$
reduced yellow enzyme

YEI
Yersinia enterocolitica infection

yel.
yellow

ye.s.
yellow spot (of retina)

YF
yellow fever

YFA
young female artertitis

YFI
yellow fever immunization

609

YHMD
yellow hyaline membrane disease

YHT
Young-Helmholtz theory (re: color
vision)

Yk
York (antibodies)

YLF
yttrium lithium fluoride

YLS
years of life saved

YM
yeast, mannitol (medium)

ym
yellow mutant (oculocutaneous
albinism—re: genetics)

YMA
yeast morphology agar

YMT
Yaba monkey tumor

YNB
yeast nitrogen base

YNS
yellow nail syndrome

YO, Y/O, y/o
year(s) old

YOB
year of birth

Y-organ
molting gland in crustacea

YP
yeast phase
yield point
yield pressure

YPA
yeast, peptone, adenine sulfate

yr.
year

YRD
Yangtze River disease

yrs.
years

YS, y.s.
yolk sac

YS, y.s., ys
yellow spot (of retina)

YSC
yoke sac carcinoma

YSIGA
Yellow Springs Instrument glucose
analyzer

YST
yolk sac tumor

Y sutures
junction lines within eye lens

Yt^a
high frequency blood group antigen

YVS
yellow vernix syndrome

Z

Z
atomic number
benzyloxycarbonyl (carbobenzoxy)
(characteristic) impedance
intermediate disk (Z line, Z disk)
ionic charge number
no effect

Z, Z.
Zuckung (Ger. contraction)

Z, Z′, Z″
increasing degrees of contraction

Z, z
standardized deviate (standardized
    score—re: statistics)
zero
zone

Z^1, Z^{11}, Z^{111}
increasing degrees of contraction

Z, Z^I, Z^{II}
increasing degrees of contraction

Z-
zusammen (Ger. together—a
    stereodescriptor—re: isomerism)

(Z)-
zusammen (Ger. together—opposite of
    (E)-; equivalent to cis- in sample
    cases)

ZAP
zymosan-activated plasma

ZAPF
zinc adequate pair—fed

ZAS
zymosan-activated autologous serum

ZAWP
zinc adequate weight—paired

"z" axis of Fick
vertical axis of Fick (re: Ophth)

ZCP
zinc chloride poisoning

ZD
zero discharge
zinc deficient

ZD, Z/D
zero defects

Z-disk
Zwischenscheibe (Ger. intermediate
    disk)

ZDO
zero differential overlap (method)

ZE, Z-E
Zollinger-Ellison (syndrome)

ZEC
Zinsser-Engman-Cole (syndrome)

ZEEP
zero end-expiratory pressure

ZES
Zollinger-Ellison syndrome

ZE syndrome
Zollinger-Ellison syndrome

ZF
zero frequency
zona fasciculata (of adrenal cortex)

ZG
zona glomerulosa (of adrenal cortex)

Z/G
zoster immune globulin

ZGM
zinc glycinate marker

ZI, z.i.
zona incerta (L. uncertain zones
    [area]—re: Neuro)

zi^a
symbol for isotope with atomic number
    Z and atomic weight A

ZIG, ZIg
zoster immune globulin

ZIP
zoster immune plasma

ZK
Zuelzer-Kaplan (syndrome)

Z line
re: myofibrils (Z disk; intermediate disk)

ZMA
zinc meta-arsenite (insecticide)

ZN
Ziehl-Neelsen (method, stain)

Zn
zinc (element)

^{65}Zn
radioactive isotope of zinc

^{69}Zn
radioactive isotope of zinc

Zn fl.
zinc flocculation (test)

ZnO
zinc oxide

ZO
Ziehen-Oppenheim (syndrome)
Zuelzer-Ogden (syndrome)

ZO$_2$
microliters of oxygen taken up per hour
(re: spermatozoa—can vary as
function of temperature)

Zool
zoological
zoology

ZPA
zone of polarizing activity

ZPC
zero point of charge

ZPG
zero population growth

ZPO
zinc peroxide (topical antiseptic;
astringent; wound deodorizer)

ZPP
zinc protoporphyrin

ZR
zona reticularis (re: adrenal cortex)

Zr
zirconium (element)

^{95}Zr
radioactive isotope of zirconium

^{97}Zr
radioactive isotope of zirconium

Z score
standardized deviate (re: statistics)
standard score (re: statistics)

ZSO
zinc suboptimal

ZSR
zeta sedimentation ratio (re: red cells)

ZT
Ziehen's test

ZTS
zymosan-treated serum

ZTT
zinc turbidity test

ZyC
zymosan complement (reagent)

Zz.
zingiber (ginger)

+   acid reaction
added to
an additional whole (if
    before) or part of a
    (if after)
    chromosome (re:
    cytogenetic
    nomenclature)
and
convex lens
decreased (re:
    reflexes)
diminished (re:
    reflexes)
excess
less than 50%
    inhibition of
    hemolysis (re:
    Wassermann)
mild
mild (re: severity)
plus
plus (slightly more
    than stated amount)
positive
positive, mildly
present
slight reaction
slight trace (noticeable
    reaction—re:
    qualitative tests)
sluggish (re: reflexes)

(+)   significant
uncommon or
    uncertain mode of
    inheritance (re:
    genetics)

(+)ive   positive

⊕   plus
positive
present

+ reaction   acid reaction

+ +   50% inhibition of
    hemolysis (re:
    Wassermann)
moderate (re: severity)
moderate pain

normally active (re:
    reflexes)
notable reaction
noticeable reaction
trace
positive moderately
trace (re: qualitative
    tests)

+ + +   increased (re:
    reflexes)
75% inhibition of
    hemolysis (re:
    Wassermann)
moderate amount
moderate reaction
moderate reaction
    (qualitative tests)
moderately
    hyperactive (re:
    reflexes)
moderately severe
moderately severe (re:
    severity)
moderately severe
    pain
positive

+ + + +   complete inhibition of
    hemolysis (re:
    Wassermann)
large amount (re:
    qualitative tests)
markedly hyperactive
    (re: reflexes)
markedly severe pain:
    spastic muscles
positive
pronounced reaction
severe
severe pain (re: pain
    and related
    disability)

−   absent
alkaline
alkaline reaction
concave lens
deficiency
deficient
minus

	missing a whole (if before) or part of a (if after) chromosome (re: cytogenetic nomenclature) negative nil no none triple point of water without
(-)	insignificant
⊖	absent minus negative
− reaction	alkaline reaction
—	mass energy conversion factor
±	doubtful either positive or negative equivocal equivocal (re: qualitative tests) equivocal (re: reflexes) flicker (re: reflexes) indefinite more or less not definite plus or minus possibly significant questionable questionable (re: reflexes) suggestive variable very slight (re: severity) very slight reaction very slight trace very slight trace (re: qualitative tests) with or without
∓	minus or plus
‡	moderate (re: severity) normally active (re: reflexes)
++	moderate (re: severity) normally active (re: reflexes) trace (re: qualitative tests)
+++	increased (re: reflexes) moderate reaction (re: qualitative tests) moderately hyperactive moderately severe (re: severity)
++++	large amount (re: qualitative tests) markedly hyperactive markedly severe pain: spastic muscles pronounced reaction
⊹	moderate pain
⊹⊹	moderately severe pain
⊹⊹⊹	severe pain
± to +	minimal pain
+ to ± ±	slight pain
=	equal equal to equals
≠	does not equal not equal not equal to unequal
≡	identical identical with
≢	not identical not identical with
≒	nearly equal to
≑	approximately equal
≅	approximately approximately equals congruent to
≐	approaches
≜	equilateral
△	equiangular
↑	above elevated elevation enlarged gas greater than

	improved increase increased increases more than rising superior (re: position) upper
↑ V	increase due to in vivo effect
↑↑	extensor response, Babinski sign positive Babinski testes undescended
↓	below decrease decreased deficiency deficit depressed depression deteriorated deteriorating diminished diminution down falling inferior less than low lower precipitate precipitates
↓ V	decrease due to in vivo effect
↓↓	down bilaterally plantar response, Babinski sign testes descended
↑↓	reversible reaction up and down
↖	direction
↗	deviated displaced increasing
↙	decreased
↘	decreasing
↓ g	decreasing diminishing falling lowering

↑	up
→	approaches limit of causes demonstrates direction of flow distal followed by implies indicates indicating "from__to__" (re: cytogenetic nomenclature) is due to leads to produces radiates to radiating to results in reveals shows to to the right toward transfer to yields
←	caused by derived from is due to produced by proximal resulting from secondary to to the left
⇋	electric current reversible reaction reversible chemical reaction
↔ or △	widened width
⇒	implication implies
)	causes demonstrates distal followed by from which is derived greater than implies indicates larger than leads to more severe than produces radiates to radiating to

	results in reveals shows to toward worse than yields	♀	copper female female sex Venus
⟨	caused by derived from less severe than less than produced by proximal smaller than	♂	earth male terra
		♂	conjunction mated mating
≯	not greater than	♂ ♀	having male and female flowers separate
≮	not less than	♂ — ♀	having male and female flowers on the same plant
≥ or ⩾	greater than or equal to		
≤ or ⩽	less than or equal to	♂ : ♀	having male and female flowers on different plants
≧	equal to or greater than equal to or more than greater than or equal to	Ⓐ	axilla
		ⓐₓ	axilla
		©	copyright
≦	equal to or less than less than or equal to	Ⓗ	hypodermic hypodermically
○	annual circle female (re: charts) full moon moon octarius (L. pint) respirations (re: anesthesia records) sex undetermined silver	ⓗ	hypodermic hypodermically
		Ⓜ	intramuscular intramuscularly
		Ⓘᵥ	intravenous intravenously
		Ⓛ	left
		Ⓜ	murmur
○○	male	ⓜ	by mouth mouth murmur
⊙	annual annual plant gold start of operation sun	√ⓜ	factitial murmur
		⊙	by mouth oral orally
⊖	normal		
⊙⊙	biennial biennial plant	Ⓡ	rectal right trademark
♂	iron Mars male male sex	Ⓡ	rectally rectum

⟳ rectally

⊗ end of anesthesia (re:
  anesthesia records)
  end of operation

∧ above
  and
  diastolic blood
    pressure (re:
    anesthesia records)
  elevated
  enlarged
  greater than
  improved
  increased
  more than
  superior (position)
  upper

∨ below
  decreased
  deficiency
  deficit
  depressed
  deteriorated
  deteriorating
  diminished
  diminution
  down
  inferior
  less than
  low
  lower
  or
  systolic blood
    pressure (re:
    anesthesia records)

∠ angle
  flexion
  flexor

∡ angle of entry

∡ angles
  flexors

∡ angle of exit

⌐ right turn (re: accident)

⌐ left turn (re: accident)

□ male
  quadrature

L factorial product
  right angle
  right lower quadrant

Γ right upper quadrant

⌐ left upper quadrant

⌐ left lower quadrant

△ anion gap
  centrad prism
  change
  delta gap
  heat
  increment
  occipital triangle
  prism diopter
  sulfur
  temperature (re:
    anesthesia records)
  trine

△+ time interval

△A change in absorbance

△ dB difference in decibels
  (re: Audio)

△P change in pressure
  (intraocular)

△pH change in pH

△ scan delta scan (CAT scan)

△t time interval

H△ Hesselbach's triangle

H's △ Hesselbach's triangle

÷ divided by
  division

~ about
  approximate
  approximately
  cycle
  difference
  proportionate to
  similar cycle

≃ approximate

≈ approximately equal
  nearly equal to

⊥ perpendicular

† one

†† two

// for
  parallel
  parallel bars

|| parallel
parallel bars

| given

| | absolute value

˙/. defecation

∪ logical sum
union

∩ intersection
logical product

⊂ is contained in

, separates
chromosome
number from sex
chromosome
constitution;
separates sex
chromosome
constitution from
description of
unusual
chromosome(s) (re:
cytogenetic
nomenclature)

/ divided by
either meaning
extension
extensor
fraction
of
organic
per
separates different
karyotypes in
mosaics and
cimaeras (re:
cytogenetic
nomenclature)
shilling
slash
solidus
to
virgule

; separates different
chromosomes (or
parts) involved in
rearrangements (re:
cytogenetic
nomenclature)

: is to
ratio

used to describe a
break (re:
cytogenetic
nomenclature)

:: as
describes breakage
and reunion (re:
cytogenetic
nomenclature)
equality between
ratios
proportion
porportionate to

... no data (in a given
category)

∴ therefore

∵ because
since

' foot
minute
primary accent
univalent

" bivalent
ditto
inch
minute
second
secondary accent

‴ line (¹/₁₂ inch)
trivalent

[ ] brackets
concentration

? doubtful
equivocal (re: reflexes)
flicker (re: reflexes)
not tested (re:
severity)
possible
questionable
question of
suggested
suggestive (re:
severity)
unknown (re:
cytogenetic
nomenclature)

! factorial product

* birth
not verified
presumed

supposed
used as a
  multiplication sign in
  describing variant or
  heteromorphic
  chromosomes (re:
  cytogenetic
  nomenclature)

†   death
    deceased

\#   following a number
    fracture
    gauge
    has been done
    has been given
    number
    pound(s)
    weight

$\sqrt{}$ radical
    root
    square root

$\sqrt[2]{}$ square root

$\sqrt[3]{}$ cube root

$\sqrt[4]{}$ fourth root

$\rightarrow$ not

$\rightleftharpoons$ reversible reaction

$\sqrt{}$ check
    observe for
    urine
    voided

$\sqrt{.}$ urine and defecation
    voided and bowels
    moved

$\sqrt{}$'d   checked
    examined
    observed

$\sqrt{}$g   checking

$\sqrt{}$ing   checking

$\sqrt{}$qs   voided sufficient
    quantity

$\sqrt{}$ c̄   check with

°   degree (temperature,
    severity,
    measurement)

hour (time — 1°, 2°,
  etc.)
measurement of
  strabismus angle
  (re: Ophth)

1°   first degree
    one hour
    primary

2°   because of
    due to
    secondary
    secondary to
    second degree
    two hours

24°   24 hours

$\frown$ combined with

$\approx$ equivalent

$\not\approx$ not equivalent to

∞ indefinitely more
    infinity
    infinity (six meters [20
    feet] or more
    distance—re:
    Ophth)
    is to

(concave

$\propto$ variant
    varies

∂ differential

MISCELLANEOUS SYMBOLS

  acinar

$\dot{\bar{1}}$ bowel movement
    (roman numeral
    indicates number of
    stools in a given
    period)

$\dfrac{4\ cm}{-2}\ \bigg|\ \dfrac{75\%}{Vtx}$ 4 cm = dilation of
    cervix
  75% = degree of
    cervical
    effacement
  Vtx = vertex;
    presentation
    of fetus (Br
    = breech)

− 2 = station; distance above (−) or below (+) the spine of the ischium measured in centimeters

circumduction

coarsening

coin-like

conical

dilated pupil

discoid

3 or 3⊤ dram, teaspoonful, 5 ml

ellipsoid

eye

encircling girdling

Erlenmeyer flask-like

ƒ3 fluid dram

3 ss̄ half ounce, tablespoonful, 15 ml

international symbol for biohazard

/ linear

mosaic

∘○◯ nodular

i̇s̄s̄ one and one-half

3 or 3⊤ ounce, 30 ml

plate-like

♉ pound

ptosis (lid lag)

▱ pyramidal

○─< recumbent position

 Э scruple

sitting position

○ spherical

spindling

thumb-printing

△ triangular

triple arthrodesis

3 ⅱ two drams, 2 teaspoonsful, 10 ml

GENETICS SYMBOLS

◦ ● abortion or stillbirth sex unspecified

(□) adopted

● affected female

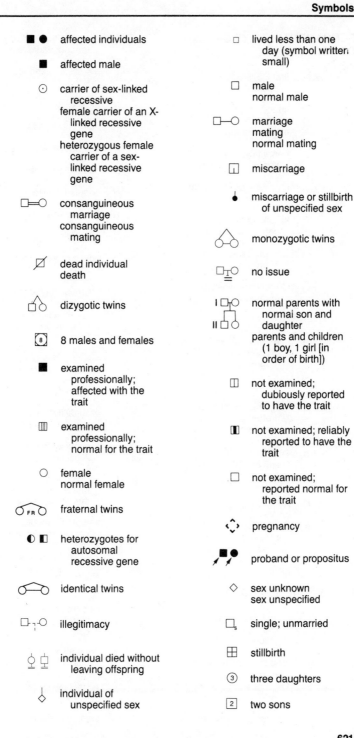

■ ● affected individuals

■ affected male

☉ carrier of sex-linked recessive
female carrier of an X-linked recessive gene
heterozygous female carrier of a sex-linked recessive gene

□═○ consanguineous marriage
consanguineous mating

▨ dead individual
death

△○ dizygotic twins

⑧ 8 males and females

■ examined professionally; affected with the trait

▥ examined professionally; normal for the trait

○ female
normal female

○FR○ fraternal twins

◑ ◧ heterozygotes for autosomal recessive gene

⌒ identical twins

□⌐○ illegitimacy

♀ ♂ individual died without leaving offspring

◇ individual of unspecified sex

□ lived less than one day (symbol written small)

□ male
normal male

□─○ marriage
mating
normal mating

▣ miscarriage

● miscarriage or stillbirth of unspecified sex

△○ monozygotic twins

□⊤○ no issue

I □○
II □ ○ normal parents with normal son and daughter
parents and children (1 boy, 1 girl [in order of birth])

▦ not examined; dubiously reported to have the trait

◧ not examined; reliably reported to have the trait

□ not examined; reported normal for the trait

⟨⟩ pregnancy

■● proband or propositus

◇ sex unknown
sex unspecified

□ₛ single; unmarried

⊞ stillbirth

③ three daughters

② two sons

621

FUNDAMENTAL PHYSICAL CONSTANTS

αa_o	first Bohr radius of hydrogen
c	speed of light
e	electron charge
ϵ_0	permittivity of free space
J	mechanical equivalent (15° calorie)
Λ	kX unit to ångström conversion factor
λ_c	Compton wavelength of proton
λ_{cp}	Compton wavelength of proton
m	electronic rest mass
μ_B	magnetic moment of electron (Bohr magneton)
M_n	neutron rest mass
μ_N	magnetic moment of proton (proton magneton)
μ_O	permeability of free space (rationalized)
M_p	proton rest mass
R	Rydberg constant
σ	Stefan-Boltzmann constant
V_O	standard volume

STATISTICAL SYMBOLS

α	probability of Type I error significance level
β	probability of Type II error
E	expected frequency in a cell of a contingency table
$E(X)$	expected value of the random variable X
F	F statistic (variance ratio)
f	frequency
H_O	null hypothesis
H_1	alternative hypothesis
μ	population mean
N	population size
n	sample size
$n!$	n factorial
$1 - \beta$	power of a statistical test
$_nC_k$; $\binom{n}{k}$	binomial coefficient number of combinations of n thing taken k at a time
O	observed frequency in a contingency table
P	probability
p	probability of success in independent trials
$P(A)$	probability that event A occurs
$P(A/B)$	conditional probability that A occurs given that B has occurred
r	sample correlation coefficient (usually Pearson product-moment correlation)
r_2	coefficient of determination
r_s	Spearman rank correlation coefficient
ρ	population correlation coefficient
s	sample standard deviation
s_2	sample variance

σ	population standard deviation standard deviation	t	student's t statistic student's test variable
σ_2	population variance	ϕ	ability continuum phi coefficient
$\sigma_{diff.}$	standard error of the difference between scores	θ	latent trait
SE	standard error of estimate	U	Mann-Whitney rank sum statistic
$\sigma_{est.}$	standard error of estimate	W	Wilcoxson rank sum statistic
$\displaystyle\sum_{i=1}^{n} x_i$	$x_1 + x_2 + \ldots x_n$	$\overline{X}$	sample mean
		$\lvert x \rvert = x$	$x \geq 0$ (absolute value) $x \leq 0$ (absolute value)
$\sigma_{meas.}$	standard error of measurement	z	standard score

CHEMOTHERAPY REGIMENS

ABC
Adriamycin, BCNU, cyclophosphamide

ABCM
Adriamycin (doxorubicin), bleomycin, cyclophosphamide, and mitomycin C

ABD
Adriamycin, bleomycin, DTIC (dacarbazine)

ABDIC
Adriamycin (doxorubicin), bleomycin, dacarbazine (DIC), CCNU (lomustine)

ABDV
Adriamycin, bleomycin, DTIC, vinblastine

ABP
Adriamycin, bleomycin, prednisone

ABV
actinomycin D, bleomycin, vincristine
Adriamycin, bleomycin, vinblastine

ABVD
Adriamycin, bleomycin, vinblastine, dacarbazine

AC
Adriamycin, CCNU
Adriamycin, cyclophosphamide

A-C
Adriamycin, cyclophosphamide

ACe
Adriamycin, cyclophosphamide (Cytoxan)

ACFUCY
actinomycin D, 5-fluorouracil, cyclophosphamide

ACM
Adriamycin (doxorubicin), cyclophosphamide, and methotrexate

ACOP
Adriamycin, cyclophosphamide, Oncovin, prednisone

ACOPP, A-COPP
Adriamycin (doxorubicin), cyclophosphamide, Oncovin (vincristine), procarbazine, and prednisone

ADBC
Adriamycin, DTIC, bleomycin, CCNU

ADOAP
Adriamycin (doxorubicin), Oncovin (vincristine), ara-C (cytarabine), and prednisone

ADOP
Adriamycin, Oncovin, prednisone

Adria-L-PAM
Adriamycin, L-phenylalanine mustard

ALOMAD
Adriamycin (doxorubicin), Leukeran (chlorambucil), Oncovin (vincristine), methotrexate, actinomycin D (dactinomycin), and dacarbazine

APC
AMSA (amsacrine; 4'-(9-acridimylamino-methanesulfon-*m*-anisidide), prednisone, chlorambucil

APO
Adriamycin, prednisone, Oncovin (vincristine)

ara-C-HU
cytosine arabinoside and hydroxyurea

AV
Adriamycin (doxorubicin) and vincristine

AVP
actinomycin D (dactinomycin), vincristine, and Platinol (cisplatin)

BACOD
bleomycin, Adriamycin, Cytoxan, Oncovin, dexamethasone (Decadron)

BACON
bleomycin, Adriamycin (doxorubicin), CCNU (lomustine), Oncovin (vincristine), and nitrogen mustard

BACOP
bleomycin, Adriamycin (doxorubicin), cyclophosphamide, Oncovin (vincristine), and prednisone

BACT
BCNU, ara-C, cyclophosphamide,
6-thioguanine

BAMON
bleomycin, Adriamycin (doxorubicin),
methotrexate, Oncovin (vincristine),
and nitrogen mustard

BAVIP
bleomycin, Adriamycin (doxorubicin),
vinblastine, imidazole carboxamide
(dacarbazine), and prednisone

BCAVe, B-CAVe
bleomycin, CCNU (lomustine),
Adriamycin (doxorubicin), velban
(vinblastine)

BCD
bleomycin, cyclophosphamide,
dactinomycin

B-CHOP
bleomycin, Cytoxan,
hydroxydaunomycin (Adriamycin),
Oncovin, prednisone

BCMF
bleomycin, cyclophosphamide,
methotrexate, and 5-fluorouracil

BCOP
BCNU (carmustine),
cyclophosphamide, Oncovin
(vincristine), and prednisone

BCP
BCNU (carmustine),
cyclophosphamide, prednisone

BCVP
BCNU (carmustine),
cyclophosphamide, vincristine, and
prednisone

BCVPP
BCNU (carmustine),
cyclophosphamide, vinblastine,
procarbazine, and prednisone

B-DOPA
bleomycin, DTIC, Oncovin, prednisone,
Adriamycin

BEP
bleomycin, etoposide, Platinol

BHD
BCNU (carmustine), hydroxyurea, and
dacarbazine

BHDV, BHD-V
BCNU (carmustine), hydroxyurea,
dacarbazine, and vincristine

BLEO-COMF
bleomycin, cyclophosphamide, Oncovin
(vincristine), methotrexate, and
5-fluorouracil

B-MOPP
bleomycin, nitrogen mustard, Oncovin,
procarbazine, prednisone

BMP
BCNU, methotrexate, procarbazine

BOAP
bleomycin, Oncovin, Adriamycin,
prednisone

BOLD
bleomycin, Oncovin (vincristine),
lomustine, and dacarbazine

BONP
bleomycin, Oncovin, Natulan
(procarbazine hydrochloride),
prednisolone

BOP
BCNU, Oncovin, prednisone

BOPAM
bleomycin, Oncovin (vincristine),
prednisone, Adriamycin (doxorubicin),
mechlorethamine (nitrogen mustard),
and methotrexate

BOPP
BCNU, Oncovin, procarbazine,
prednisone

BVAP
BCNU (carmustine), vincristine,
Adriamycin (doxorubicin), and
prednisone

BVCPP
BCNU (carmustine), vinblastine,
cyclophosphamide, procarbazine,
and prednisone

BVDS
bleomycin, Velban, doxorubicin
(Adriamycin), streptozotocin

BVPP
BCNU, vincristine, procarbazine,
prednisone

CABOP, CA-BOP
Cytoxan (cyclophosphamide),
Adriamycin (doxorubicin), bleomycin,
Oncovin (vincristine), and prednisone

CABS
CCNU, Adriamycin, bleomycin,
streptozotocin

CAD
cyclophosphamide, Adriamycin,
dacarbazine
cytosine arabinoside (cytarabine) and
daunorubicin

CAF
cyclophosphamide (Cytoxan),
Adriamycin (doxorubicin), and
5-fluorouracil (5-FU)

CAFP
cyclophosphamide (Cytoxan),
Adriamycin (doxorubicin),
5-fluorouracil, and prednisone

CAFVP
cyclophosphamide (Cytoxan),
Adriamycin (doxorubicin),
5-fluorouracil, vincristine (Oncovin),
and prednisone

CAM
cyclophosphamide (Cytoxan),
Adriamycin (doxorubicin), and
methotrexate

CAMB
Cytoxan (cyclophosphamide),
Adriamycin (doxorubicin),
methotrexate, bleomycin

CAMELEON
cytosine arabinoside (cytarabine),
methotrexate, Leukovorin (citrovorum
factor), and Oncovin (vincristine)

CAMEO
cyclophosphamide, Adriamycin,
methotrexate, etoposide, Oncovin

CAMF
cyclophosphamide (Cytoxan),
Adriamycin (doxorubicin),
methotrexate, and folinic acid
(citrovorum factor)

CAMP
Cytoxan (cyclophosphamide),
Adriamycin (doxorubicin),
methotrexate (MTX), procarbazine
hydrochloride (Matulane)

CAO
cyclophosphamide, Adriamycin,
Oncovin

CAP
cyclophosphamide (Cytoxan),
Adriamycin (doxorubicin), and Platinol
(cisplatin)
cyclophosphamide (Cytoxan),
Adriamycin (doxorubicin), and
prednisone

CAP-I
cyclophosphamide (Cytoxan),
Adriamycin (doxorubicin), and Platinol
(cisplatin)

CAP-II
cyclophosphamide (Cytoxan),

Adriamycin (doxorubicin), and high
dose Platinol (cisplatin)

CAP-BOP
cyclophosphamide (Cytoxan),
Adriamycin (doxorubicin),
procarbazine (Matulane), bleomycin,
Oncovin (vincristine), and prednisone

CAT
cytosine arabinoside, Adriamycin,
6-thioguanine

CAV
cyclophosphamide (Cytoxan),
Adriamycin (doxorubicin), and
vincristine (Oncovin)
Cytoxan, Adriamycin, Velban

CAVe, CA-Ve
CCNU (lomustine), Adriamycin
(doxorubicin), and Velban
(vinblastine)

CBVD
CCNU, bleomycin, vinblastine,
dexamethasone

CCM
cyclophosphamide (Cytoxan), CCNU
(lomustine), and methotrexate

CCV-AV
CCNU (lomustine), cyclophosphamide
(Cytoxan), vincristine (Oncovin)
alternating with Adriamycin
(doxorubicin) and vincristine

CCVPP
CCNU, cyclophosphamide, Velban,
procarbazine, prednisone

CEP
CCNU, etoposide (VP-16-213),
prednimustine

CFP
cyclophosphamide (Cytoxan),
5-fluorouracil, and prednisone

CHAD
cyclophosphamide (Cytoxan),
hexamethylmelamine, Adriamycin
(doxorubicin), and cis-
diamminedichloroplatinum (cisplatin)

CHEX-UP, ChexUP, Chex-Up
cyclophosphamide,
hexamethylmelamine, 5-fluorouracil,
Platinol

CHF
cyclophosphamide,
hexamethylmelamine, 5-fluorouracil,

CHO
cyclophosphamide (Cytoxan),

hydroxydaunomycin (doxorubicin),
and Oncovin (vincristine)

CHOB
cyclophosphamide, Adriamycin,
Oncovin, bleomycin

CHOP
cyclophosphamide,
hydroxydaunomycin/doxorubicin
(Adriamycin), Oncovin, prednisone

CHOP-BLEO
cyclophosphamide,
hydroxydaunomycin/doxorubicin
(Adriamycin), Oncovin, prednisone,
bleomycin

CHOR
cyclophosphamide, hydroxydaunomycin
(doxorubicin), Oncovin (vincristine),
and radiation therapy

CHVP
cyclophosphamide, hydroxydaunomycin
(doxorubicin), VM-26 (teniposide),
and prednisone

CH1VPP, Ch1VPP
chlorambucil, vinblastine, procarbazine,
prednisone

CIA
CCNU (lomustine), isophosphamide,
and Adriamycin (doxorubicin)

CISCA, CisCA
cisplatin, Cytoxan, Adriamycin

CIVPP
chlorambucil, vinblastine, procarbazine,
prednisone

CMC
cyclophosphamide, methotrexate,
CCNU

CMC-VAP
cyclophosphamide (Cytoxan),
methotrexate, CCNU (lomustine),
vincristine (Oncovin), Adriamycin
(doxorubicin), and procarbazine

CMF
Cytoxan (cyclophosphamide),
methotrexate, 5-fluorouracil (5-FU)

CMF/AV
cyclophosphamide (Cytoxan),
methotrexate, 5-fluorouracil,
Adriamycin (doxorubicin), and
Oncovin (vincristine)

CMFAVP
cyclophosphamide, methotrexate,
5-fluorouracil, Adriamycin, vincristine,
prednisone

CMFP, CMF-P
cyclophosphamide (Cytoxan),
methotrexate, 5-fluorouracil, and
prednisone

CMFT
cyclophosphamide, methotrexate,
5-fluorouracil, tamoxifen

CMFVAT
cyclophosphamide, methotrexate,
5-fluorouracil, vincristine, Adriamycin,
testosterone

CMFVP
Cytoxan, methotrexate, 5-fluorouracil,
vincristine (Oncovin), prednisone

CMOP
cyclophosphamide, Oncovin,
procarbazine, prednisone

C-MOPP
cyclophosphamide (Cytoxan),
mechlorethamine (Mustargen),
Oncovin (vincristine), procarbazine,
and prednisone (a modification of
standard MOPP chemotherapy
regimen in which Cytoxan is
substituted for the M [Mustargen]—
also called COPP)

COAP
cyclophosphamide (Cytoxan), Oncovin
(vincristine), ara-C (cytarabine), and
prednisone

COAP-BLEO
cyclophosphamide (Cytoxan), Oncovin
(vincristine), ara-C (cytarabine),
prednisone, and bleomycin

COM
cyclophosphamide, Oncovin
(vincristine), and MeCCNU
(semustine)
cyclophosphamide, Oncovin,
methotrexate

COMA-A
cyclophosphamide (Cytoxan), Oncovin
(vincristine), methotrexate/citrovorum
factor, Adriamycin (doxorubicin), and
ara-C (cytarabine)

COMB
cyclophosphamide (Cytoxan), Oncovin
(vincristine), MeCCNU (semustine),
and bleomycin
Cytoxan, Oncovin, methotrexate,
bleomycin

COMe
Cytoxan, Oncovin, methotrexate

COMF
cyclophosphamide (Cytoxan), Oncovin

(vincristine), methotrexate, and
5-fluorouracil

COMLA
cyclophosphamide (Cytoxan), Oncovin
(vincristine), methotrexate,
leucovorin, ara-C (cytarabine)

COMP
CCNU, Oncovin, methotrexate,
procarbazine
cyclophosphamide (Cytoxan), Oncovin
(vincristine), methotrexate, and
prednisone

CONPADRI, CONPADRI-I
cyclophosphamide, Oncovin
(vincristine), L-phenylalanine
mustard, and Adriamycin
(doxorubicin)

COP
Cytoxan (cyclophosphamide), Oncovin
(vincristine sulfate), prednisone

COPA
Cytoxan (cyclophosphamide), Oncovin
(vincristine sulfate), prednisone,
Adriamycin (doxorubicin)

COPA-BLEO
cyclophosphamide (Cytoxan), Oncovin
(vincristine), prednisone, Adriamycin
(doxorubicin), and bleomycin

COPAC
CCNU (lomustine), Oncovin
(vincristine), prednisone, Adriamycin
(doxorubicin), and cyclophosphamide
(Cytoxan)

COPB
cyclophosphamide, Oncovin,
prednisone, bleomycin

COP-BLAM
cyclophosphamide, Oncovin,
prednisone, bleomycin, Adriamycin,
Matulane (procarbazine)

COP-BLEO
cyclophosphamide (or chlorambucil),
Oncovin (vincristine), prednisone,
and bleomycin

COPP
CCNU, Oncovin, procarbazine,
prednisone
cyclophosphamide (Cytoxan), Oncovin
(vincristine), procarbazine,
prednisone

CP
cyclophosphamide and prednisone

CPM
CCNU, procarbazine, methotrexate

CPOB
cyclophosphamide, prednisone,
Oncovin, bleomycin

CROP
cyclophosphamide, Rubidazone,
Oncovin (vincristine), and prednisone

Ctx-Plat
cyclophosphamide, Platinol

CVA
cyclophosphamide, vincristine,
Adriamycin

CVA-BMP, CVA + BMP
cyclophosphamide (Cytoxan),
vincristine, Adriamycin (doxorubicin),
BCNU (carmustine), methotrexate,
and procarbazine

CVB
CCNU, vinblastine, bleomycin

CVM
cyclophosphamide, vincristine,
methotrexate

CVP
Cytoxan (cyclophosphamide),
vincristine, prednisone

CVPP
CCNU (lomustine), vinblastine,
prednisone, and procarbazine
cyclophosphamide, Velban,
procarbazine, prednisone

CVPP-CCNU
cyclophosphamide, vinblastine,
procarbazine, prednisone, CCNU

CyADIC
cyclophosphamide, Adriamycin
(doxorubicin), and DIC (dacarbazine)

CY-VA-DACT
cyclophosphamide, vincristine,
Adriamycin (doxorubicin), and
dactinomycin

CYVADIC, CY-VA-DIC, CyVADIC
Cytoxan (cyclophosphamide),
vincristine, Adriamycin, and dimethyl
imidazole carboxamide
(DTIC = dimethyl triazene imidazole
carboxamide; DIC)

CYVMAD
cyclophosphamide, vincristine,
methotrexate, Adriamycin, DTIC
(dimethyl triazene imidazole
carboxamide; DIC)

DA
daunomycin and ara-C (cytarabine)

DAP-II
dianhydrogalactitol, Adriamycin
(doxorubicin), and Platinol (cisplatin)

DAT
daunomycin, ara-C, 6-thioguanine

DAVH
dibromodulcitol, Adriamycin
(doxorubicin), vincristine, and
Halotestin (fluoxymesterone)

DCCMP
daunorubicin, cyclocytidine,
6-mercaptopurine, and prednisone

DCMP
daunorubicin, cytarabine,
6-mercaptopurine, and prednisone

DCV
DTIC, CCNU, vincristine

DOAP
daunorubicin, Oncovin (vincristine), ara-
C (cytarabine), and prednisone

DTIC-ACT-D
DTIC (dacarbazine), actinomycin D
(dactinomycin)

DVB
cis-diamminedichloroplatinum,
vindesine, bleomycin

DZAPO
daunorubicin, azacytidine, ara-C
(cytarabine), prednisone, and
Oncovin (vincristine)

ECHO
etoposide, cyclophosphamide,
hydroxydaunomycin (doxorubicin),
and Oncovin (vincristine)

FAC
5-fluorouracil, Adriamycin (doxorubicin),
and cyclophosphamide (Cytoxan)

FAC-LEV
5-fluorouracil, Adriamycin (doxorubicin),
cyclophosphamide (Cytoxan), and
levamisole

FACP
ftorafur, Adriamycin (doxorubicin),
cyclophosphamide (Cytoxan), and
Platinol (cisplatin)

FAM
5-fluorouracil, Adriamycin (doxorubicin),
and mitomycin C

FAME
5-fluorouracil, Adriamycin (doxorubicin),
and MeCCNU (semustine)

FAMMe
5-fluorouracil, Adriamycin, mitomycin C,
semustine

FAM-S
5-fluorouracil, Adriamycin, mitomycin C,
streptozotocin

FCP
5-fluorouracil, cyclophosphamide, and
prednisone

FIME
5-fluorouracil, ICRF-159 (razoxane), and
MeCCNU (methyl-CCNU—
semustine)

FOAM
5-FU, Oncovin, Adriamycin,
mitomycin C

FOMI
5-fluorouracil, Oncovin (vincristine), and
mitomycin

FUM
5-fluorouracil and methotrexate

FURAM
ftorafur, Adriamycin (doxorubicin), and
mitomycin C

HAD
hexamethylmelamine, Adriamycin
(doxorubicin), and cis-
diamminedichloroplatinum (cisplatin)

HAM
hexamethylmelamine, Adriamycin
(doxorubicin), and melphalan
hexamethylmelamine, Adriamycin,
methotrexate

H-CAP
hexamethylmelamine,
cyclophosphamide, Adriamycin,
Platinol

HDMTX-CF
high-dose methotrexate-citrovorum
factor

HDMTX/LV
high-dose methotrexate and leucovorin

HexaCAF, Hexa-CAF
hexamethylmelamine,
cyclophosphamide, methotrexate,
5-fluorouracil

HOAP-BLEO
hydroxydaunomycin (doxorubicin),
Oncovin (vincristine), ara-C
(cytarabine), prednisone, and
bleomycin

HOP
hydroxydaunomycin (doxorubicin), Oncovin (vincristine), and prednisone

LAPOCA
L-asparaginase, prednisone, Oncovin (vincristine), cytarabine, and Adriamycin (doxorubicin)

LMF
Leukeran (chlorambucil), methotrexate, and 5-fluorouracil

MABOP
Mustargen (nitrogen mustard), Adriamycin, bleomycin, Oncovin, prednisone

MAC
methotrexate, actinomycin D, cyclophosphamide
mitomycin C, Adriamycin (doxorubicin), and cyclophosphamide

MACC
methotrexate, Adriamycin (doxorubicin), cyclophosphamide, and CCNU (lomustine)

MAD
MeCCNU (semustine) and Adriamycin (doxorubicin)

M-BACOD
methotrexate/citrovorum factor, bleomycin, Adriamycin (doxorubicin), cyclophosphamide (Cytoxan), Oncovin (vincristine), and dexamethasone

MBD
methotrexate, bleomycin, diamminedichloroplatinum (cisplatin)

MCBP
melphalan, cyclophosphamide, BCNU, prednisone

MCP
melphalan, cyclophosphamide, prednisone

MECY
methotrexate, cyclophosphamide

MF
mitomycin, 5-fluorouracil

MFP
melphalan, 5-fluorouracil, medroxyprogesterone acetate

MIFA
mitomycin C, 5-fluorouracil, and Adriamycin (doxorubicin)

Mini-COAP
cyclophosphamide, Oncovin (vincristine), ara-C (cytarabine), and prednisone

MOB
(nitrogen) mustard, Oncovin, bleomycin

MOB-III
mitomycin C, Oncovin (vincristine), bleomycin, and cisplatin

MOF
MeCCNU (semustine), Oncovin (vincristine), and 5-fluorouracil

MOF-STREP, MOF-Strep
MeCCNU (semustine), Oncovin (vincristine), 5-fluorouracil, and streptozotocin

MOMP
mechlorethamine, Oncovin (vincristine), methotrexate, and prednisone

MOP
Mustargen (nitrogen mustard), Oncovin, prednisone

MOP-BAP
mechlorethamine (nitrogen mustard), Oncovin (vincristine), procarbazine, bleomycin, Adriamycin (doxorubicin), and prednisone

MOPP
(nitrogen) mustard, Oncovin (vincristine), procarbazine, and prednisone
Mustargen hydrochloride (mechlorethamine hydrochloride), Oncovin (vincristine), procarbazine, and prednisone
Mustine hydrochloride (mechlorethamine hydrochloride), Oncovin (vincristine), procarbazine, and prednisone

MOPP/ABV hybrid
nitrogen mustard, Oncovin, procarbazine, prednisone, Adriamycin, bleomycin, vinblastine

MOPP-BLEO, MOPP-Bleo
mechlorethamine (nitrogen mustard), Oncovin (vincristine), procarbazine, prednisone, and bleomycin

MOPPHDB
(nitrogen) mustard, Oncovin, procarbazine, prednisone, and high-dose bleomycin

MOPPLDB
(nitrogen) mustard, Oncovin, procarbazine, prednisone, and low-dose bleomycin

MOPr
(nitrogen) mustard, Oncovin,
  procarbazine

MP
melphalan and prednisone

MVPP
(nitrogen) mustard, vinblastine,
  procarbazine, prednisone

MVVPP
(nitrogen) mustard, vincristine,
  vinblastine, procarbazine, prednisone

NAC
nitrogen mustard, Adriamycin
  (doxorubicin), and CCNU (lomustine)

OAP
Oncovin (vincristine), ara-C
  (cytarabine), and prednisone

O-DAP
Oncovin (vincristine),
  dianhydrogalactitol, Adriamycin
  (doxorubicin), and Platinol (cisplatin)

OMAD
Oncovin (vincristine), methotrexate (and
  citrovorum factor), Adriamycin
  (doxorubicin), and dactinomycin
  (actinomycin D)

OPAL
Oncovin (vincristine), prednisone,
  L-asparaginase

OPP
Oncovin (vincristine), procarbazine, and
  prednisone

PAC
Platinol (cisplatin), Adriamycin
  (doxorubicin), and cyclophosphamide

PATCO
prednisone, ara-C (cytarabine),
  thioguanine, cyclophosphamide, and
  Oncovin (vincristine)

PAVe
procarbazine, Alkeran, Velban

PBV
Platinol, bleomycin, vinblastine

PEP
Procytox (cyclophosphamide),
  epipodophyllotoxin derivative
  (VM-26), and prednisolone

PFT
phenylalanine mustard (melphalan),
  fluorouracil, tamoxifen

POC
procarbazine, Oncovin, CCNU

POCA
prednisone, Oncovin (vincristine),
  cytarabine, and Adriamycin
  (doxorubicin)

POCC
procarbazine, Oncovin (vincristine),
  cyclophosphamide, and CCNU
  (lomustine)

POMP
prednisone, Oncovin (vincristine),
  methotrexate, and Purinethol
  (6-mercaptopurine)

PRIME
procarbazine, isophosphamide, and
  methotrexate

ProMACE
prednisone, methotrexate, Adriamycin,
  cyclophosphamide, etoposide
  (VP-16-213)

PROMACE-MOPP
procarbazine, methotrexate,
  Adriamycin, Cytoxan, etoposide
  (VP-16-213), Mustargen, Oncovin,
  procarbazine, prednisone

Pulse VAC
vincristine, actinomycin D
  (dactinomycin), and
  cyclophosphamide

PVB
Platinol (cisplatin), vinblastine, and
  bleomycin

ROAP
Rubidazone, Oncovin (vincristine),
  ara-C (cytarabine), and prednisone

RUBIDIC
Rubidazone/DTIC

SMF
streptozotocin, mitomycin C, and
  5-fluorouracil

STEAM
streptonigrin, thioguanine,
  cyclophosphamide, actinomycin,
  mitomycin C

TAD
6-thioguanine, ara-C (cytarabine), and
  daunorubicin

T-CAP III
triazinate, cyclophosphamide,
  Adriamycin (doxorubicin), and Platinol
  (cisplatin)

TOAP
thioguanine, Oncovin (vincristine),
  cytosine arabinoside (cytarabine),
  and prednisone

VAB
vinblastine, actinomycin D
(dactinomycin), and bleomycin

VAB-I
vinblastine, actinomycin D, bleomycin

VAB-II
vinblastine, actinomycin D
(dactinomycin), bleomycin, and
cisplatin

VAB-III
vinblastine, actinomycin D
(dactinomycin), bleomycin, cisplatin,
chlorambucil, and cyclophosphamide

VAB-V
vinblastine, actinomycin D
(dactinomycin), bleomycin,
cyclophosphamide, and cisplatin

VABCD
vinblastine, Adriamycin, bleomycin,
CCNU, DTIC

VAC
vincristine, actinomycin D
(dactinomycin), and
cyclophosphamide
vincristine, Adriamycin (doxorubicin),
and cyclophosphamide

VAFAC
vincristine, amethopterin
(methotrexate), 5-fluorouracil,
Adriamycin (doxorubicin), and
cyclophosphamide

VAM
VP-16-213 (etoposide), Adriamycin
(doxorubicin), and methotrexate

VAMP
vincristine, amethopterin
(methotrexate), 6-mercaptopurine,
and prednisone

VAP
vinblastine, actinomycin D
(dactinomycin), and Platinol
(cisplatin)
vincristine, Adriamycin (doxorubicin),
and prednisone
vincristine, Adriamycin, procarbazine

VATD, VAT-D
vincristine, ara-C (cytarabine),
6-thioguanine, and daunorubicin

VATH
vinblastine, Adriamycin (doxorubicin),
and thiotepa
vinblastine, Adriamycin (doxorubicin),
thiotepa, Halotestin
(fluoxymesterone)

VAV
VP-16-213 (etoposide), Adriamycin
(doxorubicin), and vincristine

VB
vinblastine, bleomycin

VBA
vincristine, BCNU, Adriamycin

VBAP
vincristine, BCNU (carmustine),
Adriamycin (doxorubicin), and
prednisone

VBD
vinblastine, bleomycin, and cis-
diamminedichloroplatinum (cisplatin)

VBM
vincristine, bleomycin, methotrexate

VBMCP
vincristine, BCNU (carmustine),
melphalan, cyclophosphamide,
prednisone

VBP
vinblastine, bleomycin, and Platinol
(cisplatin)

VCAP
vincristine, cyclophosphamide,
Adriamycin (doxorubicin), and
prednisone

V-CAP III
VP-16-213 (etoposide),
cyclophosphamide, Adriamycin
(doxorubicin), and Platinol (cisplatin)

VCF
vincristine, cyclophosphamide, and
5-fluorouracil

VCMP
vincristine, cyclophosphamide,
melphalan, prednisone

VCP
vincristine, cyclophosphamide,
prednisone

VDP
vincristine, daunorubicin, prednisone

VENP
vincristine, Endoxan
(cyclophosphamide), Natulan,
prednisone

VEPA
vincristine, Endoxan
(cyclophosphamide), prednisolone,
Adriamycin

VLP
vincristine, L-asparaginase, and
prednisone

VMAD
vincristine, methotrexate, Adriamycin,
actinomycin D

VMCP
vincristine, melphalan,
cyclophosphamide, prednisone

VM-26PP
VM-26 (teniposide), procarbazine,
prednisone

VOCAP
VP-16-213 (etoposide), Oncovin
(vincristine), cyclophosphamide,
Adriamycin (doxorubicin), Platinol
(cisplatin)

VP
vincristine and prednisone

VPB
vinblastine, Platinol, bleomycin

VPBCPr
vincristine, prednisone, vinblastine,
chlorambucil, procarbazine

VPCMF
vincristine, prednisone,
cyclophosphamide, methotrexate,
and 5-fluorouracil

A
acetum (L. vinegar)
acidum (L. acid)
annus (L. year)

A, a
aqua (L. water)

A, a, a.
arteria (L. artery)

a.
ante (L. before)
auris (L. ear)

ā
before (L. ante)

aa.
arteria (L. arteries)

absc.
abscissa (L. torn or wrenched away;—
the x-coordinate value of a point on a
graph)

abs. feb.
absente febre (L. in the absence of
fever)

AC, a.c., āc.
ante cibum (L. before a meal)

a.c.
ante cibos (L. before meals)

accur.
accuratissime (L. most carefully,
accurately)

acet.
acetum (L. vinegar)

AC&HS
ante cibum et hora somni (L. before a
meal and at the hour of sleep—at
bedtime)

AD
atrio dextro (L. in the right atrium)
atrium dextra (L. hall or entrance room
+ right)

AD, a.d.
auris dextra (L. right ear)
aurio dextra (L. in the right ear)

ad.
adde (L. add)
addetur (L. let there be added)

ad baln.
ad balneum (L. to the bath)

add.
addantur (L. let them be added)
addatur (L. let it be added)
adde (L. add)
addendo (L. by adding)
addendum (L. to be added)
addetur (L. let there be added)

add. c. trit.
adde cum tritu (L. add with a rubbing
[triturition])

ad def. an.
ad defectionem animi (L. to the point of
fainting)

ad deliq.
ad deliquium (L. to fainting)

addend.
addendum (L. to be added)

ad duas vic.
ad duas vices (L. to two doses [for two
doses])

ad effect.
ad effectum (L. to effect)

ad. feb.
adstante febre (L. fever being present)

ad gr. acid.
ad grata aciditatem (L. to an agreeable
acidity)

ad grat. acid.
ad grata aciditatem (L. to an agreeable
acidity)

ad grat. gust.
ad gratum gustum (L. to an agreeable
taste)

ad gr. gust.
ad gratum gustum (L. to an agreeable
taste)

adhib.
adhibendus (L. to be administered)

ad int.
ad interim (L. to meanwhile)

Ad lib., ad lib.
ad libitum (L. freely; at pleasure)

adm.
admove (L. apply, add)

ad man. med.
ad manus medici (L. [to be delivered] into the hands of the [prescribing] physician)

admov.
admove (L. apply; add)
admoveantur (L. let them be added)
admoveatur (L. let there be added; let it be applied)

ad naus.
ad nauseam (L. to the extent of producing nausea)

ad neut.
ad neutralisandum (L. to neutralization)
ad neutrum (L. to neither [neutralize; neutralized; neutralization])

ad part. dolent.
ad partes dolentes (L. to the aching parts)

ad pond. om.
ad pondus omnium (L. to the weight of the whole)

ad rat.
ad rationem (L. to ratio)

ad sat.
ad saturandum (L. to saturation)

ad satur.
ad saturandum (L. to saturation)

adst. feb.
adstante febre (L. when fever is present; while fever is present)

ad tert. vic.
ad tertium vicem (L. to the third time [to three doses])

ad us.
ad usum (L. according to custom)

ad us. ext.
ad usum externum (L. for external use)

ad us. exter.
ad usum externum (L. for external use)

ad us. med.
ad usum medicinalem (L. for medicinal use)

ad us. propr.
ad usum proprium (L. according to proper use)

ad us. vet.
ad usum veterinarium (L. for veterinary use)

adv.
adversum (L. against; adverse to; opposed to)

ad 2 vic.
ad duas vices (L. at two times; for two doses)

ae.
aetatis (L. of age)

AEG, aeg.
aeger; aegra (L. the sick one [male, female])

aeq.
aequales (L. equals)

aet.
aetas (L. age)
aetatis (L. of age)

aetat.
aetatis (L. of age)

aff.
affinis (L. having an affinity with [but not identical with])

Ag
argentum (L. silver)

ag. feb.
aggrediente febre (L. when the fever increases)

AGIT, agit.
agita (L. shake; stir)

agit. ante sum.
agita ante sumendum (L. shake before taking)

agit. a. us.
agita ante usum (L. shake before using)

agit. bene
agita bene (L. shake well)

agit. vas.
agitato vase (L. the vial having been shaken)

AL, a.l.
auris laeva (L. left ear)

alb.
albus (L. white)

aliq.
aliquot (L. some; several)

alt. die.
alternis diebus (L. every other day)

alt. dieb.
alternis diebus (L. every other day)

alt. h.
alternis horis (L. every other hour)

alt. hor.
alternis horis (L. every other hour)

alt. noc.
alterna nocte (L. every other night)

alt. noct.
alterna nocte (L. every other night)

alv. adst.
alvo adstricto (L. when the bowels are
    constricted)

alv. deject.
alvi dejectiones (L. throwing down of the
    bowel— [pertaining to the bowel or
    intestine; bowel movement])

AM, A.M., a.m.
ante meridiem (L. before noon [in the
    morning])

a.m.
ante menstruationem (L. before
    menstruation)

ampl.
amplus (L. large)

ampul.
ampulla (L. ampule; ampoule)

ant. jentac.
ante jentaculum (L. before breakfast)

ant. prand.
ante prandium (L. before dinner)

AP, A/P
ante partum (L. before + to bring forth
    [before onset of labor—re: the
    mother])
antepartum (L. before parturition—re:
    the mother)

a p.
a priori (L. first; before)

a.p.
ante prandium (L. before dinner)

APH
ante partum hemorrhage (L. before
    onset of labor—re: the mother)
antepartum hemorrhage (L. before
    onset of childbirth—re: the mother)

applan.
applanatus (L. flattened; flat)

applicand.
applicandus (L. to be applied)

AQ, aq.
aqua (L. water)
aqueous (watery)

aq. astr.
aqua astricta (L. frozen water)

aq. bul.
aqua bulliens (L. boiling water)

aq. bull.
aqua bulliens (L. boiling water)

aq. cal.
aqua calida (L. hot water)

aq. com.
aqua communis (L. common water)

aq. comm.
aqua communis (L. common water)

aq. dest.
aqua destillata (L. distilled water)

aq. ferv.
aqua fervens (L. boiling water)

aq. fluv.
aqua fluvialis (L. flowing water [river
    water]

aq. font.
aqua fontis (L. spring water [fountain
    water])

aq. frig.
aqua frigida (L. cold water)

aq. mar.
aqua marina (L. sea water)

aq. menth. pip.
aqua menthae piperitae (L. peppermint
    water)

aq. niv.
aqua nivalis (L. snow water)

aq. pluv.
aqua pluvialis (L. rain water)

aq. pur.
aqua pura (L. pure water)

aq. tep.
aqua tepida (L. lukewarm water)

arg.
argentum (L. silver)

AS, A.S., a.s.
auris sinistra (L. left ear)

ascr.
ascriptum (L. ascribed to)

AU, A.U., a.u.
aures unitae (L. both ears together)
aures utrae (L. both ears)
auris utraque (L. each ear)

Au
aurum (L. gold—element)

a.u.
ad usum (L. according to custom)

auct.
auctorum (L. of authors)

aug.
augere (L. to increase)

aur.
aures (L. ears)
auris (L. ear)
aurum (L. gold)

aurin.
aurinarium (L. ear cone)

aurist.
auristillae (L. ear drops)

B, b.
balneum (L. bath)
bis (L. twice, two times)

BA
balneum arenae (L. sand bath)

BAL, bal.
balneum (L. bath)

bal. arenae
balneum arenae (L. sand bath)

bal. mar.
balneum maris (L. salt or sea-water bath)

bals.
balsamum (L. balsam)

bal. sin.
balneum sinapsis (L. mustard bath)

bal. vap.
balneum vaporis (L. steam or vapor bath)

BD, b.d.
bis die (L. twice a day)

b.d.s.
bis in die summendus (L. to be taken twice a day)

ben.
bene (L. well)

bib.
bibe (L. drink)

b.i.d.
bis in die (L. twice daily; twice a day)

bihor.
bihorium (during two hours [perhaps a contraction of Latin bis = twice + horium = hourly])

b.i.n.
bis in noctus (L. twice a night)

bis in 7d.
bis in septem diebus (L. twice a week)

b.l.
balneum luti (L. mud bath)

BM, B.M., b.m.
balneum maris (L. sea-water bath)

bol.
bolus (L. pill)

bull.
bulliant (L. let them boil)
bulliat (L. let it boil)
bulliens (L. boiling)

but.
butyrum (L. butter)

b.v.
balneum vaporis (L. vapor bath)

C
carbon (element—L. charcoal)
compositus (L. compound)
congius (L. gallon)
contusus (L. bruised)
costa (L. rib)

C, c.
centum (L. one hundred)
cibus (L. meal)
circa (L. about)

C̄, c, c., c̄
cum (L. with)

c.
cornu (L. horn)

Ca
calcium (L. calx; limestone—[element])

ca.
circa (L. about, approximately)

caerul.
caeruleus (L. sky blue)

calef.
calefac (L. make warm)
calefactus (L. warmed)

c. amplum
cocleare amplum (L. [spoon shaped like a snail's shell] heaping spoonful; also spelled cochleare)

CaO
calcium oxide (L. calx, quicklime [plus oxide])

CAP, Cap, cap.
capsula (L. a little chest—capsule)

CAP, cap.
capiat (L. let the patient take)

cap.
caput (L. head)

capiend.
capiendus (L. to be taken)

cap. moll.
capsula mollis (L. soft capsule)

cap. quant. vult
capiat quantum vult (L. let [the patient] take as much as he wants)

caps.
capsula (L. a little box—capsule)

capsul.
capsula (L. a little box—capsule)

cat.
cataplasma (L. a poultice)

CATH, Cath, cath.
catharticus (L. cathartic)

cc, c.c., c̄c
cum correctione (L. with correction—re: Ophth)

CD, cd
candela (L. candle—SI base unit of luminous intensity)

CD, c.d.
conjugata diagonalis (L. diagonal conjugate—diameter of pelvic inlet)

Ce
celeriter (L. quickly)

cerat.
ceratum (L. wax ointment)

CF, cf, cf.
confer (L. compare, confer, bring together, compare with, or refer to)

CH
chirugia (L. surgery)

CHART, Chart, chart.
charta (L. paper [a powder in paper])

chart.
chartula (L. a small [medicated] paper)

chart. bib.
charta bibula (L. blotting paper)

chart. cerat.
charta cerata (L. waxed paper; parchment paper)

chirurg.
chirurgicalis (L. surgical)

chord. chirurg.
chorda chirurgicalis (L. surgical cord—re: suture)

cht.
chartula (L. a small [medicated] paper)

cib.
cibus (L. food; meal)

cito disp.
cito dispensetur (L. let it be dispensed quickly)

CM
causa mortis (L. cause of death)

c.m.
cras mane (L. tomorrow morning)

c. magnum
cocleare magnum (L. [spoon shaped like a snail's shell] large spoonful—also spelled cochleare)

c. medium
cocleare medium (L. a half spoonful)

c.m.s.
cras mane sumendus (L. to be taken tomorrow morning)

c.n.
cras nocte (L. tomorrow night)

c.n.s.
cras nocte sumendus (L. to be taken tomorrow night)

co.
compositus (L. a compound, compounded)

coch.
cochleare (L. [spoon shaped like a snail's shell] by the spoonful)

coch. amp.
cochleare amplum (L. [spoon shaped like a snail's shell] a heaping spoonful)

cochl.
cochleare (L. [spoon shaped like a snail's shell] by the spoonful)

cochl. amp.
cochleare amplum (L. [spoon shaped like a snail's shell] a heaping spoonful)

cochleat.
cochleatum (L. [spoon shaped like a snail's shell] spoonful)

cochl. mag.
cochleare magnum (L. [spoon shaped like a snail's shell] a large spoonful)

cochl. med.
cochleare medium (L. [spoon shaped like a snail's shell] a half spoonful)

cochl. parv.
cochleare parvum (L. [spoon shaped like a snail's shell] a teaspoonful)

coch. mag.
cochleare magnum (L. [spoon shaped like a snail's shell] a large spoonful)

coch. med.
cochleare medium (L. [spoon shaped like a snail's shell] half spoonful)

coch. mod.
cochleare modicum (L. [spoon shaped like a snail's shell] a medium-size spoonful [dessert spoonful])

coch. parv.
cochleare parvum (L. [spoon shaped like a snail's shell] a teaspoonful)

Coct, coct.
coctio (L. boiling)

COL, col.
cola (L. filter, strain [imperative])

col.
colatus (L. strained, filtered)

colat.
colatus (L. strained, filtered)

colen.
colentur (L. let them be strained, filtered)

colet.
coletur (L. let it be strained, filtered)

coll.
collyrium (L. eyewash—a soothing eye water; originally any eye preparation—poultice, salve)

collun.
collunarium (L. a nose wash)

collut.
collutorium (modified L. col- + past participle of luo-, to wash [lutus]; washed thoroughly [mouthwash])

collyr.
collyrium (L. an eyewash—a soothing eye water; originally any eye preparation—poultice, salve)

color.
coloretur (L. let it be colored)

comm. cer.
commotio cerebri (L. violent movement of cerebrum [cerebral concussion])

comp.
compositus (L. compound, compounded, compounded [of])

con.
contra (L. against)

conc.
concisus (L. cut, brief)

CONCIS, concis.
concisus (L. cut; brief)

conf.
confectio (L. a confection)

cong.
congius (L. gallon)

cons.
conserva (L. keep, save)
consonans (L. sounding with [tinkling])

consperg.
consperge (L. dust, sprinkle [imperative])
conspergere (L. to dust or sprinkle)
conspergitur (L. it is being sprinkled)

cont.
contra (L. against)
contusus (L. bruised)

conter.
contere (L. rub together)

contin.
continuetur (L. let it be continued)

cont. rem.
continuentur remedia (L. let the medicines be continued)

contrit.
contritus (L. broken; ground)

contus.
contusus (L. bruised)

coq.
coquatur (L. let it be boiled)
coque (L. boil)

coq. in s.a.
coque in sufficiente aqua (L. boil in sufficient water)

coq. s.a.
coque secundum artem (L. boil properly)

coq. simul
coque simul (L. boil at the same time)

COR
corpus (L. body)

cort.
cortex (L. bark, rind)

c. parvum
cochleare parvum (L. [spoon shaped like a snail's shell] a teaspoonful)

cr.
cras (L. tomorrow)

crast.
crastinus (L. for tomorrow)

cr. vesp.
cras vespere (L. tomorrow evening)

CS
corpus striatum (L. the striate body—re: Neuro)

CTa, Cta, cta.
catamenia (L. according to the month [menstruation])

c. tant.
cum tanto (L. with the same amount [of])

Cu
cuprum (L. copper—[an element])

cuj.
cujus (L. of which, of any)

cuj. lib.
cujus libet (L. of any you please; of whatever you please)

curat.
curatio (L. a taking care of [a dressing)])

CV
conjugata vera (L. true conjugate [diameter of pelvic inlet])

CV, c.v.
cras vespere (L. tomorrow evening)

CVO
conjugata vera obstetrica (L. true obstetric conjugate [diameter of pelvic inlet])

cwt
cent (L. centum [+ weight—hundredweight])

cyath.
cyathus (L. ladle for removing wine from the bowl [wineglass])

cyath. vin.
cyathus vinarius (L. a wineglass)

cyath. vinos.
cyathus vinosus (L. wineglass)

D, d
dentur (L. let [such] be given)

D, d.
da (L. give)
detur (L. let it be given)
dexter (L. right)
dosis (L. dose)

d
dies (L. day)

dand.
dandus (L. to be given)

d.c.f.
detur cum formula (L. let it be given with set form "prescribed rule")

dct.
decoctum (L. boiled [down to concentrate or extract an active principle by boiling thoroughly])

d.d.
de die (L. daily)
detur ad (L. let it be given to)

d. d. in d.
de die in diem (L. from day to day)

d.e.
dosis effectiva (L. effective dose)

dearg. pil.
deargentur pilulae (L. let the pills be silvered)

deaur. pil.
deaurentur pilulae (L. let the pills be gilded)

deb. spis.
debita spissitudine (L. of the proper consistency)

deb. spiss.
debita spissitudo (L. proper consistency)

dec.
decanta (L. pour off)
decoctum (L. boiled down [to extract an active principle or to concentrate by boiling thoroughly])

decoct.
decoctum (L. boiled [down to extract an

active principle or to concentrate by boiling thoroughly])

decub.
decubitus (L. lying down)

de d. in d.
de die in diem (L. from day to day)

D eff.
dosis efficax (L. efficacious dose)

deglut.
deglutia (L. swallow [imperative])
deglutiatur (L. let it be swallowed)

dent.
dentur (L. give; let them be given)

dent. tal. dos.
dentur tales doses (L. let such doses be given)

dep.
depuratus (L. purified)

dest.
destilla (L. distil)
destillatus (L. distilled)

destil.
destilla (L. distil)

det.
detur (L. give)
detur (L. let it be given)

det. in dup.
detur in duplo (L. let twice as much be given)

det. in 2 plo.
detur in duplo (L. let twice as much be given)

d. et s.
detur et signetur (L. let it be given and labeled)

dext.
dexter (L. right)
dextra (L. right)
dextro (L. right)

dieb. alt.
diebus alternis (L. on alternate days)

dieb. secund.
diebus secundis (L. every second day)

dieb. tert.
diebus tertiis (L. every third day)

dig.
digeratur (L. let it be digested)

dil.
dilue (L. dilute or dissolve)
dilutus (L. dilute, diluted)

diluc.
diluculo (L. at daybreak)

dilut.
dilutus (L. diluted, dilute)

DIM
dosis infectiosis media (L. medium infectious dose)

DIM, dim.
dimidius (L. halved)

dim.
diminutus (L. diminished)

d. in dup.
detur in duplo (L. let twice as much be given)

d. in p. aeq.
dividatur in partes aequales (L. divide into equal parts)

dir.
directione (L. by direction)

direct. prop.
directione propria (L. with proper direction; with the proper directions)

dir. prop.
directione propria (L. with proper direction; with the proper directions)

disp.
dispensa (L. dispense)
dispensetur (L. let it be dispensed)

div.
dividatur (L. divide)

divid.
dividatur (L. divide)

div. in p. aeq.
dividatur in partes aequales (L. let it be divided into equal parts)

div. in par. aeq.
dividatur in partes aequales (L. let it be divided into equal parts)

DL
dosis letalis (L. lethal dose)

do.
dicto (L. the same, as before, repeat)

dol.
dolor (L. pain)

don.
donec (L. until)

donec alv. sol. ft.
donec alvus soluta fuerit (L. until the bowels are open)

donec alv. sol. fuerit
donec alvus soluta fuerit (L. until the bowels are open)

dos.
dosis (L. dose)

d.p.
directione propria (L. with proper direction)

d.s.n.
detur suo nomine (L. let it be given in his/her name)

D tal. dos.
dentur tales doses (L. let such doses be given)

d.t.d.
dentur tales doses (L. give such doses; let such doses be given)
detur talis dosis (L. give such a dose; let such a dose be given)
dosis therapeutica die (L. daily therapeutic dose)

d.t.d. No. iv
dentur tales doses No. iv (L. let four such doses be given)

Dtox
dosis toxica (L. toxic dose)

dulc.
dulcis (L. sweet)

dur.
durante (L. duration; during)
durus (L. hard)

dur. dol.
durante dolore (L. while the pain lasts)

dur. dolor.
durante dolore (L. while the pain lasts)

dwt
denarius weight (L. denarius—a Roman coin which was also used as a measure of weight [pennyweight])

e, e.
ex (L. from, out of)

ead.
eadem (L. the same)

e.g.
exempli gratia (L. for example)

ejusd.
ejusdem (L. of the same)

elect.
electuarium (L. electuary—a medium which melts in the mouth; a confection)

emend.
emendatis (L. emended)

emp.
emplastrum (L. a plaster)

e.m.p.
ex modo praescripto (L. in [or] after the manner prescribed; as directed)

emp. vesic.
emplastrum vesicatorium (L. a blistering plaster)

emuls.
emulsio (L. an emulsion)

ES
enema saponis (L. soap enema)

et al.
et alibi (L. and elsewhere)
et alii (L. and others)

etc.
et cetera (L. and others; and so forth)

et seq.
et sequens (L. and the following)
et sequentes (L. and those that follow)

ex aff.
ex affinibus (L. of the neighboring [affinity])

exhib.
exhibeatur (L. let it be displayed [shown])

expect.
expectoratium (L. expectorant)

exsicc.
exsiccatus (L. dried out)

ext.
extendere (L. to spread; to extend)
extractum (L. extract)

F, f
fiat (L. let it be made)
forma (L. form, figure, shape)

f
fac (L. make)
fiant (L. let them be made)

fac.
facere (L. to make; to form; construct; create)

fasc.
fasciculus (L. small bundle)

Fe
ferrum (L. iron [an element])

feb.
febris (L. fever)

feb. dur.
febre durante (L. while the fever lasts)
febris durantibus (L. while the fevers
  last)

FEM
femoris (L. of the thigh)

Fem Intern., fem. intern.
femoribus internus (L. at the inner side
  of the thighs)

Fer
ferrum (L. iron)

ferv.
fervens (L. boiling)

f.h.
fiat haustus (L. let a draught be made)

filt.
filtra (L. filter [imperative form])

fl.
fluidus (L. fluid)

f.l.a.
fiat lege artis (L. let it be done according
  to rule of the art)

flav.
flavus (L. yellow)

fldext.
fluidius extractus (L. fluidextract)
fluidum extractum (L. fluidextract)

fldxt.
fluidius extractus (L. fluidextract)
fluidum extractum (L. fluidextract)

flor.
flores (L. flowers)

fluid.
fluidus (L. fluid [adj.])

F.M., f.m.
fiat mistura (L. let a mixture be made)

fol.
folia (L. leaves)
folium (L. a leaf)

fort.
fortis (L. strong)

f.p.
fiat potio (L. let a potion be made)
fiat pulvis (L. let a powder be made)

f. pil.
fiant pilulae (L. let pills be made)
fiat pilula (L. let a pill be made)

f. pil. xi
fac pilulas xi (L. make 11 pills [lower-
case letter Roman numerals for
  number of pills])

FR
fructus (L. fruit, enjoyment)

fract. dos.
fracta dosi (L. in a divided dose)

frem.
fremitus vocalis (L. vocal + roaring,
  murmuring, growling [a thrill caused
  by speaking—on auscultation])

frig.
frigidus (L. cold)

frust.
frustillatim (L. by small pieces)

f.s.a.
fiat secundum artem (L. let it be made
  skillfully)

f.s.a.r.
fiat secundum artis regulas (L. let it be
  made according to the rules of the
  art)

ft.
fac (L. make)
fiant (L. let them be made)
fiat (L. let it be made)

ft. catapl.
fiat cataplasma (L. let a poultice be
  made)

ft. cataplasm.
fiat cataplasma (L. let a poultice be
  made)

ft. cerat.
fiat ceratum (L. let a cerate be made
  [medicinal topical formulation made
  with wax for ease of spreading
  without liquifying])

ft. chart. vi
fiant chartulae vi (L. let six powders be
  made [use small letter Roman
  numerals for number])

ft. collyr.
fiat collyrium (L. let an eyewash be
  made)

ft. emuls.
fiat emulsio (L. let an emulsion be
  made)

ft. enem.
fiat enema (L. let an enema be made)

ft. garg.
fiat gargarisma (L. let a gargle be made)

ft. infus.
fiat infusum (L. let an infusion be made)

ft. injec.
fiat injectio (L. let an injection be made)

ft. linim.
fiat linimentum (L. let a liniment be made)

ft. mas.
fiat massa (L. let a mass be made)

ft. mas. div. in pil.
fiat massa dividenda in pilulae (L. let a mass be made and divided into pills)

ft. mass. div. in pil. xiv
fiat massa et divide in pilulae xiv (L. let a mass be made and divide into 14 pills [lower-case Roman numerals for number of pills])

ft. mist.
fiat mistura (L. let a mixture be made)

ft. pil. xxiv
fiant pilulae xxiv (L. let 24 pills be made [lower-case Roman numerals for number of pills])

ft. pulv.
fiat pulvis (L. let a powder be made)

ft. sol.
fiat solutio (L. let a solution be made)

ft. solut.
fiat solutio (L. let a solution be made)

ft. suppos.
fiat suppositorium (L. let a suppository be made)

ft. troch.
fiant trochisci (L. let lozenges be made)

ft. ung.
fiat unguentum (L. let an ointment be made)

f. vs., f.v.s.
fiat venae sectio (L. let there be a cutting of a vein [venisection])

g.
gramma (L. gram)

GARG, garg.
gargarisma (L. a gargle)

gel. quav.
gelatina quavis (L. in any kind of jelly)

gen.
genus (L. kind)

gen. et sp. nov.
genus et species nova (L. new genus and species)

gen. nov.
genus novum (L. new genus)

ging.
gingiva (L. gum)

GL
glandula (L. gland)

gl.
glandula(e) (L. gland[s])

gland.
glandula (L. gland)

glyc.
glyceritum (L. glycerite)

Gm
gramma (L. gram)

gr.
grana (L. grains)
granum (L. grain)
gravida (L. heavy; pregnant)

GRAD, grad.
gradatim (L. by degrees; gradually)

gran.
granulatus (L. granulated)

Grav, grav.
gravida (L. heavy; pregnant)

grav. I
gravida una (L. heavy; pregnant once)
primigravida (L. first heavy; first pregnancy)

gravid.
gravida (L. heavy; pregnant)

grav. †
primigravida (L. first heavy; first pregnancy)

grav. †/Ab. †
gravida 1, aborta 1 (L. one pregnancy, one abortion)

gr.m.p.
grosso modo pulverisatum (L. ground in a coarse way)

gros.
grossus (L. coarse)

gt.
gutta (L. drop)

gtt.
guttae (L. drops)

gtts.
guttae (L. drops)

gutt.
gutturi (L. to the throat)

guttat.
guttatim (L. drop by drop)

gutt. quibusd.
guttis quisbusdam (L. with a few drops)

H, h.
haustus (L. a draught; a drink)
hora (L. hour)

habt.
habeatur (L. let the patient have)

haust.
haustus (L. a draught; a drink)

HD
heloma durum (L. hard core [re: Podiatry])

h.d.
hora decubitus (L. at bedtime)

HE
hic est (L. this, that is)
hoc est (L. this, that is)

herb. recent.
herbarium recentium (L. of fresh herbs)

Hg
hydrargyrum (New Latin from Greek hydrarguros—silver water [the element mercury])

HM
heloma molle (L. soft corn [re: Podiatry])

h.n.
hoc nocte (L. tonight)

hoc vesp.
hoc vespere (L. this evening)

hor. decu.
hora decubitus (L. at bedtime)

hor. decub.
hora decubitus (L. at bedtime)

hor. interm.
hora intermedia (L. at the intermediate hour)
horis intermediis (L. at the intermediate hours)

hor. som.
hora somni (L. hour of sleep; bedtime)

hor. 1 spat.
horae unius spatio (L. one hour's time)

hor. un. spatio
horae unius spatio (L. one hour's time)

HS, h.s.
hora somni (L. hour of sleep; bedtime)

h. som.
hora somni (L. hour of sleep; bedtime)

ht.
haustus (L. a draught; a drink)

h.v.
hoc vespere (L. this evening)

I
incisivus (L. cut into)

ib.
ibidem (L. in the same place)

ibid.
ibidem (L. in the same place)

i.c.
inter cibos (L. between meals)

id.
idem (L. the same)

i.d.
in diem (L. during the day)

id. ac
idem ac (L. the same as)

idon. vehic.
idoneo vehiculo (L. in a suitable vehicle)

i.e.
id est (L. that is)

illic. lag. obturat.
illico lagena obturatur (L. let the bottle be closed at once)

incid.
incide (L. cut)

in d.
in die (L. in a day)
in dies (L. daily)

in extrem.
in extremis (L. in the last [hours of life])

INF, inf.
infunde (L. pour in)
infusum (L. an infusion)

in f.
in fine (L. finally; at the end)

infund.
infunde (L. pour in)

inhal.
inhalatio (L. inhalation)

inj.
injectio (L. an injection)

inj. enem.
injiciatur enema (L. let an enema be injected)

in litt.
in litteris (L. in correspondence)

in loc. cit.
in loco citato (L. in the place cited)

in pulm.
in pulmento (L. in gruel)

insuf.
insufflatio (L. an insufflation)

int.
intime (L. to the innermost)

int. cib.
inter cibos (L. between meals)

int. noct.
inter noctem (L. during the night)

involv.
involve (L. roll on [coat])

i.q.
idem quod (L. the same as)

IS, i.s.
in situ (L. in [original] place)

i.s.q.
in statu quo (L. unchanged)

IU
in utero (L. in the uterus)

IV
in vitro (L. in a glass [test tube])
in vivo (L. in the alive [body])

jentac.
jentaculum (L. breakfast)

jucund.
jucunde (L. pleasantly)

JUXT, juxt.
juxta (L. near)

Kal
kalium (L. potassium; from Arabic—qali [potash]— an element)

L
liber (L. book)
lues (L. plague—syphilis)

L, l
libra (L. pound; balance)

l.a.
lege artis (L. according to the art)

laev.
laevus (L. left)

lag.
lagena (L. a flask, bottle)

lapid.
lapideum (L. stony)

lat. admov.
lateri admoveatum (L. let it be applied to the side)

lat. dol.
lateri dolenti (L. to the painful side)

lb, lb.
libra (L. "pound"; balance [about 12 troy ounces])

lb ap.
libra apothecary (L. apothecary [pound])

lb av.
libra avoirdupois (L. avoirdupois [pound])

lbs
librae (L. pounds)

lb t.
libra troy (L. pound[s] troy)

l.c.
loco citato (L. in the place cited)

lenit.
leniter (L. gently)

lev.
levis (L. light)

levit.
leviter (L. lightly)

lib.
libra (L. balance; "pound" [about 12 troy ounces])

LIM
limes (L. boundary)

lin.
linimentum (L. a liniment)

liq.
liquor (L. a liquor; a solution)

loc. cit.
loco citato (L. in the place cited)

loc. dol.
loco dolenti (L. to the painful spot)

long.
longus (L. long)

lot.
lotio (L. a lotion)

l.q.
lege quaeso (L. I ask by law)

LT
lues test (L. plague—re: syphilis)

luc. prim.
luce prima (L. at first light [daybreak])

lut.
luteum (L. yellow)

M
macerare (L. to soften)
mentum (L. chin)
meridies (L. noon)
mille (L. thousand)
misce (L. mix)
mistura (L. a mixture)
mitte (L. send)
morbus (L. disease, sickness)
mors (L. death)
mortuus (L. dead)
multipara (L. many labors—births)
mutitas (L. dumbness)

M, m.
manipulus (L. handful)

M, m, m.
milli- (L. one thousand)

m.
mane (L. in the morning)
minimum (L. least)

ma.
macera (L. soften)

mac.
macera (L. soften)
macerare (L. to soften)

m. accur.
misce accuratissme (L. mix very
   accurately)

mag.
magnus (L. large)

magn.
magnus (L. large)

mal.
malanando (L. by blistering)
malandria (L. blisters)

man.
mane (L. morning, in the morning)
manipulus (L. a handful)

MANIP, manip.
manipulus (L. a handful)

man. pr.
mane primo (L. first thing in the
   morning)

man. prim.
mane primo (L. first thing in the
   morning)

mas.
massa (L. a mass)

mas. pil.
massa pilularum (L. pill mass)

mass.
massa (L. a mass)

matut.
matutinus (L. in the morning)

m.b.
misce bene (L. mix well)

m. caute
misce caute (L. mix cautiously)

m. dict.
more dicto (L. in the manner directed)

M.D.S.
misce, da, signa (L. mix, give, label)

med.
medicamentum (L. a medicine)

M et f. pil.
misce et fiant pilulae (L. mix and let pills
   be made)

M et f. pulv.
misce et fiat pulvis (L. mix and let a
   powder be made)

m. et n.
mane et nocte (L. morning and night)

M et sig., m. et sig.
misce et signa (L. mix and label)

M flac., m. flac.
membrana flaccida (L. flaccid
   membrane [pars flaccida membrana
   tympani—Shrapnell's membrane])

m.f. pil.
misce, fiant pilulae (L. mix, let pills be
   made)

m. ft.
mistura fiat (L. let a mixture be made)

mic. pan.
mica panis (L. bread crumb)

MIN, min.
minimum (L. minimum)

mist.
mistura (L. a mixture)

mit.
mitte (L. let go)

mitt.
mitte (L. let go)

mitte sang.
mitte sanguinem (L. let go the blood [blood letting procedure])

mitt. tal.
mitte tales (L. send such)

mitt. x tal.
mitte decem tales (L. send ten like this)

mixt.
mixtura (L. mixture)

mod.
modicus (L. moderate-sized)
modulus (L. a little measure)

mod. praesc.
modo praescripto (L. in the manner prescribed)

moll.
mollis (L. soft)

mor. dict.
more dicto (L. in the manner directed)

mor. sol.
more solito (L. in the usual way, manner, as accustomed)

MP, m.p.
modo praescripto (L. in the manner prescribed)

MTAD
membrana tympana auris dextrae (L. tympanic membrane of the right ear)

MTAS
membrana tympana auris sinistrae (L. tympanic membrane of the left ear)

MTAU
membranae tympani aures unitae (L. tympanic membranes of both ears)

m.t.d.
mitte tales doses (L. send such doses)

MUC, muc.
mucilago (L. mucilage)

N, n
natus (L. born)

n
naris (L. nostril)

Na
natrium (L. sodium—an element)

Natr
natrium (L. sodium)

NB, n.b.
nota bene (L. note well; take notice)

nebul.
nebula (L. a cloud [as a nebulizer])

n. et m.
nocte et mane (L. night and morning)

ne. tr. s. num.
ne tradas sine nummo (L. deliver not without the money [do not deliver unless paid])

nig.
niger (L. black)

nil.
nihil (L. nothing)

n.l.
non licet (L. it is not permitted; it is not lawful)
non liquet (L. it is not clear)

nm
nocte et mane (L. night and morning)

n & m
nocte et mane (L. night and morning)

nn.
nervi (L. nerves)
nomen novum (L. new name)

n. nov.
nomen novum (L. new name)

no.
numero (L. to the number of)
numerus (L. number)

nob.
nobis (L. to us [as a new species])

noc.
noctis (L. of the night—[nocturnal])

Noct, noct.
nocte (L. at night)

noct.
noctis (L. of the night—[nocturnal])
nox (L. night)

noct. maneq.
nocte maneque (L. night and morning)

nom. dub.
nomen dubium (L. a doubtful name)

nom. nov.
nomen novum (L. new name)

nom. nud.
nomen nudum (L. a naked name
  [without designation])

non rep.
non repetatur (L. do not repeat—[no
  refills])

non repet.
non repetatur (L. do not repeat—[no
  refills])

NON REPETAT, non repetat.
non repetatur (L. do not repeat—[no
  refills])

nov.
novum (L. new)

nov. n.
novum nomen (L. new name)

nov. sp.
nova species (L. new species)

n.p.
nomen proprium (L. proper name [label
  with])

NPO, n.p.o.
non per os (L. nothing through the
  mouth)

NPO/HS, n.p.o./h.s., npo.hs
nulla per os hora somni (L. nothing
  through the mouth at bedtime)

NR, n.r.
non repetatur (L. do not repeat—[no
  refills])

ns
non sequelae (L. no following
  [consequences])

O
oculus (L. eye)

O, o.
octarius (L. pint)

OB, ob.
obiit (L. he died; she died)

o.c.
opere citato (L. in the work cited)

octup.
octuplus (L. eight-fold)

OD, O.D.
oculo dextro (L. in the right eye)
oculus dexter (L. right eye)

o.d.
omni die (L. every day)

odoram.
odoramentum (L. a perfume)

odorat.
odoratus (L. odorous, smelling,
  perfuming)

OH, o.h.
omni hora (L. every hour)

OI
otitis interna (L. inflammation of the
  inner ear)

OL, O.L.
oculus laevus (L. left eye)

Ol, ol.
oleum (L. oil)

OL OLIV, ol. oliv.
oleum olivae (L. oil of the olive)
oleum olivarium (L. olive oil)

o.m.
omni mane (L. every morning)

om. ¼ h.
omni quadranta hora (L. every fifteen
  minutes)

om. mane vel. noc.
omni mane vel nocte (L. every morning
  or night)

omn. hor.
omni hora (L. every hour)

omn. 2 hor.
omni secunda hora (L. every second
  hour)

omn. man.
omni mane (L. every morning)

omn. noct.
omni nocte (L. every night)

omn. quad. hor.
omni quadrante hora (L. every quarter
  of an hour)

omn. sec. hor.
omni secunda hora (L. every second
  hour)

om. quad. hor
omni quadrante hora (L. every quarter
  of an hour)

ON, On, o.n.
omni nocte (L. every night)

op.
opus (L. work)

op. cit.
opus citatum (L. the work cited)

opt.
optimus (L. best)

OS, O.S.
oculo sinistro (L. in the left eye)
oculus sinister (L. left eye)

OU, O.U.
oculi unitas (L. both eyes together)
oculo utro (L. in each eye)

ov.
ovum (L. egg)

P
parte (L. part)
pater (L. father)
pondere (L. by weight)
pondus (L. weight)
proximum (L. near)

P, p
per (L. by; through; excessive)
post (L. after)

P, p.
pugillus (L. handful)

p.a.
per annum (L. by the year; yearly)
post applicationem (L. after [the]
    application)
pro analysi (L. analysis)
pro anno (L. for the year)

Paa, p.a.a
parti affectae applicandus (L. apply to
    the affected parts)

p.a.a.
parti affectase applicetur (L. let it be
    applied to the affected region)

p. ae.
partes aequales (L. equal parts)

Par aff., par. aff.
pars affecta (L. to the part affected)

part.
partim (L. partly)
partis (L. of a part)

part. aeq.
partes aequales (L. equal parts)

part. dolent.
partes dolentes (L. painful parts)

part. vic.
partitis vicibus (L. in divided doses)

parv.
parvus (L. small)

pass.
passim (L. here and there)

Pb
plumbum (L. lead—element)

PC, P.C., p.c.
pondus civile (L. citizen weight
    [avoirdupois])

p.c.
post cibos (L. after meals)
post cibum (L. after a meal)

Pcb
puncta convergentis basalis (L. point of
    convergence to the baseline—re:
    Ophth)

p.d.
per diem (L. by the day)
pro die (L. for the day)

p.e.
per exemplum (L. for example)

penic. cam.
penicillum camelinum (L. camel's tail
    [camel's hair brush])

per. op. emet.
peracta operatione emetici (L. when the
    action of the emetic is over)

p. ex.
per exemplum (L. for example)

PI
post infectionem (L. after infection)

pigm.
pigmentum (L. paint)

pil.
pilula(e) (L. pill[s])

ping.
pinguis (L. fat)

plumb.
plumbum (L. lead)

PM
post mortem (L. after death)

PM, P.M., p.m.
post meridiem (L. after noon—used as
    evening, night)

p.m.
punctum maximum (L. largest point)

PO, P.O., p.o.
per os (L. through the mouth [by mouth;
    orally])

pocill.
pocillum (L. a small cup)

pocul.
poculum (L. cup)

POHS
per os hora somni (L. through the

mouth at the hour of sleep [by mouth at bedtime])

POLL
pollex (L. thumb)

pond.
pondere (L. by weight)
ponderosus (L. heavy)

POST, post.
post mortem (L. after death)

post cib.
post cibos (L. after meals)
post cibum (L. after a meal)

post part.
post partum (L. occurring after childbirth)

post sing. sed. liq.
post singulas sedes liquidas (L. after every loose stool)

POT, pot.
potus (L. a drink, draught)

PP
per pro (L. instead of)

PP, P.P.
per primam (intentionem—L. by first [intention]—re: healing by first intention; fibrous adherence of wound without suppuration or granulation tissue formation)

PP, pp
postprandium (L. after an early meal)

pp
postpartum (L. occurring after childbirth or delivery [adj.—re: the mother])
post partum (L. after childbirth or delivery [noun])

PPA, Ppa, p.p.a.
phiala prius agitata (L. the bottle having first been shaken)

Ppt, ppt
praeparatus (L. prepared)

ppt.
praecipitatus (L. precipitated)

PR, P.R., Pr., pr.
punctum remotum (L. farthest point [of accommodation—re: Ophth])

PR, pr., p.r.
per rectum (L. through the rectum)

prand.
prandium (L. late breakfast or lunch; an early meal)

p. rat. aetat.
pro ratione aetatis (L. in proportion to age)

p. rec.
per rectum (L. through the rectum)

prim. luc.
prima luce (L. at first light [early in the morning])

prim. m.
primo mane (L. first [thing] in the morning)

p.r.n.
pro re nata (L. according as circumstances may require; as required; whenever necessary; as occasion arises; as needed)

pro dos.
pro dose (L. for a dose)

prolong.
prolongatus (L. prolonged)

pro rat. aet.
pro ratione aetatis (L. according to [patient's] age, in proportion to age)

pro rect.
pro recto (L. by rectum)

pro us. ext.
pro usu externo (L. for external use)

prox. luc.
proxima luce (L. the next morning)

PSA
pone (ad) situm affectum (L. apply to the affected parts)

PSI
per secundam intentionem (L. by second intention [re: healing by second intention—two granulating surfaces uniting with suppuration and delayed closure])

PSt
punctum sternale (L. sternal puncture)

PT
post transfusionem (L. after transfusion)

pt.
perstetur (L. let it be continued)

pul.
pulvinar (L. pulvinus—cushion—re: nucleus lateralis thalamus)

pul. gros.
pulvis grossus (L. a coarse powder)

PULM, pulm.
pulmentum (L. gruel)

pul. tenu.
pulvis tenuis (L. a fine powder)

PULV, pulv.
pulveres (L. powders)
pulvis (L. powder)

pulv. gros.
pulvis grossus (L. a coarse powder)

pulv. subtil.
pulvis subtilis (L. a smooth powder)

pulv. tenu.
pulvis tenuis (L. a fine powder)

purg.
purgativus (L. cathartic, purgative)

PV
post vaccinationem (L. after vaccination)

PV, p.v.
per vaginam (L. through the vagina)

p.v.n.
per vias naturales (L. by natural ways)

Q, q.
quaque (L. each, every)

Qa.m., q.a.m.
quaque ante meridiem (L. every morning)

Qd, q.d.
quaque die (L. every day)

Q2d, q2d, q. 2 d.
quaque secunda die (L. every second day)

q.d.s.
quater die sumendum (L. to be taken four times a day)

QED
quod erat demonstrandum (L. that which is to be demonstrated)

Qh, q.h.
quaque hora (L. every hour)

Q2h, q2h, q. 2 h.
quaque secunda hora (L. every second hour)

Q3h, q3h, q. 3 h.
quaque tertia hora (L. every three hours)

Q4h, q4h, q. 4 h.
quaque quater hora (L. every four hours)

QHS, q.h.s.
quaque hora somni (L. every hour of sleep; each bedtime)

q.l.d.
quater in die (L. four times a day)

q.l.
quantum libet (L. as much as you please; as much as wanted)

Qm, q.m.
quaque mane (L. every morning)

Qn, q.n.
quaque nocte (L. every night)

QNS, q.n.s.
quantum non sufficiat (L. quantity would not suffice)

Qod, q.o.d.
quaque (other) die (L. q.a.d.—quaque altera die—every other day)

Qoh, q.o.h.
quaque (other) hora (L. q.a.h.—quaque altera hora— every other hour)

Qon, q.o.n.
quaque (other) nocte (L. q.a.n.— quaque altera nocte— every other night)

q.p.
quantum placeat (L. as much as desired)

Qpm., q.p.m.
quaque post meridiem (L. each evening)

q.q.
quaque (L. each or every)
quoque (L. also)

Qqh, q.q.h.
quaque quarta hora (L. every fourth hour)

Qq hor., qq. hor.
quaque hora (L. every hour)

QR
quantum rectum (L. quantity is correct)

q.s.
quantum satis (L. a sufficient quantity)
quantum sufficiat (L. as much as may suffice)
quantum sufficit (L. as much as suffices)

q.s. ad
quantum satis ad (L. to a sufficient quantity)

q. suff.
quantum sufficit (L. as much as suffices)

quadrupl.
quadruplicato (L. four times as much)

quart.
quartus (L. fourth)

quat.
quater (L. four times)
quattuor (L. four)

quinq.
quinque (L. five)

quint.
quintus (L. fifth)

quor.
quorum (L. of which)

quot.
quoties (L. as often [as necessary; as needed])

QUOTID, quotid.
quotidie (L. daily)

quot. op. sit
quoties opus sit (L. as often as necessary)

quot. o. s.
quoties opus sit (L. as often as needed)

q.v.
quantum vis (L. as much as you please; as much as you wish)
quantum volueris (L. as much as you wish)

q.v., *qv*
quod vide (L. which see)

R
recipe (L. take)

R, r
remotum (L. far)

rad.
radix (L. root)

ras.
rasurae (L. scrapings or filings)

rec.
recens (L. fresh; recent)

rect.
rectificatus (L. rectified)

redig. in pulv.
redigatur in pulverem (L. let it be reduced to powder)

red. in pulv.
redactus in pulverem (L. reduced to [a] powder)
redige in pulverem (L. reduce to a powder [imperative])

reliq.
reliquus (L. remainder)

ren.
renoveatur (L. renew)

ren. sem.
renoveatum semis (L. renewed only once)
renoveatur semel (L. renew once; shall be renewed [only] once)

REP, rep.
repetatur (L. let it be repeated)

rep.
repetendum (L. to be repeated)

repetat.
repetatus (L. repeated)

rept.
repetatur (L. let it be repeated)

rub.
ruber (L. red)

RX, Rx, R$_x$
recipe (L. take)

S
signa (L. mark; write on [label])
signetur (L. let it be written, labeled; it shall be written [as instruction to the patient])

S, s
semis (L. half)
sinister (L. left)

S, s, $\bar{s}$
sine (L. without)

$\dot{\bar{s}}$, $\dot{s}$., š
sine (L. without)

SA, S.A., s.a.
secundum artem (L. according to the art; by skill)

S.A.L., s.a.l.
secundum artis legis (L. according to the rules of the art)

sat.
saturatus (L. saturated)

SC
scrupulus (L. scruple [a weight])

SC, sc.
scilicet (L. it is permitted to know [namely])

SC, s.c.
sine correctione (L. without correction)

scat.
scatula (L. box)

scat. orig.
scatula originalis (L. original package [manufacturer's package and label])

SEC
secundum (L. according to)

sec. a.
secundum artem (L. according to the art [by skill])

sed.
sedes (L. stool)

sem.
semen (L. seed)
semi; semis (L. one-half)

semel in d.
semel in die (L. once a day)

semih.
semihora (L. half an hour)

sens. lat.
sensu lato (L. in the broad sense)

sens. str.
sensu stricto (L. in the strict sense)

SEP
sepultus (L. buried)

separ.
separatim (L. separately)

sept.
septem (L. seven)

seq.
sequela (L. that which follows)

seq. luce
sequenti luce (L. the following morning)

seqq.
sequentiae (L. the following)

serv.
serva (L. keep, preserve)

sesquih.
sesquihora (L. an hour and a half)

sesquiunc.
sesquiuncia (L. an ounce and a half)

s. expr.
sine expressione (L. without expressing or pressing)

s. fr.
spiritus frumenti (L. spirit of grain [whiskey])

sic.
siccus (L. dry, dried)

s.i.d.
semel in die (L. once a day)

Sig, sig.
signa (L. write; label)
signetur (L. let it be written, labeled [as instruction to patient])

sig. n. pro.
signum nomine proprio (L. label with the proper name)

simp.
simplex (L. simple, single)

sin.
sine (L. without)

sine conf.
sine confectione (L. without sweetness)

sing.
singuli (L. each)
singulorum (L. of each)

si non val.
si non valeat (L. if it is not strong enough)

si n. val.
si non valeat (L. if it is not strong enough)

si op. sit
si opus sit (L. if it is necessary; if necessary)

si vir. perm.
si vires permittant (L. if the strength will permit)

s.l.
secundum legem (L. according to the rules)
sensu lato (L. in the broad sense)

Sn
stannum (L. tin—element)

s.n.
secundum naturam (L. according to nature)

sol.
solubilis (L. soluble)
solutio (L. a solution)

SOLV, solv.
solve (L. dissolve)

S. op. s., s. op. s.
si opus sit (L. if it is necessary)

S OP SIT, s. op. sit
si opus sit (L. if it is necessary)

SOS, s.o.s.
si opus sit (L. if it is necessary)

SP, S/P
status post (L. no change after)

sp.
spiritus (L. spirit)

sp. indet.
species indeterminata (L. species indeterminate)

sp. inquir.
species inquirenda (L. species of doubtful status)

spir.
spiritus (L. spirit)

spiss.
spissus (L. dried)

sp. n.
species novum (L. new species)

sp. nov.
species novum (L. new species)

spt.
spiritus (L. spirit)

sq.
sequentia (L. the following)

sqq, sqq.
sequentia (L. and following)

s.s.
sensu stricto (L. in the strict sense)

ss, $\overline{ss}$, $\overline{\overline{ss}}$.
semi- (L. a half [prefix])
semisse (L. a half)
semissem (L. one-half)

$\dot{\overline{ss}}$, $\overline{ss}$, $\overset{..}{ss}$
semis (L. one-half)

$\dot{s}$ seq.
sine sequela (L. without sequela)

s.s.n.
signetur suo nomine (L. let it be labeled with its own name)

sss, s.s.s.
stratum super stratum (L. layer upon layer)

s. str.
sensu stricto (L. in the strict sense)

SSV, s.s.v.
sub signo veneni (L. under a poison label)

St, st.
stent (L. let them stand)
stet (L. let it stand)

stat.
statim (L. immediately)

stillat.
stillatim (L. by drops [in small quantities])

St pr.
status praesens (L. present status)

su.
sumat (L. let the patient take)

sub fin. coct.
sub finem coctionis (L. toward the end of cooking)

subind.
subinde (L. immediately after)

suc.
succus (L. juice)

sum.
sumantur (L. let them be taken)
sumat (L. let [the patient] take)
sume (L. take)
sumendum (L. to be taken)

sum. tal.
sumat talem (L. let [the patient] take one like this)

sup.
supra (L. above; over)

supp.
suppositorium (L. that which is placed under [suppository])

suppos.
suppositorium (L. that which is placed under [suppository])

supra cit.
supra citato (L. cited above)

s.v.
spiritus vini (L. alcoholic spirit)

s.v.g.
spiritus vini gallici (L. brandy)

s.v.r.
spiritus vini rectificatus (L. rectified spirit of wine [distilled])

s.v.t.
spiritus vini tenuis (L. thin spirit of wine [diluted])

s.v.v.
spiritus vini vitus (L. brandy)

t, t.
ter (L. three times)

TAB, tab.
tabella (L. a [medicated] tablet)
tabellae (L. [medicated] tablets)

tal.
tales (L. such ones)
talia (L. such)
talis (L. such a one)

Tct
tinctura (L. tincture)

t.d.
ter die (L. three times daily)

t.d.s.
ter die sumendum (L. to be taken three times a day)

temp. dext.
tempori dextro (L. to the right temple)
tempus dextrum (L. the right temple)

temp. sinist.
tempori sinistro (L. to the left temple)
tempus sinistrum (L. the left temple)

ter.
tere (L. rub)

ter. sim.
tere simul (L. rub at the same time [together])

t.i.d.
ter in die (L. three times a day)

t.i.n.
ter in nocte (L. three times nightly; three times a night)

tinct.
tinctura (L. tincture)

TO, to
tinctura opii (L. tincture of opium)

TR, Tr, tr.
tinctura (L. tincture)

trid.
triduum (L. three days)

TRIT, trit.
tritura (L. triturate)

tus.
tussis (L. a cough)

tuss.
tussis (L. a cough)

U
ulcus (L. ulcer)
utendus (L. to be used)

u.a.
usque ad (L. up to; as far as)

u.a.f.
ut aliquid fiat (L. that something be done)

u.d.
ut dictum (L. as directed)

ult.
ultime (L. lastly)
ultimus (L. ultimately, last)

ult. praes.
ultimus praescriptus (L. the last ordered or prescribed)

unct.
unctus (L. anointed [smeared])

UNG, ung.
unguentum (L. ointment)

ungt.
unguentum (L. ointment)

up ad lib.
up ad libitum (L. at pleasure [out of bed or ambulatory as desired])

up OOB ad lib.
up out of bed ad libitum (L. as desired)

u.s.
ut supra (L. as above)

ust.
ustus (L. burnt)

ut dct.
ut dictum (L. as directed)

ut dict.
ut dictum (L. as directed)

utend.
utendus (L. to be used)

utend. mor. sol.
utendus more solito (L. to be used in the usual manner)

ut supr.
ut supra (L. as above)

ux.
uxor (L. wife)

V
visus (L. seeing; sight)

V, v
versus (L. turn, towards, in that direction)

v.
vel (L. or [take what you will; one or the other])
vena (L. vein)
vide (L. see)

vas vit.
vas vitreum (L. a glass vessel)

VD
ventriculo dextro (L. in the left ventricle)

vdg. q.s.
voiding sufficient quantity (L. quantum sufficiat)

vehic.
vehiculum (L. vehicle)

VES, ves.
vesica (L. bladder)

vesic.
vesicula (L. a little bladder [blister])

vesp.
vesper (L. evening)

ves. ur.
vesica urinaria (L. urinary bladder)

v. et.
vide etiam (L. see also)

VI
virgo intacta (L. untouched girl)

v.i.
via intermedia (L. intermediate way)

vic.
vices (L. times)

vid.
vide (L. see)

vin.
vinum (L. wine)

vir.
viridis (L. green)

vit.
vitellus (L. yolk of an egg)

vitel.
vitellus (L. yolk of an egg)

vit. ov. sol.
vitello ovi solutus (L. dissolved in yolk of egg)

vitr.
vitreum (L. glass)

viz.
videlicet (L. namely)

VM
ventralis medialis (L. middle belly)

VOD
visio, oculus dexter (L. sight, right eye)

vol.
volatilis (L. volatile)
volvendus (L. to be rolled)

VOS
visus, oculus sinister (L. sight, left eye)

v.o.s.
vitello ovi solutus (L. dissolved in yolk of egg)

VOU
visio oculi utriusque (L. vision of each eye)

Vs
venae sectio (L. venesection [venisection])

vs.
versus (L. a turning toward)

v.s.
vide supra (L. see above)

VsB
venae sectio brachii (L. a cutting of a vein of the arm [to draw blood from a vessel in the arm])

vv.
venae (L. veins)

ZI, z.i.
zona incerta (L. uncertain zones [area]—re: Neuro)

CANCER STAGING ABBREVIATIONS

The following is an overview of the TNM (tumor, node, metastasis) system of staging for cancer as adapted from the American Joint Committee on Cancer's publication, *Manual for Staging of Cancer, 2nd Edition,* edited by Oliver H. Beahrs, M.D., and Max H. Myers, Ph.D., and published by the J. B. Lippincott Company, 1983. This outline is intended as a reference only to the many different definitions inherent within a specific classification. Each classification is applicable only to certain organs/nodes/areas of the body; therefore, the following appendix is not recommended or suggested as a definitive source for clinical practice or transcription. For specific area of involvement relating to cancer staging, we strongly urge you to consult the above publication.

General Abbreviations

a
autopsy (re: chronology of classification)

aTNM
autopsy (staging) tumor, node, metastases

c
clinical-diagnostic (re: chronology of classification)

cTNM
clinical (diagnostic staging) tumor, node, metastases

GX
grade cannot be assessed (re: histologic type of cancer)

G1
well differentiated (re: histologic type of cancer)

G2
moderately well differentiated (re: histologic type of cancer)

G3-G4
poorly to very poorly differentiated (re: histologic type of cancer)

H
the physical state (performance scale) of the patient, considering all cofactors determined at the time of stage classification and subsequent follow-up examinations (re: host performance scale)

H0
normal activity (re: host performance scale)

H1
symptomatic and ambulatory; cares for self (re: host performance scale)

H2
ambulatory more than 50% of time; occasionally needs assistance (re: host performance scale)

H3
ambulatory 50% or less of time; nursing care needed (re: host performance scale)

H4
bedridden; may need hospitalization (re: host performance scale)

L0
no evidence of lymphatic invasion (re: lymphatic invasion)

L1
evidence of invasion of superficial lymphatics (re: lymphatic invasion)

L2
evidence of invasion of deep lymphatics (re: lymphatic invasion)

LX
lymphatic invasion cannot be assessed (re: lymphatic invasion)

M
distant metastasis

N
regional lymph nodes

p
postsurgical treatment—pathologic (re: chronology of classification)

pTNM
postsurgical (resection-pathologic staging) tumor, node, metastases

R0

no residual tumor (re: residual tumor following surgical treatment)

R1

microscopic residual tumor (re: residual tumor following surgical treatment)

R2

macroscopic residual tumor, specify _____(re: residual tumor following surgical treatment)

r

retreatment (re: chronology of classification)

rTNM

retreatment (staging) tumor, node, metastases

s

surgical-evaluative (re: chronology of classification)

sTNM

surgical (-evaluative staging) tumor, node, metastases

T

primary tumor

V0

veins do not contain tumor (re: venous invasion)

V1

efferent veins contain tumor (re: venous invasion)

V2

distant veins contain tumor (re: venous invasion)

VX

venous invasion cannot be assessed (re: venous invasion)

TNM (Tumor, Node, Metastasis) Abbreviations

TX

Minimum requirements to assess the primary tumor cannot be met

Minimum requirements to assess the primary tumor cannot be met (In the absence of orchiectomy, TX must be used.)

No evidence of primary tumor (unknown primary or primary tumor removed and not histologically examined)

Presence of tumor cannot be assessed

Tumor either proven by the presence of malignant cells in bronchopulmonary secretions but not visualized roentgenographically or bronchoscopically or cannot be assessed

Tumor is present but cannot be assessed

T0

Atypical melanocytic hyperplasia (Clark Level I); not a malignant lesion

No demonstrable tumor

No evidence of primary tumor

No evidence of tumor

No primary tumor present

Primary tumor is undetectable

Tis

Carcinoma in situ

Carcinoma in situ (no invasion of lamina propria)

Carcinoma in situ (If used without subscript, Tis indicates bladder alone.)

b	Bladder
u	Ureter
pr.u.	Prostatic urethra
p.d.	Prostatic ducts

In situ cancer (in situ lobular, pure intraductal, and Paget's disease of the nipple without palpable tumor)

Preinvasive carcinoma (carcinoma in situ)

Tumor limited to mucosa without penetration into the lamina propria

Ta

Papillary noninvasive carcinoma

T1

Carcinoma without microscopic invasion beyond the lamina propria. On bimanual examination, a freely mobile mass may be felt; this should not be felt after complete transurethral resection of the lesion

Greatest diameter 3 cm or less; confined to one side (re: infratentorial tumor)

Greatest diameter 5 cm or less; confined to one side (re: supratentorial tumor)

Greatest diameter of primary tumor 2 cm or less

Greatest diameter of primary tumor 3 cm or less

Invasion of papillary dermis (Level II) or 0.75 mm thickness or less

Invasion limited to the submucosa or to the muscle layer

Invasion limited to wall

Limited to body of testis

No direct extension of the primary tumor beyond the pancreas

Small solitary tumor (3 cm) confined to one lobe

Small tumor; minimal renal and calyceal

distortion or deformity; circumscribed neovasculature surrounded by parenchyma

Tumor 1.5 cm or less

Tumor 2 cm or less in greatest diameter.

Tumor 2 cm or less in greatest diameter without significant local extension (Significant local extension is defined as evidence of tumor involvement of skin, soft tissues, bone, or the lingual or facial nerves)

Tumor 2 cm or less in greatest dimension

Tumor 2 cm or less in its largest dimension, strictly superficial or exophytic

A tumor that is 3 cm or less in greatest diameter, surrounded by lung or visceral pleura, and without evidence of invasion proximal to a lobar bronchus at bronchoscopy

Tumor 5 cm or less in diameter

Tumor confined to the antral mucosa of the infrastructure with no bone erosion or destruction

Tumor confined to the mucosa or submucosa (e.g., carcinoma de novo or carcinomatous adenoma, either polypoid or papillary/villous)

Tumor confined to one site

Tumor confined to one site of nasopharynx or no tumor visible (positive biopsy only)

Tumor confined to region of origin with normal mobility

Tumor confined to the subglottic region

Tumor confined to vocal cord(s) with normal mobility (includes involvement of anterior or posterior commissures)

Tumor confined within the cortex of the bone

Tumor limited to mucosa or mucosa and submucosa regardless of its extent (or location)

A tumor that involves 5 cm or less of esophageal length, that produces no obstruction, and that has no circum-ferential involvement and no extraesophageal spread

T1a

No fixation to underlying pectoral fascia or muscle

No palpable tumor; on histologic section no more than three high-power fields of carcinoma found

T1b

Fixation to underlying pectoral fascia or muscle

   i tumor $\leq$ 0.5 cm
   ii tumor $0.5 \leq 1.0$ cm
   iii tumor $1.0 \leq 2.0$ cm

No palpable tumor; histologic sections

revealing more than three high-power fields of prostatic carcinoma

T2

Extension beyond the tunica albuginea

Extension of tumor to adjacent region or site without fixation of hemilarynx

Greatest diameter of primary tumor more than 2 cm but not more than 4 cm

Greatest diameter of primary tumor more than 3 cm

Greatest diameter more than 3 cm; confined to one side (re: infratentorial tumor)

Greatest diameter more than 5 cm; confined to one side (re: supratentorial tumor)

Invasion limited to periductal connective tissues

Invasion limited to perimuscular connective tissue; no extension beyond serosa or into liver

Invasion of the papillary-reticular-dermal interface (Level III) or 0.76- to 1.5 mm thickness

Large tumor (3 cm) confined to one lobe

Large tumor with deformity or enlargement of kidney or collecting systems

Limited direct extension to duodenum, bile ducts, or stomach, still possibly permitting tumor resection

Microscopic invasion of superficial muscle of the bladder. On bimanual examination, there may be induration of the bladder wall, which is mobile. There is usually no residual induration after complete transurethral resection of the lesion.

Supraglottic or subglottic extension of tumor with normal or impaired cord mobility, or both

Tumor confined to the suprastructure mucosa without bone destruction or to the infrastructure, with destruction of medial or inferior bony walls only

Tumor extending beyond the cortex of the bone

Tumor extension to vocal cords with normal or impaired cord mobility

Tumor involves the mucosa and the submucosa (including the muscularis propria), and extends to or into the serosa but does not penetrate through the serosa

Tumor involving adjacent supraglottic site(s) or glottis without fixation

Tumor involving two sites (both posterosuperior and lateral walls)

Tumor limited to wall of colon or rectum but not beyond—viz, invasion into muscularis propria or subserosa (colon and proximal rectum) and into muscularis propria but not beyond (distal rectum)

Tumor more than 1.5 cm

Tumor more than 2 cm but not more than 4 cm in greatest diameter

Tumor more than 2 cm but not more than 4 cm in greatest diameter without significant local extension

Tumor more than 2 cm but not more than 5 cm in its greatest dimension

Tumor more than 2 cm but not more than 5 cm in its largest dimension or with minimal infiltration of the dermis, irrespective of size

A tumor more than 3 cm in greatest diameter or a tumor of any size that either invades the visceral pleura or has associated atelectasis or obstructive pneumonitis extending to the hilar region. At bronchoscopy, the proximal extent of demonstrable tumor must be within a lobar bronchus or at least 2 cm distal to the carina. Any associated atelectasis or obstructive pneumonitis must involve less than an entire lung, and there must be no pleural effusion.

Tumor more than 5 cm in diameter

A tumor that involves more than 5 cm of esophageal length without extraesophageal spread or a tumor of any size that produces obstruction or that involves the entire circumference but without extraesophageal spread

T2a

No fixation to underlying pectoral fascia or muscle

Palpable nodule less than 1.5 cm in diameter with compressible, normal-feeling tissue on at least three sides

Single tumor nodule

Tumor extending into muscularis propria but not penetrating through it

T2b

Fixation to underlying pectoral fascia or muscle

Multiple tumor nodules (any size)

Palpable nodule more than 1.5 cm in diameter or nodule or induration in both lobes

Tumor extending through the wall with complete penetration of the muscularis propria

T3

Any tumor with evidence of extraesophageal spread

Clear radiographic evidence of destruction of cortical bone, with invasion; histopathologic confirmation of invasion of major artery or nerve

Diffuse involvement of the orbital tissues and/or bony walls

Extension of tumor into nasal cavity or oropharynx

Extension of tumor to adjacent region or site with fixation of hemilarynx

Further direct extension (incompatible with surgical resection)

Greatest diameter of primary tumor more than 4 cm

Invades or encroaches upon the ventricular system; greatest diameter 3 cm or less (re: infratentorial tumor)

Invades or encroaches upon the ventricular system; greatest diameter 5 cm or less (re: supratentorial tumor)

Invasion of the reticular dermis (Level IV) or 1.51- to 4.0 mm thickness

Involvement of all layers and direct extension beyond serosa or into one adjacent organ, or both (must be less than 2 cm into the liver)

Involvement of all layers and direct extension into one adjacent major vessel or organ

Involvement of the rete testis or epididymis

More extensive tumor invading skin of cheek, orbit, anterior ethmoid sinuses, or pterygoid muscle

Multiple intraglandular foci of primary tumor

On bimanual examination, there may be induration or a nodular mobile mass palpable in the bladder wall that persists after transurethral resection (T3 may not be used alone).

Palpable tumor extending into or beyond the prostatic capsule

Tumor confined to the larynx with cord fixation

Tumor invades all layers of bowel wall including serosa (colorectal) with or without extension to adjacent or contiguous tissues. Fistula may or may not be present.

Tumor involving both major lobes

Tumor limited to larynx with fixation or extension to involve postcricoid area, medial wall of piriform sinus, or preepiglottic space

Tumor more than 4 cm but not more than 6 cm in greatest diameter without significant local extension

Tumor more than 4 cm in greatest diameter

Tumor more than 5 cm in its greatest dimension

Tumor more than 5 cm in its largest dimension or with deep infiltration of the dermis, irrespective of size

A tumor of any size with direct extension into an adjacent structure such as the parietal pleura or chest wall, the diaphragm, or the mediastinum and its contents; a tumor bronchoscopically demonstrable to involve a main bronchus less than 2 cm distal to the carina; any tumor associated with atelectasis or obstructive pneumonitis of an entire lung or pleural effusion

Tumor penetrates through the serosa without invading contiguous structures

T3a

Large tumor involving perinephric tissues

Microscopic invasion of deep muscle is defined as histologic evidence of tumor clearly extending through muscle bundles to both edges of a resected specimen

No fixation to underlying pectoral fascia or muscle

Palpable tumor extending into the periprostatic tissues or involving one seminal vesicle

Single tumor nodule (with direct extension)

T3b

Fixation to underlying pectoral fascia or muscle

Invasion into perivesical fat

Multiple tumor nodules

Palpable tumor extending into the periprostatic tissues, involving one or both seminal vesicles; tumor size more than 6 cm in diameter

Tumor involving vein

T3c

Tumor involving renal vein and infradiaphragmatic vena cava

T4

Crosses the midline, invades the opposite hemisphere, or extends infratentorially (re: supratentorial tumor)

Crosses the midline, invades the opposite hemisphere, or extends supratentorially (re: infratentorial tumor)

Fixation of primary tumor, direct invasion through thyroid capsule

Invasion of subcutaneous tissue (Level V) or 4.1 mm or greater thickness, or satellite(s) within 2 cm of any primary melanoma

Involvement of all layers and direct extension beyond secondary ductal bifurcation or into two or more adjacent organs including the following: liver, pancreas, duodenum,

stomach, colon, omentum, gallbladder

Involvement of all layers and direct extension 2 cm or more into liver or into two or more adjacent organs (includes stomach, duodenum, colon, pancreas, omentum, extrahepatic bile ducts, and any involvement of liver)

Massive tumor extending beyond the larynx to involve oropharynx, soft tissues of neck, or destruction of thyroid cartilage

Massive tumor invading bone or soft tissues of neck

Massive tumor more than 4 cm in diameter with deep invasion to involve antrum, pterygoid muscles, base of tongue, skin of neck

Massive tumor more than 4 cm in diameter with invasion of bone, soft tissues of neck, or root (deep musculature) of tongue

Massive tumor with cartilage destruction or extension beyond the confines of the larynx, or both

Massive tumor with invasion of cribriform plate, posterior ethmoids, sphenoid, nasopharynx, pterygoid plates, or base of skull

Massive tumor with thyroid cartilage destruction or extension beyond the confines of the larynx or both

Microscopic evidence of muscle invasion; tumor is fixed or invades neighboring structures

Spread beyond the orbit to the adjacent sinuses and/or to the cranium

Tumor extending into neighboring organs or abdominal wall

Tumor fixed or involving neighboring structures

Tumor has spread by direct extension beyond contiguous tissue or the immediately adjacent organs

Tumor invading adjacent organs

Tumor invasion of skull, cranial nerve involvement, or both

Tumor involving other structures such as cartilage, muscle, or bone

Tumor of any size with direct extension to chest wall or skin (Chest wall includes ribs, intercostal muscles, and serratus anterior muscle, but not pectoral muscle.)

T4a

Fixation to chest wall

Invasion of spermatic cord

Tumor invading substance of prostate (microscopically proven), uterus, or vagina

Tumor over 6 cm in greatest diameter without significant local extension

Tumor penetrates through the serosa

and involves immediately adjacent tissues such as lesser omentum, perigastric fat, regional ligaments, greater omentum, transverse colon, spleen, esophagus, or duodenum by way of intraluminal extension

T4b

Edema (including peau d'orange), ulceration of the skin of the breast, or satellite skin nodules confined to the same breast

Invasion of scrotal wall

Tumor fixed to the pelvic wall or infiltrating the abdominal wall

Tumor of any size with significant local extension (Significant local extension is defined as evidence of tumor involvement of skin, soft tissues, bone, or the lingual or facial nerves)

Tumor penetrates through the serosa and involves the liver, diaphragm, pancreas, abdominal wall, adrenal glands, kidney, retroperitoneum, small intestine or esophagus, or duodenum by way of serosa

T4c

Edema (including peau d'orange), ulceration of the skin of the breast, and satellite skin nodules confined to the same breast

NX

Minimum requirements to assess the regional nodes cannot be met

Nodes cannot be assessed

N0

No clinically or histologically positive node(s)

No clinically palpable nodes

No clinically positive node

Nodes not involved

No evidence of involvement of regional lymph nodes

No evidence of regional lymph node involvement

No histological evidence of metastasis to regional or distant lymph nodes

No histologic evidence of metastasis to regional lymph nodes

No histologically verified metastases to lymph nodes

No involvement of regional lymph nodes

No metastases to regional lymph nodes

No regional lymph node involvement

Regional lymph nodes do not contain metastatic deposits

Regional nodes not involved

N1

Clinically positive or histologically positive node(s)

Evidence of involvement of movable homolateral regional lymph nodes

Evidence of regional lymph node involvement

Histologically confirmed spread to regional lymph nodes in porta hepatis

Histologically proven metastasis to first station regional lymph nodes

Histologically verified lymph node involvement

Histologically verified regional lymph node metastasis

Involvement of only one regional lymph node station; node(s) movable and not over 5 cm in diameter, or negative regional lymph nodes and the presence of less than five in-transit metastases beyond 2 cm from the primary site

Involvement of perigastric lymph nodes within 3 cm of the primary tumor along the lesser or greater curvature

Involvement of a single homolateral regional lymph node

Involvement of a single homolateral regional lymph node that, if inguinal, is mobile

Metastasis to lymph nodes in the peribronchial or the ipsilateral hilar region, or both, including direct extension

Movable, unilateral, palpable nodes

One to three involved regional nodes adjacent to primary lesion

Regional lymph nodes contain metastatic deposits

Regional nodes involved

Single, clinically positive homolateral node 3 cm or less in diameter

Single, homolateral regional nodal involvement

N2

Any one of the following: (1) involvement of more than one regional lymph node station; (2) regional node(s) over 5 cm in diameter or fixed; (3) five or more in-transit metastases or any in-transit metastases beyond 2 cm from the primary site with regional lymph node involvement

Evidence of involvement of movable contralateral or bilateral regional lymph nodes

Histologically confirmed spread to lymph nodes beyond porta hepatis

Histologically proven metastasis to second station regional lymph nodes

Invasion of multiple regional or of contralateral or bilateral nodes.

Involvement of contralateral, bilateral, or multiple regional lymph nodes

Involvement of contralateral or of

bilateral or multiple regional lymph nodes that, if inguinal, are mobile (specify number)

Involvement of the regional lymph nodes more than 3 cm from the primary tumor, that are removed or removable at operation, including those located along the left gastric, splenic, celiac, and common hepatic arteries

Metastasis to lymph nodes in the mediastinum

Movable, bilateral, palpable nodes

Regional nodes involved extending to line of resection or ligature of blood vessels

Single clinically positive homolateral node more than 3 cm but not more than 6 cm in diameter or multiple clinically positive homolateral nodes, none more than 6 cm in diameter

N2a

Single clinically positive homolateral node more than 3 cm but not more than 6 cm in diameter

N2b

Multiple clinically positive homolateral nodes, none more than 6 cm in diameter

N3

Evidence of involvement of fixed regional lymph nodes

A fixed mass present on the pelvic wall with a free space between this and the tumor

Fixed nodes

Fixed regional nodes (assessable only at surgical exploration)

Involvement of other intra-abdominal lymph nodes such as the para-aortic, hepatoduodenal, retropancreatic, and mesenteric nodes

Massive homolateral node(s), bilateral nodes, or contralateral node(s)

Nodes contain metastasis, location not identified. Specify number examined; number involved. (Case cannot be properly staged.)

Palpable abdominal mass present or fixed inguinal lymph nodes

N3a

Clinically positive homolateral node(s), one more than 6 cm in diameter

N3b

Bilateral clinically positive nodes (in this situation, each side of the neck should be staged separately; i.e., N3b: right, N2a; left, N1)

N3c

Contralateral clinically positive node(s) only

MX

Minimum requirements to assess the presence of distant metastasis cannot be met

Not assessed

M0

No (known) distant metastasis

No evidence of distant metastasis

No known distant metastasis

No known metastasis

M1

Distant metastasis present
Specify _____

Distant metastasis present (including extra-abdominal nodes; intra-abdominal nodes proximal to mesocolon and inferior mesenteric artery (juxtaregional); peritoneal implants, liver, lungs, and bones).
Specify _____

Involvement of skin or subcutaneous tissue beyond the site of primary lymph node drainage.
Specify _____

ELEMENTS

The following elements are listed alphabetically rather than by atomic weight.

Ac
actinium

Ag
argentum (silver)

Al
aluminum

Am
americium

Ar
argon

As
arsenic

At
astatine

Au
aurum (gold)

B
boron

Ba
barium

Be
beryllium

Bi
bismuth

Bk
berkelium

Br
bromine

C
carbon

Ca
calcium

Cd
cadmium

Ce
cerium

Cf
californium

Cl
chlorine

Cm
curium

Co
cobalt

Cr
chromium

Cs
cesium

Cu
copper

Dy
dysprosium

Element 104
rutherfordium; dubnium

Element 105
hahnium

Element 106
preparation of isotope (mass no. 263) by bombardment of ^{249}Cf with ^{18}O ions

Er
erbium

Es
einsteinium

Eu
europium

F
fluorine

Fe
ferrum (iron)

Fm
fermium

Fr
francium

Ga
gallium

Gd
gadolinium

Ge
germanium

H
hydrogen

He
helium

Hf
hafnium

Hg
hydrargyrum (mercury)

Ho
holmium

I
iodine

In
indium

Ir
iridium

K
kalium (potassium)

Kr
krypton

La
lanthanum

Li
lithium

Lr
lawrencium (formerly Lw)

Lu
lutetium

Md
mendelevium

Mg
magnesium

Mn
manganese

Mo
molybdenum

N
nitrogen

Na
natrium (sodium)

Nb
niobium

Nd
neodymium

Ne
neon

Ni
nickel

No
nobelium

Np
neptunium

O
oxygen

Os
osmium

P
phosphorus

Pa
protactinium

Pb
plumbum (lead)

Pd
palladium

Pm
promethium

Po
polonium

Pr
praseodymium

Pt
platinum

Pu
plutonium

Ra
radium

Rb
rubidium

Re
rhenium

Rh
rhodium

Rn
radon

Ru
ruthenium

S
sulfur

Sb
stibium (antimony)

Sc
scandium

Se
selenium

Si
silicon

Sm
samarium

Sn
stannum (tin)

Sr
strontium

Ta
tantalum

Tb
terbium

Tc
technetium

Te
tellurium

Th
thorium

Ti
titanium

Tl
thallium

Tm
thulium

U
uranium

V
vanadium

W
wolfram; wolframium (tungsten)

Xe
xenon

Y
yttrium

Yb
ytterbium

Zn
zinc

Zr
zirconium

SUGGESTED REFERENCES

American Society of Hospital Pharmacists. Drug Information '84. American Hospital Formulary Service, 1984.

Anastasi A. Psychological Testing. 5th ed. Macmillan, 1982.

Austrin M. Young's Learning Medical Terminology Step by Step. 5th ed. St Louis, CV Mosby, 1983.

Bennington JL (ed). Saunders Dictionary and Encyclopedia of Laboratory Medicine and Technology. Philadelphia, WB Saunders, 1984.

Beth Israel Hospital. Respiratory Intensive Care Nursing. 2nd ed. Boston, Little Brown and Company, 1979.

Billups NF (ed). American Drug Index. 30th ed. Philadelphia, JB Lippincott, 1986.

Blakiston's Gould Medical Dictionary, 4th ed. McGraw-Hill, 1979.

Blauvelt CT and Nelson FRT. Manual of Orthopedic Terminology. 2nd ed. St Louis, CV Mosby, 1983.

Blessum WT and Sippl CJ. Computer Glossary for Medical and Health Sciences. Funk and Wagnalls, 1972.

Boyes JH (ed). Bunnell's Surgery of the Hand, 5th ed. Philadelphia, JB Lippincott, 1970.

Buros OK (ed). The Eighth Mental Measurements Yearbook. Gryphon Press, 1978.

Cassin B and Solomon S. Dictionary of Eye Terminology. Triad Publishing Company, 1984.

The Charles Press Handbook of Current Medical Abbreviations. Bowie, Maryland, The Charles Press, 1976.

Chicago Manual of Style. 13th ed. revised and expanded. University of Chicago Press, 1982.

Cloherty JP and Stark AB. Manual of Neonatal Care. Boston, Little Brown and Company, 1980.

DeVita VT et al. Cancer, Principles and Practice of Oncology. 2nd ed. Philadelphia, JB Lippincott, 1985.

Dorland's Illustrated Medical Dictionary. 26th ed. Philadelphia, WB Saunders, 1981.

Dunmore CW and Fleischer RM. Medical Terminology: Exercises in Etymology. Edition II. Philadelphia, FA Davis Company, 1985.

Dupayrat J. Dictionary of Biomedical Acronyms and Abbreviations. John Wiley, 1984.

Emery AH and Rimon DL (ed). Principles and Practice of Medical Genetics. Churchill Livingstone, 1983.

Etter LE. Glossary of Words and Phrases Used in Radiology, Nuclear Medicine and Ultrasound. 2nd ed. Charles C Thomas, 1970.

Farm Chemicals Handbook. Meister Publishing, 1984.

Garb S. Abbreviations and Acronyms in Medicine and Nursing. New York, Springer Publishing, 1976.

Glanze WD (ed). Mosby's Medical and Nursing Dictionary. 2nd ed. St. Louis, CV Mosby, 1986.

Godman A. Barnes and Noble Thesaurus of Chemistry. Barnes and Noble, 1982.

References

Guidos B and Hamilton B (ed). MASA: Medical Acronyms, Symbols and Abbreviations. Neal-Schuman Publishing Inc, 1984.

Hutchinson L. Standard Handbook for Secretaries. 8th ed. McGraw-Hill, 1969.

Jablonski S. Illustrated Dictionary of Eponymic Syndromes and Diseases and their Synonyms. Philadelphia, WB Saunders, 1969.

Jerrard HG and McNeill DB. A Dictionary of Scientific Units including dimensionless numbers and scales. 4th ed. Chapman and Hall in association with Methuen Inc, 1980.

Johnson CE. Medical Spelling Guide: A Reference Aid. Charles C Thomas, 1966.

Joint Commission on Accreditation of Hospitals. Accreditation Manual for Hospitals. 1985 ed.

Kamenetz HL. Physiatric Dictionary: Glossary of Physical Medicine and Rehabilitation. Charles C Thomas, 1965.

Kerr AH. Medical Hieroglyphs, Abbreviations and Symbols. Enterprise Publications, 1970.

King R and Stansfield WD. A Dictionary of Genetics. 3rd ed. Oxford University Press, 1985.

Lorenzini J. Medical Phrase Index. Medical Economics, 1978.

Merritt HH. A Textbook of Neurology. 6th ed. Philadelphia, Lea and Febiger, 1979.

Miller BF and Keane CB. Encyclopedia and Dictionary of Nursing and Allied Health. 3rd ed. Philadelphia, WB Saunders, 1983.

Milunsky A. Prevention of Genetic Disease and Mental Retardation. Philadelphia, WB Saunders, 1975.

Modell W et al. Applied Pharmacology. Philadelphia, WB Saunders, 1976.

Morris W (ed). American Heritage Dictionary of the English Language. American Heritage Publishing Company and Houghton Mifflin, 1981.

Newell F. Ophthalmology, Principles and Concepts. 5th ed. St Louis, CV Mosby, 1982.

Patient Care Magazine. Medical Abbreviations Handbook. 2nd ed. Medical Economics, 1983.

Peyman GA et al (ed). Principles and Practice of Ophthalmology. Philadelphia, WB Saunders, 1981.

Preston JD et al. Cancer Chemotherapeutic Agents: Handbook of Clinical Data. 2nd ed. Boston, GK Hall, 1982.

Schertel A. Abbreviations in Medicine. 3rd ed. Karger Publishing, 1984.

Simpson DP. Cassell's Latin Dictionary. MacMillan, 1963.

Skeel RT et al. Manual of Cancer Chemotherapy. Boston, Little Brown and Company, 1982.

Sloane SB. Medical Abbreviations and Eponyms. Philadelphia, WB Saunders, 1985.

Sloane SB. Medical Word Book. 2nd ed. Philadelphia, WB Saunders, 1982.

Sloane SB and Dusseau J. A Word Book in Pathology and Laboratory Medicine. Philadelphia, WB Saunders, 1984.

Smith DW et al (ed). Recognizable Patterns of Human Malformation: Genetic, Embryologic, and Clinical Aspects. 3rd ed. Philadelphia, WB Saunders, 1982.

Sodee DB and Early PJ. Technology and Interpretation of Nuclear Medicine Procedures. 2nd ed. St Louis, CV Mosby, 1975.

Stedman's Medical Dictionary. 24th ed. Baltimore, Maryland, Williams and Wilkins, 1982.

Steen EB. Abbreviations in Medicine. 4th ed. London, Balliere Tindall/ WB Saunders, 1978.

Steen EB. Balliere's Abbreviations. 5th ed. Balliere Tindall, 1984.

Thomas CL (ed). Taber's Cyclopedic Medical Dictionary. 15th ed. Philadelphia, FA Davis Company, 1985.

Tietz, NW (ed). Clinical Guide to Laboratory Tests. Philadelphia, WB Saunders, 1983.

United States Pharmacopeial Convention Inc. USAN and the USP Dictionary of Drug Names (through June 15, 1984). 1983.

Waters K and Murphy G. Medical Records in Health Information. Aspen, 1979.

Windholz M et al (ed). The Merck Index. 10th ed. Merck and Company Inc, 1983.

Warkany J. Congenital Malformations, Notes and Comments. Year Book Publishing, 1971.

Do you use abbreviations daily that are not found in this book? If so, we would be most grateful if you would fill out the form below, and we will include them in the next edition of this text. Please type or print your entries. Thank you.

Abbreviation	Definition	Specialty in which used

Your name _____

Medical affiliation/Occupation _____

Comments _____

_____

_____

_____

Send form to: **Carolynn M. Logan**
℅ Nursing Division
J. B. Lippincott Company
East Washington Square
Philadelphia, PA 19105